Dr Ian Morton graduated with a First Class [Honours B.Sc. in Pharmacology] from Chelsea College, University of London. [He went on to obtain a Ph.D. at] University College London, where he was app[ointed Lecturer in] Pharmacology in 1965. He then moved to Kin[g's College London where he] became Senior Lecturer in Pharmacology unti[l ......]. He is now a consultant editor and writer in pharmacology. He is the author of more than one hundred research papers, books and monographs.

Dr Judith Hall graduated with a First Class Honours B.Sc. in Pharmacology from King's College London where she went on to obtain a Ph.D. She has occupied postdoctoral positions at King's College since 1988, and in 1995 she was awarded a personal Wellcome Trust Medical Research Fellowship at the University of Surrey. She is the author of more than fifty research papers, reviews, books and monographs and is the Editor of the *British Journal of Pharmacology*.

MEDICINES
THE COMPREHENSIVE GUIDE
FOURTH EDITION

DR IAN MORTON AND **DR JUDITH HALL**

BLOOMSBURY

This completely revised edition first published 1995

Text and database copyright © 1995, 1997
Dr I K M Morton, Dr J M Hall
and Book Creation Services Limited, London

Dr I K M Morton and Dr J M Hall assert their moral rights to be identified as the authors of this work.

Bloomsbury Publishing Limited,
38 Soho Square, London W1V 5DF

British Library Cataloguing in Publication Data

A CIP catalogue for this book is available from the British Library

ISBN 0 7475 3342 3

10 9 8 7 6 5 4 3 2 1

Editor: Sam Merrell

Designed and typeset by
Book Creation Services Limited
21 Carnaby Street
London W1V 1PH

Printed and bound by
Clays Ltd, St Ives plc

CONTENTS

PREFACE

This is the fourth edition of *Medicines: The Comprehensive Guide* – a dictionary-style reference source-book for the range of medicines that are available in the UK today. The text has been extensively revised – to take account of the many new drugs, both generic and proprietary, that have been developed and marketed since publication of the third edition in 1995, along with changes in details of those that remain on the market. Earlier editions of this book, as with all constantly updated books of this type, should be discarded since they contain superseded information. In response to requests from readers, this edition also sees the introduction of a glossary of medical terms, which we hope will help readers to understand some of the more technical terms.

The purpose of the book is to give straightforward information on constituent drug components of medicines, describing their actions, explaining how they work and what side-effects they may have. It has been our aim to provide as full a list as is possible and practical, in such a changeable industry, of the generic drugs and most of the proprietary preparations available.

There are some categories of preparations we have not felt it was either possible or appropriate to include, however. In particular: [1] preparations of vitamins and minerals that are part of a normal balanced diet are not included, although there are entries on medicines where vitamins or minerals are used medically to correct clinical dificiencies (for example, iron preparations for anaemia, folic acid vitamin supplements in pregnancy); [2] homeopathic or herbal remedies do not fall within the scope of the book, but nevertheless there are many entries on drugs of plant and natural origin, and standardized plant extracts that are part of everyday medicine; [3] the 'social' and non-medical use of drugs is also not covered, although some medicines used to treat drug-overdose and drug-dependence (addiction) are included.

Finally, it is important to note that this book is not intended to be a guide to the prescription or administration of drugs, and it gives neither doses nor recommendations regarding which drugs to use in particular circumstances. A qualified practitioner should always be consulted before any medicine is taken.

IKMM
JMH
King's College London & University of Surrey

How to use this book

The layout of this book was designed to be sufficiently clear for it to be used without further instructions, but some words of explanation may be helpful.

The main section of this book contains entries on the medicinal drugs available in the UK, listed A to Z. Drugs are listed under their generic and proprietary names. There are also entries covering the major drug families that explain in more detail how they work and what they are used for. These are indicated by an ⧆ after the name. The A to Z is cross-referenced within the text of one entry to further related entries. These cross-references are indicated when the drug name is printed in the text in SMALL CAPITALS. The side-effects and warnings to be borne in mind when taking a drug are indicated by symbols – ✚ for side-effects and ▲ for warnings – in entries about generic drugs. At the end of these articles there is a list of related entries – indicated by a ✪ – which are the proprietary preparations that contain that drug.

Following common practice, drugs are listed in two ways:

The generic name, without an initial capital letter, is the official (simplified) chemical name of a drug, which unambiguously describes an active constituent of a medicine. The generic name is now routinely used in everyday medicine, and doctors are encouraged to refer to and prescribe drugs by this name, because this is less likely to be misunderstood and generic forms of drugs are often cheaper.

The proprietary name, always with an initial capital letter, is a brand name which is a preparation of a drug, or a mixture of drugs, that represents a particular formulation from a particular manufacturer.

For instance, paracetamol is the generic name of an established and familiar drug. In the case of a particular generic formulation, such as paracetamol tablets, even details concerning purity, the time taken for the tablets to dissolve and accuracy of doses are subject to strict control as laid out in the British Pharmacopoeia, or other official standards.

A doctor may prescribe paracetamol simply as 'paracetamol'. In practice, however, common non-prescription drugs such as paracetamol are available not just under their generic name, but also as proprietary preparations under a variety of brand names. Drugs are often prescribed or sold in a variety of forms (tablets, capsules, effervescent tablets, powders for solution, suppositories, etc.) and sometimes in different strengths (the stronger ones usually have a distinguishing name like Forte, Extra or Ultra).

To add to these complexities, an analgesic (painkiller) such as paracetamol is also readily available for non-prescription (OTC; over-the-counter) sale, alone or in combination with other drugs, ie as a 'compound preparation'. For example, there are compound analgesic preparations that contain two or more analgesics (such as paracetamol and codeine) or compound cold-cures (such as paracetamol with a decongestant or a cough suppressant).

This potentially confusing system of describing and marketing medicines can be understood through the system of entry types and cross-references used in this book.

STEP BY STEP

The following examples highlight the most common points where confusion can arise and serve to illustrate how this book can help. For example, you have bought a proprietary medicine – *Nurofen* – and want to learn more about its constituents, their other uses, possible side-effects and when such a drug should not be used. Take the following steps:

[1] Discover the generic name(s) of the constituent(s)

This information can be obtained by reading the label or packet, or by looking the proprietary (brand) name up in this book. A proprietary entry will list the generic or generics it contains, the pharmacological class they belong to (eg analgesics or antibiotics), the form it is available in (eg tablets or nasal spray) and a word or two about its uses. It also provides the manufacturer's name in brackets at the beginning of the entry, which is a useful cross-check of the identity of the preparation. Major pharmaceutical companies, however, may label particular medicines either under their own familiar name or that of a subsidiary. The latter is especially common with OTC (over-the-counter) 'healthcare' products.

[2] Turn to the generic names or names

Generic entries contain substantially more detail; eg '...is a non-narcotic analgesic with antipyretic properties which is used to treat... '. It also has further information about the drug which detail its main side-effects (✚) and warnings (▲) relating to its administration.

The list of possible side-effects is extensive, starting with the common and most-often experienced ones, followed by relatively infrequent reactions and finishing with rarely reported effects.

The 'warning' information describes the circumstances when the drugs may be unsafe to use or used with extreme caution. Two common examples would be during pregnancy or when breast-feeding. Other circumstances may relate to certain diseases, such as kidney or liver disorders which could prevent the drug from being metabolized and excreted normally, or rare but important inherited disorders, such as porphyria, which may cause adverse reactions. These warnings do not necessarily apply to all but they do emphasize the importance of seeking professional medical advice.

[3] For more information read the cross-references

Certain terms or names in SMALL CAPITALS indicates that related or further information can be found at that term's entry. For example, antirheumatic leads to an article that discusses other classes of drugs that are used in treating rheumatoid arthritis and osteoarthritis. Non-narcotic analgesic leads to an entry explaining that the drugs called analgesics are used to treat pain, and they can be split (on the basis of the way they work and whether or not they cause drug-dependence) into the (opioid) narcotic analgesic and (NSAID) non-narcotic analgesic classes; the NSAID entry is the most important because it will detail the information concerning side-effects and warnings for all the analgesics of this class.

[4] Going from generic drug names to proprietary preparations

At the end of every generic entry there is a **Related entry/entries** subheading which lists all the proprietaries in this book that contain the generic drug in question. Using the A to Z in this way is particularly useful when you are familiar with the generic drug and want an appropriate brand to go and buy.

If you are concerned whether the generic constituents included in, for example, a cold-cure have adverse effects in your particular situation, then a glance at the entries would remind you that, say, a sympathomimetic vasoconstrictor should under no circumstances be taken on top of a course of a prescribed monoamine-oxidase inhibitor (MAOI) antidepressant; or that an antihistamine can cause drowsiness to the extent that it would be advisable not to operate machinery or drive a car, and is best taken last thing at night.

These examples illustrate, we hope, that gaining an understanding of how prescribed drugs work is not necessarily difficult, and that such an understanding can greatly assist you in getting the most out of the modern healthcare system.

INTRODUCTION

The sweeping changes that have occurred – and are still occurring – in the ways the pharmaceutical industry develops and promotes its products in the UK have meant that this new edition, of what has become one of the most successful books on this subject ever published, had to be updated so extensively that a substantial proportion of entries have changed from the third edition. What are these changes and why have they occurred? And most significantly, what do they mean for those of us who buy and use these medicines?

The pharmaceutical industry and drug development

The drug industry is one of the most rapidly expanding areas of commerce. Although pharmaceutical companies are increasingly international in their organization, many (whether British- or foreign-owned) have a strong base in the UK. In research and development, scientists in the UK have an enviable record of innovation. Also, in the later stages of drug development involving clinical trials, and ultimately the approval and continuing licensing of drugs for use in patients, our Committee on Safety of Medicines and other parts of the Medicines Control Agency set world standards for authoritative assessment of safety and efficacy of drugs.

Currently, we have one of the most restrictive legislations in relation to limiting the majority of drugs to prescription-only use – although this is now beginning to move towards European practice and standards as discussed below. One outcome of the last couple of decades, the most dynamic period in the history of the pharmaceutical industry, has been the emergence of many new generic drugs. These have not simply been further examples of existing drugs or drug types (often derogatorily called 'me-too' drugs), but entirely new classes of drugs. Some of these have now become famous, such as the beta-blocker 'heart-drugs' and the ulcer-healing H_2-antagonist drugs, which are both British inventions.

In this fourth edition, development work within the pharmaceutical industry has now yielded considerable numbers of different generic drugs, each with its individual virtues, within these and other groups. For instance, there are described in this book some 18 different generic beta-blockers, which are marketed in over one hundred different proprietary preparations.

This edition also sees the full introduction of several promising new types of drug, including angiotensin-receptor blockers and potassium-channel activators, which are used to treat cardiovascular disorders. There have been welcome advances in the development of antiviral drugs; some, such as the protease inhibitors, have an entirely new mode of action, and are valuable drugs in the treatment of AIDS.

The impact of biotechnology – the application of biological techniques to the manufacture of biopharmacetical drugs (normally complex polypeptides) – becomes apparent in this edition. Many drugs that previously required difficult extraction from materials of animal or human origin, can now be manufactured by recombinant DNA technology (genetic engineering). Such drugs include recombinant versions of such vital drugs as insulin, hepatitis B vaccine, somatropin (human growth hormone), erythropoietins and interferons.

Although production by genetic engineering can be costly, in the long-term it will become cheaper. In some cases literally life-prolonging therapy – for instance, for cancer, AIDS, bleeding and hormone-deficiency diseases – may well become economically as well as theoretically possible. A bonus of these biosynthetically manufactured drugs is their enhanced safety, especially in preventing infection, immune reactions and other biological complications. For example, human growth hormone, used to treat short stature (dwarfism) in children, was at one time isolated from the pituitary glands of cadavers and so brought with it the risk of acquiring Creutzfeldt-Jakob disease due to infecting contamination, however, it has now been replaced in the UK by somatropin, which is a biosynthetic form that has no risk of contamination.

Another encouraging trend, which is set to continue, is the success of pharmacology and medicinal chemistry in discovering lead compounds in nature. In the second-half of the 20th century, hundreds of valuable antibiotics have been developed from ferments of fungal moulds. These are used not only for infections by micro-organisms but also in cancer treatment, and as leads in discovery of novel chemicals for a variety of purposes. This edition sees a number of new types of drugs developed from natural compounds, notably the taxanes, which are anticancer compounds derived from the yew tree.

Future developments

Will this rapid progess continue? Many people within the industry are not optimistic because of escalating costs of drug development; to produce just one new drug can take years and cost millions. However, new research strategies, many involving the emerging science of molecular biology, may prove cheaper and more effective.

There are also several major targets for drug therapy towards which progress has been slow. For instance, it was once dreamed that a 'magic bullet' could be developed whereby the cause of disease was 'hit' leaving the patient unharmed. Although antibiotics have realized this dream in the treatment of infections caused by bacteria and other micro-organisms, the battle against malignant cells or viruses has yet to be won. There are some 60 generic anticancer drugs and 18 antiviral drugs listed in this book, but unfortunately most of these leave a lot to be desired in terms of efficacy and freedom from side-effects. Overall, however, there is more cause for hope than pessimism.

Partnerships between patients, doctors and pharmacists

Successful medical therapy has always depended on a partnership between the patient and medical professionals. Every patient is different and requires individual treatment – a truth that is often easy to forget in a world where mass production and standardization of products and practice is regarded as the norm. Medicines are prepared and tested according to the most rigorous criteria of standardization, for the sake of safety as well as for economic efficiency. But because people are all likely to be different to some degree, either in their basic genetic make-up or in the circumstances surrounding the condition they are seeking to treat, an individual's response to a certain drug must therefore be taken into account.

Where prescribed medicines are concerned, the doctor can help interpret specific needs and situations, and prescribe accordingly. But an increasingly wide range of medicines are now becoming available without prescription and can be purchased directly from a pharmacy.

Associated with this is a growing trend to give an increasing share of the advisory role to the pharmacist. However, the doctor will know important details of a patient's history and present condition, which is privileged information that the pharmacist will not have access to. Consequently, this trend towards making more medicines available without prescription places a substantial responsibility for choosing the correct medication on the patient, or on carers in the case of children, the elderly and those who are too ill to cooperate. This book should therefore be of considerable value in making sensible choices.

The move to non-prescription drugs

The number of drugs switched each year from prescription-only to an OTC, over-the-counter (non-prescription), status is increasing at a remarkable rate. There were only 11 such changes in individual generic drugs or their indicated uses during the nine-year period from 1983 to 1992, there were 15 between 1993 and 1994, and another 14 joined these in 1995. This switch has perhaps its greatest overall effect in the area of the marketing of proprietary medicines. For example, the analgesic ibuprofen was one of the 11 prescription drugs that changed status between 1983 and 1992, and now there are 38 proprietary preparations of it listed in this book.

Types of drugs are also affected; in the last two editions of this guide, members of several major drug groups have changed their status from prescription-only to over-the-counter. For example, the ulcer-healing drugs of the H_2-antagonist group (although only for the treatment of dyspepsia), a number of corticosteroids for topical use and antifungal antibiotic treatments for thrush infections.

As more medicines become readily available without prescription, authorities in the UK expect patients to become more skilled at knowing when they should seek expert advice. For much the same reasons, the list of drugs that may be prescribed by nurses and dentists has also been extended, and it is likely that various healthcare workers will be empowered in future either to prescribe or to recommend medication.

Not all healthcare professionals welcome this trend towards deregulation, and are worried that aspects of it will be detrimental both to the health of an individual and the community as a whole. For instance, in other parts of the world the excessive and often inappropriate use of antibiotics obtained without prescription (OTC) is a major reason for the now widespread emergence of antibiotic-resistant strains of bacteria that cause major diseases, such as tuberculosis and gonorrhoea.

It is hoped that in the UK, with cooperation and appropriate health education, some of these dangers can be avoided.

Cost considerations

In part, these changes from prescription-only to OTC medicines are motivated by financial objectives. On the one hand, the cost of drugs is the biggest single item of the National Health Service annual bill, so the government is looking to shed some of this load. On the other hand, nearly half of all prescriptions actually cost less than the standard prescription charge.

The move to European practices

These changes are part of a gradual evolution towards a common standard in Europe. Currently, the UK has one of the most restrictive pharmaceutical legislations in the world, and those who travel widely may already be aware that a very high proportion of the drugs listed in this dictionary as prescription-only are available over-the-counter in Europe, and to an even greater extent in the Americas and in the East.

Drugs and the traveller

The traveller should note that generic names of drugs differ little between countries. This dictionary lists the new European standard names, and major American names, both as separate cross-indexes and in brackets after the UK generic name.

Because it is cheaper in some cases to buy proprietary drugs in Europe and dispense them here – so called 'parallel imports' – it is not uncommon to have a prescription for a generic drug supplied by the pharmacist in packaging showing an unfamiliar foreign spelling of the usual British proprietary name.

Proprietary names used by a manufacturer for the same generic drug are today less likely to be totally different according to the country in which it is marketed, although there may be minor variations in spelling to accommodate local requirements. A pharmacist should always be consulted in cases of doubt.

The protective shield: what should the patient know?

It is clear from consideration of these changing circumstances that patients and carers will be playing an increasingly large role in drug therapy. This is also the case in other branches of medicine and is seen by most people as a welcome democratization of medical practice.

In the case of drugs, however, the lowering of this protective shield afforded by the older scheme – where virtually all the drugs that were potentially harmful were available only on prescription – has obvious dangers. Therefore the public will need to understand more and more about the medicines they are prescribed or purchase. However, drugs today are far safer than their forebears. The strictest safety criteria must now be satisfied before a new drug can be introduced into medical use, and indeed many of the more dangerous drugs that were in everyday use not so very long ago have been withdrawn or are reserved for special circumstances.

This dictionary is emphatically not a guide to self-medication, but it is intended to help in this process by providing a comprehensive source of understandable information about the medicines themselves.

What are side-effects and why do they occur?

One of the biggest problems associated with taking medicines relates to the side-effects they may have. Drugs act by having specific effects on the body, usually to attack the cause or relieve the symptoms of an illness. However, while dealing with the conditions they were designed to treat, many drugs may also affect the body in other, undesirable ways that are incidental to their primary purpose. These adverse reactions, or side-effects, may be so mild as to be barely noticeable, or so severe as to be life-threatening, depending on the drug and the person taking it.

Adverse drug reactions that result in side-effects can be categorized into one of two basic kinds:

◆ **'Type A' reactions** are inherent in the way the drug acts pharmacologically, and may be largely inevitable and very difficult to circumvent. For instance, the side-effects of drowsiness and sedation (due to actions on the brain) is so common with antihistamines that it is accepted by most sufferers as inevitable. However, the pharmaceutical industry is aware of the inconvenience of side-effects and attempts are continually being made to minimize them. For example, newer antihistamines are altered chemically to restrict the drug's access to the brain. It is important to be aware that such developments are occurring so that, where undesirable side-effects are experienced, discussion with a physician may result in finding a more individually acceptable treatment.

◆ **'Type B' reactions** are less predictable, and are often referred to as 'idiosyncratic'. A major cause of these idiosyncratic reactions is a true allergic reaction to a drug by the body's immune system. A sensitivity reaction of this kind can present a serious threat to the patient, and the dangers can only be minimized if the patient is aware of the danger because of an earlier reaction to a drug of that class. Physicians routinely ask whether the patient is allergic to antibiotics or local anaesthetics before prescribing them – and each individual must know his or her own idiosyncratic (allergic) responses. However, some antibiotics, local anaesthetics, and other drugs that cause allergic reactions, are now available over-the-counter for non-prescription use, so it is vitally important to read the Patient Information Leaflet (PIL) that comes with the medicine.

Reporting adverse drug reactions

Both doctors and the pharmaceutical industry are constantly aware of the challenge to safe and acceptable medication posed by the incidence of side-effects of drugs. When information is available about the incidence of a particular drug's adverse reactions – perhaps in relation to dose and duration of treatment, interactions with other drugs or foodstuffs, or the medical history and individual characteristics of patients exhibiting adverse reactions – then it becomes easier to treat individual patients more safely.

Armed with such information, a doctor will be in a position to decide whether to use that drug for a given individual, to adjust the dose so side-effects are tolerable, to watch out for potentially serious adverse reactions, or to switch to a similar drug that may be better tolerated.

In practice, much information about adverse reactions to drugs is gained during the pre-marketing, clinical-trial phase of testing, and at this stage it is often possible to identify factors that predispose towards individual side-effects.

Once a drug is in use, there are various forms of reporting that continue to track patients on a particular medication. In addition, the UK has a 'yellow card' reporting system, whereby all medical practitioners are issued with supplies of cards which they use to report to the Committee on Safety of Medicines any adverse effects in any drug as they are noticed. Such later procedures help identify rarer adverse reactions and lead to specific warnings being issued about the type of patient for whom the drug should not be prescribed.

How safe are drugs?

Questions about drug safety only make sense on a risks-to-benefit basis. In other words, does the severity of the condition warrant risking certain known side-effects? At one end of the scale, is a certain individual's headache sufficiently severe that it is worth risking the known side-effects of the humble aspirin tablet? If the individual is in good health with no history of intolerance to NSAID drugs, and no form of stomach upset, then the answer may well be Yes. On the other hand if the individual is a child, or has a predisposition towards gastric ulcers or asthma, then the answer will be No.

At the other end of the risks-to-benefit scale is the patient who has a life-threatening infection or cancer, then the physician may discuss with the patient whether to treat the condition with drugs that would be too toxic to use for less serious conditions.

How serious is serious?

Looking at the list of side-effects and warnings for some generic drugs the reader may feel that he or she would be ill-advised to take any of them. At one extreme, certainly, on the basis of the risk-to-benefit ratio, it is true that any unnecessary taking of drugs should always be avoided. Nevertheless, most people accept that in some circumstances the use of drugs is unavoidable. For example, the risks or undesirability of an unplanned pregnancy may outweigh the known risks of taking the Pill. The seasonal hay-fever sufferer may be willing to endure any side-effects of antihistamines to gain relief from the misery of sneezing and rhinitis. And when it comes to serious illness, benefits can outweigh risks by a considerable margin.

A short course of antibiotics may achieve a complete and permanent cure of infections that without them could prove fatal (eg meningitis), and the side-effects of such a course may be no worse than occasional diarrhoea.

Vaccination can, by treating the most vulnerable sectors of the population, completely eliminate some infectious diseases. Smallpox infection no longer exists in the world population, and poliomyelitis may soon be eliminated, both as a result of global vaccination programmes. In the UK, MMR vaccination of children has been introduced with the intention of eliminating mumps, measles and rubella (German measles). Although there may be very rare incidences of serious adverse reactions, most people accept that these risks are far outweighed by the considerable threat to children of contracting the infections themselves. And in any vaccination programme, it is important that all children, rather than just a selection, are vaccinated, or the diseases may regenerate in the unvaccinated group and so become re-established in the population.

When interpreting the listed side-effects of individual drugs, it is important to understand that the longer the period a drug has been in use, the longer the list of possible side-effects is likely to be. Conversely, new drugs may appear to be free of side-effects because relatively little is known about them as they are still going through the yellow card and other reporting processes. In the listings provided in this book, the most frequently experienced side-effects appear first, while those at the end of the list are likely to be seen less often.

Similarly, the 'warnings' are based on doctors' accumulated experience in using that drug. As already mentioned, many drugs need to be used with special care where there may be greater sensitivity; for instance, where the drug is not metabolized or excreted as rapidly as normal, causing it to build up to toxic levels. This is most likely to happen in patients with certain kidney or liver disorders, and in the elderly: when the physician is aware of the circumstances, using a lower dosage often avoids any potential problems.

It can also be seen that the majority of the drugs in this book should be avoided by women who are pregnant or breast-feeding, because, although it is not known for certain that they are dangerous, the lessons of the thalidomide disaster have not been forgotten.

Individuals at risk of adverse reaction

People suffering from the following conditions are particularly susceptible to certain drugs or forms of drug therapy. Although the conditions are generally rare, it is very important to be aware of them, and reminders to this effect appear throughout the book under the lists of 'warnings'.

Inherited conditions

◆ **Porphyria** appears as a 'should not use' warning in many entries. This fairly rare inherited condition, which causes abnormal metabolism of blood pigments, is serious in its own right, but is potentially lethal in combination with a wide range of drugs – some of which are commonly available and otherwise harmless. Normally, individuals who have porphyria know so, but the condition is sufficiently serious that relatives of patients should also be screened.

◆ **G6PD deficiency** (glucose 6-phosphate dehydrogenase enzyme deficiency) is a genetically inherited condition, and is relatively common in African, Indian and some Mediterranean peoples. Serious adverse reactions occur in those affected when they take quite a few drugs; for instance, the antimalarial drug primaquine causes blood red cell haemolysis in 5–10% of black males, leading to severe anaemia.

◆ **Slow acetylators** are mentioned only a few times. Similar to G6PD deficiency, this describes an inherited condition where an enzyme that breaks down drugs within the body has low activity, and so it is therefore important that lower doses of such drugs (eg isoniazid) are taken by people with this disorder.

Non-inherited conditions

◆ **Age** needs to be taken into account as a factor in drug doses. The elderly metabolize drugs slowly, so lower doses usually need to be used; the elderly are also more likely to become confused with many drugs that act on the brain. Children are especially at risk, and doctors have special ways of working out appropriate doses when it is necessary to prescribe for the young. The manufacturers of OTC medicines always take care to indicate the age-groups and doses for those of their products appropriate for children, and the labelling should be read carefully. Although this book does provide the manufacturers' instructions for OTC medicines, it is important to remember that only the current labelling on these products is definitive.

◆ **Kidney disorders** slow down the excretion of drugs and so active constituents may remain in the body for longer than is intended, therefore doses should be adjusted.

◆ **Liver disorders** slow down the body's metabolism of drugs, so lower doses may be required.

◆ **Alcoholism** is likely to have caused damage to the liver, so the same considerations apply as to liver disorders.

◆ **Heart disease** requires special care when drugs are prescribed, and more usually patients need special advice in the safe use of medicines.

◆ **Pregnancy** requires special care and, as mentioned already, it is probably best to avoid taking any drugs during pregnancy if this is possible. Even before becoming pregnant it is a good idea to discontinue use of some drugs as well as alcohol to avoid any residual effects. Not all drugs are damaging in pregnancy, however, and the Department of Health now agree that supplements of the vitamin folic acid help prevent neural tube defects (eg spinal bifida) when taken before and during the first three months of pregnancy.

◆ **In breast-feeding**, specific information is now available on which drugs are of concern because they pass to the baby in the mother's milk or effect milk production. Here, too, as a general rule it is best to avoid all drugs if possible, and if this is not possible then, of course, a doctor should be consulted in every case.

Drug interactions: good or bad?

One of the greatest inherent dangers in the use of either prescription or non-prescription drugs lies in the unpredictability of the interactions between two or more different drugs, or even in the interaction between drugs and foodstuffs or environmental factors.

The risk of serious interactions between monoamine-oxidase inhibitor (MAOI) antidepressants and certain foodstuffs and decongestants is well known. Most people will be aware of the additive or potentiating action of alcohol has on the sedative or sleep-enhancing effects of many drugs, such as benzodiazepine anxiolytics, antihistamines and components of 'cold-cures'. It is a legal requirement that medicines are labelled in standard ways to warn the user of such hazards.

There is a widely held belief that antibiotics and alcohol 'do not mix'. This is true for some but not for all. For example, certain antibiotics (eg azole antimicrobials such as metronidazole) interfere with the metabolism of alcohol so that it produces a toxic metabolite, called acetaldehyde, in the body, and this may make the subject feel very ill indeed (see the entry on disulfiram).

Details of some of the more worrying drug interactions are given under individual generic entries. However, by no means all interactions between two drugs are detrimental, and two drugs may be specifically prescribed to be taken together for a variety of reasons. For example, one of a pair of drugs may inhibit the break down or excretion of the other drug, so prolonging its beneficial effects (eg clavulanic acid prolongs the duration of action of antibiotics such as amoxycillin by inhibiting bacterial penicillinase enzymes which break down many penicillin antibiotics). Another reason for taking two drugs simultaneously is where one drug counteracts the adverse effects of the other; this can occur in the treatment of Parkinson's disease and other diseases of the central nervous system.

In general, however, drug interactions are complex and sometimes difficult to predict. The doctor or pharmacist will have detailed charts of known interactions, and in all cases should be consulted if the patient is worried, and expert opinion should always be taken if more than one drug is to be used at a time.

In summary

Deregulation is lowering the protective shield afforded by the older prescription-only approach to drug therapy, and as a result greater responsibility is being thrown on the individual. We must therefore become conversant with some basic facts about our own individual reactions to the basic types of drugs. We must know when to seek advice from the healthcare professionals and what to ask them.

Good medical therapy depends on a partnership between the patient and medical professionals.

Other publications

Healthcare professionals use a number of similar guides. The British National Formulary (BNF) – issued twice a year by the British Medical Association and the Pharmaceutical Society of Great Britain – is the standard, impartial and authoritative guide. Along with MIMS (Monthly Index of Medical Specialities, a commercial compendium), the BNF is circulated to prescribing medical practitioners. Over-the-counter drugs are covered by the OTC Directory, published by PAGB (Proprietary Association of Great Britain) and issued to healthcare professionals.

Detailed information on proprietary drugs is also available to professionals from manufacturers, and is published annually in the ABPI Handbook (Association of British Pharmaceutical Industry). Independent comment on drug-related matters is available to everyone in the *Drug and Therapeutics Bulletin* published by the Consumers Association.

The *Guide to Drugs and Medicines*, published by the British Medical Association, and *Which Medicine?*, from the Consumers Association, deal with drugs under disease-related headings, and this book can act as a complementary reference source to these.

Readers' letters

The authors would welcome any comments, suggestions or criticisms, regarding the scope, structure and ease of use of this book, as it is their aim to constantly review and improve the guide during the compiling and revision of each new edition. If you do wish to contact them, please write to the publishers who will then pass on any correspondence. However, the authors are unable comment on an individual's course of treatment.

IKMM
JMH
King's College London & University of Surrey

May 1997

MEDICINES

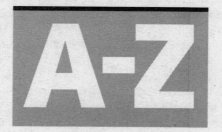

A-Z

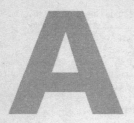

Abelcet

(Liposome Company) is a proprietary, prescription-only preparation of the ANTIFUNGAL and ANTIBIOTIC amphotericin, which has an unusual formulation as a lipid colloidal dispersion (with α dimyristoylphosphatidylcholine and α dimyristoylphosphatidylglycerol) that is intended to minimize toxicity (particularly to the kidney), so that it can be used for severe systemic or deep-seated fungal infections (for example, in patients with severe invasive candidiasis and in AIDS patients). It is available in a form for infusion.

✛▲ Side-effects/warning: See AMPHOTERICIN.

abortifacients ▣

are drugs which are used to induce abortion or miscarriage. There are a number of drug types that have been used to procure therapeutic abortion, but commonly used is the progestogen HORMONE ANTAGONIST drug MIFEPRISTONE (administered orally) and/or a prostaglandin (eg GEMEPROST or DINOPROSTONE; administered either by pessary or local injection, dependng on the stage of pregnancy). Sometimes OXYTOCIN or ERGOMETRINE MALEATE are used as part of the procedure (eg to help stop bleeding following abortion). A variety of other synthetic or natural agents, and certain microbial toxins, may cause abortion (depending on dose and route of administration).

AC Vax

(SmithKline Beecham) is a proprietary, prescription-only VACCINE preparation. It can be used to give protection against the organism meningococcus (*Neisseria meningitidis* groups A and C), which can cause serious infection such as meningitis. It is available in a form for injection.

✛▲ Side-effects/warning: See MENINGOCOCCAL POLYSACCHARIDE VACCINE.

acarbose

is an ENZYME INHIBITOR that interferes with the conversion in the intestine of starch and sucrose (sugar) to glucose and is used in DIABETIC TREATMENT. It has recently been introduced for the treatment of Type II diabetes (non-insulin-dependent diabetes mellitus; NIDDM; maturity-onset diabetes). It may be of value in patients where other drugs, or diet control, have not been successful. It is available as tablets to be taken immediately before food.

✛ Side-effects: Gastrointestinal disturbances, including diarrhoea, flatulence and distension.

▲ Warning: Because of side-effects it should not be used if there are certain types of intestinal disease. Do not use in pregnancy and when breast-feeding, or when there are certain kidney or liver disorders. Monitor blood glucose and enzymes.

✪ Related entry: Glucobay.

Accupro

(Parke-Davis) is a proprietary, prescription-only preparation of the ACE INHIBITOR quinapril. It can be used as an ANTIHYPERTENSIVE and in HEART FAILURE TREATMENT, and is available as tablets.

✛▲ Side-effects/warning: See QUINAPRIL.

Accuretic

(Parke-Davis) is a proprietary, prescription-only COMPOUND PREPARATION of the ACE INHIBITOR quinapril and the THIAZIDE DIURETIC hydrochlorothiazide. It can be used as an ANTIHYPERTENSIVE, and is

A

available as tablets.

+▲ Side-effects/warning: See HYDROCHLOROTHIAZIDE; QUINAPRIL.

ACE inhibitors ☒

(angiotensin-converting enzyme inhibitors) are used as ANTIHYPERTENSIVES and in HEART FAILURE TREATMENT. They work by inhibiting the conversion of the natural circulating HORMONE angiotensin I to angiotensin II; and because the latter is a potent VASOCONSTRICTOR, the overall effect is vasodilation (see VASODILATOR) with a HYPOTENSIVE action. This action is of value when the blood pressure is raised (as in hypertension) and also in the treatment of heart failure. There has been a considerable increase recently in the use of ACE inhibitors in moderate hypertension and in severe hypertension when other treatments are not suitable or successful. They are usually used in conjunction with other antihypertension treatments, especially DIURETICS. See CAPTOPRIL; CILAZAPRIL; ENALAPRIL MALEATE; FOSINOPRIL; LISINOPRIL; PERINDOPRIL; QUINAPRIL; RAMIPRIL; TRANDOLAPRIL.

acebutolol

is a BETA-BLOCKER. It can be used as an ANTIHYPERTENSIVE for raised blood pressure, as an ANTI-ANGINA drug to relieve symptoms and to improve exercise tolerance and as an ANTI-ARRHYTHMIC to regularize heartbeat and to treat myocardial infarction (damage to heart muscle, usually due to a heart attack). Administration is oral. It is also available, as an antihypertensive, in the form of COMPOUND PREPARATIONS with DIURETICS.

+▲ Side-effects/warning: See PROPRANOLOL HYDROCHLORIDE.

✪ Related entries: Secadrex; Sectral.

acemetacin

is a (NSAID) NON-NARCOTIC ANALGESIC and ANTIRHEUMATIC. It is used to treat serious rheumatic and arthritic complaints, musculoskeletal pain and postoperative

pain. Chemically, it is closely related to indomethacin (it is its glycolic acid ester), and is administered orally.

+▲ Side-effects/warning: See INDOMETHACIN. It should not be administered to patients who are breast-feeding.

✪ Related entry: Emflex.

acenocoumarol

see NICOUMALONE

acetaminophen

is the standard name used in the USA for PARACETAMOL.

acetazolamide

is a CARBONIC ANHYDRASE INHIBITOR with quite wide-ranging actions in the body. It can be used in GLAUCOMA TREATMENT because it reduces the formation of aqueous humour in the eye. It acts as a DIURETIC and so can be used to treat oedema, especially when associated with congestive heart failure.It has also been used as an ANTI-EPILEPTIC to assist in the prevention of certain types of epileptic seizures, especially in children. Additionally, it can be used to treat the symptoms of premenstrual syndrome and to prevent motion sickness. Administration is either oral or by injection.

+ Side-effects: There may be numbness and tingling of the hands and feet. Rarely, there may be blood disorders or lowered blood potassium.

▲ Warning: It should be administered with caution to patients who are pregnant; and avoid its use in patients with certain severe kidney disorders.

✪ Related entry: Diamox.

acetylcholine

is a NEUROTRANSMITTER in the body. It has a number of important roles in both the central and peripheral nervous systems, relaying messages between nerves or from nerve to innervated organs. In medicine it is rarely used as a drug treatment because it is rapidly broken down in the body by cholinesterase enzymes.

However, in the form of ACETYLCHOLINE CHLORIDE it can be administered in solution to the eyes for cataract surgery and other ophthalmic procedures requiring rapid constriction of the pupil. Although acetylcholine itself is not used therapeutically, a considerable number of drugs work by mimicking, exaggerating or blocking its actions.

PARASYMPATHOMIMETICS have effects similar to those of the parasympathetic nervous system and mimick the actions of acetylcholine. Important parasympatho-mimetic actions include slowing of the heart, vasodilation, constriction of the pupil and altered focusing of the eye. *Direct-acting* parasympathomimetics ANTICHOLINESTERASES act at *muscarinic* RECEPTORS for acetylcholine (eg CARBACHOL and PILOCARPINE). *Indirect-acting* parasympathomimetics prolong the duration of action of naturally released acetylcholine by inhibiting cholinesterase enzymes (eg NEOSTIGMINE).

Certain SKELETAL MUSCLE RELAXANTS act to interfere with neurotransmission by acetylcholine at so-called *nicotinic* receptors, which lie at the junction between nerves and voluntary (skeletal) muscles and are called *neuromuscular blocking drugs*. They are used in surgical operations to paralyse skeletal muscles that are normally under voluntary nerve control and so allow lighter levels of anaesthesia to be administered. These drugs are of one or two sorts: *non-depolarizing* skeletal muscle relaxants (eg GALLAMINE TRIETHIODIDE and TUBOCURARINE CHLORIDE); or *depolarizing* skeletal muscle relaxants (eg SUXAMETHONIUM CHLORIDE). The action of the non-depolarizing blocking drugs can be reversed at the end of an operation by administering an anticholinesterase drug.

GANGLION-BLOCKERS block the transmission of acetylcholine in the peripheral autonomic nervous system at the junctions called ganglia. The ganglion-blockers are now rarely used in medicine because they have very widespread actions.

However, TRIMETAPHAN CAMSYLATE is used as a HYPOTENSIVE for controlling blood pressure during bloodless surgery.

Drugs that mimic acetylcholine through the stimulation of nicotinic receptors also have only a limited use in medicine, because their actions have unacceptable side-effects and are too widespread. Indeed, NICOTINE, as adsorbed into the body by the use of tobacco products, causes widespread and generally undesirable effects, such as an increase in blood pressure, heart rate and blood sugar levels and also a release of adrenaline (which contributes to many of these effects).

In the brain, nicotine acts at nicotinic receptors and causes further stimulation and euphoria, which are all factors in making it such a powerfully habituating (addictive) drug.

Although some ANTICHOLINERGICS act at nicotinic receptors, there is an important group that work by blocking the actions of acetylcholine at muscarinic receptors. The ANTIMUSCARINIC drugs have extensive uses in medicine and it is because they are used so extensively that the term *antimuscarinic* is often used synonymously for *anticholinergic* (even though this is incorrect). Antimuscarinics tend to relax smooth muscle, reduce the secretion of saliva, digestive juices and sweat and dilate the pupils of the eyes. They can also be used as ANTISPASMODICS and ANTIPARKINSONISM drugs (in the treatment of some of the symptoms of Parkinson's disease), or as ANTINAUSEANTS, or ANTI-EMETICS, in the treatment of motion sickness, peptic ulcers, in ophthalmic examinations and in antagonizing adverse effects of anticholinestrases (in medicine, agricultural accidental poisoning or warfare). Examples of antimuscarinic (anticholinergic) drugs include ATROPINE SULPHATE, BENZHEXOL HYDROCHLORIDE and HYOSCINE HYDROBROMIDE.

acetylcholine chloride

is a PARASYMPATHOMIMETIC which is rarely

used therapeutically because it is rapidly broken down in the body. However, it can be applied in solution to the eye for cataract surgery, iridectomy and other types of surgery requiring rapid miosis (constriction of the pupil). Administration is by topical application as a solution. (ACETYLCHOLINE is the natural NEUROTRANSMITTER released from cholinergic nerves in the body.)

+▲ Side-effects/warning: See PILOCARPINE.
✪ Related entry: Miochol.

acetylcysteine

is a MUCOLYTIC drug which reduces the viscosity of sputum and so can be used as an EXPECTORANT in patients with disorders of the upper respiratory airways, such as chronic asthma and bronchitis. It is also used to treat abdominal complications associated with cystic fibrosis and in the eye to increase lacrimation (the production of tears) and mucus secretion.

It is also used as an ANTIDOTE to treat overdose poisoning by the NON-NARCOTIC ANALGESIC paracetamol. The initial symptoms of poisoning usually settle within 24 hours, but they then give way to a serious toxic effect on the liver which takes some days to develop. It is to prevent these latter effects that treatment is directed and is required immediately after overdose, and is normally administered in hospital.

Administration as an antidote is by injection, and for other purposes it is either topical or oral.

+ Side-effects: The type and severity of any side-effects depends on the route of administration, but there may be headache, tinnitus (ringing in the ears) and gastrointestinal irritation.

▲ Warning: Administer with caution to patients with asthma.

✪ Related entries: Ilube; Parvolex.

Acezide

(Squibb) is a proprietary, prescription-only COMPOUND PREPARATION of the ACE INHIBITOR quinapril and the (THIAZIDE) DIURETIC hydrochlorothiazide. It can be used as an ANTIHYPERTENSIVE, and is available as tablets.

+▲ Side-effects/warning: See QUINAPRIL; HYDROCHLOROTHIAZIDE.

Achromycin

(Lederle) is a proprietary, prescription-only preparation of the broad-spectrum ANTIBACTERIAL and (TETRACYCLINE) ANTIBIOTIC tetracycline (as hydrochloride). It can be used to treat many types of infection, and is available as tablets, capsules, an ointment (for skin, eye or ear) and in a form for infusion.

+▲ Side-effects/warning: See TETRACYCLINE.

Aci-Jel

(Cilag) is a proprietary, non-prescription ANTIMICROBIAL preparation of acetic acid. It can be used to treat non-specific vaginal infections and to restore acidity to the vagina. It is available as a jelly, which is supplied with a special applicator.

aciclovir

see ACYCLOVIR

acipimox

is used as a LIPID-LOWERING DRUG in hyperlipidaemia to reduce the levels, or change the proportions, of various lipids in the bloodstream. It is thought to act in a similar way to NICOTINIC ACID, by inhibiting synthesis of lipids in the liver. Generally, it is administered only to patients in whom a strict and regular dietary regime, alone, is not having the desired effect. Administration is oral.

+ Side-effects: There may be flushing, itching, rashes and reddening of the skin; nausea and abdominal pain; diarrhoea; malaise; headache.

▲ Warning: It should not be administered to patients who are pregnant, or have peptic ulcers; and should be administered with caution to those with impaired kidney function.

✪ Related entry: Olbetam.

A

acitretin

is chemically a retinoid (it is a metabolite of etretinate, which is a derivative of RETINOL or vitamin A) and has a marked effect on the cells that make up the skin epithelium. It can be administered over a period of weeks to relieve a severe case of psoriasis that is resistant to other treatments, and also for certain other skin conditions (including severe Darier's disease). Treatment is under strict medical supervision. Administration is oral.
✚ Side-effects: These include dryness of skin, cracked lips and mucous membrane, muscle and joint ache, hair loss, reversible visual disturbances, nausea, headache, sweating, changes in liver function, blood upsets, mood changes and drowsiness.
▲ Warning: Do not use in patients who are pregnant (and exclude pregnancy before starting and after treatment) or breast-feeding, or who have certain liver or kidney disorders. Avoid excessive exposure to sunlight.
✪ Related entry: Neotigason.

Aclacin

(Lundbeck) is a proprietary, prescription-only preparation of the (CYTOTOXICS) ANTICANCER drug aclarubicin. It is used to treat certain leukaemias, and is available in a form for injection.
✚▲ Side-effects/warning: See ACLARUBICIN.

aclarubicin

is a recently introduced CYTOTOXIC drug (in fact, an ANTIBIOTIC in origin) with properties similar to doxorubicin. It is used as an ANTICANCER treatment, particularly to treat acute non-lymphocytic leukaemia in patients who have not responded to, or who have relapsed from, other forms of chemotherapy. Administration is by injection.
✚▲ Side-effects/warning: See CYTOTOXICS. Administer with caution to patients with kidney or liver impairment; it is irritant to tissues.
✪ Related entry: Aclacin.

Acnecide

(Novex) is a proprietary, non-prescription preparation of the KERATOLYTIC and ANTIMICROBIAL benzoyl peroxide. It can be used to treat acne, and is available as a gel.
✚▲ Side-effects/warning: See BENZOYL PEROXIDE.

Acnegel

(Stiefel) is a proprietary, non-prescription preparation of the KERATOLYTIC and ANTIMICROBIAL benzoyl peroxide (5%). It can be used to treat acne, and is available as a gel. It is not normally used for children under 12 years, except on medical advice.
✚▲ Side-effects/warning: See BENZOYL PEROXIDE.

Acnegel Forte

(Stiefel) is a proprietary, non-prescription preparation of the KERATOLYTIC and ANTIMICROBIAL benzoyl peroxide (10%). It can be used to treat acne, and is available as a gel. It is not normally used for children under 12 years, except on medical advice.
✚▲ Side-effects/warning: See BENZOYL PEROXIDE.

Acnidazil

(Cilag) is a proprietary, non-prescription COMPOUND PREPARATION of the ANTIFUNGAL miconazole (as nitrate) and the KERATOLYTIC and ANTIMICROBIAL benzoyl peroxide. It can be used to treat acne, and is available as a cream.
✚▲ Side-effects/warning: See BENZOYL PEROXIDE; MICONAZOLE.

Acnisal

(Euroderma) is a proprietary, non-prescription preparation of the KERATOLYTIC agent salicylic acid. It can be used to treat acne, and is available as a solution for topical application.
✚▲ Side-effects/warning: See SALICYLIC ACID.

acrivastine

is an ANTIHISTAMINE which has only recently

A

been developed and has less sedative side-effects than some of the older antihistamines. It can be used for the symptomatic relief of allergic conditions, such as hay fever and urticaria. Administration is oral.

+▲ Side-effects/warning: See ANTIHISTAMINES; but the incidence of sedative and anticholinergic effects is low. Avoid its use in patients with kidney impairment.
۞ Related entry: Semprex.

Act-HIB

(Mérieux) is a proprietary, prescription-only VACCINE preparation for influenza (*Haemophilus influenzae*) infection, and is available in a form for injection.
+▲ Side-effects/warning: See HAEMOPHILUS INFLUENZAE TYPE B VACCINE.

Actal Tablets

(SmithKline Beecham) is a proprietary, non-prescription preparation of the ANTACID alexitol sodium. It can be used for the relief of hyperacidity, dyspepsia and indigestion. It is available as tablets and is not normally given to children, except on medical advice.
+▲ Side-effects/warning: See ALEXITOL SODIUM.

Actifed Compound Linctus

(Warner Wellcome) is a proprietary, non-prescription preparation of the ANTIHISTAMINE triprolidine hydrochloride, the SYMPATHOMIMETIC and DECONGESTANT pseudoephedrine hydrochloride and the (OPIOID) NARCOTIC ANALGESIC and ANTITUSSIVE dextromethorphan hydrobromide. It can be used for the symptomatic relief of unproductive cough and congestion of the upper respiratory tract, including such symptoms caused by allergic conditions. It is available as a liquid, and is not normally given to children under two years, except on medical advice.
+▲ Side-effects/warning: See DEXTROMETHORPHAN HYDROBROMIDE; PSEUDOEPHEDRINE HYDROCHLORIDE; TRIPROLIDINE HYDROCHLORIDE.

Actifed Expectorant

(Warner Wellcome) is a proprietary, non-prescription COMPOUND PREPARATION of the ANTIHISTAMINE triprolidine hydrochloride, the SYMPATHOMIMETIC and DECONGESTANT pseudoephedrine hydrochloride and the EXPECTORANT agent GUAIPHENESIN. It can be used for the symptomatic relief of upper respiratory tract disorders accompanied by productive cough. It is available as a liquid, and is not normally given to children under two years, except on medical advice.
+▲ Side-effects/warning: See PSEUDOEPHEDRINE HYDROCHLORIDE; TRIPROLIDINE HYDROCHLORIDE.

Actifed Junior Cough Relief

(Warner Wellcome) is a proprietary, non-prescription COMPOUND PREPARATION of the ANTIHISTAMINE triprolidine hydrochloride and the ANTITUSSIVE dextromethorphan hydrobromide. It can be used for the symptomatic relief of upper respiratory tract disorders accompanied by unproductive cough and other cold symptoms in children. It is available as a liquid, and is not normally given to children under one year, except on medical advice.
+▲ Side-effects/warning: See DEXTROMETHORPHAN HYDROBROMIDE; TRIPROLIDINE HYDROCHLORIDE.

Actifed Syrup

(Warner Wellcome) is a proprietary, non-prescription COMPOUND PREPARATION of the ANTIHISTAMINE triprolidine hydrochloride and the SYMPATHOMIMETIC and DECONGESTANT pseudoephedrine hydrochloride. It can be used for congestion of the upper airways and sinuses, and for the symptomatic treatment of colds, hay fever and rhinitis. It is available as a liquid, and is not normally given to children under two years, except on medical advice.
+▲ Side-effects/warning: See PSEUDOEPHEDRINE HYDROCHLORIDE; TRIPROLIDINE HYDROCHLORIDE.

Actifed Tablets

(Warner Wellcome) is a proprietary, non-prescription COMPOUND PREPARATION of the ANTIHISTAMINE triprolidine hydrochloride and the SYMPATHOMIMETIC and DECONGESTANT pseudoephedrine hydrochloride. It can be used for congestion of the upper airways and sinuses, and for the symptomatic treatment of colds, hayfever and rhinitis. It is available as a liquid, and is not normally given to children under 12 years, except on medical advice.

+▲ Side-effects/warning: See PSEUDOEPHEDRINE HYDROCHLORIDE; TRIPROLIDINE HYDROCHLORIDE.

Actilyse

(Boehringer Ingelheim) is a proprietary, prescription-only preparation of the FIBRINOLYTIC alteplase. It can be used to treat myocardial infarction, and is available in a form for injection.

+▲ Side-effects/warning: See ALTEPLASE.

Actinac

(Roussel) is a proprietary, prescription-only COMPOUND PREPARATION of the broad-spectrum ANTIBACTERIAL and ANTIBIOTIC chloramphenicol and the ANTI-INFLAMMATORY and CORTICOSTEROID hydrocortisone (as acetate). It can be used by topical application to treat acne, and is available as a lotion.

+▲ Side-effects/warning: See CHLORAMPHENICOL; HYDROCORTISONE.

actinomycin D

see DACTINOMYCIN

activated charcoal

is an adsorbent material. Its primary use is for soaking up poisons in the stomach or small intestine, especially drug overdoses in cases where only a small quantity of the drug may be extremely toxic (eg some ANTIDEPRESSANTS). It can help prevent the effects of drug overdose by increasing the elimination of certain drugs even after they have been absorbed (eg ASPIRIN and

BARBITURATES). It is available as a powder to be taken in solution as often as necessary. It can also be used as a constituent in ANTIDIARRHOEAL preparations – it is effective in binding together faecal matter – and can relieve flatulence.

✪ Related entries: Carbomix; Medicoal.

Actron

(Bayer) is a proprietary, non-prescription COMPOUND PREPARATION of the (NSAID) NON-NARCOTIC ANALGESIC paracetamol, the (NSAID) non-narcotic and ANTIRHEUMATIC aspirin, the ANTACID sodium bicarbonate, citric acid and the STIMULANT caffeine. It can be used for general aches and pains and for headache with upset stomach. It is available as effervescent tablets, and is not normally given to children under 12 years, except on medical advice.

+▲ Side-effects/warning: See ASPIRIN; CAFFEINE; PARACETAMOL; SODIUM BICARBONATE.

Acular

(Allergan) is a proprietary, prescription-only preparation of the (NSAID) NON-NARCOTIC ANALGESIC ketorolac trometamol. It can be used to prevent and reduce inflammation following eye surgery, and is available as eye-drops.

+▲ Side-effects/warning: See KETOROLAC TROMETAMOL.

Acupan

(3M) is a proprietary, prescription-only preparation of the NON-NARCOTIC ANALGESIC nefopam hydrochloride. It can be used to treat moderate pain, and is available as tablets and in a form for injection.

+▲ Side-effects/warning: See NEFOPAM HYDROCHLORIDE.

acyclovir

(aciclovir) is an ANTIVIRAL which is used specifically to treat infection by the herpes viruses (eg shingles, chickenpox, cold sores, genital herpes and herpes infections of the eye and mouth). It works by inhibiting the action of enzymes in human

A

cells that are used by the virus to replicate itself. To be effective, however, treatment must begin early. It can be valuable in immunocompromised patients. The drug can also be used prophylactically to prevent individuals at risk from contracting a herpes disease. Administration can be oral, as a variety of topical preparations (ointments and creams) or by injection.

+ Side-effects: When applied topically, there may be a temporary burning or stinging sensation; some patients experience a localized drying of the skin. When taken orally, it may give rise to gastrointestinal disturbance and various blood-cell deficiencies. There may also be fatigue, rash, headache, tremor and effects on mood.

▲ Warning: Administer with caution to patients who are pregnant or breast-feeding; or who have impaired kidney function. Adequate fluid intake must be maintained.

✪ Related entry: Zovirax; Zovirax Cold Sore Cream.

Adalat

(Bayer) is a proprietary, prescription-only preparation of the CALCIUM-CHANNEL BLOCKER nifedipine. It can be used as an ANTI-ANGINA treatment in the prevention of attacks, as an ANTIHYPERTENSIVE and as a VASODILATOR in peripheral vascular disease (Raynaud's phenomenon). It is available as capsules.

+▲ Side-effects/warning: See NIFEDIPINE.

Adalat LA

(Bayer) is a proprietary, prescription-only preparation of the CALCIUM-CHANNEL BLOCKER nifedipine. It can be used as an ANTIHYPERTENSIVE, and is available as modified-release tablets in two doses: *Adalat LA 30* and *Adalat LA 60*.

+▲ Side-effects/warning: See NIFEDIPINE.

Adalat Retard

(Bayer) is a proprietary, prescription-only preparation of the CALCIUM-CHANNEL BLOCKER nifedipine. It can be used as an ANTIHYPERTENSIVE and an ANTI-ANGINA treatment in the prevention of attacks. It

is available as modified-release tablets in two doses: *Adalat Retard 10* and *Adalat Retard 20*.

+▲ Side-effects/warning: See NIFEDIPINE.

Adcortyl

(Squibb) is a proprietary, prescription-only preparation of the CORTICOSTEROID and ANTI-INFLAMMATORY triamcinolone acetonide. It can be used to treat skin conditions, such as eczema and psoriasis, that are unresponsive to other corticosteroids. It is available as a cream and an ointment.

+▲ Side-effects/warning: See TRIAMCINOLONE ACETONIDE.

Adcortyl in Orabase

(Bristol-Myers Squibb) is a proprietary, prescription-only preparation of the CORTICOSTEROID and ANTI-INFLAMMATORY triamcinolone acetonide. (A version called *Adcortyl in Orabase for Mouth Ulcers* is available without prescription). It can be used to treat mouth ulcers and inflammation, and is available as an oral paste.

+▲ Side-effects/warning: See TRIAMCINOLONE ACETONIDE.

Adcortyl Intra-articular/Intradermal

(Squibb) is a proprietary, prescription-only preparation of the CORTICOSTEROID and ANTI-INFLAMMATORY triamcinolone acetonide. It can be administered by intradermal injection to relieve some skin lesions, or by injection directly into soft tissue or a joint to relieve pain, swelling and stiffness (eg tennis elbow).

+▲ Side-effects/warning: See TRIAMCINOLONE ACETONIDE.

Adcortyl with Graneodin

(Squibb) is a proprietary, prescription-only COMPOUND PREPARATION of the ANTI-INFLAMMATORY and CORTICOSTEROID triamcinolone acetonide and the ANTIBACTERIAL and ANTIBIOTIC drugs neomycin sulphate and gramicidin. It can

be used to treat inflammatory skin conditions with infection, such as psoriasis and eczema, and is available as a cream.
+▲ Side-effects/warning: See GRAMICIDIN; NEOMYCIN SULPHATE; TRIAMCINOLONE ACETONIDE.

Adenocor

(Sanofi Winthrop) is a proprietary, prescription-only preparation of the ANTI-ARRHYTHMIC adenosine. It can be used to correct heart irregularities, and is available as tablets and in a form for injection.
+▲ Side-effects/warning: See ADENOSINE.

Adenoscan

(Sanofi Winthrop) is a proprietary, prescription-only preparation of the ANTI-ARRHYTHMIC adenosine. It can be used in conjunction with radionuclide myocardial perfusion imaging in patients who cannot exercise adequately as a diagnostic procedure. Administration is by injection.
+▲ Side-effects/warning: See ADENOSINE.

adenosine

can be used as an ANTI-ARRHYTHMIC to correct certain abnormal rhythms (eg Wolff-Parkinson-White syndrome) and help in the diagnosis of certain arrhythmias (complex supraventricular tachycardias). Administration is by injection.
+ Side-effects: Flushes of the face; shortness of breath, choking and bronchospasm; nausea and light-headedness; extreme slowing of the heart and chest pain.
▲ Warning: It should be administered with caution in certain heart conditions, and is not to be given to patients with asthma.
✪ Related entries: Adenocor; Adenoscan.

ADH (antidiuretic hormone)

see VASOPRESSIN

Adifax

(Servier) is a proprietary, prescription-only preparation of the APPETITE SUPPRESSANT dexfenfluramine hydrochloride. It can be used in obesity, and is available as capsules.

+▲ Side-effects/warning: See DEXFENFLURAMINE HYDROCHLORIDE.

Adizem-60

(Napp) is a proprietary, prescription-only preparation of the CALCIUM-CHANNEL BLOCKER diltiazem hydrochloride. It can be used as an ANTIHYPERTENSIVE and as an ANTI-ANGINA drug. It is available as modified-release tablets.
+▲ Side-effects/warning: See DILTIAZEM HYDROCHLORIDE.

Adizem-SR

(Napp) is a proprietary, prescription-only preparation of the CALCIUM-CHANNEL BLOCKER diltiazem hydrochloride. It can be used as an ANTIHYPERTENSIVE and as an ANTI-ANGINA drug. It is available as modified-release tablets and capsules.
+▲ Side-effects/warning: See DILTIAZEM HYDROCHLORIDE.

Adizem-XL

(Napp) is a proprietary, prescription-only preparation of the CALCIUM-CHANNEL BLOCKER diltiazem hydrochloride. It can be used as an ANTIHYPERTENSIVE and as an ANTI-ANGINA drug. It is available as modified-release capsules.
+▲ Side-effects/warning: See DILTIAZEM HYDROCHLORIDE.

Adizem-XL Plus

(Napp) is a proprietary, prescription-only COMPOUND PREPARATION of the CALCIUM-CHANNEL BLOCKER diltiazem hydrochloride with the DIURETIC hydrochlorothiazide. It can be used as an ANTIHYPERTENSIVE, and is available as modified-release capsules.
+▲ Side-effects/warning: See DILTIAZEM HYDROCHLORIDE; HYDROCHLOROTHIAZIDE.

adrenaline

is chemically called a catecholamine (in the USA it is known as *epinephrine* or *Adrenalin*). It is secreted into the bloodstream (along with the closely related substance NORADRENALINE) as an endocrine

A

HORMONE by the adrenal glands, from the region called the medulla (the central core; hence *adrenomedullary hormone*).

The adrenal glands constitute an important part of the sympathetic nervous system. Together with noradrenaline (which also acts as a NEUROTRANSMITTER, being released from nerve-endings by electrical signals travelling from the central nervous system via nerves in the body), adrenaline activates or inhibits a wide variety of muscles, exocrine glands and metabolic processes in the body.

The responses of the body to stimulation of the sympathetic nervous system are primarily concerned with reactions to stress. In the face of stress, or the need for exertion, the body uses adrenaline and noradrenaline to cause constriction of some blood vessels while dilating others, with the net effect that the two catecholamines increase blood flow to the skeletal muscles and heart. The heart rate is raised and there is relaxation of the smooth muscles of the intestine and bronchioles.

There is also a rise in concentration of energy-supplying glucose and free fatty-acids in the bloodstream. The actions of noradrenaline and adrenaline are similar. Adrenaline itself is not greatly used therapeutically because its actions are so widespread.

In emergencies, however, it may be injected (in the form of adrenaline acid tartrate) in cardiac arrest, to treat the circulatory collapse and bronchoconstriction of anaphylactic shock and in angio-oedema. More commonly, adrenaline is included in several LOCAL ANAESTHETIC preparations, because its pronounced VASOCONSTRICTOR actions considerably prolong anaesthesia by preventing the local anaesthetic from being removed in the bloodstream. Also, it is administered in solution in eye-drops to treat glaucoma. Administration of adrenaline is by injection (as well as various specialized methods with local anaesthetics), by inhalation or topically as eye-drops.

✚ Side-effects: Depending on the route of administration, there may be an increase in heart rate and irregular rhythms; dry mouth, anxiety or fear and coldness in the fingertips and toes. High dosage may lead to tremor, the accumulation of fluid in the lungs and cerebral haemorrhage. Adrenaline in eye-drops may cause redness and smarting of the eye.

▲ Warning: It should be administered with caution to patients who suffer from ischaemic heart disease or hypertension, diabetes or over-activity of the thyroid gland (hyperthyroidism). There may be severe drug interactions in patients who are already taking a number of other drugs, particularly antidepressants and beta-blockers.

✪ Related entries: Epifen; Eppy; Ganda; Marcain with Adrenaline; Medihaler-epi; Min-I-Jet Adrenaline; Min-I-Jet Lignocaine Hydrochloride with Adrenaline; Simplene.

adrenergic-neurone blockers ⊠

act to prevent the release of NORADRENALINE from the nerves of the sympathetic nervous system, which is involved in controlling involunary functions, such as blood pressure, heart rate and the activity of muscles of internal organs (eg blood vessels, intestines and glandular secretions).

Noradrenaline is the main NEUROTRANSMITTER of the sympathetic nervous system and therefore adrenergic-neurone blockers cause an overall ANTISYMPATHETIC action with a fall in blood pressure. Consequently, the main therapeutic use of such drugs is as ANTIHYPERTENSIVES. However, because of their quite marked side-effects, adrenergic-neurone blockers are not the drugs-of-choice in the treatment of moderate to severe high blood pressure. See BETHANIDINE SULPHATE; BRETYLIUM TOSYLATE; DEBRISOQUINE; GUANETHIDINE MONOSULPHATE.

adrenocorticotrophic hormone (ACTH)

see CORTICOTROPHIN

Adsorbed Diphtheria and Tetanus Vaccine

(District Health Authorities) (DT/Vac/Ads) is a non-proprietary, prescription-only VACCINE preparation that combines (toxoid) vaccines for diphtheria and tetanus vaccine adsorbed onto a mineral carrier. It is available in a form for injection.

+▲ Side-effects/warning: See DIPHTHERIA VACCINES; TETANUS VACCINE.

adsorbed diphtheria and tetanus vaccine

(DT/Vac/Ads) is a VACCINE used for IMMUNIZATION against diphtheria and tetanus and is adsorbed onto a mineral carrier. This combination of DIPHTHERIA VACCINE and TETANUS VACCINE is used for the primary immunization of children and as an alternative to ADSORBED DIPTHERIA, TETANUS AND PERTUSSIS VACCINE (DTPer/Vac/Ads), for children who can not be given the pertussis vaccine. It is also used as a reinforcing vaccination at school entry. Administration is by injection.

+▲ Side-effects/warning: See DIPHTHERIA VACCINE; TETANUS VACCINE.

✪ Related entries: Adsorbed Diphtheria and Tetanus Vaccine; Adsorbed Diphtheria and Tetanus Vaccine for Adults and Adolescents; Diftavax.

Adsorbed Diphtheria and Tetanus Vaccine for Adults and Adolescents

(District Health Authorities) (DT/Vac/Ads for Adults) is a non-proprietary, prescription-only VACCINE preparation which combines (toxoid) vaccines for diphtheria and TETANUS VACCINE adsorbed onto a mineral carrier. It is available in a form for injection.

+▲ Side-effects/warning: See DIPHTHERIA VACCINES; TETANUS VACCINE.

Adsorbed Diphtheria, Tetanus and Pertussis Vaccine

(District Health Authorities) (DTPer/Vac/Ads) is a non-proprietary, prescription-only VACCINE preparation, commonly referred to as *triple vaccine*, which combines (toxoid) vaccines for diphtheria and pertussis (whooping cough) with TETANUS VACCINE adsorbed onto a mineral carrier. It is available in a form for injection.

+▲ Side-effects/warning: See DIPHTHERIA VACCINES; PERTUSSIS VACCINE; TETANUS VACCINE.

adsorbed diphtheria, tetanus and pertussis vaccine

(DTPer/Vac/Ads) is a VACCINE used for IMMUNIZATION against diphtheria, tetanus and pertussis (whooping cough). It consists of DIPHTHERIA VACCINE, TETANUS VACCINE and PERTUSSIS VACCINE adsorbed onto a mineral carrier. This *triple vaccine* is used for the primary immunization of children, and is administered by injection.

+▲ Side-effects/warning: See DIPHTHERIA VACCINE; PERTUSSIS VACCINE; TETANUS VACCINE.

✪ Related entries: Adsorbed Diphtheria, Tetanus and Pertussis Vaccine; Trivac-AD.

Adsorbed Diphtheria Vaccine

(District Health Authorities) (Dip/Vac/Ads) is a non-proprietary, prescription-only VACCINE preparation of (toxoid) vaccines for diphtheria adsorbed onto a mineral carrier. It is available in a form for injection.

+▲ Side-effects/warning: See DIPHTHERIA VACCINES.

adsorbed diphtheria vaccine

(Dip/Vac/Ads) is a VACCINE used for IMMUNIZATION against diphtheria and is adsorbed onto a mineral carrier. This form of DIPHTHERIA VACCINE is administered to those who come into contact with someone who has diphtheria or is a carrier.

A

Administration is by injection.

+▲ Side-effects/warning: See DIPHTHERIA VACCINE.

✪ Related entries: Adsorbed Diphtheria Vaccine; Adsorbed Diphtheria Vaccine for Adults.

Adsorbed Diphtheria Vaccine for Adults

(District Health Authorities) (Dip/Vac/Ads for Adults) is a non-proprietary, prescription-only VACCINE preparation of (*toxoid*) vaccines for diphtheria adsorbed onto a mineral carrier. It is available in a form for injection.

+▲ Side-effects/warning: See DIPHTHERIA VACCINES.

Adsorbed Tetanus Vaccine

(Evans) (Tet/Vac/Ads) is a non-proprietary, prescription-only VACCINE preparation of adsorbed tetanus vaccine. It can be used for active IMMUNIZATION against tetanus, and is available in a form for injection.

+▲ Side-effects/warning: See ADSORBED TETANUS VACCINE.

adsorbed tetanus vaccine

(Tet/Vac/Ads) is a VACCINE used for IMMUNIZATION against tetanus and is adsorbed onto a mineral carrier. This form of TETANUS VACCINE is used where a combined vaccine, such as *triple vaccine*, has not been given or as a booster in later life. Administration is by injection.

✪ Related entries: Adsorbed Tetanus Vaccine.

AeroBec

(3M) is a proprietary, prescription-only preparation of the CORTICOSTEROID and ANTI-ASTHMATIC drug beclomethasone dipropionate. It can be administered to prevent asthmatic attacks, and is available in aerosols for inhalation in two forms: *AeroBec 50 Autohaler* and *AeroBec 100 Autohaler*.

+▲ Side-effects/warning: See BECLOMETHASONE DIPROPIONATE.

AeroBec Forte

(3M) is a proprietary, prescription-only preparation of the CORTICOSTEROID and ANTI-ASTHMATIC drug beclomethasone dipropionate. It can be used to prevent asthmatic attacks, and is available in an aerosol for inhalation.

+▲ Side-effects/warning: See BECLOMETHASONE DIPROPIONATE.

Aerocrom

(Fisons) is a proprietary, prescription-only COMPOUND PREPARATION of the ANTI-ALLERGIC sodium cromoglycate and the BETA-RECEPTOR STIMULANT salbutamol (as salbutamol sulphate), which is used as an ANTI-ASTHMATIC. It is important that it is used for the prevention (prophylaxis) of asthma symptoms, rather than the acute treatment of asthma attacks. It is available as an aerosol.

+▲ Side-effects/warning: See SALBUTAMOL; SODIUM CROMOGLYCATE.

Aerolin Autohaler

(3M) is a proprietary, prescription-only preparation of the BETA-RECEPTOR STIMULANT salbutamol (as salbutamol sulphate). It can be used as a BRONCHODILATOR in reversible obstructive airways disease, as an ANTI-ASTHMATIC in the treatment of severe acute asthma or for the alleviation of symptoms of chronic bronchitis and emphysema. It is available as a breath-actuated metered aerosol inhalant.

+▲ Side-effects/warning: See SALBUTAMOL.

Afrazine

(Schering-Plough) is a proprietary, non-prescription preparation of the NASAL DECONGESTANT oxymetazoline hydrochloride. It can be used for the relief of nasal congestion associated with a wide variety of upper respiratory tract disorders. It is available as a nasal spray and is not normally given to children under five years, except on medical advice.

+▲ Side-effects/warning: See OXYMETAZOLINE HYDROCHLORIDE.

Agarol

(Warner Wellcome) is a proprietary, non-prescription COMPOUND PREPARATION of the (*stimulant*) LAXATIVE phenolphthalein and the (*faecal softener*) laxative liquid paraffin. It can be used to relieve temporary constipation and is available as an emulsion. It is not normally given to children under five years, except on medical advice.

+▲ Side-effects/warning: See LIQUID PARAFFIN; PHENOLPHTHALEIN.

Airomir

(3M) is a proprietary, prescription-only preparation of the BETA-RECEPTOR STIMULANT salbutamol. It can be used as a BRONCHODILATOR in reversible obstructive airways disease, as an ANTI-ASTHMATIC in severe acute asthma and for the alleviation of symptoms of chronic bronchitis and emphysema. It is available in an aerosol inhalant.

+▲ Side-effects/warning: See SALBUTAMOL.

Akineton

(Knoll) is a proprietary, prescription-only preparation of the ANTICHOLINERGIC biperiden. It can be used in the treatment of parkinsonism, and is available as tablets and in a form for injection.

+▲ Side-effects/warning: See BIPERIDEN.

Aknemin

(Merck) is a proprietary, prescription-only preparation of the ANTIBACTERIAL and (TETRACYCLINE) ANTIBIOTIC minocycline. It can be used to treat a wide range of infections, and is available as capsules.

+▲ Side-effects/warning: See MINOCYCLINE.

albendazole

is an ANTHELMINTIC which is used to provide cover during surgery for the removal of cysts caused by the tapeworm *Echinococcus* and as treatment when surgery is not possible. Administration is oral.

+ Side-effects: There may be headache,

dizziness, gastrointestinal disturbances, hair loss, rash and fever. Blood disorders have been reported.

▲ Warning: It is not to be given to anyone who is pregnant and administer with care to those who are breast-feeding. Blood and liver function tests are advisable.

○ Related entry: Eskazole.

alclometasone dipropionate

is a CORTICOSTEROID with ANTI-INFLAMMATORY properties. It is used in the treatment of inflammatory skin disorders, particularly eczema. Administration is by topical application.

+▲ Side-effects/warning: See HYDROCORTISONE.

○ Related entry: Modrasone.

Alcobon

(Roche) is a proprietary, prescription-only preparation of the ANTIFUNGAL flucytosine. It can be used to treat systemic fungal infections (eg candidiasis), and is available in a form for infusion.

+▲ Side-effects/warning: See FLUCYTOSINE.

Alcoderm

(Novex) is a proprietary, non-prescription preparation of liquid paraffin and a number of other EMOLLIENT agents. It can be used for dry or itchy skin, and is available as a lotion.

+▲ Side-effects/warning: See LIQUID PARAFFIN.

alcohol

is the name of a class of compounds that are derived from hydrocarbons. The best-known alcohol is ethyl alcohol, or ethanol. Although not normally used as a medicine, the actions of ethanol are similar to a number of drugs that depress the central nervous system and is therefore similar to SEDATIVES or HYPNOTICS. The apparent stimulation experienced by many users is usually due to the loss of social inhibitions. Although it *can* be used as a hypnotic drug,

A

it can also cause rebound wakefulness during the night.

Ethanol has quite a strong DIURETIC action, which can also lead to a disrupted night's sleep. There is also a marked dilation of blood vessels (particularly of the face) which can lead to a profound and potentially dangerous loss of body heat in cold weather. An equally dangerous and sometimes lethal side-effect, is that vomiting is stimulated at higher doses and a protective reflex is inhibited which can lead to the inhalation of vomit. For medical purposes, a strong solution of ethanol can be used as an ANTISEPTIC (particularly to prepare skin before injection) or as a preservative.

Aldactide 25

(Searle) is a proprietary, prescription-only COMPOUND PREPARATION of the (*aldosterone-antagonist* and *potassium-sparing*) DIURETIC spironolactone and the (THIAZIDE) diuretic hydroflumethiazide (a combination called co-flumactone 25/25). It can be used for congestive HEART FAILURE TREATMENT, and is available as tablets.

✚▲ Side-effects/warning: See HYDROFLUMETHIAZIDE; SPIRONOLACTONE.

Aldactide 50

(Searle) is a proprietary, prescription-only COMPOUND PREPARATION of the (*aldosterone-antagonist* and *potassium-sparing*) DIURETIC spironolactone and the (THIAZIDE) diuretic hydroflumethiazide (a combination called co-flumactone 50/50). It can be used for congestive HEART FAILURE TREATMENT, and is available as tablets.

✚▲ Side-effects/warning: See HYDROFLUMETHIAZIDE; SPIRONOLACTONE.

Aldactone

(Searle) is a proprietary, prescription-only preparation of the (*aldosterone-antagonist* and *potassium-sparing*) DIURETIC spironolactone, which can be used in conjunction with other types of diuretic, such as the THIAZIDES, that cause loss of potassium. It can be used to treat oedema associated with aldosteronism, for congestive HEART FAILURE TREATMENT, kidney disease and fluid retention, and ascites caused by cirrhosis of the liver. It is available as tablets.

✚▲ Side-effects/warning: See SPIRONOLACTONE.

aldesleukin

(recombinant interleukin-2), is a one of the cytokine inflammatory mediators called interleukins, produced naturally by cells called macrophages in response to infection or antigenic challenge. Synthetic (recombinant) versions can be used as IMMUNOMODULATORS (or IMMUNOSTIMULANTS). Aldesleukin can be used as an ANTICANCER drug, mainly for metastatic renal cell carcinoma. Administration is by injection.

✚▲ Side-effects/warning: It has widespread toxicity, including oedema and hypotension, and adverse actions on the bone marrow, kidneys, liver, thyroid gland and central nervous system.

○ Related entry: Proleukin.

Aldomet

(Merck Sharp & Dohme) is a proprietary, prescription-only preparation of the ANTISYMPATHETIC methyldopa. It can be used as an ANTIHYPERTENSIVE, and is available as tablets, an oral suspension and in a form for injection (as methyldopate hydrochloride).

✚▲ Side-effects/warning: See METHYLDOPA.

alendronate sodium

see ALENDRONIC ACID

alendronic acid

is a drug (a biphosphonate) used (as alendronate sodium) to treat disorders of bone metabolism due to HORMONE imbalance. It reduces calcium release from the bone, and can be used for treating postmenopausal osteoporosis. Administration is oral.

✚ Side-effects: Oesophageal reactions

(characterized by oesophagitis, erosions and ulcers), abdominal pain, distension and flatulence, diarrhoea or constipation, muscle pain, headache; rash and erythema; transient decreases in blood calcium and phosphate reported.

▲ Warning: Not to be administered to patients with certain abnormalities of the oesophagus or other structures, low blood calcium or renal impairment. It is not for use in pregnancy or when breast-feeding.
✪ Related entry: Fosamax.

alexitol sodium

is an aluminium-containing salt which is used as an ANTACID for the relief of hyperacidity, dyspepsia and indigestion. Administration is oral.
✪ Related entries: Actal Tablets; Magnatol.

alfacalcidol

(1α-hydroxycholecalciferol) is a synthesized form of CALCIFEROL (VITAMIN D). It is used to make up vitamin D deficiency, particularly in the treatment of types of hypoparathyroidism and rickets. Administration is oral.
✪ Related entry: One-Alpha.

alfentanil

is an (OPIOID) NARCOTIC ANALGESIC which is used for short surgical operations, outpatient surgery, in combination to enhance the effect of GENERAL ANAESTHETIC and to suppress breathing in patients on artificial ventilation. Administration is by injection. Its proprietary form is on the Controlled Drugs List.
✚▲ Side-effect/warning: See OPIOIDS.
✪ Related entry: Rapifen.

alfuzosin

is a selective ALPHA-ADRENOCEPTOR BLOCKER which can be used to treat urinary retention in benign prostatic hypertrophy. Administration is oral.
✚▲ Side-effects/warning: See PRAZOSIN HYDROCHLORIDE.
✪ Related entry: Xatral.

Algesal

(Duphar) is a proprietary, non-prescription preparation of diethylamine salicylate, which has a COUNTER-IRRITANT, or RUBEFACIENT, action. It can be applied to the skin for the symptomatic relief of musculoskeletal rheumatic conditions, and is available as a cream.
✚▲ Side-effects/warning: See DIETHYLAMINE SALICYLATE.

Algicon

(Rhône-Poulenc Rorer) is a proprietary, non-prescription COMPOUND PREPARATION of the ANTACID aluminium hydroxide combined with magnesium carbonate, potassium bicarbonate, magnesium alginate (a DEMULCENT protectant in reflux oesophagitis) and sucrose (as a sweetener). It can be used for the symptomatic relief of heartburn associated with gastric reflux, reflux oesophagitis, hiatus hernia and hyperacidity (it can be used to relieve these symptoms in pregnancy). It is available as tablets and a suspension.
✚▲ Side-effects/warning: See ALUMINIUM HYDROXIDE; MAGNESIUM CARBONATE.

alginic acid

usually in the form of alginate (magnesium alginate or sodium alginate), is extracted from seaweed. It has a viscous, sticky consistency and is used as a DEMULCENT in certain ANTACID preparations to protect against reflux oesophagitis. It is also incorporated in some mouthwashes or gargles to protect and soothe mucous membranes within the mouth.
✪ Related entries: Algitec; Bisodol Heartburn; Gastrocote; Gaviscon 250; Gaviscon 500; Gaviscon Liquid; Pyrogastrone; Tagamet Dual Action Liquid; Topal.

Algipan Rub

(Whitehall) is a proprietary, non-prescription COMPOUND PREPARATION of capsicum oleoresin, methyl nicotinate and

A

GLYCOL SALICYLATE, which all have COUNTER-IRRITANT, or RUBEFACIENT, actions. It can be applied to the skin for the symptomatic relief of muscle pain and stiffness in backache, lumbago, sciatica and fibrosis rheumatic pain. It is available as a cream.
+▲ Side-effects/warning: See CAPSICUM OLEORESIN; METHYL NICOTINATE.

Algitec

(SmithKline Beecham) is a proprietary COMPOUND PREPARATION of the H$_2$-ANTAGONIST cimetidine and the DEMULCENT alginic acid. It is usually only available on prescription, but it can be obtained without one in a limited amount and for short-term use only. It is used as an ULCER-HEALING drug for benign peptic ulcers, gastro-oesophageal reflux, dyspepsia and associated conditions. It is available as chewable tablets (*Chewtab*) and a suspension.
+▲ Side-effects/warning: See CIMETIDINE.

alglucerase

is an ENZYME which is used as a replacement in the specialist treatment of Gaucher's disease (a genetically determined enzyme deficiency disease affecting the spleen, liver, bone marrow and lymph nodes). Administration is by intravenous infusion.
+ Side-effects: Nausea and vomiting, abdominal pain, diarrhoea; irritation or pain at injection site; reports of hypersensitivity reactions.
▲ Warning: It should not be used in androgen-sensitive tumours; administer with care to patients who are pregnant or breast-feeding; specialist monitoring is required.
✪ Related entry: Ceredase.

alimemazine tartrate

see TRIMEPRAZINE TARTRATE

Alimix

(Cilag) is a proprietary, prescription-only preparation of the MOTILITY STIMULANT cisapride. It can be used to stimulate the stomach and intestine in a number of conditions, and is available as tablets.
+▲ Side-effects/warning: See CISAPRIDE.

Alka-Seltzer Original

(Bayer) is a proprietary, non-prescription COMPOUND PREPARATION of the (NSAID) NON-NARCOTIC ANALGESIC and ANTIRHEUMATIC aspirin, citric acid and the ANTACID sodium bicarbonate. It can be used for general aches and pains and for headache with upset stomach. It is available as effervescent tablets and also as *Alka-Seltzer Lemon Flavour*. It is not normally given to children under 12 years, except on medical advice.
+▲ Side-effects/warning: See ASPIRIN; SODIUM BICARBONATE.

alkaloids 🗓

are chemically a group of compounds that are used as drugs. The majority of alkaloids were originally extracted from plants and are chemically heterocyclic, often complex, organic compounds with basic (alkali) properties and in medicine they are usually administered in the form of their salts. Examples still in medical use today include the BELLADONNA ALKALOIDS from the *Atropa belladonna* plant and related species (eg ATROPINE SULPHATE and HYOSCINE HYDROBROMIDE); the alkaloids of opium from the poppy *Papaver somniferum* (eg CODEINE PHOSPHATE, MORPHINE SULPHATE and PAPAVERINE); ERGOT ALKALOIDS (eg ERGOMETRINE MALEATE and ERGOTAMINE TARTRATE); the CINCHONA ALKALOIDS (QUINIDINE and QUININE) from the bark of the cinchona tree; the VINCA ALKALOIDS (eg VINBLASTINE SULPHATE, VINCRISTINE SULPHATE and VINDESINE SULPHATE); EPHEDRINE HYDROCHLORIDE from Chinese plants of the *Ephedra* species; NICOTINE from *Nicotiana tabacum*; TUBOCURARINE CHLORIDE, originally a South American arrow-poison from *Chondrodendron tomentosum* and other species; PILOCARPINE from a South American *Pilocarpus* shrub; and IPECACUANHA, which contains emetine and cephaeline from ipecac ('Brazil root').

Alkeran

(Wellcome) is a proprietary, prescription-only preparation of the (CYTOTOXIC) ANTICANCER drug melphalan. It can be used in the treatment of myelomatosis, and is available as tablets and in a form for injection.

✚▲ Side-effects/warning: See MELPHALAN.

Allegron

(Dista) is a proprietary, prescription-only preparation of the (TRICYCLIC) ANTIDEPRESSANT nortriptyline hydochloride. It can be used to treat depressive illness and also to stop children bed-wetting. It is available as tablets.

✚▲ Side-effects/warning: See NORTRIPTYLINE HYDROCHLORIDE.

Aller-eze

(Intercare) is a proprietary, non-prescription preparation of the ANTIHISTAMINE clemastine (as hydrogen fumarate). It can be used to treat the symptoms of allergic disorders, such as hay fever and urticaria. It is available as tablets and is not normally given to children under three years, except on medical advice.

✚▲ Side-effects/warning: See CLEMASTINE.

Aller-eze Clear

(Intercare) is a proprietary, non-prescription preparation of the ANTIHISTAMINE terfenadine. It can be used to treat the symptoms of allergic disorders, such as hay fever and urticaria. It is available as tablets and is not normally given to children.

✚▲ Side-effects/warning: See TERFENDINE.

Aller-eze Plus

(Intercare) is a proprietary, non-prescription COMPOUND PREPARATION of the ANTIHISTAMINE clemastine (as hydrogen fumarate) and the SYMPATHOMIMETIC and DECONGESTANT phenylpropanolamine. It can be used to treat the symptoms of allergic disorders, such as hay fever, urticaria and nasal congestion. It is available as tablets and is not normaly given to children, except on medical advice.

✚▲ Side-effects/warning: See CLEMASTINE; PHENYLPROPANOLAMINE HYDROCHLORIDE.

allopurinol

is an ENZYME INHIBITOR. It is a XANTHINE-OXIDASE INHIBITOR that inhibits the action of the enzyme xanthine oxidase, which produces uric acid and so can be used to treat excess uric acid in the blood (hyperuricaemia). It is used to prevent attacks of gout and to treat uric acid and calcium oxalate stones in the urinary tract (renal stones). Administration is oral.

✚ Side-effects: A rash (which may mean that treatment should be stopped), gastrointestinal disorders, fever, skin reactions; rarely, malaise, headache, vertigo, drowsiness, hypertension, taste disturbance, xanthine deposits in muscle, hair loss, liver toxicity and peripheral nerve disorders.

▲ Warning: It is not to be used in patients with acute gout; concurrent treatment is required with other drugs (eg colchicine and a NSAID, but not aspirin) and an adequate fluid intake must be maintained.

⊙ Related entries: Caplenal; Cosuric; Rimapurinol; Xanthomax.

Almevax

(Evans) is a proprietary, prescription-only VACCINE preparation for the prevention of rubella (German measles). It is available in a form for injection.

✚▲ Side-effects/warning: See RUBELLA VACCINE.

Almodan

(Berk) is a proprietary, prescription-only preparation of the broad-spectrum ANTIBACTERIAL and (PENICILLIN) ANTIBIOTIC amoxycillin. It can be used to treat systemic bacterial infections, infections of the upper respiratory tract, of the ear, nose and throat, and of the urinogenital tracts. It is available as capsules and as an oral suspension.

✚▲ Side-effects/warning: See AMOXYCILLIN.

A

aloin

is a (*stimulant*) LAXATIVE which is
incorporated into some proprietary
preparations intended for the relief of
constipation.

+▲ Side-effects/warning: See SENNA.

**✪ Related entries: Alophen Pills; Beecham
Pills; Carter's Little Pills.**

Alophen Pills

(Warner Wellcome) is a proprietary, non-
prescription COMPOUND PREPARATION of the
(*stimulant*) LAXATIVES aloin and
phenolphthalein. It can be used to relieve
constipation, and is available as tablets. It is
not normally given to children, except on
medical advice.

+▲ Side-effects/warning: See ALOIN;
PHENOLPHTHALEIN.

aloxiprin

is a (NSAID) NON-NARCOTIC ANALGESIC and
ANTIRHEUMATIC which is incorporated into
some proprietary COMPOUND ANALGESIC
preparations.

✪ Related entries: Askit Powders.

Alpha Keri Bath

(Bristol-Myers) is a proprietary, non-
prescription COMPOUND PREPARATION of liquid
paraffin and lanolin oils, which have
EMOLLIENT properties. It can be used for dry
or itchy skin, and is available as a bath oil.

+▲ Side-effects/warning: See LANOLIN;
LIQUID PARAFFIN.

alpha tocopheryl acetate

is a form of vitamin E (TOCOPHEROL). It is
used to treat deficiency due to
malabsorption, such as in
abetalipoproteinaemia in young children
with congenital cholestasis or cystic fibrosis
and as a vitamin supplement.
Administration is oral.

+ Side-effects: Diarrhoea, abdominal pain.

▲ Warning: Use with care if there is a
predisposition to thrombosis (clot
formation).

✪ Related entry: Vitamin E Suspension.

Alpha VIII

(Alpha) is a proprietary, prescription-only
preparation of dried human factor VIII
fraction, which acts as a HAEMOSTATIC drug
to reduce or stop bleeding. It can be used
in the treatment of disorders in which
bleeding is prolonged and potentially
dangerous (mainly haemophilia A). It is
available in a form for infusion or injection.

+▲ Side-effects/warning: See FACTOR VIII
FRACTION, DRIED.

alpha-adrenoceptor antagonists ▨

see ALPHA-ADRENOCEPTOR BLOCKERS

alpha-adrenoceptor blockers ▨

(alpha-blockers; alpha-adrenoceptor
antagonists) inhibit some actions of the
alpha receptor-stimulant drugs, such as the
HORMONE ADRENALINE (released from the
adrenal gland) and the NEUROTRANSMITTER
NORADRENALINE (which is released from
sympathetic nerves). They also inhibit some
actions of the SYMPATHOMIMETICS that are
used therapeutically (some are chemically
catecholamines). The alpha-adrenoceptor
blocking drugs work by blocking the
receptor sites called alpha-adrenoceptors,
thereby preventing the action of adrenaline-
like agents. A major use of alpha-blockers
is as ANTIHYPERTENSIVES, because they lower
blood pressure by preventing
VASOCONSTRICTOR actions of noradrenaline
and adrenaline (including in the treatment
of phaeochromocytoma). They are also
used to treat urinary retention in benign
prostatic hyperplasia (through an action on
the blood circulation within the prostate).
See INDORAMIN; PHENOXYBENZAMINE
HYDROXIDE; PHENTOLAMINE MESYLATE; PRAZOSIN
HYDROCHLORIDE; TERAZOSIN.

alpha-blockers

see ALPHA-ADRENOCEPTOR BLOCKERS

Alphaderm

(Procter & Gamble) is a proprietary,

prescription-only COMPOUND PREPARATION of the CORTICOSTEROID and ANTI-INFLAMMATORY hydrocortisone and the HYDRATING AGENT urea. It can be used to treat mild inflammation of the skin, such as eczema, and is available as a cream for topical application.
+▲ Side-effects/warning: See HYDROCORTISONE.

Alphanine
(Alpha) is a proprietary, prescription-only preparation of factor IX fraction, dried, which is prepared from human blood plasma. It can be used in treating patients with a deficiency in factor IX (haemophilia B), and is available in a form for infusion.
+▲ Side-effects/warning: See FACTOR IX FRACTION, DRIED.

Alphaparin
(Alpha) is a proprietary, prescription-only preparation of the ANTICOAGULANT certoparin sodium, which is a low molecular weight version of heparin. It can be used for prophylaxis of deep-vein thrombosis, and is available in a form for injection.
+▲ Side-effects/warning: See CERTOPARIN SODIUM.

Alphavase
(Ashbourne) is a proprietary, prescription-only preparation of the ALPHA-ADRENOCEPTOR BLOCKER prazosin hydrochloride. It can be used as an ANTIHYPERTENSIVE, and is available as tablets.
+▲ Side-effects/warning: See PRAZOSIN HYDROCHLORIDE.

Alphosyl
(Stafford-Miller) is a proprietary, non-prescription preparation of coal tar (with allantoin). It can be used to treat eczema and psoriasis, and is available as a cream and a lotion.
+▲ Side-effects/warning: See COAL TAR.

Alphosyl 2 in 1 Shampoo
(Stafford-Miller) is a proprietary, non-

prescription preparation of coal tar. It can be used for the treatment of psoriasis, seborrhoeic dermatitis, scaling, dandruff and itching.
+▲ Side-effects/warning: See COAL TAR.

Alphosyl HC
(Stafford-Miller) is a proprietary, prescription-only COMPOUND PREPARATION of the CORTICOSTEROID and ANTI-INFLAMMATORY hydrocortisone and coal tar (with allantoin). It can be used to treat eczema and psoriasis, and is available as a cream.
+▲ Side-effects/warning: See COAL TAR; HYDROCORTISONE.

alprazolam
is a BENZODIAZEPINE which is used as an ANXIOLYTIC in the short-term treatment of anxiety. Administration is oral.
+▲ Side-effects/warning: See BENZODIAZEPINES.
✪ Related entry: Xanax.

alprostadil
is a PROSTAGLANDIN (PGE$_1$) which is used to maintain babies born with congenital heart defects (to maintain patency of ductus arteriosus), while emergency preparations are being made for corrective surgery and intensive care; administration is by infusion. In men, it is used to treat erectile dysfunction when it is given by intracavernosal injection into the penis.
+ Side-effects: In babies, breathing difficulties (particularly if small); fever, flushing, diarrhoea, blood-clotting problems, convulsions. In men, testicular pain during erection (especially where there is deformation), haematoma at the injection site and a variety of local actions. Other effects have been reported on the cardiovascular system, as well as dizziness and headache.
▲ Warning: In babies, monitoring of arterial pressure is essential; a close watch must also be kept for haemorrhage, hypotension and slow or fast heart rate, high temperature and flushing. Prolonged

A

use may cause bone deformity and damage to the pulmonary artery. It should not be administered to babies whose lungs are imperfectly expanded (hyaline membrane disease). In men, it should not be given when there is a predisposition to prolonged erection (myeloma, sickle-cell anaemia, leukaemia); it should not be given to men who have deformed penises.

✪ Related entries: Caverject; Prostin V; Viridal.

Altacite Plus

(Roussel) is a proprietary, non-prescription COMPOUND PREPARATION of the ANTACID hydrotalcite and the ANTIFOAMING AGENT dimethicone. It can be used for the relief of hyperacidity, flatulence, gastritis and dyspepsia, and is available as a liquid.

✚▲ Side-effects/warning: See DIMETHICONE; HYDROTALCITE.

Altacite Suspension

(Roussel) is a proprietary, non-prescription preparation of the ANTACID hydrotalcite. It can be used for the relief of hyperacidity, gastritis and dyspepsia, and is available as an oral suspension.

✚▲ Side-effects/warning: See HYDROTALCITE.

Altacite Tablets

(Roussel) is a proprietary, non-prescription preparation of the ANTACID hydrotalcite. It can be used for the relief of hyperacidity, gastritis and dyspepsia, and is available as chewable tablets.

✚▲ Side-effects/warning: See HYDROTALCITE.

alteplase

(tissue-type plasminogen activator; rt-PA) is used therapeutically as a FIBRINOLYTIC, because it has the property of breaking up blood clots. It is used in serious conditions such as myocardial infarction (damage to heart muscle, usually after a heart attack). Administration is by injection.

✚ Side-effects: Nausea, vomiting and

bleeding. There may be allergic reaction, such as a rash and a high temperature.

▲ Warning: It should not be administered to patients with disorders of coagulation, or after recent surgery; who are liable to bleed (vaginal bleeding, peptic ulceration, recent trauma or surgery); with acute pancreatitis, or oesophageal varices. Administer with caution to patients who are pregnant.

✪ Related entry: Actilyse.

Alu-Caps

(3M) is a proprietary, non-prescription preparation of the ANTACID aluminium hydroxide. It is used for the relief of hyperacidity and dyspepsia, and is available as capsules. It is not normally given to children, except on medical advice.

✚▲ Side-effects/warning: See ALUMINIUM HYDROXIDE .

Aludrox Liquid

(Pfizer) is a proprietary, non-prescription preparation of the ANTACID aluminium hydroxide. It can be used for hyperacidity and dyspepsia, and is available as a liquid gel. It is not normally given to children under six years, except on medical advice.

✚▲ Side-effects/warning: See ALUMINIUM HYDROXIDE.

Aludrox Tablets

(Pfizer) is a proprietary, non-prescription COMPOUND PREPARATION of the ANTACIDS aluminium hydroxide and magnesium hydroxide. It can be used for the relief of hyperacidity and dyspepsia, and is available as tablets. It is not normally given to children under six years, except on medical advice.

✚▲ Side-effects/warning: See ALUMINIUM HYDROXIDE; MAGNESIUM CARBONATE.

aluminium acetate

is an ASTRINGENT which is used primarily to clean sites of infection and inflammation, particularly weeping or suppurating wounds or sores, eczema and infections of the outer ear. Administration is topical.

aluminium chloride

is a powerful ANTIPERSPIRANT with ASTRINGENT properties. It can be used to treat hyperhidrosis (excessive sweating). Administration is topical.

✚ Side-effects: There may be skin irritation.

▲ Warning: Keep away from the eyes; do not shave the armpits or use hair-removing creams for 12 hours after application.

✪ Related entries: Anhydrol Forte; Driclor.

aluminium hydroxide

is an ANTACID which, because it is relatively insoluble in water, has a long duration of action when retained in the stomach. It can be used to for the symptomatic relief of dyspepsia, hyperacidity, gastritis, peptic ulcers and oesophageal reflux. It can also be used to treat elevated levels of phosphates in the blood (hyperphosphataemia). Administration is oral.

▲ Warning: It should not be administered to patients with hypophosphataemia (low blood phosphates); and use with caution in those with porphyria.

✪ Related entries: Algicon; Alu-Caps; Aludrox Liquid; Aludrox Tablets; Asilone Liquid; Asilone Suspension; Asilone Tablets; Caved-S; Dijex Suspension; Dijex Tablets; Diovol; Gastrocote; Gaviscon 250; Gaviscon 500; Kolanticon Gel; Maalox Plus Suspension; Maalox Plus Tablets; Maalox Suspension; Maalox TC Suspension; Maalox TC Tablets; Maclean Indigestion Tablets; Mucaine; Mucogel Suspension; Pyrogastrone; Topal.

Alupent

(Boehringer Ingelheim) is a proprietary, prescription-only preparation of the BETA-RECEPTOR STIMULANT orciprenaline sulphate. It can be used as a BRONCHODILATOR in reversible obstructive airways disease, as an ANTI-ASTHMATIC treatment in severe acute asthma, or for the alleviation of symptoms of chronic bronchitis and emphysema. It is available as tablets, as an aerosol spray (*Alupent Aerosol*) or as a sugar-free syrup (*Alupent Syrup*).

✚▲ Side-effects/warning: See ORCIPRENALINE SULPHATE.

Alvercol

(Norgine) is a proprietary, non-prescription COMPOUND PREPARATION of the ANTISPASMODIC alverine citrate and the (*bulking-agent*) LAXATIVE sterculia. It can be used to treat irritable bowel syndrome, and is available as oral granules.

✚▲ Side-effects/warning: See ALVERINE CITRATE; STERCULIA.

alverine citrate

is an ANTISPASMODIC which is used to treat spasm in the gastrointestinal tract and in dysmenorrhoea (menstrual discomfort). Administration is oral.

✚ warning: It should not be administered to patients who suffer from paralytic ileus; and administer with care to pregnant women.

✪ Related entries: Alvercol; Relaxyl; Spasmonal.

amantadine hydrochloride

is a prescription-only ANTIPARKINSONISM drug, but is not used to treat the parkinsonian symptoms induced by drugs. It also has some ANTIVIRAL activity and has been used orally to prevent infection with the influenza A_2 virus (but not other influenza viruses) and in the treatment of herpes zoster (shingles). Administration is oral.

✚ Side-effects: Restlessness and inability to concentrate; there may also be dizziness and insomnia, gastrointestinal disturbances, oedema, blood disorders, skin discolouration, anorexia, hallucinations and blurred vision.

▲ Warning: It should not be administered to patients with gastric ulcers or epilepsy. Administer with care to patients with certain heart, liver or kidney disorders, psychosis or long-term eczema; who are pregnant or breast-feeding; who are in a state of confusion; or who are elderly. Withdrawal of

A

treatment in Parkinson's disease must be gradual. It may effect performance of skilled tasks, such as driving.
○ Related entry: Symmetrel.

Ambaxin

(Upjohn) is a proprietary, prescription-only preparation of the broad-spectrum ANTIBACTERIAL and (PENICILLIN) ANTIBIOTIC bacampicillin hydrochloride. It can be used to treat systemic bacterial infections, infections of the upper respiratory tract, of the ear, nose and throat and of the urinogenital tracts. It is available as tablets.
✚▲ Side-effects/warning: See BACAMPICILLIN HYDROCHLORIDE.

AmBisome

(Vestar) is a proprietary, prescription-only preparation of the ANTIFUNGAL and ANTIBIOTIC drug amphotericin, which is in an unusual lipid formulation (encapsulated in liposomes) that is intended to minimize toxicity (particularly to the kidney) so that it can be used for severe systemic or deep-seated fungal infections. It is available in a form for infusion.
✚▲ Side-effects/warning: See AMPHOTERICIN.

amethocaine hydrochloride

is a LOCAL ANAESTHETIC which is used to treat localized pain and irritation and in ophthalmic treatments. Administration is by topical application.
✚▲ Side-effects/warning: See LIGNOCAINE HYDROCHLORIDE. Also, hypersensitivity reactions have been reported. It is absorbed rapidly through mucous membranes and so should not be applied to inflamed, traumatized or highly vascular surfaces.
○ Related entries: Ametop; Eludril Spray; Minims Amethocaine Hydrochloride.

Ametop

(Smith & Nephew) is a proprietary, non-prescription preparation of the LOCAL ANAESTHETIC amethocaine. It can be used by topical application to thr site of

venepuncture or venous cannulation, and is available as a gel.
✚▲ Side-effects/warning: See AMETHOCAINE HYDROCHLORIDE.

Amfipen

(Yamanouchi) is a proprietary, prescription-only preparation of the broad-spectrum ANTIBACTERIAL and (PENICILLIN) ANTIBIOTIC ampicillin. It can be used to treat systemic bacterial infections, infections of the upper respiratory tract, of the ear, nose and throat and of the urinogenital tracts. It is available as capsules and an oral suspension.
✚▲ Side-effects/warning: See AMPICILLIN.

amifostine

is a recently introduced specialist CHELATING AGENT used to reduce neutropenia-related risk of infection due to treatment of ovarian carcinoma with CYCLOPHOSPHAMIDE or CISPLATIN. Administration is by injection.
✚ Side-effects: Hypotension, nausea and vomiting, flushing, chills, dizziness, sleepiness, hiccups and sneezing; rarely low blood calcium; allergic reactions.
○ Related entry: Ethyol.

amikacin

is a broad-spectrum ANTIBACTERIAL and (AMINOGLYCOSIDE) ANTIBIOTIC. Although it does have activity against Gram-positive bacteria, it is used primarily against serious infections caused by Gram-negative bacteria that prove to be resistant to the more widely used aminoglycoside GENTAMICIN. Administration is by injection.
✚▲ Side-effects/warning: See GENTAMICIN.
○ Related entry: Amikin.

Amikin

(Bristol-Myers) is a proprietary, prescription-only preparation of the ANTIBACTERIAL and (AMINOGLYCOSIDE) ANTIBIOTIC amikacin (as sulphate). It can be used to treat several serious bacterial infections, particularly those that prove to be resistant to the more widely used aminoglycoside GENTAMICIN. It is available in forms for injection and infusion.

✚▲ Side-effects/warning: See AMIKACIN.

Amil-Co

(Baker Norton) is a proprietary, prescription-only COMPOUND PREPARATION of the (*potassium-sparing*) DIURETIC amiloride hydrochloride and the THIAZIDE diuretic hydrochlorothiazide (a combination called co-amilozide 5/50). It can be used to treat oedema and as an ANTIHYPERTENSIVE. It is available as tablets.

✚▲ Side-effects/warning: See AMILORIDE HYDROCHLORIDE; HYDROCHLOROTHIAZIDE.

amiloride hydrochloride

is a weak, *potassium-sparing* DIURETIC which retains potassium in the body and is therefore used as an alternative to, or commonly in combination with, other diuretics such as the THIAZIDE and *loop diuretics* (which normally cause a loss of potassium from the body). It can be used to treat oedema, ascites in liver cirrhosis (fluid in the abdomen), as an ANTIHYPERTENSIVE (in combination with other drugs such as the BETA-BLOCKERS) and in congestive HEART FAILURE TREATMENT. Administration is oral.

✚ Side-effects: Gastrointestinal upsets, skin rashes, dry mouth, confusion (particularly in the elderly), postural hypotension (fall in blood pressure on standing); raised blood potassium and lowered blood sodium.

▲ Warning: It should not be administered to patients who have high blood potassium levels, who are taking potassium supplements or who have kidney failure. Administer with care to patients who are pregnant, have diabetes or are elderly.

⊙ Related entries: Amil-Co; Amilospare; Berkamil; Delvas; Fru-Co; Frumil; Frumil Forte; Frumil LS; Kalten; Lasoride; Moducren; Moduret-25; Moduretic; Navispare.

Amilospare

(Ashbourne) is a proprietary, prescription-

only preparation of the (*potassium-sparing*) DIURETIC amiloride hydrochloride. It can be used to treat oedema, ascites in cirrhosis of the liver, congestive heart failure (in conjunction with other diuretics) and as an ANTIHYPERTENSIVE. It is available as tablets.

✚▲ Side-effects/warning: See AMILORIDE HYDROCHLORIDE.

aminacrine hydrochloride

is an ANTISEPTIC incorporated into preparations that are used to treat mouth ulcers.

⊙ Related entries: Bonjela Antiseptic Pain-Relieving Pastilles; Medijel Gel.

aminobenzoic acid

is an unusual drug, sometimes classed as one of the B complex vitamins. It is also used as a SUNSCREEN because it helps to protect the skin from ultraviolet radiation. For this reason, aminobenzoic acid is present in many suntan lotions and also in some barrier preparations to ward off the harmful effects of repeated radiotherapy. Administration is topical.

▲ Warning: Protection is temporary, so creams and lotions must be reapplied every so often. It has been suggested that some preparations containing aminobenzoates may cause photosensitivity reactions.

⊙ Related entries: Spectraban Lotion; Spectraban Ultra; Sun E45.

aminoglutethimide

is used to treat breast cancer. It is thought to work as an indirect HORMONE ANTAGONIST, by inhibiting the conversion of ANDROGENS to OESTROGENS (both groups of sex hormones). It may also be used to treat Cushing's disease caused by cancer of the adrenal gland, which results in the excessive release of CORTICOSTEROID hormones in the body, by inhibiting the formation of corticosteroids. Administration is oral.

✚ Side-effects: There may be drowsiness, lethargy, unsteadiness, rashes and allergic manifestations, nausea and diarrhoea,

A

thyroid gland disturbances and blood disorders.

▲ Warning: It should not be given to pregnant or breast-feeding women; administer with caution to patients with porphyria.

✪ Related entry: Orimeten.

aminoglycosides ▨

make up a chemical class of ANTIBIOTICS that have ANTIBACTERIAL activity and are all *bactericidal* (that is, they kill bacteria rather than merely inhibiting their growth). Although they can be used against some Gram-positive bacteria, aminoglycosides are administered primarily to treat serious infections caused by Gram-negative bacteria.

Aminoglycosides are not absorbed from the gut (unless there is damage), so they must be administered by injection, or by topical application in the case of the toxic members (eg NEOMYCIN SULPHATE). However, they all share a number of common toxic properties (ie side-effects) and, because they are excreted via the kidneys, a potentially dangerous accumulation can occur in patients with impaired kidney function. Toxic effects are related to the dose and one of the most serious is ototoxicity (impaired hearing and balance). See AMIKACIN; GENTAMICIN; KANAMYCIN; METILMICIN; STREPTOMYCIN; TOBRAMYCIN.

aminophylline

is a BRONCHODILATOR which is used as an acute ANTI-ASTHMATIC or bronchitis treatment for severe acute attacks. It is chemically classed as a xanthine and is a chemical combination of theophylline (with ethylenediamine to make it more water-soluble). Administration is either oral or by injection.

✚▲ Side-effects/warning: See THEOPHYLLINE; but the ethylenediamine can cause allergic reactions in the skin.

✪ Related entries: Amnivent; Min-I-Jet Aminophylline; Pecram; Phyllocontin Continus.

aminosalicylates ▨

are a chemical class of drugs that contain a 5-aminosalicylic acid component. They are used primarily to treat active Crohn's disease and to induce and maintain remission of the symptoms of ulcerative colitis, and also sometimes to treat rheumatoid arthritis.

The drugs in this group include MESALAZINE, which is 5-aminosalicylic acid itself, OLSALAZINE SODIUM, which is two molecules of 5-aminosalicylic acid joined together, and SULPHASALAZINE, which combines within the one chemical both 5-aminosalicylic acid and the (SULPHONAMIDE) ANTIBACTERIAL sulphapyridine.

The aminosalicylate component causes characteristic side-effects, such as diarrhoea, salicylate hypersensitivity and kidney effects (interstitial nephritis); whereas sulphasalazine also has sulphonamide-related side-effects, including rashes, blood disorders, azoospermia (lack of sperm) and lupoid syndrome. The sensitivity of individual patients to one or other chemical component partly determines the most suitable treatment.

amiodarone hydrochloride

is a potentially toxic drug which is used as an ANTI-ARRHYTHMIC to treat certain severe irregularities of the heartbeat, especially in cases where, for one reason or another, alternative drugs cannot be used. Administration can be either oral or by injection.

✚ Side-effects: These are many and include: photosensitivity, deposits on the cornea; neurological effects; nausea, vomiting; blood disturbances, rashes and impaired vision.

▲ Warning: It should not be administered to patients with certain heart irregularities; thyroid disorders; certain liver and kidney disorders; or to those who are pregnant or breast-feeding. There should be regular testing of thyroid, liver and lung function.

✪ Related entry: Cordarone X.

amitriptyline hydrochloride

is an ANTIDEPRESSANT of the TRICYCLIC class. It has quite marked SEDATIVE properties, which may be of benefit to agitated or violent patients. Along with other members of this class, it has pronounced ANTICHOLINERGIC side-effects. An alternative use is to prevent bed-wetting by children. Administration can be either oral or by injection.

✚ Side-effects: Common effects include loss of intricacy in movement or thought (affecting driving ability), dry mouth, blurred vision and constipation; there may also be difficulty in urinating, sweating, irregular heartbeat, behavioural disturbances, a rash, a state of confusion and changes in appetite and libido. Rarely, there may also be blood disorders.

▲ Warning: It should not be administered to patients who suffer from certain heart disorders, severe liver disorders, psychosis or mania. It should be administered with caution to patients who suffer from diabetes, epilepsy, liver or thyroid disease, closed-angle glaucoma or urinary retention; or who are pregnant or breast-feeding. Withdrawal of treatment must be gradual.
✪ Related entries: Domical; Elavil; Lentizol; Triptafen; Tryptizol.

Amix

(Ashbourne) is a proprietary, prescription-only preparation of the broad-spectrum ANTIBACTERIAL and (PENICILLIN) ANTIBIOTIC amoxycillin. It can be used to treat systemic bacterial infections, infections of the upper respiratory tract, of the ear, nose and throat and of the urinogenital tracts. It is available as capsules and an oral suspension.
✚▲ Side-effects/warning: See AMOXYCILLIN.

amlodipine besylate

is a CALCIUM-CHANNEL BLOCKER which can be used as an ANTIHYPERTENSIVE and as an ANTI-ANGINA drug in the prevention of attacks. Administration is oral.
✚ Side-effects: Flushing, dizziness, headache, oedema and fatigue. There may

be an excessive growth of the gums and blood upsets.
▲ Warning: Administer with caution to patients with certain liver disorders, or who are pregnant or breast-feeding.
✪ Related entry: Istin.

Ammonia and Ipecacuanha Mixture, BP

is a non-proprietary non-prescription COMPOUND PREPARATION of the EXPECTORANTS ammonium bicarbonate and ipecacuanha tincture (together with liquorice liquid extract). It can be used to promote the expulsion of excess bronchial secretions, and is administered orally as a liquid preparation.
✚▲ Side-effects/warning: See IPECACUANHA.

ammonium chloride

is used as an EXPECTORANT and is sometimes incorporated into cough treatments, though evidence of its efficacy is lacking. It can cause metabolic acidosis and so can be used to correct metabolic alkalosis. It has been used as a DIURETIC and has some use in the therapeutic acidification of urine, which increases the rate of the excretion of some drugs and poisons and is therefore effectively an ANTIDOTE.
✪ Related entries: BN Liniment; Bronalin Expectorant Linctus; Bronalin Junior Linctus; Penetrol Catarrh Lozenges.

ammonium salicylate

is a soluble (NSAID) NON-NARCOTIC ANALGESIC and ANTIRHEUMATIC. It is used to treat rheumatic and other musculoskeletal disorders. Administration is oral. See also SALICYLATES; SALICYLIC ACID.
✚▲ Side-effects/warning: See NSAID.
✪ Related entries: Aspellin; Radian B Heat Spray; Radian B Muscle Lotion.

Amnivent

(Ashbourne) is a proprietary, non-prescription preparation of the BRONCHODILATOR aminophylline. It can be used as an ANTI-ASTHMATIC and to treat

A

bronchitis, and is available as modified-release tablets.

✚▲ Side-effects/warning: See AMINOPHYLLINE.

amoebicidals 🔲

are ANTIMICROBIAL drugs that are used to treat infection by the microscopic protozoan organisms known as amoebae, which cause such disorders as amoebic dysentery and hepatic amoebiasis. The best-known and most-used amoebicidal is the (AZOLE) METRONIDAZOLE. See also DILOXANIDE FUROATE; TINIDAZOLE.

Amoram

(Eastern) is a proprietary, prescription-only preparation of the broad-spectrum ANTIBACTERIAL and (PENICILLIN) ANTIBIOTIC amoxycillin. It can be used to treat systemic bacterial infections, infections of the upper respiratory tract, of the ear, nose and throat and of the urinogenital tracts. It is available as capsules and an oral suspension.

✚▲ Side-effects/warning: See AMOXYCILLIN.

amorolfine

is a recently introduced ANTIFUNGAL drug that differs chemically from other antifungals. It can be used topically to treat fungal skin infections, such as foot mycosis. It is available as a cream and a nail lacquer.

✪ Related entry: Loceryl.

amoxapine

is an ANTIDEPRESSANT of the TRICYCLIC class, and can be used to treat depressive illness. Administration is oral.

✚▲ Side-effects/warning: See AMITRIPTYLINE HYDROCHLORIDE; but has less sedative actions. There may also be menstrual irregularities, breast enlargement in men, change in libido and, rarely, tardive dyskinesia.

✪ Related entry: Asendis.

amoxicillin

see AMOXYCILLIN

Amoxil

(Bencard) is a proprietary, prescription-only preparation of the broad-spectrum ANTIBACTERIAL and (PENICILLIN) ANTIBIOTIC amoxycillin. It can be used to treat systemic bacterial infections, infections of the upper respiratory tract, of the ear, nose and throat and of the urinogenital tracts. It is available as capsules, sugar-free soluble tablets, chewable tablets, a syrup for dilution, an oral suspension for children, a powder in sachets, a sugar-free powder in sachets and in a form for injection.

✚▲ Side-effects/warning: See AMOXYCILLIN.

amoxycillin

(amoxicillin) is a broad-spectrum, penicillin-like ANTIBACTERIAL and ANTIBIOTIC drug, which is closely related to AMPICILLIN. It is readily absorbed orally (better than ampicillin) and is used to treat many infections (due to both Gram-positive and Gram-negative bacteria), especially infections of the urinogenital tracts, the upper respiratory tract and the middle ear. It is also sometimes used to prevent infection following dental surgery, to prevent endocarditis, to treat Lyme disease in children and (in combination with other drugs) to treat long-standing *Helicobacter pylori* infection associated with peptic ulcers.

However, it is not *penicillinase-resistant*, as it is inactivated by penicillinase enzymes produced by Gram-positive bacteria such as *Stapylococcus aureus* and common Gram-negative bacteria such as *Escherichia coli*. For this reason, it is sometimes combined with CLAVULANIC ACID, which is an inhibiter of penicillinase enzymes. Administration can be either oral or by injection.

✚▲ Side-effects/warning: See AMPICILLIN.

✪ Related entries: Almodan; Amix; Amoram; Amoxil; Amoxymed; Amrit; Augmentin; Galenamox; Rimoxallin.

Amoxymed

(Medipharma) is a proprietary,

prescription-only preparation of the broad-spectrum ANTIBACTERIAL and (PENICILLIN) ANTIBIOTIC amoxycillin. It can be used to treat systemic bacterial infections, infections of the upper respiratory tract, of the ear, nose and throat and of the urinogenital tracts. It is available as capsules and an oral suspension.

+▲ Side-effects/warning: See AMOXYCILLIN.

Amphocil

(Zeneca) is a proprietary, prescription-only preparation of the ANTIFUNGAL and ANTIBIOTIC amphotericin, which has an unusual formulation as a lipid colloidal dispersion (with sodium cholesteryl sulphate) that is intended to minimize toxicity (particularly to the kidney) so that it can be used for severe systemic or deep-seated fungal infections. It is available in a form for infusion.

+▲ Side-effects/warning: See AMPHOTERICIN.

amphotericin

(amphotericin B) is a broad-spectrum ANTIFUNGAL which is one of the (*polyene*) ANTIBIOTICS. It can be used particularly to treat infection by most fungi and yeasts and is an extremely important drug in the treatment of systemic fungal infections. However, it is a toxic drug and side-effects are common. There have been recent attempts to minimize toxicity (particularly to the kidney) by making a lipid formulation (encapsulated in liposomes; *AmBisome*) and a colloidal dispersion (with sodium cholesteryl sulphate; *Amphocil*) so that it can be used for severe systemic or deep-seated fungal infections. Administration is either oral or by injection.

+ Side-effects: Treatment by infusion may cause nausea, vomiting, anorexia, abdominal pain, headache, muscle and joint pain, kidney, heart, hearing, liver and blood disorders; and rash.

▲ Warning: During treatment by infusion, tests on kidney and blood function are essential. Administer with care to patients

who are pregnant or breast-feeding.

✪ Related entries: Abelcet; AmBisome; Amphocil; Fungilin; Fungizone.

amphotericin B

see AMPHOTERICIN

ampicillin

is a broad-spectrum, penicillin-type ANTIBACTERIAL and ANTIBIOTIC drug. It is taken orally (though absorption is reduced by the presence of food in the stomach or intestines) and is used to treat many infections (due to both Gram-positive and Gram-negative bacteria), especially infections of the urinogenital tracts, the upper respiratory tract, the middle ear and also gonorrhoea and invasive salmonellosis. It is sometimes given as a COMPOUND PREPARATION with CLOXACILLIN, which is a combination called CO-FLUAMPICIL. Administration is either oral or by injection.

+ Side-effects: Diarrhoea is common; nausea; rarely, sensitivity reactions such as rashes (particularly in patients suffering from glandular fever, leukaemia or with HIV infection), high temperature and joint pain. Allergic patients may suffer anaphylactic shock.

▲ Warning: It should not be administered to patients who are known to be allergic to penicillin-type antibiotics in case anaphylactic shock ensues. It should be administered with caution to those with impaired kidney function.

✪ Related entries: Amfipen; Ampiclox; Ampiclox Neonatal; Flu-Amp; Magnapen; Penbritin; Rimacillin; Vidopen.

Ampiclox

(Beecham) is a proprietary, prescription-only COMPOUND PREPARATION of the broad-spectrum ANTIBACTERIAL and (PENICILLIN) ANTIBIOTIC ampicillin and the *penicillinase-resistant*, antibacterial and (penicillin) antibiotic cloxacillin. It can be used to treat systemic bacterial infections, infections of the upper respiratory tract, of the ear, nose and throat and of the urinogenital tracts. It

A

is available as capsules, a syrup and in a form for injection.

+▲ Side-effects/warning: See AMPICILLIN; CLOXACILLIN.

Ampiclox Neonatal

(Beecham) is a proprietary, prescription-only COMPOUND PREPARATION of the broad-spectrum ANTIBACTERIAL and (PENICILLIN) ANTIBIOTIC ampicillin and the *penicillinase-resistant*, antibacterial and (penicillin) antibiotic cloxacillin. It can be used to treat systemic bacterial infections, infections of the upper respiratory tract, of the ear, nose and throat and of the urinogenital tracts. It is available as capsules, an oral suspension and in a form for injection.

+▲ Side-effects/warning: See AMPICILLIN; CLOXACILLIN.

Amrit

(BHR) is a proprietary, prescription-only preparation of the broad-spectrum ANTIBACTERIAL and (PENICILLIN) ANTIBIOTIC amoxycillin. It can be used to treat systemic bacterial infections, infections of the upper respiratory tract, of the ear, nose and throat and of the urinogenital tracts. It is available as capsules and an oral suspension.

+▲ Side-effects/warning: See AMOXYCILLIN.

amsacrine

is a (CYTOTOXIC) ANTICANCER drug which is used specifically in the treatment of acute myeloid leukaemia. Administration is by injection.

+▲ Side-effects/warning: See CYTOTOXICS; there may also be heartbeat irregularities.
○ Related entry: Amsidine.

Amsidine

(Parke-Davis) is a proprietary, prescription-only preparation of the (CYTOTOXIC) ANTICANCER drug amsacrine. It can be used to treat acute myeloid leukaemia, and is available in a form for intravenous infusion.

52 | **+▲** Side-effects/warning: See AMSACRINE.

amylobarbitone

is a BARBITURATE which is used as a HYPNOTIC, but only when absolutely necessary, to treat severe and intractable insomnia in patients who are already taking barbiturates. Administration is either oral or by injection. Preparations containing amylobarbitone are on the Controlled Drugs List.

+▲ Side-effects/warning: See BARBITURATES.
○ Related entries: Amytal; Sodium Amytal; Tuinal.

Amytal

(Lilly) is a proprietary, prescription-only preparation of the BARBITURATE amylobarbitone and is on the Controlled Drugs List. It can be used as a HYPNOTIC to treat persistent and intractable insomnia, and is available as tablets.

+▲ Side-effects/warning: See AMYLOBARBITONE.

Anabact

(ASTA Medica) is a proprietary, prescription-only preparation of the ANTIMICROBIAL metronidazole, which has both ANTIPROTOZOAL and ANTIBACTERIAL properties. It can be used to deodorize and treat fungating, malodorous tumours. It is available as a gel for topical application.

+▲ Side-effects/warning: See METRONIDAZOLE.

Anacal Rectal Ointment

(Panpharma) is a proprietary, non-prescription preparation of heparinoid (with lauromacrogol). It can be used for the symptomatic relief of haemorrhoids, perianal eczema, itching and anal fissure. It is available as an ointment and is not normally used for children under five years, except on medical advice.

+▲ Side-effects/warning: See HEPARINOID.

Anacal Suppositories

(Panpharma) is a proprietary, non-prescription preparation of heparinoid (with lauromacrogol). It can be used for the symptomatic relief of haemorrhoids, perianal eczema, itching and anal fissure. It is available as suppositories and is not normally used for children under five years, except on medical advice.

+▲ Side-effects/warning: See HEPARINOID.

Anadin Analgesic Capsules, Maximum Strength

(Whitehall) is a proprietary, non-prescription COMPOUND PREPARATION of the (NSAID) NON-NARCOTIC ANALGESIC and ANTIRHEUMATIC aspirin and the STIMULANT caffeine. It can be used to treat of mild to moderate pain and for symptomatic relief of colds and flu. It is available as capsules and is not normally given to children under 12 years, except on medical advice.

+▲ Side-effects/warning: See ASPIRIN; CAFFEINE.

Anadin Analgesic Tablets

(Whitehall) is a proprietary, non-prescription COMPOUND PREPARATION of the (NSAID) NON-NARCOTIC ANALGESIC and ANTIRHEUMATIC aspirin and the STIMULANT caffeine. It can be used for mild to moderate pain, and the symptoms of feverish colds and flu. It is available as tablets and is not normally given to children, except on medical advice.

+▲ Side-effects/warning: See ASPIRIN; CAFFEINE.

Anadin Extra

(Whitehall) is a proprietary, non-prescription COMPOUND PREPARATION of the (NSAID) NON-NARCOTIC ANALGESIC and ANTIRHEUMATIC aspirin, the non-narcotic analgesic paracetamol and the STIMULANT caffeine. It can be used for the treatment of pain, especially headaches, period, dental and rheumatic pain, and also to relieve cold and flu symptoms. It is available as capsules and is not normally given to children, except on medical advice.

+▲ Side-effects/warning: See ASPIRIN; CAFFEINE; PARACETAMOL.

Anadin Extra Soluble Tablets

(Whitehall) is a proprietary, non-prescription COMPOUND PREPARATION of the (NSAID) NON-NARCOTIC ANALGESIC and ANTIRHEUMATIC aspirin, the non-narcotic analgesic paracetamol and the STIMULANT caffeine. It can be used to treat mild to moderate pain, relieve swelling, stiffness and cold and flu symptoms. It is available as soluble tablets and is not normally given to children under 12 years, except on medical advice.

+▲ Side-effects/warning: See ASPIRIN; CAFFEINE; PARACETAMOL.

Anadin Paracetamol Tablets

(Whitehall) is a proprietary, non-prescription preparation of the NON-NARCOTIC ANALGESIC paracetamol. It can be used for the treatment of headache, migraine, period pain and dental pain, and to relieve the symptoms of colds and flu. It is available as tablets.

+▲ Side-effects/warning: See PARACETAMOL.

anaemia treatment ▨

involves the use of drugs to correct a deficiency of the oxygen-carrying blood pigment haemoglobin (anaemia). The type of treatment depends on the cause of the anaemia. For example, the drugs administered to treat iron-deficient anaemia are mainly salts of IRON and are used where there is deficiency of iron in the form of haemoglobin in blood and a similar oxygen-carrier in muscles.

Dietary deficiency of iron in the diet, and disease states that prevent its proper absorption, can both lead to forms of anaemia. Iron supplements may be administered orally in one of several forms, as FERROUS FUMARATE, FERROUS GLUCONATE, FERROUS GLYCINE SULPHATE or FERROUS SULPHATE (and other salts), or by injection or intravenous infusion in the form of iron dextran and other preparations. Iron supplements are also used where there is deficiency of iron during pregnancy.

anaesthetics ▣

are used to reduce sensations, especially pain. LOCAL ANAESTHETICS (eg LIGNOCAINE HYDROCHLORIDE) affect a specific area and do not cause a loss of consciousness. GENERAL ANAESTHETICS (eg HALOTHANE) do cause a loss of consciousness and the loss of sensation is a result of this. Local anaesthetics are a logical choice for minor and local surgical procedures, such as in dental surgery, because their duration of action can be short and there is less discomfort and medical risk.

However, local anaesthetics can also achieve a more extensive loss of sensation with nerve block (eg injected near to the nerve supplying a limb), or with spinal anaesthesia (eg epidural injection in childbirth) where loss of sensation in whole areas of the body allows major surgery. Local anaesthetics are particularly valuable in situations where general anaesthesia carries a high risk, or the conscious cooperation of the patient is required. General anaesthetics are normally used for more extensive surgical procedures. In modern anaesthetic practice, ANALGESICS, SEDATIVES or SKELETAL MUSCLE RELAXANTS are used in premedication or during the operation so that quite low doses of general anaesthetic are needed. See also NARCOTIC ANALGESICS.

Anaflex

(Geistlich) is a proprietary, non-prescription preparation of the ANTIFUNGAL and ANTIBACTERIAL polynoxylin. It can be used topically to treat minor skin infections, and is available as a cream.
➕▲ Side-effects/warning: SEE POLYNOXYLIN.

Anafranil

(Geigy) is a proprietary, prescription-only preparation of the (TRICYCLIC) ANTIDEPRESSANT clomipramine hydrochloride. It can be used to relieve the symptoms of depressive illness and as an additional treatment in phobic and obsessional states. It is available as

capsules, modified-release tablets (*Anafranil SR*), a syrup and in a form for injection.
➕▲ Side-effects/warning: See CLOMIPRAMINE HYDROCHLORIDE.

analeptics

see RESPIRATORY STIMULANTS

analgesics ▣

are drugs that relieve pain, which can be achieved in many ways. In this book the term analgesic is restricted to two main classes of drug. The first class is the NARCOTIC ANALGESICS (eg MORPHINE SULPHATE), which have powerful actions on the central nervous system and alter the perception of pain. Because of the numerous possible side-effects, the most important of which is drug dependence (habituation or addiction), this class is usually used under strict medical supervision and preparations are normally available only on prescription. Other notable side-effects include depression of respiration, nausea and vomiting, sometimes hypotension, constipation, inhibition of coughing (ANTITUSSIVE action) and constriction of the pupils (miosis). Narcotic analgesics are used for different types and severities of pain. It is now recognized that the characteristic pharmacology of the narcotic analgesics follows from their action as mimics of the natural opioid NEUROTRANSMITTERS (enkephalins, endorphins, dynorphins) in nerves in the brain.

Other members of this class, also known as OPIOIDS (or OPIATES), include CODEINE PHOSPHATE, DIAMORPHINE HYDROCHLORIDE (heroin), METHADONE HYDROCHLORIDE, PENTAZOCINE and PETHIDINE HYDROCHLORIDE.

The second class is the NON-NARCOTIC ANALGESICS, which are drugs that have no tendency to produce dependence, for example ASPIRIN, but are by no means free of side-effects. This class is referred to by many names, including *weak analgesics*

A

(something of a misnomer in view of their powerful actions in treating inflammatory pain); and, in medical circles, a very large number are referred to as *non-steroidal, anti-inflammatory drugs*, abbreviated to NSAID (see NSAID). The latter term refers to the valuable anti-inflammatory action of some members of this class. These drugs are used for a variety of purposes, ranging from mild aches and pains (at lower dosages) to the treatment of rheumatoid arthritis (at higher dosages).

PARACETAMOL does not have strong anti-inflammatory actions, but is non-narcotic and, along with other drugs in this class, has ANTIPYRETIC action (the ability to lower raised body temperature). The non-narcotic analgesics work by altering the synthesis of prostaglandins (natural LOCAL HORMONES within the body) that tend to enhance pain.

Although this class of drugs has important actions and uses, all its members have side-effects of concern, which for aspirin-like drugs include gastrointestinal upsets ranging from dyspepsia to serious haemorrhage. Other examples of non-narcotic analgesics include IBUPROFEN and INDOMETHACIN. Drugs in this class are often used in combination with other analgesics (eg paracetamol with codeine) or with drugs of other classes (eg caffeine).

Apart from these two main classes, there are other drugs that are sometimes referred to as analgesic because of their ability to relieve pain. For example, LOCAL ANAESTHETICS are referred to as *local analgesics* in the USA; and RUBEFACIENTS, or COUNTER-IRRITANTS, are sometimes called analgesics.

Anapolon 50

(Syntex) is a proprietary, prescription-only preparation of the (*anabolic*) STEROID oxymetholone. It can be used to treat aplastic anaemia in particular, and is available as tablets.
✚▲ Side-effects/warning: See OXYMETHOLONE.

anastrozole

is an ANTICANCER drug which is used to treat advanced breast cancer in postmenopausal women. It is a non-steroidal compound that works as an indirect HORMONE ANTAGONIST by inhibiting the conversion of the male SEX HORMONES the androgens to the female sex hormones the OESTROGENS. Administration is oral.
✚ Side-effects: There may be drowsiness, sleepiness and lethargy (which at first may affect the ability to drive or operate machinery); rashes, vomiting and diarrhoea; hot flushes and headache; vaginal dryness, hair thinning; a slight increase in cholesterol levels and loss of appetite has been reported.
▲ Warning: It should not be used in pre-menopausal women or in those who are pregnant or breast-feeding, or with impaired kidney function or liver disease.
✪ Related entry: Arimidex.

Anbesol Adult Strength Gel

(Whitehall) is a proprietary, non-prescription COMPOUND PREPARATION of the LOCAL ANAESTHETIC lignocaine hydrochloride and the ANTISEPTIC cetylpyridinium chloride (with chlorocresol). It can be used for the temporary relief of pain caused by mouth ulcers and denture irritation. It is available as a gel for topical application.
✚▲ Side-effects/warning: See CETYLPYRIDINIUM CHLORIDE; LIGNOCAINE HYDROCHLORIDE.

Anbesol Liquid

(Whitehall) is a proprietary, non-prescription COMPOUND PREPARATION of the LOCAL ANAESTHETIC drug lignocaine hydrochloride and the ANTISEPTIC cetylpyridinium chloride (with chlorocresol). It can be used for the temporary relief of pain caused by teething, mouth ulcers and denture irritation. It is available as a liquid for topical application.
✚▲ Side-effects/warning: See CETYLPYRIDINIUM CHLORIDE; LIGNOCAINE HYDROCHLORIDE.

A

Anbesol Teething Gel

(Whitehall) is a proprietary, non-prescription COMPOUND PREPARATION of the LOCAL ANAESTHETIC lignocaine hydrochloride and the ANTISEPTIC cetylpyridinium chloride (with chlorocresol). It can be used for the temporary relief of pain caused by teething, mouth ulcers and denture irritation. It is available as a gel for topical application.

+▲ Side-effects/warning: See CETYLPYRIDINIUM CHLORIDE; LIGNOCAINE HYDROCHLORIDE.

ancrod

is an effective ANTICOAGULANT that is an ENZYME derived from a constituent of the venom of the Malaysian pit viper. It works by depleting the protein fibrinogen, which is necessary for the formation of blood clots. It is used in the treatment of deep-vein thrombosis (blood clots), especially the sort that occur following surgery, or to prevent thrombosis. It is no longer commonly used and is available only on a 'named-patient' basis. Administration is by injection.

○ Related entry: Arvin.

Andrews Antacid

(SmithKline Beecham) is a proprietary, non-prescription COMPOUND PREPARATION of the ANTACIDS calcium carbonate and magnesium carbonate. It can be used for the relief of upset stomach, heartburn, indigestion and trapped wind. It is available as chewable tablets and also in a flavoured version called *Andrews Antacid Fruit Flavour*. It is not normally given to children, except on medical advice.

+▲ Side-effects/warning: See CALCIUM CARBONATE; MAGNESIUM CARBONATE.

Androcur

(Schering) is a proprietary, prescription-only preparation of the ANTI-ANDROGEN cyproterone acetate, which is a sex HORMONE ANTAGONIST. It can be administered to treat patients suffering from severe hypersexuality and also for sexual deviation in men, and is available as tablets.

+▲ Side-effects/warning: See CYPROTERONE ACETATE.

androgen antagonists

see ANTI-ANDROGENS

androgens ▣

are a group of predominantly male (STEROID) SEX HORMONES, which stimulate the development of male sex organs and male secondary sexual characteristics. In men, they are produced primarily by the testes and the main form is called TESTOSTERONE. However, androgens are produced in both men and women by the adrenal glands and in women small quantities are also secreted by the ovaries. An excessive amount of androgens in women causes masculinization. Forms of the natural hormones and a number of synthetic androgens are administered therapeutically (eg forms of testosterone and MESTEROLONE) to correct hormonal deficiency, for example, in those with delayed puberty, and can also be used as ANTICANCER treatments for cancers linked to sex hormones (eg breast cancer in women). ANTI-ANDROGENS are a class of drugs that inhibit the actions of androgens and are also used in medicine.

+ Side-effects: Oedema, leading to weight gain. Increased levels of calcium in the body may cause bone growth (and in younger patients may fuse bones before fully grown), there may be enlargement of the prostate gland, reduced production of sperm, priapism in men and masculinization in women.

▲ Warning: They should not be administered to male patients who suffer from nephrosis, cancer of the prostate gland or cancer of the breast; or to patients who are pregnant or breast-feeding. Administer with caution to those with impaired function of the heart, liver or kidney; or certain circulatory disorders and/or hypertension, epilepsy or diabetes, thyroid disorders or migraine.

Andropatch

(SmithKline Beecham) is a proprietary, prescription-only preparation of the ANDROGEN (male SEX HORMONE) testosterone. It can be used to treat testosterone deficiency in men, and is available in the form form of skin patches.

✚▲ Side-effects/warning: See TESTOSTERONE.

Anectine

(Wellcome) is a proprietary, prescription-only preparation of the (*depolarizing*) SKELETAL MUSCLE RELAXANT suxamethonium chloride. It can be used to induce muscle paralysis during surgery, and is available in a form for injection.

✚▲ Side-effects/warning: See SUXAMETHONIUM CHLORIDE.

Anestan Bronchial Tablets

(Seton) is a proprietary, non-prescription COMPOUND PREPARATION of the SYMPATHOMIMETIC and DECONGESTANT ephedrine hydrochloride and the BRONCHODILATOR theophylline (anhydrous). It can be used as an ANTI-ASTHMATIC for reversible bronchospasm. It is not normally given to children under 12 years, except on medical advice.

✚▲ Side-effects/warning: See EPHEDRINE HYDROCHLORIDE; THEOPHYLLINE.

Anexate

(Roche) is a proprietary, prescription-only preparation of the BENZODIAZEPINE antagonist flumazenil. It can be used to reverse the effects of benzodiazepines, and is available in a form for intravenous injection or infusion.

✚▲ Side-effects/warning: See FLUMAZENIL.

Angettes 75

(Bristol-Myers) is a proprietary, non-prescription preparation of the ANTIPLATELET aggregation agent aspirin. It can be used to help prevent the formation of thrombi (blood clots) and is used particularly for problems relating to blocked blood vessels, such as following and to prevent heart attacks. It is available as tablets.

✚▲ Side-effects/warning: See ASPIRIN.

Angilol

(DDSA) is a proprietary, prescription-only preparation of the BETA-BLOCKER propranolol hydrochloride. It can be used as an ANTIHYPERTENSIVE for raised blood pressure, as an ANTI-ANGINA treatment to relieve symptoms and to improve exercise tolerance and as an ANTI-ARRHYTHMIC to regularize heartbeat and to treat myocardial infarction. It may also be used as an ANTITHYROID drug for short-term treatment of thyrotoxicosis, as an ANTIMIGRAINE treatment to prevent attacks, as an ANXIOLYTIC, particularly for symptomatic relief of tremor and palpitations, and, with an ALPHA-ADRENOCEPTOR BLOCKER, in the acute treatment of phaeochromocytoma. It is available as tablets.

✚▲ Side-effects/warning: See PROPRANOLOL HYDROCHLORIDE.

Angiopine

(Ashbourne) is a proprietary, prescription-only preparation of the CALCIUM-CHANNEL BLOCKER nifedipine. It can be used as an ANTI-ANGINA treatment in the prevention of attacks, as an ANTIHYPERTENSIVE and as a VASODILATOR in peripheral vascular disease (Raynaud's phenomenon). It is available as capsules.

✚▲ Side-effects/warning: See NIFEDIPINE.

angiotensin-receptor blockers ▣

are drugs that work by blocking angiotensin receptors. Angiotensin II is a circulating HORMONE that is a powerful VASOCONSTRICTOR and so blocking its effects leads to a fall in blood pressure. LOSARTAN POTASSIUM and VALSARTAN are recently introduced drugs of this type and can be used as ANTIHYPERTENSIVE agents. The general actions are similar to those of ACE INHIBITORS, but without the tendency of the latter to cause a persistent dry cough.

A

angiotensin-converting enzyme inhibitors

See ACE INHIBITORS

Angiozem

(Ashbourne) is a proprietary, prescription-only preparation of the CALCIUM-CHANNEL BLOCKER diltiazem hydrochloride. It can be used as an ANTIHYPERTENSIVE and as an ANTI-ANGINA drug, and is available as modified-release tablets.

+▲ Side-effects/warning: See DILTIAZEM HYDROCHLORIDE.

Anhydrol Forte

(Dermal) is a proprietary, non-prescription preparation of aluminium chloride (as hexahydrate), which can be used as an ANTIPERSPIRANT to treat hyperhidrosis (excessive sweating). It is available in a roll-on applicator.

+▲ Side-effects/warning: See ALUMINIUM CHLORIDE.

anistreplase

is used therapeutically as a FIBRINOLYTIC because it has the property of breaking up blood clots. It is used rapidly in serious conditions such as myocardial infarction. Administration is by injection.

+▲ Side-effects/warning: See ALTEPLASE.

✪ Related entry: Eminase.

Anodesyn

(Seton) is a proprietary, non-prescription preparation of the LOCAL ANAESTHETIC lignocaine hydrochloride (with allantoin). It can be used for the symptomatic relief of the pain and itching of haemorrhoids, and is available as suppositories and an ointment. It is not normally given to children, except on medical advice.

+▲ Side-effects/warning: See LIGNOCAINE HYDROCHLORIDE.

Anquil

(Janssen) is a proprietary, prescription-only preparation of the ANTIPSYCHOTIC benperidol. It can be used to treat and tranquillize psychotic patients, especially those with antisocial and deviant sexual behaviour, and is available as tablets.

+▲ Side-effects/warning: See BENPERIDOL.

Antabuse 200

(Dumex) is a proprietary, prescription-only preparation of the ENZYME INHIBITOR disulfiram. It can be used to assist in the treatment of alcoholism, because, in combination with the consumption of even small quantities of alcohol, it causes unpleasant reactions: flushing, headache, palpitations, nausea and vomiting. It is available as tablets.

+▲ Side-effects/warning: See DISULFIRAM.

antacids ▨

are used to neutralize the hydrochloric acid that the stomach produces as part of the normal digestion of food. Over-production of acid (hyperacidity) can cause the symptoms of dyspepsia (indigestion), which can be exacerbated by alcohol and NSAID drugs. Antacids give symptomatic relief of the dyspepsia and gastritis associated with peptic ulcers (gastric or duodenal ulcer), but allow little actual healing of ulcers. A further painful condition is when there is regurgitation of acid and enzymes into the oesophagus (oesophageal reflux), which in the short term causes heartburn and in the long term can result in inflammation (reflux oesophagitis: common in hiatus hernia and pregnancy). Antacids taken alone effectively reduce acidity, but they are commonly combined with other drugs, such as ANTIFOAMING AGENTS, DEMULCENTS and ULCER-HEALING DRUGS. Antacids themselves have side-effects; bicarbonates and carbonates tend to cause flatulence and some aluminium-containing antacids cause constipation, whereas magnesium-containing antacids can cause diarrhoea (and therefore are often used in combination). See ALUMINIUM HYDROXIDE; CALCIUM CARBONATE; MAGNESIUM CARBONATE; MAGNESIUM HYDROXIDE; MAGNESIUM TRISILICATE; SODIUM BICARBONATE.

A

antagonists ☐

are drugs that have no pharmacological actions in their own right, but have profound actions because they actually block (physically occupy) RECEPTORS that normally allow natural mediators, or sometimes synthetic drugs, to have an effect. Many of the most widely used drugs in medicine are antagonists. Their most important property is that they can be used to prevent the actions of mediators within the body, including within the brain and can therefore be used to 'switch-off' systems that are not functioning correctly, for instance in a disease state caused by excessive amounts of NEUROTRANSMITTERS, LOCAL HORMONES and HORMONES. This very valuable property can be used in a range of applications from changing mood and psychological states of mind, through to preventing allergic responses. Some examples will illustrate this point.

BETA-BLOCKERS (beta-adrenoceptor blockers) are antagonists that prevent the action of ADRENALINE and NORADRENALINE by blocking the receptors called beta-adrenoceptors. They may be used as ANTIHYPERTENSIVES, in ANTI-ARRHYTHMIC and ANTI-ANGINA treatment for the heart, as ANXIOLYTICS and ANTITHYROID agents, and in GLAUCOMA TREATMENT. The best-known and most-used beta-blockers include ACEBUTOLOL, OXPRENOLOL HYDROCHLORIDE, PROPRANOLOL HYDROCHLORIDE and SOTALOL HYDROCHLORIDE, and as a class they are probably the single most-used drugs in medicine.

ANTIHISTAMINES (H_1-antagonists) are drugs that inhibit the effects in the body of the local hormone histamine by blocking receptors called H_1 receptors. Histamine is released as an allergic reaction to a substance, for example, pollen, insect bites and stings, contact with certain metal objects or certain foods. Antihistamines can be given by mouth or applied topically to block many of the unpleasant or dangerous actions of histamine.

There is a second group of drugs that also inhibit histamine effects, but block a quite different class of receptor called the (H_2) receptor, which is involved in (stomach) gastric acid secretion. This group is referred to as H_2-ANTAGONISTS and they are used as ULCER-HEALING DRUGS, for example, in the treatment of peptic ulcers. The H_2-antagonist drug RANITIDINE is probably the most prescribed individual drug in the world.

Other examples of antagonist drugs include ANTICHOLINERGICS, ANTI-ANDROGENS, ANTI-OESTROGENS and OPIOID ANTAGONISTS.

antazoline

is an ANTIHISTAMINE which can be used for the symptomatic relief of allergic symptoms, such as allergic conjunctivitis in the eye. Administration is topical.
✚▲ Side-effects/warning: See ANTIHISTAMINES. Avoid its use in patients with kidney impairment.
✪ Related entry: Otrivine-Antistin.

Antepsin

(Wyeth) is a proprietary, prescription-only preparation of the CYTOPROTECTANT drug sucralfate. It can be used to treat gastric and duodenal ulcers, and is available as tablets.
✚▲ Side-effects/warning: See SUCRALFATE.

anthelmintics ☐

are used to treat infections by parasitic organisms of the helminth (worm) family. The threadworm, roundworm and tapeworm are the most common helminths responsible for infection in the UK. In warmer countries illnesses caused by helminths are a major problem, eg hookworm disease (caused by hookworms), bilharziasis (caused by schistosomes) and elephantiasis (caused by filaria). Most worms infest the intestines and diagnosis is often made by finding the worms in the faeces. Drugs can then be administered and the worms are killed or anaesthetized and then excreted. Complications arise if the worms migrate

A

within the body, in which case the treatment becomes very unpleasant for the patient. In the case of threadworms, medication should be combined with hygienic measures (eg short fingernails) and the whole family should be treated. Among the most useful and best-known anthelmintics are NICLOSAMIDE, PIPERAZINE, MEBENDAZOLE and THIABENDAZOLE.

Anthranol

(Stiefel) is a proprietary, non-prescription COMPOUND PREPARATION of dithranol and salicylic acid. It can be used for subacute and chronic psoriasis, and is available as an ointment.

+▲ Side-effects/warning: See DITHRANOL; SALICYLIC ACID.

Anthrax Vaccine

(Public Health Laboratory Service) is a non-proprietary, prescription-only VACCINE preparation, which can be used to protect individuals exposed to anthrax-infected materials. It is available in a form for injection.

anthrax vaccine

for IMMUNIZATION is required only by individuals who are exposed to anthrax-infected hides and carcasses, or who handle imported bone meal, fish meal and other feedstuffs. The VACCINE is a precipitate of antigen from *Bacillus anthracis*, which causes anthrax and can be administered by injection.

anti-allergic ▣

drugs relieve the symptoms of an allergic reaction that follows exposure to specific substances to which a patient is allergic. These substances may be either endogenous (in the patient's body) or exogenous (present in the environment). Because allergic reactions generally cause the release of the natural LOCAL HORMONE histamine within the body, ANTIHISTAMINES are often extremely effective for providing symptomatic relief.

For example, allergic skin reactions to foreign proteins, contact dermatitis and insect stings and bites, show characteristic symptoms – including pruritus (itching), urticaria (an itchy skin rash) and erythema (reddening of the skin) – and these often respond well to treatment with antihistamines (including local application in a cream). However, because allergic responses cause an inflammatory effect, many anti-allergic drugs also have ANTI-INFLAMMATORY properties. For example, in the treatment of atopic (allergic) bronchial asthma, chronic (long-term) inhalation of CORTICOSTEROIDS may prevent asthma attacks and the associated bronchoconstriction and congested airways. Similar anti-inflammatory protection from the symptoms of allergic asthma may be achieved by chronic inhalation of SODIUM CROMOGLYCATE, which prevents the release of histamine and other substances (though exactly how it works is not clear). In the acute treatment of anaphylactic shock immediate treatment with three types of drugs is often required: an injection of a SYMPATHOMIMETIC, such as ADRENALINE, to dilate the bronchioles and stimulate the cardiovascular circulation; and administration of corticosteroids and antihistamines to counter other serious allergic reactions. In general, corticosteroids will suppress or mask inflammatory responses at most sites (including the skin), but these drugs have quite marked and serious side-effects and are only given systemically in serious conditions and are normally used topically only for short-term alleviation of symptoms.

anti-androgens ▣

(androgen antagonists) are a class of drugs that are HORMONE ANTAGONISTS, which usually act directly to prevent the actions of the male sex hormone TESTOSTERONE at its target tissues. Other anti-androgens act indirectly to prevent the formation, or inhibit the release, of the hormones and are known as indirect hormone antagonists. Examples of drugs acting by the direct mechanism include CYPROTERONE ACETATE and FLUTAMIDE; and those that act through the indirect mechanism include BUSERELIN.

anti-angina ⬚

drugs are used to relieve the pain of angina pectoris, which is an intense pain originating from the heart and due to ischaemia (insufficient blood supply to the heart muscle) and is especially pronounced in *exercise angina*. The disease state often results from atheroma, which is a degeneration of the lining of the arteries of the heart due to a build up of fatty deposits. The objective of drug treatment is to reduce the heart's workload and to prevent spasm or to dilate the arteries of the heart (the coronary arteries). Unloading can be achieved by stopping exercise, preventing the speeding of the heart and by dilating the coronary arteries.

BETA-BLOCKERS prevent the normal increase in heart rate seen in exercise by blocking the effect of ADRENALINE and NORADRENALINE on the heart, and are very effective in preventing anginal pain. Examples of beta-blockers include: ACEBUTOLOL, ATENOLOL, METOPROLOL TARTRATE, NADOLOL, OXPRENOLOL HYDROCHLORIDE, PINDOLOL, PROPRANOLOL HYDROCHLORIDE, SOTALOL HYDROCHLORIDE and TIMOLOL MALEATE.

VASODILATORS are drugs (many of which are SMOOTH MUSCLE RELAXANTS) that dilate blood vessels and thereby increase blood flow. For the acute treatment of anginal pain (and to a lesser extent in preventing angina attacks) the NITRATES (eg GLYCERYL TRINITRATE, ISOSORBIDE DINITRATE, ISOSORBIDE MONONITRATE and PENTAERYTHRITOL TETRANITRATE) are widely used.

CALCIUM-CHANNEL BLOCKERS are a more recently introduced anti-angina treatment. They dilate the coronary arteries and peripheral small arteries, which helps to reduce the workload on the heart. If drug treatment is not sufficient, then a coronary bypass operation may be needed. See also AMLODIPINE BESYLATE; DILTIAZEM HYDROCHLORIDE; NICARDIPINE HYDROCHLORIDE; NIFEDIPINE; VERAPAMIL HYDROCHLORIDE.

anti-arrhythmics ⬚

(antidysrrhythmics) strengthen and regularize a heartbeat that has become unsteady and is not showing its usual 'patter' of activity. But because there are many ways in which the heartbeat can falter – atrial tachycardia, ventricular tachycardia, atrial flutter or fibrillation and the severe heartbeat irregularity that may follow a heart attack (myocardial infarction) – there is a variety of drugs available, each for a fairly specific use. The best-known and most-used anti-arrhythmics include DIGOXIN (a CARDIAC GLYCOSIDE), VERAPAMIL HYDROCHLORIDE (a CALCIUM-CHANNEL BLOCKER) and LIGNOCAINE HYDROCHLORIDE (a LOCAL ANAESTHETIC, especially used for ventricular arrhythmia); also extremely effective are the BETA-BLOCKERS (which are also used to treat high blood pressure and angina pectoris).

anti-asthmatic ⬚

drugs relieve the symptoms of bronchial asthma or prevent recurrent attacks. The symptoms of asthma include bronchoconstriction (a narrowing of the bronchioles of the airways, with consequent difficulty in exhaling), often with over-secretion of fluid by glands within the bronchioles, with coughing and breathing difficulties. Two main types of drugs are used: one group treat acute attacks; and the second prevent attacks (as prophylaxis). BRONCHODILATORS, which are SMOOTH MUSCLE RELAXANTS, work by dilating and relaxing the bronchioles. The most commonly used are the BETA-RECEPTOR STIMULANTS (which are SYMPATHOMIMETICS), notably SALBUTAMOL and TERBUTALINE SULPHATE. The beta-receptor stimulants, normally inhaled, are mostly used for treating acute attacks (or immediately before exertion in patients with exercise asthma) and are largely of a type that does not normally adversely stimulate the heart. Other bronchodilator

A

drugs that work directly on the bronchioles include smooth muscle relaxants such as THEOPHYLLINE.

The second group of anti-asthmatic drugs do not directly cause bronchodilation, but because of their ANTI-INFLAMMATORY action they prevent the release of local inflammatory mediators, which contribute to attacks; so preventing asthma attacks and providing symptomatic relief. Examples of this group of anti-inflammatory drugs include the CORTICOSTEROIDS and SODIUM CROMOGLYCATE. These drugs are almost always taken over a period of time, both to prevent attacks and to reverse pathological changes, and preferably are inhaled so as to deliver the drug to where it is required and which helps limit side-effects. Indeed, a great deal of research has been done to design devices that are able to more efficiently deliver the inhaled droplets, or particles, of bronchodilator or anti-inflammatory drugs into the airways, particularly in an attempt to reach the narrower bronchioles.

There are some other drugs, such as KETOTIFEN and IPRATROPIUM BROMIDE, that are occasionally used to treat asthma (for instance, when the other types of drug are ineffective for some reason). ANTIHISTAMINES, however, are now thought to be of no value, but are useful as ANTI-ALLERGIC treatments for hay fever or rashes.

anti-D (Rh₀) immunoglobulin

(anti-D immunoglobulin) for IMMUNIZATION is a SPECIFIC IMMUNOGLOBULIN which is used to prevent rhesus-negative mothers from making antibodies against foetal rhesus-positive cells that may pass into the mother's circulation during childbirth or abortion, so protecting a future child from haemolytic disease of the newborn. Anti-D (Rh₀) immunoglobulin should be injected within a few days of birth.

✚▲ Side-effects/warning: See IMMUNIZATION.

62 | ○ **Related entry: Partobulin.**

antibacterials ?

are used to treat infections caused by bacteria, on which they have a selective toxic action. They can be used both topically (eg, on the skin or the eye) to treat infections of superficial tissues or systemically (carried by the blood after being swallowed or injected to the site of the infection). Many are ANTIBIOTICS.

A distinction can be made between *bacteriostatic* drugs, which act primarily by arresting bacterial growth (eg SULPHONAMIDES, TETRACYCLINES and CHLORAMPHENICOL) and the *bactericidal* agents, which act primarily by killing bacteria (eg AMINOGLYCOSIDES, CEPHALOSPORINS, ISONIAZID, PENICILLINS and RIFAMPICIN). As bacteria are the largest and most diverse group of pathogenic (disease-causing) micro-organisms, antibacterials form the major constituent group of ANTIMICROBIALS.

antibiotics ?

are, strictly speaking, natural products secreted by micro-organisms into their environment where they inhibit the growth of competing micro-organisms of different types. But in common usage the term is often applied to any drug, natural or synthetic, that has a selectively toxic action on bacteria or similar non-nucleated, single-celled micro-organisms (including chlamydia, rickettsia and mycoplasma) – but they are not effective against viruses.

However, the more accurate term for these drugs is ANTIMICROBIALS. Most modern antibiotics are, in fact, either completely or partly synthetic and not produced by natural organisms, but nevertheless they are generally modelled on natural substances.

When administered by an appropriate route, whether topically (eg to the skin or eyes) orally, by injection or by infusion, antibiotics kill micro-organisms such as bacteria – *bactericidal action* – or inhibit their growth – *bacteriostatic action*. The selectively toxic action on invading micro-organism exploits differences between bacteria and their human host cells. Major target sites for antibiotics are the bacterial cell wall located outside the cell membrane (animal cells have only a cell membrane) or the bacterial ribosome (the protein-synthesizing organelle within its cell), which in micro-organisms is different to human cells. Families of antibiotics, such as the PENICILLINS and CEPHALOSPORINS (collectively known as BETA-LACTAMS), attack the bacterial cell wall, whereas other groups, such as the AMINOGLYCOSIDES and TETRACYCLINES, attack the ribosomes.

Viruses lack both cell walls and ribosomes and are therefore resistant to these and other types of antibiotics. Because there is such a diversity of pathogenic (disease-causing) micro-organisms, it is not at all surprising that specific infections are best treated using specific antibiotics which were developed to combat them.

Unfortunately, because of the widespread use of antibiotics certain strains of common bacteria have developed resistance to antibiotics that were once effective against them and this has become a major problem. A mechanism by which bacteria become resistant is through the development of enzymes called *penicillinases*, which break down penicillins and so limit an antibiotic's action. It has proved possible, however, both to use drugs that inhibit these enzymes and, more directly, to develop *penicillinase-resistant* antibiotics.

Another problem is the occurrence of *superinfections*, in which the administration of a broad-spectrum antibiotic disturbs the normal, harmless bacterial population in a patient's body, as well as the pathogenic ones. In mild cases this may allow, for example, an existing but latent oral or vaginal thrush infection to become worse, or mild (usually) diarrhoea to develop. In rare cases the superinfection that develops is more serious than the original disorder.

anticancer ▨

drugs are used to treat cancer and most of them are CYTOTOXICS, that is, they work by interfering with cell replication or production, so preventing the growth of new cancerous tissue. Inevitably, this means that normal cell production is also affected, which causes serious side-effects. They are usually administered in combination in a group of treatments known collectively as *chemotherapy*.

In cases where the growth of a tumour is linked to the presence of a sex hormone (as with some cases of breast cancer or cancer of the prostate gland), treatment with sex hormones opposite to the patient's own sex can be extremely beneficial – though side-effects may be psychologically stressful. The CORTICOSTEROID drug PREDNISONE is also used as an anticancer drug in the treatment of the lymphatic cancer Hodgkin's disease and other forms of lymphoma, and may also be helpful in halting the progress of hormone-linked breast cancer.

anticholinergics ▨

inhibit the action, release or production of the NEUROTRANSMITTER ACETYLCHOLINE, which plays an important part in the nervous system. The term is commonly used synonymously with ANTIMUSCARINIC (drugs that block the actions of acetylcholine at *muscarinic* receptors). Anticholinergic drugs (of the antimuscarinic type) tend to relax smooth (involuntary) muscle, reduce the secretion of saliva, digestive juices and sweat and dilate the pupil of the eye (mydriasis). They can therefore be used as ANTISPASMODICS in the treatment of parkinsonian symptoms, peptic ulcer and to dilate the pupil for ophthalmic examinations. Other uses include reversal of the adverse effects of overdose with anticholinesterases (in medicine, agricultural accidental poisoning or warfare). However, the administration of these drugs is usually accompanied by side-effects, including dry mouth, dry skin,

A

A

blurred vision, increased heart rate, constipation and difficulty in urinating.

A number of other types of drug, for instance, ANTIHISTAMINES, can also cause *anticholinergic side-effects*.

Examples of drugs used in medicine for their antimuscarinic anticholinergic actions include: ATROPINE SULPHATE, BENZHEXOL HYDROCHLORIDE, BENZTROPINE MESYLATE, BIPERIDEN, CO-PHENOTROPE, CYCLOPENTOLATE HYDROCHLORIDE, FLAVOXATE HYDROCHLORIDE, GLYCOPYRRONIUM BROMIDE, HYOSCINE BUTYLBROMIDE, HYOSCINE HYDROBROMIDE, IPRATROPIUM BROMIDE, MEBEVERINE HYDROCHLORIDE, MEPENZOLATE BROMIDE, ORPHENADRINE CITRATE, ORPHENADRINE HYDROCHLORIDE, PIPENZOLATE BROMIDE, PIRENZEPINE, POLDINE METHYLSULPHATE, PROCYCLIDINE HYDROCHLORIDE, PROPANTHELINE BROMIDE and TROPICAMIDE.

The other main types of anticholinergic drugs work at sites where acetylcholine interacts with *nicotinic* receptors (such as in the autonomic ganglia, skeletal neuromuscular junction and central nervous system) and have quite different actions. See GANGLION-BLOCKERS and SKELETAL MUSCLE RELAXANTS.

anticholinesterases ▣

are ENZYME INHIBITORS. They inhibit certain enzymes (called cholinesterases) that are normally involved in the rapid break down of the natural NEUROTRANSMITTER acetylcholine. Acetylcholine is released from *cholinergic* nerves and has many actions in the body. Consequently, since anticholinesterase drugs enhance the effects of acetylcholine on its release from these nerves, they may have a very wide range of actions and can be used for a variety of purposes.

In respect of their actions at the junction of nerves with skeletal (voluntary) muscles, anticholinesterases are used in the diagnosis and treatment of the muscle-weakness disease myesthenia gravis. At the end of surgical operations in which certain SKELETAL MUSCLE RELAXANTS have been used,

the anaesthetist is able to reverse the muscle paralysis by injecting an anticholinesterase.

In organs that are innervated by parasympathetic division of the autonomic nervous system, anticholinesterases cause an exaggeration of the nerves' actions – referred to as PARASYMPATHOMIMETIC actions – and they can be used for a number of purposes. These include stimulation of the bladder (in urinary retention), the intestine (in paralytic ileus) and the pupil of the eye (on local application in GLAUCOMA TREATMENT). However, anticholinesterases have a number of undesirable side-effects, such as slowing of the heart, constriction of the airways with excessive production of secretions and actions in the brain.

In anticholinesterase poisoning, their diverse actions can be life-threatening. Chemicals with anticholinesterase properties are used as insecticides (and in chemical warfare), so ANTIDOTES are required (eg PRALIDOXIME MESYLATE and ATROPINE SULPHATE). See DISTIGMINE BROMIDE; NEOSTIGMINE; PHYSOSTIGMINE SULPHATE; PYRIDOSTIGMINE.

anticoagulants ▣

prevent the clotting of blood and help break up blood clots that have formed. The blood's own natural anticoagulant is HEPARIN, which is probably the most effective anticoagulant known. Synthetic anticoagulants, such as WARFARIN SODIUM, NICOUMALONE and PHENINDIONE, take longer to act.

Therapeutically, anticoagulants are used to prevent the formation of and to treat blood clots in conditions such as thrombosis and embolism, especially following surgery. They are also used to prevent blood clots in patients fitted with a heart pacemaker or who have certain heart disorders.

anticonvulsants ▣

are used to prevent the onset of epileptic seizures, or to reduce their severity if they do occur. The best-known and most-used anticonvulsant is SODIUM VALPROATE, which is used to treat all forms of epilepsy. Other examples include CARBAMAZEPINE and PHENYTOIN, which are used to treat grand mal forms of epilepsy, and ETHOSUXIMIDE, which is used to treat petit mal. In every case, dosage must be adjusted to the requirements of each individual patient. Anticonvulsant drugs may also be used to treat other types of convulsions, for instance, in drug or chemical poisoning. However, some of these drugs, such as CHLORPROMAZINE HYDROCHLORIDE and DIAZEPAM, are not effective or suitable for treating epilepsy. See ANTI-EPILEPTICS.

antidepressants

are used to relieve the symptoms of depressive illness and are divided into three main groups. The first and oldest, group are the TRICYCLIC antidepressants (named after the chemical structure of the original members), such as AMITRIPTYLINE HYDROCHLORIDE, IMIPRAMINE HYDROCHLORIDE and DOXEPIN. They are effective in alleviating a number of depressive symptoms, but have ANTICHOLINERGIC side-effects. Most drugs of this class also have SEDATIVE properties, which in some is quite pronounced (especially amitriptyline hydrochloride, which may be beneficial in some anxious and agitated patients).

The second group consists of the MONOAMINE-OXIDASE INHIBITORS (MAOIs), eg ISOCARBOXAZID, PHENELZINE and TRANYLCYPROMINE, which are now used less frequently because they have severe side-effects, particularly through interaction with constituents of foodstuffs.

The third type of antidepressant, and the most recently developed, is the SSRIS, for example FLUOXETINE, which are named after their mechanisms of action (Selective Serotonin Re-uptake Inhibitors).

Also used is the amino acid TRYPTOPHAN, which may be used when other classes of antidepressant have not been effective, and LITHIUM, which is used to treat manic-

depression and related illnesses and also for preventing certain types of recurrent depression. The ANTIPSYCHOTIC drug FLUPENTHIXOL is occasionally used (at a much lower dose) as an antidepressant.

Treatment with antidepressants often takes some weeks to show maximal beneficial effects. (See individual class entries for more detail.)

antidiarrhoeals

prevent the onset of diarrhoea, or assist in treating it if already present. The main medical treatment while diarrhoea lasts, however, is always the replacement of fluids and minerals. However, because there is a perceived need on the part of the general public, antidiarrhoeal preparations are generally available without prescription. Many are adsorbent mixtures that bind faecal material into solid masses.

These mixtures include preparations containing KAOLIN or METHYLCELLULOSE, which may also be useful in controlling faecal consistency for patients who have undergone colostomy or ileostomy. Other antidiarrhoeals, such as antimotility drugs, work by reducing peristalsis (the movement of the intestine), which slows down the movement of faecal material. OPIOIDS, such as CODEINE PHOSPHATE and MORPHINE SULPHATE, are efficient at this.

Diarrhoea caused by inflammatory disorders, such as irritable bowel syndrome, ulcerative colitis and Crohn's disease may be relieved by treatment with CORTICOSTEROIDS or AMINOSALICYLATES.

antidiuretic hormone

see VASOPRESSIN

antidotes

are used to counteract poisons or overdose with other drugs. They are used in a wide variety of circumstances and can work in many ways. First, the most straightforward and commonly used method is where the poison works by stimulating, or over-stimulating, a distinct pharmacological

A

RECEPTOR, because here the appropriate receptor ANTAGONIST can be used to reduce or completely block the effects of the poison. For example, NALOXONE HYDROCHLORIDE is an OPIOID ANTAGONIST and can be used as an antidote to an overdose of an (OPIOID) NARCOTIC ANALGESIC (including DIAMORPHINE HYDROCHLORIDE; heroin) and being quick-acting it effectively reverses the respiratory depression, coma or convulsions that result from such an overdose. It can also be used at the end of operations to reverse respiratory depression caused by narcotic analgesics, and in newborn babies where mothers have been administered large amounts of opioid (such as pethidine) for pain-relief.

Second, poisoning by some agents is best counteracted by using an antidote that binds to the poison, rendering it relatively inert and facilitating its excretion from the body. For example, a CHELATING AGENT is used as an antidote to metal poisoning because it chemically binds to certain metallic ions and other substances, making them less toxic and allowing their excretion from the body. Chelating agents are used to treat too high levels of metals of external origin (either accidental or environmental), abnormal metabolism (eg high levels of copper in Wilson's disease) or disease states (eg penicillamine in rheumatoid arthritis). Examples of chelating agents are: DESFERRIOXAMINE MESYLATE, DICOBALT EDETATE, DIMERCAPROL, PENICILLAMINE and SODIUM CALCIUMEDETATE.

An ANTIVENOM is an antidote to the poison in a snakebite, a scorpion's sting or a bite from any other poisonous creature (such as a spider). Normally, it is an ANTISERUM and is injected into the bloodstream for immediate relief (though it has its own adverse side-effects).

DIGIBIND is a proprietary drug that comprises antibody fragments that react with the glycosides and is used in the emergency treatment of an overdose of CARDIAC GLYCOSIDES, eg DIGOXIN and DIGITOXIN.

ACETYLCYSTEINE and METHIONINE are used as antidotes to treat overdose poisoning by the ANALGESIC paracetamol. The initial symptoms of paracetamol poisoning usually settle within 24 hours, but give way to a serious toxic effect on the liver which takes some days to develop. It is to prevent these later effects that treatment is directed and is required immediately after overdose. The antidotes work by chemically reacting with toxic products made by the liver from paracetamol when it is taken in excessive amounts.

A different principle is used with ANTICHOLINESTERASE poisoning. These ENZYME INHIBITORS are used in medicine, as insecticides and in chemical warfare. PRALIDOXIME MESYLATE is an antidote that actually reactivates the cholinesterase enzyme after it has been poisoned and is highly effective (taken in conjunction with other drugs) in preventing the life-endangering chemical changes to certain anticholinesterases.

In all cases of poisoning, prompt action in using an antidote is necessary.

antidysrrhythmic drugs
see ANTI-ARRHYTHMICS

anti-emetics ☙
are drugs that prevent vomiting, whereas ANTINAUSEANTS are used to reduce or prevent the *sensation* of nausea that very often precedes the physical process of vomiting. Anti-emetics are used to help reduce the vomiting that accompanies radiotherapy and chemotherapy and may help by actually preventing vomiting and aiding the passage of food out of the stomach; that is, they act as gastric MOTILITY STIMULANTS (eg METOCLOPRAMIDE HYDROCHLORIDE and CISAPRIDE).

anti-epileptics ☙
are used to prevent the occurrence of epileptic seizures. In order to achieve this, an effective concentration of the drug must be maintained in the plasma and so the

dose varies according to each patient's requirements. Generally, only one drug is required at any one time and the drug of choice depends on the type and severity of the epilepsy. CARBAMAZEPINE, PHENYTOIN and SODIUM VALPROATE are the drugs of choice for *tonic-clonic seizures* (grand mal) as part of a syndrome of primary generalized epilepsy; ETHOSUXIMIDE and sodium valproate are used for *absence seizures* (petit mal); and CLONAZEPAM, ethosuximide and sodium valproate for *myoclonic seizures*.

For other types of seizure, such as atypical absence, atonic and tonic seizures (often in childhood), phenytoin, sodium valproate, clonazepam, PHENOBARBITONE or ethosuximide are often used. See also ANTICONVULSANTS.

antifoaming agents ▫

are chemicals incorporated into ANTACID preparations in order to lower surface tension so that small bubbles of froth coalesce into large bubbles, which allows the remedy to pass more easily through the intestine. The most effective are silicone polymers such as DIMETHICONE.

antifungals ▫

are ANTIMICROBIAL drugs that are used to treat infections caused by fungal micro-organisms, and are often ANTIBIOTICS that are produced naturally or synthetically. Fungal infections are usually not a major problem in healthy, well-nourished individuals. However, superficial, localized infections, such as thrush (caused by *Candida albicans*), athlete's foot and ringworm (caused by fungi of the dermatophyte group) are common. Severe infections occur most frequently in situations where the host's immunity is low, for example, following immunosuppression for transplant surgery.

Under such conditions fungi that are not normally pathogenic (disease-causing) can exploit their host's altered state and cause infection. Unfortunately, the most

potent antifungal drugs also tend to be highly toxic and therefore severe systemic fungal infections remain an ever-present danger. NYSTATIN and IMIDAZOLES, such as CLOTRIMAZOLE, are often used for local treatment. AMPHOTERICIN and FLUCYTOSINE are reserved for systemic fungal infections. The commonest form of fungal infection in childhood is thrush, which usually occurs in the mouth and nappy area of infants and is generally treated with the topical application of MICONAZOLE.

antihistamines ▫

are drugs of the H_1-antagonist type that inhibit the effects of histamine in the body. Histamine is released naturally as the result of a patient coming into contact with a substance to which he or she is allergically sensitive (ie allergic to) and causes various symptoms, such as hay fever, urticaria, itching (pruritus) or even asthma-like bronchoconstriction.

Many agents can act as triggers for histamine release, including inhalation of pollen, insect bites and stings, contact with some metal objects, food constituents, food dye additives, a number of drug types (notably PENICILLIN type ANTIBIOTICS, LOCAL ANAESTHETICS, MORPHINE and, potentially, all drugs of a protein or peptide nature) and many environmental factors. Consequently, antihistamines may be used for many purposes, but particularly for the symptomatic relief of allergy, such as hay fever and urticaria, and in the acute treatment of anaphylactic shock.

Many antihistamines also have ANTI-EMETIC properties and are therefore used to prevent vomiting associated with travel sickness, vertigo or the effects of chemotherapy. All but some recently developed antihistamines produce drowsiness and this SEDATIVE action may be used to help induce sleep.

Conventionally, only the long established antihistamine drugs, which act on histamine H_1-receptors, are referred to by the general name *antihistamines*

A

without qualification. However, somewhat confusingly, the newer and extensively prescribed drugs that can be used as ULCER-HEALING DRUGS (eg CIMETIDINE and RANITIDINE) are also antihistamines, but they act on H_2-receptors that are involved in gastric secretion and so are referred to as H_2-ANTAGONISTS.

See ACRIVASTINE; ASTEMIZOLE; AZATADINE MALEATE; AZELASTINE HYDROCHLORIDE; BROMPHENIRAMINE MALEATE; BUCLIZINE HYDROCHLORIDE; CETIRIZINE; CHLORPHENIRAMINE MALEATE; CINNARIZINE; CLEMASTINE; CYCLIZINE; CYPROHEPTADINE HYDROCHLORIDE; DIMENHYDRINATE; DIPHENHYDRAMINE HYDROCHLORIDE; DIPHENYLPYRALINE HYDROCHLORIDE; DOXYLAMINE SUCCINATE; HYDROXYZINE HYDROCHLORIDE; KETOTIFEN; LORATADINE; MECLOZINE HYDROCHLORIDE; MEQUITAZINE; OXATOMIDE; PHENINDAMINE TARTRATE; PHENIRAMINE MALEATE; PIZOTIFEN; PROMETHAZINE HYDROCHLORIDE; PROMETHAZINE THEOCLATE; TERFENADINE; TRIMEPRAZINE TARTRATE; TRIPROLIDINE HYDROCHLORIDE.

✚ Side-effects: With oral or systemic administration, commonly drowsiness, headache, impaired muscular coordination or dizziness, anticholinergic effects (dry mouth, blurred vision, urinary retention, gastrointestinal disturbances), occasional rashes and photosensitivity, palpitations and heart arrhythmias. Rarely, there may be paradoxical stimulation, especially in children, hypersensitivity reactions, blood disorders, liver disturbances, depression, sleep disturbances and hypotension.

▲ Warning: Administer with caution to patients with epilepsy, hypertrophy of the prostate gland, glaucoma, liver disease or porphyria; or who are pregnant or breast-feeding. Those antihistamines with sedative actions may impair the performance of skilled tasks, such as driving; and the sedative effect is enhanced by alcohol.

antihypertensives ▣
reduce hypertension (an elevation of arterial blood pressure above the normal range expected in a particular age group and sex due to several different causes) and so reduce a patient's risk of heart attacks, kidney failure or stroke. Many are also used to treat angina pectoris (heart pain). There are several large groups of drugs used as antihypertensives, each with a specific mode of action, but before any drugs are administered a check should be made on the patient's diet and lifestyle to see if therapy without drugs can be advised. DIURETICS act as antihypertensives and often a mild diuretic may be all that is required.

If further treatment is necessary, any of the BETA-BLOCKERS may be used, with or without simultaneous administration of a diuretic. Other treatments include the use of a VASODILATOR, such as a CALCIUM-CHANNEL BLOCKER (eg NIFEDIPINE) or HYDRALAZINE HYDROCHLORIDE. Some antihypertensive drugs act on the brain centre responsible for controlling blood pressure (eg METHYLDOPA) and ADRENERGIC-NEURONE BLOCKERS (eg DEBRISOQUINE) reduce the release of noradrenaline from sympathetic nerves, which are involved in controlling blood pressure. More recently introduced treatments include ACE INHIBITORS, ANGIOTENSIN-RECEPTOR BLOCKERS and POTASSIUM-CHANNEL ACTIVATORS.

anti-inflammatory ▣
drugs are used to reduce inflammation – the body's response to injury. Although inflammation is essentially a normal defensive mechanism (eg a reaction to tissue injury, infection or inhalation of foreign proteins), the manifestations may be so serious and inappropriate, or involve such discomfort, that treatment with anti-inflammatory drugs is required. Inflammatory conditions can be acute (eg insect strings) or chronic (eg chronic asthma, dermatitis and other skin conditions).

The NSAID (non-steroidal anti-inflammatory) drugs, such as ASPIRIN and IBUPROFEN, can give effective relief from inflammatory pain, tissue swelling, joint immobilization and can also lower raised body temperature, which means that they are often the first choice of treatment. They work by inhibiting the production and release in the body of pro-inflammatory LOCAL HORMONE mediators (the PROSTAGLANDINS) and, used with care, can be relatively free of side-effects. For more serious conditions CORTICOSTEROIDS may be required, but they can cause so many complications that they are normally only given by local application (eg as creams, or by inhalation into the lungs for asthma) with systemic injection reserved for emergencies, such as *anaphylactic shock*.

There are a number of other types of anti-inflammatory drugs, including SODIUM CROMOGLYCATE, the ANTIRHEUMATICS (which are used to relieve the pain and inflammation of rheumatoid arthritis and osteoarthritis) and gold (in the form of PENICILLAMINE and SODIUM AUROTHIOMALATE).

The IMMUNOSUPPRESSANTS (eg CYCLOPHOSPHAMIDE, CYCLOSPORIN and METHOTREXATE) are reserved for the prevention of tissue rejection (eg in transplants) and are sometimes used to treat autoimmune diseases, such as rheumatoid arthritis and lupus, when they are unresponsive to less toxic drugs.

antimalarials ⏣

are used to treat or prevent malaria. Malaria is caused by infection of the red blood cells by a small organism called a protozoan (of the genus *Plasmodium*), which is carried by several species of mosquito of the genus *Anopheles*. Infection occurs as a result of a mosquito's bite. The class of drug most commonly used to treat or prevent infection is the quinidines, of which CHLOROQUINE is the standard. However, in some parts of the world certain forms of the protozoan that causes malaria are resistant to chloroquine. In such cases, QUININE, the traditional remedy for malaria, is used. It may also be used in patients who cannot tolerate chloroquine. Although the prevention of malaria by drugs cannot be guaranteed, administration of antimalarial drugs before, during and for a period after a trip to a tropical place is recommended for protection. See HALOFANTRINE HYDROCHLORIDE; MEFLOQUINE; PRIMAQUINE; PROGUANIL HYDROCHLORIDE; PYRIMETHAMINE.

antimania ⏣

drugs are used to treat manic-depressive illness, which is characterized by periods of mood normality punctuated by episodes of *mania* and bouts of *depression*. Because of these mood swings around the norm, the disorder is sometimes called *bipolar disorder*. The manic phase most often requires acute treatment and initially ANTIPSYCHOTICS (eg PHENOTHIAZINES) are usually administered. Thereafter LITHIUM, a very different psychoactive drug, may gradually be substituted in most patients and this can prevent or reduce the frequency and severity of attacks.

antimicrobials ⏣

are used to treat infections caused by microbes (micro-organisms), which includes the major classes of pathogenic (disease-causing) micro-organisms covered in this book – viruses, mycoplasma, rickettsia, chlamydia, protozoa, bacteria and fungi (but not helminths; worms). The term therefore embraces ANTIBACTERIALS, ANTIBIOTICS, ANTIFUNGALS, ANTIPROTOZOALS and ANTIVIRALS.

antimigraine ⏣

drugs are used to treat migraine, which is a specific, clinically recognized form of headache and not simply a particularly severe headache. Migraine attacks vary in form, but common characteristics include a throbbing confined to one side of the head (*unilateral headache*), nausea and vomiting, and a forewarning of an attack (an *aura*) consisting of visual disturbances and weakness or numbness of the limbs.

Drugs are administered (and also for the related condition called 'cluster headache') in two quite distinct ways.

A

One group of drugs is given chronically (ie long-term) in order to help prevent attacks (prophylactic use), for example, CALCIUM-CHANNEL BLOCKERS (eg NIFEDIPINE and VERAPAMIL HYDROCHLORIDE), BETA-BLOCKERS (eg METOPROLOL TARTRATE, NADOLOL, PROPRANOLOL HYDROCHLORIDE and TIMOLOL MALEATE), CYPROHEPTADINE HYDROCHLORIDE and METHYSERGIDE. All these drugs affect blood vessels in some way. In migraine attacks, blood vessels in the head and scalp are thought to narrow (constrict) before an attack and then widen (dilate), causing the pain. A second group of drugs may be used either at the *aura* stage or during the attack, and for maximum effect the speed of administration and subsequent absorption of the drug is an all-important factor. A number of ANALGESICS can be used to offset the pain of an attack (eg ASPIRIN, CODEINE PHOSPHATE and PARACETAMOL) and are often incorporated into COMPOUND PREPARATIONS together with a variety of drugs and drug types (eg CAFFEINE, BUCLIZINE HYDROCHLORIDE, DOXYLAMINE SUCCINATE, ISOMETHEPTENE MUCATE and PIZOTIFEN).

Sometimes drugs with ANTINAUSEANT or ANTI-EMETIC properties are included (eg CYCLIZINE and METOCLOPRAMIDE HYDROCHLORIDE). Drugs that affect blood vessels can also be used during the attack stage, including the extensively used drug ERGOTAMINE TARTRATE and the recently introduced SUMATRIPTAN, which can be self-injected to achieve a rapid onset of action. In all cases, the appropriate combination of drugs will vary from individual to individual and a certain amount of experimentation may be necessary to identify the factors that trigger a migraine attack (eg certain foods).

antimuscarinics ▤

are one of the main classes that make up the ANTICHOLINERGIC group of drugs. All the anticholinergic drugs act by inhibiting the action, release or production of the NEUROTRANSMITTER ACETYLCHOLINE, which plays an important part in the central and peripheral nervous systems. The term *anticholinergic* is commonly, and incorrectly, used synonymously with antimuscarinic as so many antimuscarinics are used in medicine.

Drugs that block the actions of acetylcholine at *muscarinic* RECEPTORS (ie antimuscarinic drugs) tend to relax smooth muscle, reduce the secretion of saliva, digestive juices and sweat, and dilate the pupil of the eye. They may be used as ANTISPASMODICS, ANTIPARKINSONISM drugs (in the treatment of some symptoms of parkinsonian disease), ANTINAUSEANTS or ANTI-EMETICS in the treatment of motion sickness, to treat peptic ulcers, in ophthalmic examinations and in antagonizing adverse effects of ANTICHOLINESTERASES (in medicine, agricultural accidental poisoning or warfare).

Examples of antimuscarinic anticholinergic drugs include: ATROPINE SULPHATE, BENZHEXOL HYDROCHLORIDE, BENZTROPINE MESYLATE, BIPERIDEN, CO-PHENOTROPE, CYCLOPENTOLATE HYDROCHLORIDE, FLAVOXATE HYDROCHLORIDE, GLYCOPYRRONIUM BROMIDE, HYOSCINE BUTYLBROMIDE, HYOSCINE HYDROBROMIDE, IPRATROPIUM BROMIDE, MEPENZOLATE BROMIDE, ORPHENADRINE CITRATE, ORPHENADRINE HYDROCHLORIDE, PIPENZOLATE BROMIDE, PIRENZEPINE, POLDINE METHYLSULPHATE, PROCYCLIDINE HYDROCHLORIDE, PROPANTHELINE BROMIDE and TROPICAMIDE.

The other main groups of anticholinergic drugs are the SKELETAL MUSCLE RELAXANTS (eg TUBOCURARINE CHLORIDE) and the GANGLION-BLOCKERS. These drugs interact with *nicotinic* cholinergic receptors (at which NICOTINE is a powerful stimulant) rather than with *muscarinic* cholinergic receptors (which are powerfully stimulated by the plant ALKALOID muscarine; derived from the poisonous mushroom *Amanita muscaria*).

antinauseants ▤

are used to prevent or minimize the feeling of nausea and to reduce any subsequent vomiting. The type of drug used and the likelihood of its success depends on the mechanism and origin of the nausea, which can be triggered in a number of ways. Motion sickness, or travel sickness, can often be prevented by taking antinauseants like HYOSCINE HYDROBROMIDE, MECLOZINE HYDROCHLORIDE and DIMENHYDRINATE before travelling.

Similar drugs may be used to treat nausea and other symptoms of labyrinthine disease (where the vestibular balance mechanisms of the inner ear are disturbed, eg Ménière's disease), though other drugs may also be necessary, such as CINNARIZINE and PHENOTHIAZINES like CHLORPROMAZINE HYDROCHLORIDE and PROCHLORPERAZINE.

A number of chemicals and drugs induce nausea and vomiting by an action involving the so-called *chemoreceptor trigger zone* within the brain; for instance, this is the most common side-effect when using the (OPIOID) NARCOTIC ANALGESIC morphine and so it may be combined with cinnarizine. The nausea and vomiting that is caused by chemotherapy and radiotherapy can be difficult to treat. However, some ANTI-EMETIC drugs, such as MOTILITY STIMULANTS (eg METOCLOPRAMIDE HYDROCHLORIDE and CISAPRIDE), may be of some use by preventing vomiting and helping food out of the stomach.

Alternatively, there are some recently developed drugs that can also be effective, for instance, certain inhibitors of the actions of the mediator SEROTONIN (5-HT$_3$ antagonists) such as GRANISETRON, ONDANSETRON and TROPISETRON. The cannabis derivative NABILONE may be administered in difficult cases.

anti-oestrogens ▣

(oestrogen antagonists) are a class of HORMONE ANTAGONISTS that usually act directly to prevent the actions of female SEX HORMONES, the OESTROGENS (OESTRADIOL and OESTRIOL), at RECEPTORS in their target tissues; although they sometimes act indirectly to prevent the formation, or

inhibit the release, of the hormones. An example of a drug that acts by the direct mechanism is TAMOXIFEN and of those that act indirectly are AMINOGLUTETHIMIDE and FORMESTANE.

antiparkinsonism ▣

drugs are used to treat parkinsonism, which is the name used to describe the symptoms of several disorders of the central nervous system, including muscle tremor and rigidity (extrapyramidal symptoms), especially in the limbs. It is caused by an imbalance in the actions the NEUROTRANSMITTERS ACETYLCHOLINE and DOPAMINE. In classic Parkinson's disease this is due to the degeneration of dopamine-containing nerves. However, what are known as parkinsonian extrapyramidal side-effects may be caused by treatment with several types of drugs, especially ANTIPSYCHOTICS (eg HALOPERIDOL).

Treatment of parkinsonism may be with ANTICHOLINERGICS (eg BENZHEXOL HYDROCHLORIDE, BENZTROPINE MESYLATE, BIPERIDEN and PROCYCLIDINE HYDROCHLORIDE) or by drugs that increase the effects of dopamine (eg LEVODOPA, BROMOCRIPTINE and PERGOLIDE). The former class is more useful for controlling fine tremor, including that induced by drugs, and the latter class for overcoming difficulty in commencing movement and slowness brought about by degenerative disease. It is a difficult and often lengthy process to achieve the optimum dose in each patient and there are certain side-effects (such as confusion in the elderly) that occur with all the various treatments.

antiperspirants ▣

help to prevent sweating. Medically, they are required only in cases of severe hyperhidrosis (excessive sweating), when some disorder of the sweat glands causes constant and streaming perspiration. In such cases, ALUMINIUM CHLORIDE solution is an effective treatment and dusting powders may also be useful to dry the skin.

A

antiplatelet ⏃

drugs (also known as antithrombotic drugs) prevent the formation of blood clots (thrombi), that is, they reduce platelet aggregation. These drugs can be used as a preventive treatment (prophylactic use), eg ASPIRIN, in patients who are at risk after a heart attack or bypass operation. However, this same action may also increase bleeding time and so patients receiving ANTICOAGULANT drugs should not normally have antiplatelet drugs as well. The antiplatelet DIPYRIDAMOLE does not act as an anticoagulant, but instead seems to work by stopping platelets sticking together (or to surgically inserted tubes or artificial heart valves). EPOPROSTENOL (prostacyclin) is a naturally occurring prostaglandin present in the walls of blood vessels which has antiplatelet activity when administered therapeutically by intravenous infusion.

Antipressan

(Berk) is a proprietary, prescription-only preparation of the BETA-BLOCKER atenolol. It can be used as an ANTIHYPERTENSIVE for raised blood pressure, as an ANTI-ANGINA treatment to relieve symptoms and improve exercise tolerance and as an ANTI-ARRHYTHMIC to regularize heartbeat and to treat myocardial infarction. It is available as tablets.

✚▲ Side-effects/warning: See ATENOLOL.

antiprotozoals ⏃

are used to treat or prevent infections caused by micro-organisms called protozoa. The most important protozoa, in terms of illness and death, are those of the genus *Plasmodium*, which cause malaria (see ANTIMALARIALS). Other major protozoal diseases found in tropical countries include trypanosomiasis, leishmaniasis and amoebic dysentery. Protozoal infections more familiar in this country include toxoplasmosis, trichomoniasis and giardiasis. A common form of pneumonia is caused in immunosuppressed patients (including those suffering from AIDS) by the protozoan *Pneumocystis carinii*. The drugs used to treat amoebic-protozoal infections are commonly referred to as AMOEBICIDALS.

antipsychotics ⏃

or neuroleptics, calm and soothe patients without impairing consciousness. They are used mainly to treat psychologically disturbed patients, particularly those who manifest the complex behavioural patterns of schizophrenia. In the short-term, they can also be used to treat severe anxiety. They may also worsen, or help to alleviate, depression because they can affect mood. Antipsychotics work by acting in the brain, especially through an effect (inhibition) involving the NEUROTRANSMITTER DOPAMINE. They can cause many side-effects, including abnormal face and body movements and restlessness, which often resemble the symptoms of the condition being treated. The use of other drugs may be required to control these side-effects. Notable examples of antipsychotic drugs include FLUPENTHIXOL, HALOPERIDOL and the PHENOTHIAZINES (especially CHLORPROMAZINE HYDROCHLORIDE and THIOTIDAZINE). BENPERIDOL is used mostly to control antisocial sexual behaviour or hyperactivity. Those antipsychotics with markedly depressant side-effects are also, though somewhat misleadingly, called *major tranquillizers*.

antipyretics ⏃

are used to reduce raised body temperature, for example in fever, but they do not lower normal body temperature. The best-known and most-used antipyretics include certain NON-NARCOTIC ANALGESICS such as ASPIRIN, PARACETAMOL and IBUPROFEN. See also NSAID.

Antirabies Immunoglobulin Injection

see RABIES IMMUNOGLOBULIN

antirheumatics ⏃

are used to relieve the pain and

inflammation of rheumatism and arthritis (particularly rheumatoid arthritis and osteoarthritis, and so they are also known as *anti-arthritic drugs*) and sometimes of other musculoskeletal disorders. The primary form of treatment is with NSAIDS (non-steroidal anti-inflammatory drugs), NON-NARCOTIC ANALGESICS such as ASPIRIN, SODIUM SALICYLATE, the aspirin-paracetamol ester BENORYLATE, FENOPROFEN, IBUPROFEN, INDOMETHACIN and PHENYLBUTAZONE. The CORTICOSTEROIDS can also be used because they are anti-inflammatory (eg PREDNISOLONE and TRIAMCINOLONE). Finally, there are some drugs that seem to halt the progression of musculoskeletal disorders, for example AURANOFIN and SODIUM AUROTHIOMALATE (which both contain gold) and PENICILLAMINE. However, some of these drugs have unpleasant side-effects and others can take up to six months to have any effect. In cases where there is an autoimmune element to the disease, IMMUNOSUPPRESSANTS (eg AZATHIOPRINE, CHLORAMBUCIL, CYCLOPHOSPHAMIDE, CYCLOSPORIN and METHOTREXATE) can also be used.

Antirubella Immunoglobulin Injection
see RUBELLA IMMUNOGLOBULIN

antiseborrhoeics ☑
are used to treat seborrhoea, which is an excessive secretion of the oily substance sebum from the sebaceous glands of the skin and the glands are often enlarged, especially beside the nose. Over-secretion is common in adolescence and often results in acne or seborrhoeic eczema. Dandruff often appears during the development of seborrhoeic eczema.

antiseptics ☑
are agents that destroy micro-organisms or inhibit their activity to such an extent that they are less, or no longer, harmful to health. Antiseptics can be applied to the skin, burns or wounds to prevent infections and to limit the spread of pathogenic

(disease-causing) micro-organisms. The term is frequently used synonymously with DISINFECTANT. However, this is not strictly correct because the latter term can also apply to agents used on inanimate objects (such as surgical equipment, catheters, etc.), as well as to agents used on the skin and other living tissue.

antiserum ☑
is a general term that is used to describe certain preparations of blood serum rich in particular antibodies. Antiserum preparations (*antisera*) provide what is known as *passive immunity* to diseases, or some measure of treatment if the disease has already been contracted.

The common term used to describe that part of a disease-causing entity which is recognized by the immune system is *antigen*. If an antigen is injected into an animal, the animal produces *antibodies* in response. An antiserum is a preparation of animal blood serum containing these antibodies. Most antisera are prepared from the blood of antigen-treated horses, which are then purified and administered to humans to immunize them against disease. However, because they are *foreign* proteins, serious hypersensitivity reactions may result and, though at the most extreme, cause anaphylactic shock. For this reason, such animal preparations are now rarely used and have to a large extent been replaced by preparations of human antibodies from human antiserum preparations, usually referred to simply as as *immunoglobulins*.

However, DIPHTHERIA ANTITOXIN prepared from horses is still used for passive immunization in circumstances where contraction of the disease is suspected.
✪ Related entry: Zagreb antivenom.

antispasmodics ☑
or spasmolytics, relieve spasm in smooth muscle (involuntary muscles, eg muscles in the respiratory tract and the intestinal walls) and form part of the group of drugs

A

known collectively as SMOOTH MUSCLE
RELAXANTS. Some are used as
BRONCHODILATORS while others are used to
relieve abdominal pain due to intestinal
colic. They include the ANTICHOLINERGICS,
such as ATROPINE SULPHATE, and agents such
as MEBEVERINE HYDROCHLORIDE which act
directly on smooth muscle.

antisympathetics ▣

act at some site or other within the
sympathetic nervous system to reduce its
overall effect. Activity within this division of
the (autonomic) nervous system controls
blood pressure and heart rate, therefore
drugs that act to reduce its activity cause a
fall in blood pressure and so the main use
of such drugs is as ANTIHYPERTENSIVES.

There are a number of sites and
mechanisms by which such drugs act. For
example, METHYLDOPA acts in the brain itself
to reduce the activity of the sympathetic
nervous system, while METIROSINE inhibits
the enzymes that produce NORADRENALINE
(the sympathetic NEUROTRANSMITTER) within
nerves. The ADRENERGIC-NEURONE BLOCKERS
(BETHANIDINE SULPHATE, BRETYLIUM TOSYLAYE,
DEBRISOQUINE and GUANETHIDINE
MONOSULPHATE) interfere with the storage
and release of noradrenaline and the
CLONIDINE HYDROCHLORIDE decreases the
amount that is released.

All these drugs have quite marked
side-effects and some of them may be
administered in conjunction with other
classes of antihypertensives, for instance
the DIURETICS.

Antitetanus
Immunoglobulin Injection
see TETANUS IMMUNOGLOBULIN

antithrombotics ▣

prevent the formation of blood clots
(thrombi). See ANTICOAGULANTS;
ANTIPLATELET.

antithyroid ▣

drugs are used in the treatment of over-

activity of the thyroid gland
(hyperthyriodism; thyrotoxicosis). In
thyrotoxicosis there is an excess secretion
of THYROID HORMONES and this results in an
exaggeration of the normal activity of the
gland, which causes increased metabolic
rate, raised body temperature, sweating,
increased sensitivity to heat, nervousness,
tremor, raised heart rate, tendency to
fatigue and sometimes loss of body weight
with an increased appetite.

How the disease is treated depends on
its origin. However, if it is severe the
surgical removal of part of the gland may be
necessary, though more commonly the
gland is treated with radioactive iodine to
reduce the number of cells.

In any event, drugs are used to either
control the symptoms in the long term, or
in the short term to prepare the gland for
more radical intervention. BETA-BLOCKERS
(eg METOPROLOL TARTRATE, NADOLOL and
PROPRANOLOL HYDROCHLORIDE) are used in
the prevention of a number of the signs and
symptoms of thyrotoxicosis. They work by
blocking the effects of over-stimulation
caused by the release of ADRENALINE and
NORADRENALINE by thyroid hormones, but do
not treat the gland itself.

Some other drugs (chemically
thionamides, eg CARBIMAZOLE and
PROPYLTHIOURACIL) act directly on the
thyroid gland to reduce the production of
the thyroid hormones, so treating the
excess of thyroid hormones in the blood.
Iodine itself, which is chemically
incorporated into the thyroid hormones
THYROXINE and TRIIODOTHYRONINE, can be
given (as AQUEOUS IODINE ORAL SOLUTION, or
Lugol's solution) to suppress gland activity
prior to thyroid surgery.

antitubercular ▣

(or antituberculous) drugs are used in
combination to treat tuberculosis. The
initial phase of treatment usually involves
three drugs (commonly ISONIAZID,
RIFAMPICIN and PYRAZINAMIDE) in order to
tackle the disease as efficiently as possible,

while reducing the risk of encountering bacterial resistance.

If, after about two months, the first phase is successful, treatment usually continues with only two of the initial three drugs (one of which is often isoniazid or rifampicin). If the first line of treatment is not successful, for example, because the patient suffered intolerable side-effects or because the disease was resistant to the drugs, then other drugs are used. Treatment of tuberculosis with drugs is only necessary where the far more effective public health measure of vaccination has, for some reason, failed (see BCG VACCINE).

antituberculous
see ANTITUBERCULAR

antitussives 🗊
assist in the treatment of coughs. The term is usually used to describe only those drugs that suppress coughing, rather than drugs used to treat the cause of coughing. Cough suppressants include OPIATES, such as DEXTROMETHORPHAN HYDROBROMIDE, CODEINE PHOSPHATE and METHADONE HYDROCHLORIDE. They tend to cause constipation as a side-effect and so should not be used for prolonged periods.

Other antitussive preparations are EXPECTORANTS and DEMULCENTS. Expectorants are used to decrease the viscosity of mucus or to increase the secretion of liquid mucus in dry, irritant, unproductive coughs. Examples of expectorants include AMMONIUM CHLORIDE, GUAIPHENESIN and IPECACUANHA; and these are incorporated into a wide range of proprietary compound cough medicines. Demulcents also help to reduce the viscosity of mucus and relieve dry, unproductive coughs. All of these drugs are used to soothe coughs rather than to treat the underlying cause, such as an infection.

Antivaricella-Zoster Immunoglobulin
see VARICELLA-ZOSTER IMMUNOGLOBULIN (VZIG)

antivenin
see ANTIVENOM

antivenom 🗊
(antivenin) is an antidote to the poison in a snakebite, a scorpion's sting or a bite from any other poisonous creature (such as a spider). Normally, it is an ANTISERUM and is injected into the bloodstream for immediate relief. Identification of the poisonous creature is important so that the right antidote can be selected.

In the UK the only indigenous poisonous snake is the adder (*Vipera berus*), the poison of which can usually be treated by medical supportive therapy, but on occasion may require treatment with ZAGREB ANTIVENOM. Antivenoms have been prepared internationally for many foreign snakes, insects and spiders. Some of these are available in the UK for emergency use from regional centres in London, Liverpool and Oxford.

➕▲ Side-effects/warning: Because antivenoms are themselves foreign proteins, hypersensitivity reactions are not uncommon and may compound the symptoms and distress caused by the bite itself, therefore antivenoms should not be used except where symptoms are severe.

antivirals 🗊
are drugs that are used to treat infections caused by viruses, which are micro-organisms much smaller than bacteria, so minute they cannot be seen under the normal (light) microscope. They can only replicate within the living cells of the host which they parasitize.

In terms of public health, prevention of viral infection is best achieved by VACCINATION (eg against poliomyelitis, rubella, measles and mumps and some types of rabies), but continual mutation of other viruses makes vaccination more difficult (eg flu, the common cold, HIV). ANTIBIOTICS are inactive against viruses, and treatment of infection is only possible with a few, relatively new, antiviral drugs. Mainly,

A the use of antivirals is restricted to preventive or disease-limitation treatment (eg ACYCLOVIR against *herpes viruses*). However, some antiviral drugs can be life-savers, especially in immunocompromised patients. A great deal of effort is currently being made to develop antivirals for use in the treatment of HIV infection, but AIDS treatment currently relies heavily on drugs active against bacterial, fungal or other microbial infections in these immunocompromised individuals.

Antivirals can be divided into groups on the basis of how they work. Some are *nucleoside analogues* (or related compounds) that resemble cellular molecules necessary to viral function or replication, often working as ENZYME INHIBITORS against an essential viral enzymes; for example, the group of antivirals that work against the enzyme *reverse transcriptase* are termed *reverse transcriptase inhibitors* (eg DIDANOSINE, LAMIVUDINE, STAVUDINE). Other antivirals that prevent viral cell replication by inhibiting nucleic acid synthesis include; CARBOVIR, DIDANOSINE, FOSCARNET, GANCICLOVIR, IDOXURIDINE, TRIBAVIRIN, ZALCITABINE, ZIDOVUDINE. The most recently introduced group of antivirals, the *protease inhibitors*, work as enzyme inhibitors acting against an enzyme (*HIV-1 protease*) that is essential for the replication of viruses. Examples of this group include INDINAVIR, RITONAVIR and SAQUINAVIR. There are a number of other types of antivirals that work in a different way. AMANTIDINE is active against influenza A virus (an action unrelated to its ANTIPARKINSONISM use), and INTERFERONS act as IMMUNOMODULATORS that help the body's immunological response to viruses.

In clinical practice, antivirals are often grouped by the types of infection against which they are effective (rather than by mechanism of action). For instance, serious cytomegaloviral infections may be contained by treatment with GANCICLOVIR and FOSCARNET. Infections due to the herpes viruses (eg cold sores, genital herpes,

shingles and chickenpox) may be contained by early treatment with acyclovir, amantadine, FAMCICLOVIR, INOSINE PRANOBEX or VALACICLOVIR. HIV infections are increasingly being treated by several drug groups in combination, for instance, *protease inhibitors* together with *nucleoside analogues*.

Anturan
(Geigy) is a proprietary, prescription-only preparation of sulphinpyrazone. It can be used to treat and prevent gout and hyperurea, and is available as tablets.
+▲ Side-effects/warning: See SULPHINPYRAZONE.

Anugesic-HC
(Parke-Davis) is a proprietary, prescription-only COMPOUND PREPARATION of the CORTICOSTEROID and ANTI-INFLAMMATORY hydrocortisone (as acetate) and the ASTRINGENT agents ZINC OXIDE and BISMUTH OXIDE, benzyl benzoate (with Peru balsam) and the LOCAL ANAESTHETIC pramoxine hydrochloride. It can be used to treat haemorrhoids and inflammation in the anal region, and is available as a cream and suppositories.
+▲ Side-effects/warning: See BENZYL BENZOATE; HYDROCORTISONE; PRAMOXINE HYDROCHLORIDE.

Anusol
(Parke-Davis) is a proprietary, non-prescription COMPOUND PREPARATION of the ASTRINGENT agents BISMUTH OXIDE and ZINC OXIDE (with Peru balsam). It can be used to treat haemorrhoids and discomfort in the anal region, and is available as a cream, an ointment and suppositories.

Anusol-HC
(Parke-Davis) is a proprietary, non-prescription COMPOUND PREPARATION of the CORTICOSTEROID and ANTI-INFLAMMATORY hydrocortisone (as acetate) and the ASTRINGENT and ANTISEPTIC agents benzyl benzoate, BISMUTH OXIDE, BISMUTH SUBGALLATE

and ZINC OXIDE (with Peru Balsam). It can be used to treat haemorrhoids and inflammation in the anal region, and is available as an ointment and suppositories.

✚▲ Side-effects/warning: See BENZYL BENZOATE; HYDROCORTISONE.

anxiolytics ▯

are used to relieve medically diagnosed anxiety states and are prescribed only for patients whose anxiety is actually hindering its resolution by other therapies, such as pyschotherapy. They are also used to relieve acute anxiety, for instance, before surgery. Treatment should be at the lowest dose effective and must not be prolonged, because psychological dependence and physical dependence (addiction) readily occurs and may make withdrawal difficult. The best-known and most-used anxiolytics are the BENZODIAZEPINES (eg CHLORDIAZEPOXIDE, CLOBAZAM, DIAZEPAM and LORAZEPAM) and other drugs such as MEPROBAMATE and some of the ANTIPSYCHOTICS (at low doses). Additionally, BETA-BLOCKERS are sometimes used to treat anxiety by preventing the physical symptoms such as palpitations of the heart, sweating and tremor, which helps the patient to stop the chain reaction of worry to fear to panic.

The benzodiazepines are occasionally administered for the relief of withdrawal symptoms of addiction to other drugs (such as alcohol). Some of these drugs take time to work and careful adjustment of the dose is required. Drugs of this class are sometimes, somewhat misleadingly, referred to as *minor tranquillizers*.

apomorphine hydrochloride

is an ANTIPARKINSONISM drug that has similar actions to BROMOCRIPTINE and is used in a patient's *off* periods, which are not controlled by the drug levodopa. It is chemically related to MORPHINE, though it is not an ANALGESIC, but has been used as an EMETIC. Administration is by injection.

✚ Side-effects: Dyskinesias (movement disorders) during *on* periods, impaired

speech and balance, nausea and vomiting, confusion, euphoria, light-headedness and hallucinations; postural hypotension, blood disorders, cognitive impairment. Pain at site of injection.

▲ Warning: It should not be administered to patients with central nervous system or respiratory depression, hypersensitivity to opioids, psychiatric disorders and dementia; or who are pregnant or breast-feeding. Administer with caution to those with respiratory, cardiovascular and hormone disorders, kidney impairment; and the elderly.

✪ Related entry: Britaject.

appetite suppressants ▯

(anorectics) is a term used to describe drugs of two main types. The first type works by acting on the brain and a number of these drugs are related to amphetamine, consequently psychological dependence readily occurs. Treatment with these drugs should be short term only, and there is also a growing doubt among experts over the medical value of such a treatment. Examples of these drugs include DEXFENFLURAMINE HYDROCHLORIDE, DIETHYLPROPION HYDROCHLORIDE, FENFLURAMINE HYDROCHLORIDE and PHENTERMINE. The proprietary preparations of these drugs are on the Controlled Drugs List. The second type works by bulking out the food eaten so that the body feels it has actually taken more than it has. Bulking agents include METHYLCELLULOSE and STERCULIA. Both types of drug are intended to assist in the medical treatment of obesity, where the primary therapy is an appropriate diet.

apraclonidine

is a SYMPATHOMIMETIC which is chemically a derivative of clonidine. It can be used to control or prevent postoperative elevation of intraocular pressure (pressure in the eyeball) after laser surgery. Administration is topical.

✚ Side-effects: Eyelid retraction,

A

hyperaemia (excess blood in vessels in the eye), whitening of the conjunctiva; dilated pupil, systemic effects (for instance, on the cardiovascular system) if a sufficient quantity of the drug is absorbed into the body.

▲ Warning: Avoid its use in patients with severe cardiovascular disease (including hypertension); administer with care to those with a history of vagovagal attacks, or who are pregnant or breast-feeding.

○ Related entry: Lopidine.

Apresoline

(Ciba) is a proprietary, prescription-only preparation of the VASODILATOR hydralazine hydrochloride. It can be used in long-term ANTIHYPERTENSIVE treatment and in hypertensive crisis. It is available as tablets and in a form for injection.

✚▲ Side-effects/warning: See HYDRALAZINE HYDROCHLORIDE.

Aprinox

(Boots) is a proprietary prescription-only preparation of the (THIAZIDE) DIURETIC bendrofluazide. It can be used, either on its own or in conjunction with other diuretics or drugs, in the treatment of oedema, congestive HEART FAILURE TREATMENT and as an ANTIHYPERTENSIVE. It is available as tablets.

✚▲ Side-effects/warning: See BENDROFLUAZIDE.

aprotinin

is an inhibitor of proteolytic enzymes and has antifibrinolytic activity, because it prevents thrombosis by an action on the blood-clot formation system. It can be used to prevent life-threatening bleeding, for instance, in open-heart surgery, removal of tumours and in surgical procedures in patients with certain blood disorders (eg hyperplasminaemias).

✚ Side-effects: Hypersensitivity reactions and occasionally inflammation of vein walls.

78 ○ Related entry: Trasylol.

Apsifen

(APS) is a proprietary, prescription-only preparation of the (NSAID) NON-NARCOTIC ANALGESIC and ANTIRHEUMATIC ibuprofen, which also has ANTIPYRETIC actions. It can be used to relieve pain, particularly of rheumatic disease and other musculo-skeletal disorders. It is available as tablets.

✚▲ Side-effects/warning: See IBUPROFEN.

Apsin

(APS) is a proprietary, prescription-only preparation of the ANTIBACTERIAL and (PENICILLIN) ANTIBIOTIC phenoxymethyl-penicillin. It is particularly effective in treating tonsillitis, infection of the middle ear, certain skin infections and in preventing recurrent streptococcal throat infection, which can lead to episodes of rheumatic fever. It is available as an oral solution and tablets (as the potassium salt).

✚▲ Side-effects/warning: See PHENOXYMETHYLPENICILLIN.

Apsolol

(APS) is a proprietary, prescription-only preparation of the BETA-BLOCKER propranolol hydrochloride. It can be used as an ANTIHYPERTENSIVE for raised blood pressure, as an ANTI-ANGINA treatment to relieve symptoms and improve exercise tolerance and as an ANTI-ARRHYTHMIC to regularize heartbeat and to treat myocardial infarction. It can also be used as an ANTITHYROID drug for the short-term treatment of thyrotoxicosis, as an ANTIMIGRAINE treatment to prevent attacks, as an ANXIOLYTIC, particularly for symptomatic relief of tremor and palpitations, and, with an ALPHA-ADRENOCEPTOR BLOCKER, in the acute treatment of phaeochromocytoma. It is available as tablets.

✚▲ Side-effects/warning: See PROPRANOLOL HYDROCHLORIDE.

Apsolox

(APS) is a proprietary, prescription-only preparation of the BETA-BLOCKER oxprenolol hydrochloride. It can be used as an ANTIHYPERTENSIVE for raised blood pressure, as an ANTI-ANGINA treatment to relieve symptoms and improve exercise tolerance and as an ANTI-ARRHYTHMIC to regularize heartbeat and to treat myocardial infarction. It can also be used as an ANTITHYROID drug for the short-term treatment of thyrotoxicosis, as an ANTIMIGRAINE treatment to prevent attacks, as an ANXIOLYTIC, particularly for symptomatic relief of tremor and palpitations, and, with an ALPHA-ADRENOCEPTOR BLOCKER, in the acute treatment of phaeochromocytoma. It is available as tablets.

✚▲ Side-effects/warning: See OXPRENOLOL HYDROCHLORIDE.

Apstil

(APS) is a proprietary, prescription-only preparation of the SEX HORMONE stilboestrol, which is a synthetic OESTROGEN. It can be used as an ANTICANCER drug to treat prostate cancer and breast cancer, and is available in the form of tablets.

✚▲ Side-effects/warning: See STILBOESTROL.

Aquadrate

(Procter & Gamble) is a proprietary, non-prescription preparation of the HYDRATING AGENT urea. It can be used for dry, scaling or itching skin, and is available as a cream.

✚▲ Side-effects/warning: See UREA.

aqueous iodine oral solution

(or Lugol's solution) is a non-proprietary, freshly made solution of iodine and potassium iodide in water. It is used by patients suffering from an excess of THYROID HORMONES in the bloodstream (thyrotoxicosis) prior to thyroid surgery. It is administered by mouth after dilution.

✚▲ Side-effects/warning: See IODINE.

arachis oil

is peanut oil and is used primarily as an EMOLLIENT in treating crusts on skin surfaces in conditions such as dandruff or cradle cap. Administration is topical. It is also used as a LAXATIVE to lubricate and soften impacted faeces in order to promote bowel movement, when it is given orally.

✚▲ Side-effects/warning: Usually considered safe (it is widely used as a cooking oil) but allergy to peanut products is quite common, to the extent of anaphylaxis, and so there is a potential risk of allergic reaction.

○ Related entries: Cerumol Ear Drops; Cetavlex; Fletchers' Arachis Oil Retention Enema; Hydromol; Kamillosan; Massé Breast Cream; Oilatum.

Aramine

(Merck Sharp & Dohme) is a proprietary, prescription-only preparation of the SYMPATHOMIMETIC and VASOCONSTRICTOR metaraminol. It is most often used to raise blood pressure in a patient under general anaesthesia, or in conditions of severe hypotensive shock. It is available in a form for injection or infusion.

✚▲ Side-effects/warning: See METARAMINOL.

Arbralene

(Berk) is a proprietary, prescription-only preparation of the BETA-BLOCKER metoprolol tartrate. It can be used as an ANTIHYPERTENSIVE for raised blood pressure, as an ANTI-ANGINA treatment to relieve symptoms and improve exercise tolreance and as an ANTI-ARRHYTHMIC to regularize the heartbeat and to treat myocardial infarction. It can also be used as an ANTITHYROID drug for short-term treatment of thyrotoxicosis and as an ANTIMIGRAINE treatment to prevent attacks. It is available as tablets.

✚▲ Side-effects/warning: See METOPROLOL TARTRATE.

Aredia

(Ciba) is a recently introduced, proprietary, prescription-only preparation of disodium

A

pamidronate. It is used to treat high calcium levels associated with malignant tumours, and is available in a form for intravenous infusion.
✚▲ Side-effects/warning: See DISODIUM PAMIDRONATE.

Arfonad

(Cambridge) is a proprietary, prescription-only, preparation of the GANGLION-BLOCKER trimetaphan camsylate. It can be used as a HYPOTENSIVE for controlled blood pressure during surgery, and is available in a form for injection and infusion.
✚▲ Side-effects/warning: See TRIMETAPHAN CAMSYLATE.

Arilvax

(Evans) is a proprietary, prescription-only VACCINE preparation. It can be used to prevent infection by yellow fever, and is available in a form for injection.
▲ Warning: See YELLOW FEVER VACCINE.

Arimidex

(Zeneca) is a proprietary, prescription-only preparation of the sex HORMONE ANTAGONIST anastrozole. It can be used as an ANTICANCER drug in the advanced stages of breast cancer in postmenopausal women, and is available as tablets.
✚▲ Side-effects/warning: See ANASTROZOLE.

Arpicolin

(RP) is a proprietary, prescription-only preparation of the ANTICHOLINERGIC procyclidine hydrochloride. It can be used in the treatment of parkinsonism, and is available as a syrup.
✚▲ Side-effects/warning: See PROCYCLIDINE HYDROCHLORIDE.

Arpimycin

(RP) is a proprietary, prescription-only preparation of the ANTIBACTERIAL and (MACROLIDE) ANTIBIOTIC erythromycin. It can be used to treat and prevent many forms of infection, and is available as a liquid oral mixture.
✚▲ Side-effects/warning: See ERYTHROMYCIN.

Arret

(Johnson & Johnson) is a proprietary, non-prescription preparation of the (OPIOID) ANTIDIARRHOEAL loperamide hydrochloride. It can be used for the relief of acute diarrhoea and its associated pain and discomfort, and is available as capsules.
✚▲ Side-effects/warning: See LOPERAMIDE HYDROCHLORIDE.

Artane

(Lederle) is a proprietary, prescription-only preparation of the ANTICHOLINERGIC benzhexol hydrochloride. It can be used in the treatment of parkinsonism and to control tremor and involuntary movement. It is available as tablets.
✚▲ Side-effects/warning: See BENZHEXOL HYDROCHLORIDE.

Arthrofen

(Ashbourne) is a proprietary, prescription-only preparation of the (NSAID) NON-NARCOTIC ANALGESIC and ANTIRHEUMATIC ibuprofen. It can be used to relieve pain, particularly that of rheumatic disease and other musculoskeletal disorders, and is available as tablets.
✚▲ Side-effects/warning: See IBUPROFEN.

Arthrosin

(Ashbourne) is a proprietary, prescription-only preparation of the (NSAID) NON-NARCOTIC ANALGESIC and ANTIRHEUMATIC naproxen. It can be used to relieve pain, particularly rheumatic and arthritic pain and to treat other musculoskeletal disorders. It is available as tablets.
✚ Side-effects/warning: See NAPROXEN.

Arthrotec

(Searle) is a proprietary, prescription-only COMPOUND PREPARATION of the powerful (NSAID) NON-NARCOTIC ANALGESIC and ANTIRHEUMATIC diclofenac sodium and an ULCER-HEALING DRUG the PROSTAGLANDIN

A

misoprostol. It can be used to treat pain and inflammation in rheumatic disease. This preparation has a novel approach to minimizing the gastrointestinal side-effects of the NSAID by adding prostaglandin, which is the LOCAL HORMONE whose production has been reduced by the NSAID. Prostaglandins are necessary for correct blood circulation in the gastrointestinal tract and if their level is reduced gastrointestinal side-effects (such as ulceration) may occur. It is available as tablets.

+▲ Side-effects/warning: See DICLOFENAC SODIUM; MISOPROSTOL.

Arthroxen

(CP) is a proprietary, prescription-only preparation of the (NSAID) NON-NARCOTIC ANALGESIC and ANTIRHEUMATIC naproxen. It can be used to relieve pain and inflammation, particularly in rheumatism, arthritis and other musculoskeletal disorders, and is available as tablets.

+ Side-effects/warning: See NAPROXEN.

artificial saliva

is used to make up a deficiency of saliva in conditions that cause a dry mouth. Common preparations include viscous constituents, such as CARMELLOSE SODIUM, SORBITOL, gastric mucin, gum acacia, MALIC ACID, and electrolytes, including potassium chloride, sodium chloride and potassium phosphates.

Artracin

(DDSA Pharmaceuticals) is a proprietary, prescription-only preparation of the (NSAID) NON-NARCOTIC ANALGESIC and ANTIRHEUMATIC indomethacin. It can be used to relieve pain and inflammation, particularly in rheumatism, arthritis and other musculoskeletal disorders, and is available as tablets.

+▲ Side-effects/warning: See INDOMETHACIN.

Arvin

(Knoll) is a proprietary, prescription-only preparation of the ANTICOAGULANT ancrod. It is not in common use and is available only on a 'named-patient' basis in a form for injection.

+▲ Side-effects/warning: See ANCROD .

Arythmol

(Knoll) is a proprietary, prescription-only preparation of the ANTI-ARRHYTHMIC propafenone hydrochloride. It can be used to prevent and treat irregularities of the heartbeat, and is available as tablets.

+▲ Side-effects/warning: See PROPAFENONE HYDROCHLORIDE.

Asacol

(SmithKline Beecham) is a proprietary, prescription-only preparation of the AMINOSALICYLATE mesalazine. It can be used to treat patients who suffer from ulcerative colitis but who are unable to tolerate the more commonly used sulphasalazine. It is available as tablets, a foam enema and as suppositories.

+▲ Side-effects/warning: See MESALAZINE.

Ascabiol Emulsion

(Rhône-Poulenc Rorer) is a proprietary, non-prescription preparation of benzyl benzoate in suspension, which is an insecticidal drug used as a PEDICULICIDAL for lice infestations, or as a SCABICIDAL for infestation by mites. It is available as an emulsion.

+▲ Side-effects/warning: See BENZYL BENZOATE.

ascorbic acid

(Vitamin C) is a VITAMIN that is essential for the development and maintenance of cells and tissues. It cannot be synthesized within the body and must be found in the diet (good food sources are vegetables and citrus fruits). Deficiency eventually leads to scurvy, but before that there is a lowered resistance to infection and other disorders may develop, particularly in the elderly. However, vitamin C supplements are rarely necessary with a normal, well-balanced

A

diet. There have been claims that pharmacological doses help prevent colds and so it is incorporated into a number of cold remedies. Administration is oral.

✚ warning: It is destroyed by over-cooking or through the action of ultraviolet light (ie sunlight).

○ Related entries: Beechams Hot Lemon; Beechams Hot Lemon and Honey; Children's Vitamin Drops; Coldrex Tablets; Ferfolic SV; Hedex Headcold Cherry Menthol Powders; Redoxon.

Asendis

(Novex) is a proprietary, prescription-only preparation of the (TRICYCLIC) ANTIDEPRESSANT amoxapine. It can be used to treat depressive illness, and is available as tablets.

✚▲ Side-effects/warning: See AMOXAPINE.

Aserbine

(Forley) is a proprietary, non-prescription COMPOUND PREPARATION of the ANTISEPTIC and KERATOLYTIC agents MALIC ACID, BENZOIC ACID and salicylic acid. It can be used as a desloughing agent in the treatment of superficial ulcers, burns and bedsores, so that natural healing can take place. It is available as an ointment and a solution.

✚▲ Side-effects/warning: See SALICYLIC ACID: also, avoid contact with the eyes.

Asilone Liquid

(Seton) is a proprietary, non-prescription COMPOUND PREPARATION of the ANTACIDS aluminium hydroxide and magnesium oxide, and the ANTIFOAMING AGENT dimethicone (as simethicone). It can be used to treat dyspepsia, flatulence and associated abdominal distension, heartburn (including heartburn that occurs with hiatus hernia, pregnancy and reflux oesophagitis) and to soothe the symptoms of peptic ulcers. It is available as tablets and is not normally given to children, except on medical advice.

✚▲ Side-effects/warning: See ALUMINIUM HYDROXIDE; DIMETHICONE.

Asilone Suspension

(Seton) is a proprietary, non-prescription COMPOUND PREPARATION of the ANTACIDS aluminium hydroxide and magnesium oxide, and the ANTIFOAMING AGENT dimethicone (as simethicone). It can be used to treat dyspepsia, flatulence and associated abdominal distension, heartburn (including heartburn that occurs with hiatus hernia, pregnancy and reflux oesophagitis) and to soothe the symptoms of peptic ulcers. It is available as a suspension and is not normally given to children, except on medical advice.

✚▲ Side-effects/warning: See ALUMINIUM HYDROXIDE; DIMETHICONE.

Asilone Tablets

(Seton) is a proprietary, non-prescription COMPOUND PREPARATION of the ANTACID aluminium hydroxide and the ANTIFOAMING AGENT dimethicone (as simethicone). It can be used to treat dyspepsia, flatulence and associated abdominal distension, heartburn (including heartburn that occurs with hiatus hernia, pregnancy and reflux oesophagitis) and to soothe the symptoms of peptic ulcers. It is available as tablets and is not normally given to children under 12 years, except on medical advice.

✚▲ Side-effects/warning: See ALUMINIUM HYDROXIDE; DIMETHICONE.

Askit Powders

(Roche) is a proprietary, non-prescription COMPOUND PREPARATION of the (NSAID) NON-NARCOTIC ANALGESIC, ANTIRHEUMATIC and ANTIPYRETIC drugs aspirin and aloxiprin (which is a buffered form of aspirin), and the STIMULANT caffeine. It can be used to relieve mild to moderate pain (including the pain experienced in rheumatic disorders), to relieve swelling, flu symptoms and other feverish conditions. It is available as a powder and is not normally given to children under 12 years, except on medical advice.

✚▲ Side-effects/warning: See ALOXIPRIN; ASPIRIN; CAFFEINE.

Asmaven

(Berk) is a proprietary, prescription-only preparation of the BETA-RECEPTOR STIMULANT salbutamol (as salbutamol sulphate). It can be used as a BRONCHODILATOR in reversible obstructive airways disease, as an ANTI-ASTHMATIC treatment in severe acute asthma, or for the alleviation of symptoms of chronic bronchitis and emphysema. It may also be used to delay premature labour. It is available as tablets.

+▲ Side-effects/warning: See SALBUTAMOL.

Aspav

(Roussel) is a proprietary, prescription-only preparation of the COMPOUND ANALGESIC containing the (NSAID) NON-NARCOTIC ANALGESIC aspirin and the mixed (OPIOID) NARCOTIC ANALGESIC alkaloids (including morphine, codeine and papaverine). It can be used to relieve pain, and is available as soluble tablets.

+▲ Side-effects/warning: See ASPIRIN; CODEINE PHOSPHATE; MORPHINE SULPHATE; PAPAVERINE.

Aspellin

(Fisons) is a proprietary, non-prescription COMPOUND PREPARATION of CAMPHOR, MENTHOL, methyl salicylate, ethyl salicylate and ammonium salicylate. It has a COUNTER-IRRITANT, or RUBEFACIENT, action and can be applied to the skin for symptomatic relief of underlying muscle or joint pain, and is available as a liniment.

+▲ Side-effects/warning: See AMMONIUM SALICYLATE; ETHYL SALICYLATE; METHYL SALICYLATE.

aspirin

or acetylsalicylic acid, is a well-known and widely used NSAID (non-steroidal anti-inflammatory drug), NON-NARCOTIC ANALGESIC and ANTIRHEUMATIC. As an analgesic it relieves mild to moderate pain, particularly headache, toothache and period pain.

It is a useful ANTIPYRETIC for reducing raised body temperature in the treatment of the common cold, fevers or flu. Aspirin reduces platelet aggregation, which allows its prophylactic (preventive) use, at a lower dose, as an ANTIPLATELET treatment in those at risk (such as patients who have already suffered a heart attack or following bypass surgery). However, this same action may also increase bleeding time, so those taking ANTICOAGULANTS must avoid aspirin. In tablet form, aspirin irritates the stomach lining and may cause bleeding and ulceration; consequently forms of soluble aspirin are preferred.

Many proprietary forms combine aspirin with such drugs as codeine, paracetamol and ibuprofen. Administration is normally oral. Medicines containing aspirin are now no longer normally given to children under 12 years (except for juvenile arthritis, Still's disease and on medical advice), because of a link with the rare, but serious, condition called Reye's syndrome (which causes inflammation of the brain and liver). Aspirin can produce the same allergic-like symptoms (including bronchospasm) that many patients often experience after taking NSAIDs. Administration can be either oral or by topical application.

+▲ Side-effects/warning: See NSAID. It should not be used by women who are breast-feeding, or those with gout or certain bleeding disorders (eg haemophilia).

✪ Related entries: Actron; Alka-Seltzer Original; Maximum Strength; Anadin Analgesic Tablets; Anadin Extra; Anadin Extra Soluble Tablets; Angettes 75; Askit Powders; Aspav; Aspro Clear; Aspro Tablets; Beechams 75 mg Aspirin; Beechams Lemon Tablets; Beechams Powders; Beechams Powders Capsules; Benoral; Caprin; co-codaprin; Codis 500; Cojene Tablets; Dispirin; Dispirin CV; Dispirin Direct; Dispirin Extra; Doloxene Compound; Dristan Decongestant Tablets; Equagesic; Femigraine; Fynnon Calcium Aspirin; Maximum Strength Aspro Clear; Migravess; Nurse Sykes Powders; Nu-Seals Aspirin; Phensic; Platet; Powerin Analgesic Tablets; Robaxisal Forte; Veganin Tablets.

A

Aspro Clear

(Roche) is a proprietary, non-prescription preparation of the (NSAID) NON-NARCOTIC ANALGESIC, ANTIRHEUMATIC and ANTIPYRETIC aspirin. It can be used to treat various aches and pains and fevers. It is available as effervescent, lemon-flavoured tablets and is not normally given to children under 12 years, except on medical advice.

✚▲ Side-effects/warning: See ASPIRIN.

Aspro Tablets

(Roche) is a proprietary, non-prescription preparation of the (NSAID) NON-NARCOTIC ANALGESIC, ANTIRHEUMATIC and ANTIPYRETIC aspirin. It can be used to treat the symptoms of flu and feverish colds and mild to moderate pain (including muscular pain). It is available as tablets and is not normally given to children under 12 years, except on medical advice.

✚▲ Side-effects/warning: See ASPIRIN.

astemizole

is a recently developed ANTIHISTAMINE with less sedative side-effects than some of the older antihistamines. It can be used for the symptomatic relief of allergic symptoms, such as hay fever and urticaria. Administration is oral.

✚▲ Side-effects/warning: See ANTIHISTAMINES; but the incidence of sedative and anticholinergic effects is low. Nevertheless, subjects should be made aware that drowsiness may impair the performance of skilled tasks, such as driving. Do not use in patients who are pregnant and avoid pregnancy for several weeks after finishing treatment. Certain serious disturbances of heart rhythm have been observed after excessive dose. Occasionally, weight gain may occur.

✪ Related entries: Hismanal; Pollon-eze.

astringents ▣

precipitate proteins and are used in lotions to harden and protect skin where there are minor abrasions. They can also be used in lozenges, mouthwashes, eye-drops and antiperspirants. Examples include ZINC OXIDE and salts of aluminium (ALUMINIUM ACETATE, ALUMINIUM CHLORIDE and ALUMINIUM HYDROXIDE).

AT 10

(Sanofi Winthrop) is a proprietary, prescription-only preparation of dihydrotachysterol, which is a VITAMIN D analogue. It can be used in the treatment of vitamin D deficiency, and is available as capsules and a solution.

✚▲ Side-effects/warning: See DIHYDROTACHYSTEROL.

Atarax

(Pfizer) is a proprietary, prescription-only preparation of the ANTIHISTAMINE hydroxyzine hydrochloride, which has some additional ANXIOLYTIC properties. It can be used for the relief of allergic symptoms, such as itching and mild rashes, and also for the short-term treatment of anxiety. It is available as tablets and a syrup.

✚▲ Side-effects/warning: See HYDROXYZINE HYDROCHLORIDE.

Atenix

(Ashbourne) is is a proprietary, prescription-only preparation of the BETA-BLOCKER atenolol. It can be used as an ANTIHYPERTENSIVE for raised blood pressure, as an ANTI-ANGINA treatment to relieve symptoms and improve exercise tolerance and as an ANTI-ARRHYTHMIC to regularize heartbeat and to treat myocardial infarction. It is available as tablets.

✚▲ Side-effects/warning: See ATENOLOL.

AtenixCo

(Ashbourne) is a proprietary, prescription-only COMPOUND PREPARATION of the BETA-BLOCKER atenolol and the DIURETIC chlorthalidone (a combination called co-tenidone). It can be used as an ANTIHYPERTENSIVE for raised blood pressure, and is available as tablets.

✚▲ Side-effects/warning: See ATENOLOL: CHLORTHALIDONE.

atenolol

is a BETA-BLOCKER which can be used as an ANTIHYPERTENSIVE for raised blood pressure, as an ANTI-ANGINA treatment to relieve symptoms and to improve exercise tolerance and as an ANTI-ARRHYTHMIC to regularize heartbeat and to treat myocardial infarction. Administration can be either oral or by injection. It is also available as an antihypertensive treatment in the form of COMPOUND PREPARATIONS with DIURETICS.
✚▲ Side-effects/warning: See PROPRANOLOL HYDROCHLORIDE.
✪ Related entries: Antipressan; Atenix; AtenixCo; Beta-Adalat; co-tenidone; Kalten; Tenchlor; Tenif; Tenoret 50; Tenoretic; Tenormin; Totamol.

Atensine

(Berk) is a proprietary, prescription-only preparation of the BENZODIAZEPINE diazepam. It can be used as an ANXIOLYTIC to treat anxiety in the short term, as a HYPNOTIC to relieve insomnia and to assist in the treatment of alcohol withdrawal symptoms, as an ANTICONVULSANT and ANTI-EPILEPTIC for status epilepticus and as a SEDATIVE and SKELETAL MUSCLE RELAXANT in preoperative medication. It is available as tablets.
✚▲ Side-effects/warning: See DIAZEPAM.

Ativan

(Wyeth) is a proprietary, prescription-only preparation of the BENZODIAZEPINE lorazepam. It can be used as an ANXIOLYTIC in the short-term treatment of anxiety, as a HYPNOTIC for insomnia, as an ANTI-EPILEPTIC in status epilepticus and as a SEDATIVE, including in postoperative premedication because it also causes a degree of amnesia and so helps the patient to forget the procedure or operation. It is available as tablets or in a form for injection.
✚▲ Side-effects/warning: See LORAZEPAM.

atovaquone

is a recently introduced ANTIPROTOZOAL. It is used to treat pneumonia caused by the protozoan micro-organism *Pneumocystis*

carinii in patients whose immune system has been suppressed (either following transplant surgery or because of a disease such as AIDS). Administration is oral.
✚ Side-effects: Diarrhoea, nausea and vomiting, headache, insomnia, fever, rash, changes in liver and blood function and anaemia.
▲ Warning: Initial gastrointestinal upsets cause difficulties. Administer with care to patients with impaired kidney or liver function, or who are pregnant. Avoid its use in patients who are breast-feeding.
✪ Related entry: Wellvone.

atracurium besilate

see ATRACURIUM BESYLATE

atracurium besylate

(atracurium besilate) is a *non-depolarizing* SKELETAL MUSCLE RELAXANT. It can be used to induce muscle paralysis during surgery, and is administered by injection.
✚▲ Side-effects/warning: See TUBOCURARINE CHLORIDE; histamine may be released; it causes little block of sympathetic or vagal nerves; and is relatively safe in patients with impaired liver or kidney function.
✪ Related entry: Tracrium.

Atromid-S

(Zeneca) is a proprietary, prescription-only preparation of clofibrate. It can be used as a LIPID-LOWERING DRUG in hyperlipidaemia to reduce the levels, or change the proportions, of various lipids in the bloodstream. Generally, it is administered only to patients in whom a strict and regular dietary regime, alone, is not having the desired effect. It is available as capsules.
✚▲ Side-effects/warning: See CLOFIBRATE.

atropine sulphate

(hyoscyamine) is a powerful ANTICHOLINERGIC (acting at muscarinic receptors, an ANTIMUSCARINIC drug),

A

sometimes referred to as a BELLADONNA ALKALOID because of its origin from the family of plants that include *Atropa belladonna* (deadly nightshade). It is able to depress certain functions of the autonomic nervous system and is therefore a useful ANTISPASMODIC. It is commonly used during operations to dry up secretions and protect the heart.

It can also be used to cause a long-lasting dilation of the pupil of the eye for ophthalmic procedures. Atropine is able to decrease the secretion of gastric acid, but it has too many side-effects to make it suitable for routine treatment of peptic ulcers. Administration can be oral, topical or by injection.

✚ Side-effects: Dry mouth, difficulty in swallowing and thirst, dilation of the pupils and loss of ability to focus, increase in intraocular pressure (pressure in the eyeball), dry skin with flushing, slowing then speeding of the heart, difficulty in urination, constipation, palpitations and heart arrhythmias. Rarely, there may be high temperature accompanied by delirium or hallucinations.

▲ Warning: It should not be administered to patients with closed-angle glaucoma; and used with caution in patients with prostate gland enlargement or urinary retention, ulcerative colitis, pyloric stenosis, or who are pregnant or breast-feeding. It may worsen gastro-oesophageal reflux.

✪ Related entries: co-phenotrope; Diarphen; Isopto Atropine; Lomotil; Minims Atropine Sulphate.

Atrovent

(Boehringer Ingelheim) is a proprietary, prescription-only preparation of the ANTICHOLINERGIC and BRONCHODILATOR ipratropium bromide. It can be used to treat the symptoms of reversible airways obstructive disease, particularly chronic bronchitis, and is available as an aerosol, a breath-actuated aerosol inhaler (*Autohaler*), a powder for inhalation (*Aerocaps*) and as a nebulizer solution.

✚▲ Side-effects/warning: See IPRATROPIUM BROMIDE.

Audax Ear Drops

(Seton) is a proprietary, non-prescription COMPOUND PREPARATION of choline salicylate and glycerin. It can be used as a local pain-reliever in the outer or middle ear and as an aid to wax removal.

✚▲ Side-effects/warning: See CHOLINE SALICYLATE.

Audicort

(Lederle) is a proprietary, prescription-only COMPOUND PREPARATION of the ANTI-INFLAMMATORY and CORTICOSTEROID triamcinolone acetonide and the ANTIBACTERIAL and (AMINOGLYCOSIDE) ANTIBIOTIC neomycin (as undeconate). It can be used to treat infections of the outer ear, and is available as ear-drops.

✚▲ Side-effects/warning: See NEOMYCIN SULPHATE; TRIAMCINOLONE ACETONIDE.

Augmentin

(Beecham) is a proprietary, prescription-only COMPOUND PREPARATION of the broad-spectrum ANTIBACTERIAL and (PENICILLIN) ANTIBIOTIC amoxycillin (as trihydrate) and the PENICILLINASE INHIBITOR clavulanic acid (which is a combination known as co-amoxclav). Clavulanic acid can inhibit the enzymes (penicillinases) that are produced by some bacteria and which break down amoxycillin, so making it ineffective. The combination is therefore active against many infections that would normally be resistant to amoxycillin alone, and so this effectively extends the range and efficiency of amoxycillin as an antibiotic. It can be used to treat infections of the skin, ear, nose and throat and also of the urinary tract. It is available in a number of forms (one under the name *Augmentin-Duo*): as tablets, dispersible tablets, an oral suspension and in a form for injection or infusion.

✚▲ Side-effects/warning: See AMOXYCILLIN; CO-AMOXCLAV.

Axid

auranofin

is a form in which gold may be used as an ANTI-INFLAMMATORY and ANTIRHEUMATIC treatment. It is used to treat severe, progressive rheumatoid arthritis when NSAID treatment alone is not adequate. Administration is oral.
+▲ Side-effects/warning: See SODIUM AUROTHIOMALATE. There may also be diarrhoea; administer with caution to patients with inflammatory bowel disease.
○ Related entry: Ridaura.

Aureocort

(Lederle) is a proprietary, prescription-only COMPOUND PREPARATION of the CORTICOSTEROID triamcinolone acetonide and the ANTIBACTERIAL and (TETRACYCLINE) ANTIBIOTIC chlortetracycline (as hydrochloride). It can be used to treat severe inflammatory skin disorders, including eczema that is resistant to less powerful corticosteroids. It is available as an ointment.
+▲ Side-effects/warning: See CHLORTETRACYCLINE; TRIAMCINOLONE ACETONIDE.

Aureomycin

(Lederle) is a proprietary, prescription-only preparation of the ANTIBACTERIAL and (TETRACYCLINE) ANTIBIOTIC chlortetracycline (as hydrochloride). It can be used to treat eye and skin infections, and is available as an ophthalmic (eye) ointment and cream.
+▲ Side-effects/warning: See CHLORTETRACYCLINE.

Aureomycin Topical

(Lederle) is a proprietary, prescription-only preparation of the ANTIBACTERIAL and (TETRACYCLINE) ANTIBIOTIC chlortetracycline (as hydrochloride). It can be used to treat skin infections, and is available as an ointment for topical application.
+▲ Side-effects/warning: See CHLORTETRACYCLINE.

Aveeno Cream

(Bioglan) is a proprietary, non-prescription preparation of colloidal oatmeal and an EMOLLIENT base. It can be used for eczema, itching and other skin complaints, and is available as a cream and a bath oil.

Aveeno Oiliated

(Bioglan) is a proprietary, non-prescription preparation of colloidal oatmeal and an EMOLLIENT base. It can be used for eczema, itching and other skin complaints, and is available as a bath additive.

Aveeno Regular

(Bioglan) is a proprietary, non-prescription preparation of colloidal oatmeal and an EMOLLIENT base. It can be used for eczema, itching and other skin complaints, and is available as a bath oil and a bath additive.

Avloclor

(Zeneca) is a proprietary, prescription-only preparation of the ANTIMALARIAL chloroquine (as phosphate). It can be used to prevent or suppress certain forms of malaria and is also used as an ANTIRHEUMATIC to treat rheumatoid disease. It is available as tablets. (This product also appears in a non-prescription form labelled for use for the prevention of malaria.)
+▲ Side-effects/warning: See CHLOROQUINE.

Avomine

(Rhône-Poulenc Rorer) is a proprietary, non-prescription preparation of the ANTIHISTAMINE promethazine theoclate. It can be used as an ANTINAUSEANT for nausea, motion sickness, vertigo and labyrinthine (ear) disorders. It is available as tablets.
+▲ Side-effects/warning: See PROMETHAZINE THEOCLATE.

Axid

(Lilly) is a proprietary, prescription-only preparation of the H_2-ANTAGONIST nizatidine. It can be used as an ULCER-HEALING DRUG for benign peptic ulcers (in the stomach or duodenum), gastro-oesophageal reflux, dyspepsia and associated conditions. It is

A available as capsules and in a form for injection.

✚▲ Side-effects/warning: See NIZATIDINE.

Axsain

(Euroderma) is a proprietary, non-prescription COMPOUND PREPARATION of capsicum oleoresin, which has a COUNTER-IRRITANT, or RUBEFACIENT, action. It can be applied to the skin for symptomatic relief of post-herpatic neuralgia, and is available as a cream.

✚▲ Side-effects/warning: See CAPSICUM OLEORESIN .

Azactam

(Squibb) is a proprietary, prescription-only preparation of the ANTIBACTERIAL and (BETA-LACTAM) ANTIBIOTIC aztreonam. It can be used to treat severe infections caused by Gram-negative bacteria, including gonorrhoea and infections of the urinary tract. It is available in a form for injection.

✚▲ Side-effects/warning: See AZTREONAM.

Azamune

(Penn) is a proprietary, prescription-only preparation of the IMMUNOSUPPRESSANT azathioprine. It can be used to treat tissue rejection in transplant patients and for a variety of autoimmune diseases. It is available as tablets.

✚▲ Side-effects/warning: See AZATHIOPRINE.

Azantac

see ZANTAC

azapropazone

is a (NSAID) NON-NARCOTIC ANALGESIC and ANTIRHEUMATIC drug. Because of its side-effects, it is used to treat only serious cases of rheumatoid arthritis, acute gout and certain rheumatic diseases of the spine (ankylosing spondylitis). Administration is oral.

✚▲ Side-effects/warning: See NSAID; but there is a high incidence of gastrointestinal disturbances, so it is restricted to use where

other drugs have proved ineffective in serious inflammatory conditions. It is not to be used if there is inflammatory bowel disease or porphyria. There is also a seriously prolonged potentiation of the bleeding time when anticoagulants are being used. It should not be given to patients with gastric ulcers or kidney disease.

○ Related entry: Rheumox.

azatadine maleate

is an ANTIHISTAMINE which can be used for the symptomatic relief of allergic symptoms, such as hay fever and urticaria. Administration is oral.

✚▲ Side-effects/warning: See ANTIHISTAMINES. Because of its sedative side-effects, the performance of skilled tasks, such as driving, may be impaired.

○ Related entry: Optimine.

azathioprine

is a powerful CYTOTOXIC and IMMUNOSUPPRESSANT. It is mainly used to reduce tissue rejection in transplant patients, but it can also be used to treat myasthenia gravis, rheumatoid arthritis, ulcerative colitis and several autoimmune diseases. Administration is either oral or by injection.

✚ Side-effects: Hypersensitivity reactions including dizziness, malaise, vomiting, fever, muscular pains and shivering, joint pain, changes in liver function, jaundice, heart arrhythmias, low blood pressure (requiring withdrawal of treatment), symptoms of bone marrow suppression, which should be reported (eg bleeding or bruising), hair loss, increased susceptibility to infections, nausea, pneumonia and pancreatitis.

▲ Warning: It is not to be given to patients with known sensitivity to azathioprine or mercaptopurine; or who are pregnant; monitoring is required throughout treatment with blood count checks.

○ Related entries: Azamune; Berkaprine; Immunoprin; Imuran.

azelaic acid

is a recently introduced drug which has mild ANTIBACTERIAL and KERATOLYTIC properties, and can be used to treat skin conditions, such as acne. Administration is topical.

✚ Side-effects: Some patients experience skin irritation and sensitivity to light.

▲ Warning: Avoid the eyes when applying. Administer with caution to patients who are pregnant or breast-feeding.

✪ Related entry: Skinoren.

azelastine hydrochloride

is an ANTIHISTAMINE which can be used for the symptomatic relief of allergic rhinitis (inflammation of the mucosal lining of the nose). Administration is topical in the form of a nasal spray.

✚▲ Side-effects/warning: See ANTIHISTAMINES; but any adverse effects are less severe when given locally. Local application to the nasal mucosa may cause irritation and taste disturbances.

✪ Related entry: Rhinolast.

azidothymidine

see ZIDOVUDINE

azithromycin

is a recently introduced ANTIBACTERIAL and ANTIBIOTIC of the MACROLIDE group. It has more activity against Gram-negative organisms compared to erythromycin (though less against Gram-positive bacteria) and is mainly used in patients allergic to penicillin. It can be used to treat infections of the middle ear, the respiratory tract, the skin and soft tissues and genital chlamydia infections. It has a long duration of action and so usually it can be taken once a day. Administration is oral.

✚▲ Side-effects/warning: See ERYTHROMYCIN. Administer with caution to patients who are pregnant or breast-feeding.

✪ Related entry: Zithromax.

azlocillin

is an ANTIBACTERIAL and (PENICILLIN)

ANTIBIOTIC. It can be used primarily to treat infections by a type of Gram-negative bacteria called *Pseudomonas*, particularly in serious infections of the urinary and respiratory tracts and for septicaemia. Administration is by injection.

✚▲ Side-effects/warning: See BENZYLPENICILLIN.

✪ Related entry: Securopen.

azoles 🗈

including the IMIDAZOLES chemical group, are a family of ANTIMICROBIAL and ANTIPROTOZOAL drugs. The group includes METRONIDAZOLE and TINIDAZOLE (which also have ANTIBACTERIAL properties), CLOTRIMAZOLE, FLUCONAZOLE and MICONAZOLE (which also have ANTIFUNGAL properties) and MEBENDAZOLE and THIABENDAZOLE (which are also used as ANTHELMINTICS). Triazole drugs are also azoles and include the antifungals FLUCYTOSINE and ITRACONAZOLE. They are all synthetic drugs.

AZT

see ZIDOVUDINE

aztreonam

is an ANTIBACTERIAL and ANTIBIOTIC drug of the BETA-LACTAM group. It can be used to treat severe infections caused by Gram-negative bacteria, including *Pseudomonas aeruginosa*, *Haemophilus influenzae*, *Neisseria meningitidis*, lung infections in cystic fibrosis, gonorrhoea, cystitis and infections of the urinary tract. Administration is by injection.

✚ Side-effects: Vomiting, nausea, diarrhoea and abdominal pain; altered taste and mouth ulcers; skin rashes; hepatitis, jaundice and blood disorders.

▲ Warning: It should not be administered to patients who are known to be sensitive to aztreonam: or who are pregnant or breast-feeding. It should be administered with caution to patients with certain liver or kidney disorders.

✪ Related entry: Azactam.

B

antibiotics in the form of an ointment or spray for topical application.
✪ Related entries: Cicatrin; Polyfax; Tribiotic.

baclofen

is a SKELETAL MUSCLE RELAXANT which is used for relaxing muscles that are in spasm, particularly when caused by an injury to or a disease of the central nervous system. It works by an action on the central nervous system. Administration is oral.

✚ Side-effects: Sedation, drowsiness, nausea; sometimes light-headedness, fatigue, disturbances of gait, headache, hallucinations, euphoria, insomnia, depression, tremor, eye-flicker, loss of sensation in the extremities, convulsions, muscle weakness and pain, depression of respiration and blood pressure, gastrointestinal and urinary disturbances; rarely, taste alterations, visual disorders, sweating, rash, altered liver function or paradoxical increase in muscle spasm.

▲ Warning: It is not to be given to patients with peptic ulcer. Administer with caution to those with psychiatric disorders, impaired cerebrovascular, liver or kidney function, epilepsy, porphyria, certain bladder dysfunction; or who are pregnant. Withdrawal of treatment should be gradual. It may affect the performance of skilled tasks, such as driving.

✪ Related entries: Baclospas; Lioresal.

bacampicillin hydrochloride

is a broad-spectrum, penicillin-type ANTIBACTERIAL and ANTIBIOTIC. It is chemically an ester derivative of ampicillin and is converted to ampicillin in the body, however, it is better absorbed and has less gastrointestinal side-effects (eg diarrhoea). It can be used to treat many infections, especially those of the urinogenital areas, upper respiratory tract, middle ear and gonorrhoea. Administration is oral.

✚▲ Side-effects/warning: See AMPICILLIN.
✪ Related entry: Ambaxin.

Bacillus Calmette-Guérin Vaccine, Dried

(District Health Authorities) (Dried Tub/Vac/BCG) is a non-proprietary, prescription-only preparation of BCG vaccine, and is available in a form for injection.

✚▲ Side-effects/warning: See BCG VACCINE.

Bacillus Calmette-Guérin Vaccine, Percutaneous

(District Health Authorities) (Tub/Vac/BCG – Perc) is a non-proprietary, prescription-only preparation of BCG vaccine. It is administered percutaneously (multiple puncture through the skin).

✚▲ Side-effects/warning: See BCG VACCINE.

bacitracin zinc

is an ANTIBACTERIAL and ANTIBIOTIC drug (a polypeptide). It is commonly used for the treatment of infections of the skin and usually in combination with other

Baclospas

(Ashbourne) is a proprietary, prescription-only preparation of the SKELETAL MUSCLE RELAXANT baclofen. It can be used to treat muscle spasm caused by an injury to or a disease of the central nervous system, and is available as tablets.

✚▲ Side-effects/warning: See BACLOFEN.

Bactrim

(Roche) is a proprietary, prescription-only COMPOUND PREPARATION of the (SULPHONAMIDE) ANTIBACTERIAL sulphamethoxazole and the antibacterial

trimethoprim, which is a combination called co-trimoxazole. It can be used to treat bacterial infections, especially infections of the urinary tract, prostatitis and bronchitis. It is available as tablets and as a sugar-free paediatric syrup.
+▲ Side-effects/warning: See CO-TRIMOXAZOLE.

Bactroban

(Beecham) is a proprietary, prescription-only preparation of the ANTIBACTERIAL and ANTIBIOTIC mupirocin. It can be used to treat infections of the skin, and is available as an ointment for topical application.
+▲ Side-effects/warning: See MUPIROCIN.

Bactroban Nasal

(Beecham) is a proprietary, prescription-only preparation of the ANTIBACTERIAL and ANTIBIOTIC mupirocin. It can be used to treat staphylococcal infections (including methoxycillin-resistant *Staphylococcus aureus*) in and around the nostrils. It is available as an ointment for topical application.
+▲ Side-effects/warning: See MUPIROCIN.

BAL (British Anti-Lewisite)

see DIMERCAPROL

Balanced Salt Solution

(Alcon; Ciba Vision) is a proprietary, non-prescription preparation of SODIUM CHLORIDE, sodium acetate, SODIUM CITRATE, calcium chloride, MAGNESIUM CHLORIDE and POTASSIUM CHLORIDE. It is a sterile solution that can be used as an eyewash for cleansing and washing out noxious substances.

Balmosa Cream

(Pharmax) is a proprietary, non-prescription COMPOUND PREPARATION of capsicum oleoresin, CAMPHOR, MENTHOL and methyl salicylate, which have COUNTER-IRRITANT, or RUBEFACIENT, actions. It can be applied to the skin for symptomatic relief of rheumatism, fibrosis, lumbago and sciatica,

and also for pain associated with unbroken chilblains. It is available as a cream.
+▲ Side-effects/warning: See CAPSICUM OLEORESIN; METHYL SALICYLATE

Balneum with Tar

(Merck) is a proprietary, non-prescription preparation of coal tar. It can be used to treat psoriasis and eczema, and is available as a bath oil.
+▲ Side-effects/warning: See COAL TAR.

Baltar

(Merck) is a proprietary, non-prescription preparation of coal tar (as distillate). It can be used for conditions such as dandruff and psoriasis of the scalp, and is available as a shampoo.
+▲ Side-effects/warning: See COAL TAR.

Bambec

(Astra) is a proprietary, prescription-only preparation of the BETA-RECEPTOR STIMULANT bambuterol hydrochloride. It can be used as a BRONCHODILATOR in reversible obstructive airways disease, as an ANTI-ASTHMATIC treatment in severe acute asthma, or for the alleviation of symptoms of chronic bronchitis and emphysema. It is available as tablets.
+▲ Side-effects/warning: See BAMBUTEROL HYDROCHLORIDE.

bambuterol hydrochloride

is a SYMPATHOMIMETIC and BETA-RECEPTOR STIMULANT which has good beta$_2$-receptor selectivity. It is mainly used as a BRONCHODILATOR in reversible obstructive airways disease, as an ANTI-ASTHMATIC treatment in severe acute asthma and for the alleviation of symptoms of chronic bronchitis and emphysema. It is a pro-drug of TERBUTALINE SULPHATE (that is, it is converted to terbutaline within the body). Administration is oral.
+▲ Side-effects/warning: See SALBUTAMOL. It is not to be used by patients with certain liver disorders or who are pregnant.
✪ Related entry: Bambec.

B

Baratol

(Monmouth) is a proprietary, prescription-only preparation of the ALPHA-ADRENOCEPTOR BLOCKER indoramin hydrochloride. It can be used as an ANTIHYPERTENSIVE, often in conjunction with other antihypertensives, and is available as tablets.

✚▲ Side-effects/warning: See INDORAMIN.

barbiturates ▣

are a chemical class of drugs that are derived from barbituric acid and have a wide range of essentially depressant actions. They are most commonly used as SEDATIVES, GENERAL ANAESTHETICS, ANTICONVULSANTS and ANTI-EPILEPTICS. They work by a direct action on the brain, depressing specific areas and may be slow- or fast-acting, but are all extremely effective. However, they can rapidly cause tolerance and then both psychological and physical dependence (addiction) may result, therefore they are used as infrequently as possible.

Moreover, prolonged use, even in small doses, can have serious toxic side-effects and in overdose they are lethal. The best-known and most-used barbiturates include the HYPNOTIC drug AMYLOBARBITONE, the anticonvulsant and anti-epileptic PHENOBARBITONE and the general anaesthetics THIOPENTONE SODIUM and METHOHEXITONE SODIUM.

✚ Side-effects: Depending on the use, dose and type; there may be hangover with drowsiness, dizziness, unsteady gait, respiratory depression, headache, hypersensitivity reactions; in the elderly there may be paradoxical excitement and confusion.

▲ Warning: Depending on the use, dose and type; in general barbiturates should be avoided wherever possible; dependence can readily occur (with withdrawal syndrome, which can include rebound insomnia, anxiety, tremor and convulsions). Administer with caution to patients with respiratory failure or certain kidney or heart disorders.

barrier creams ▣

can be used to protect the skin against irritants, chapping, urine and faeces (nappy rash), bedsores and toxic substances. They are normally applied as an ointment or a cream (commonly in a WHITE SOFT PARAFFIN or LANOLIN oily base) and often incorporating a silicone (eg DIMETHICONE).

Baxan

(Bristol-Myers) is a proprietary, prescription-only preparation of the ANTIBACTERIAL and (CEPHALOSPORIN) ANTIBIOTIC cefadroxil. It can be used to treat many infections, especially those of the urinary tract, and is available as capsules and an oral suspension.

✚▲ Side-effects/warning: See CEFADROXIL.

Baycaron

(Bayer) is a proprietary, prescription-only preparation of the (THIAZIDE-like) DIURETIC mefruside. It can be used, either alone or in conjunction with other drugs, in the treatment of oedema and as an ANTIHYPERTENSIVE. It is available as tablets.

✚▲ Side-effects/warning: See MEFRUSIDE.

BCG vaccine

(bacillus Calmette-Guérin vaccine) for IMMUNIZATION is a VACCINE produced from *live* attenuated strain of the tuberculosis bacillus *Mycobacterium bovis*, which no longer causes the disease in humans but stimulates formation of the specific antibodies that react with the tuberculosis bacillus *Mycobacterium tuberculosis* and so can be used as an ANTITUBERCULAR vaccine. It is used for routine vaccination of children and those likely to come into contact with tuberculous individuals. It is available as Tub/Vac/BCG (Dried) for intradermal injection or as Tub/Vac/BCG (Perc) for percutaneous administration and a number of other preparations.

✚▲ Side-effects/warning: See VACCINES.

✪ **Related entries:** Bacillus Calmette-Guérin Vaccine, Dried; Bacillus Calmette-Guérin Vaccine, Percutaneous.

BDP Spacehaler

(Evans) is a proprietary, prescription-only preparation of the CORTICOSTEROID and ANTI-ASTHMATIC beclomethasone dipropionate. It can be used to prevent asthmatic attacks, and is available in an aerosol for inhalation.
+▲ Side-effects/warning: See
BECLOMETHASONE DIPROPIONATE.

Beclazone

(Baker Norton) is a proprietary, prescription-only preparation of the CORTICOSTEROID and ANTI-ASTHMATIC beclomethasone dipropionate. It can be used to prevent asthmatic attacks, and is available in an aerosol for inhalation.
+▲ Side-effects/warning: See
BECLOMETHASONE DIPROPIONATE.

Becloforte

(Allen & Hanburys) is a proprietary, prescription-only preparation of the CORTICOSTEROID and ANTI-ASTHMATIC beclomethasone dipropionate. It can be used to prevent asthmatic attacks, and is available in a range of aerosols for inhalation (one form, *Becloforte VM*, comes with a *Volumatic* inhaler) and as a dry powder for inhalation (in a *Diskhaler* blister pack).
+▲ Side-effects/warning: See
BECLOMETHASONE DIPROPIONATE.

beclometasone dipropionate

see BECLOMETHASONE DIPROPIONATE

beclomethasone dipropionate

(beclometasone dipropionate) is a CORTICOSTEROID which is used primarily as an ANTI-ASTHMATIC treatment to prevent attacks and also as an ANTI-INFLAMMATORY for severe skin inflammation (eg eczema and psoriasis) and for inflammatory conditions of the nasal mucosa (eg rhinitis). Administration as an anti-inflammatory preparation is by topical application as a cream or an ointment; as an anti-asthmatic it is administered by inhalation from an aerosol, nasal spray, as a powder for insufflation or as a suspension for nebulization.
+▲ Side-effects/warning: See
CORTICOSTEROIDS; but systemic effects are unlikely with the low-doses used. As a nasal spray it may cause sneezing and dryness and irritation of the nose and throat. As a cream or ointment, there may be local skin effects. When inhaled, it may cause hoarseness and candidiasis of the throat and mouth.
✪ Related entries: AeroBec; AeroBec Forte; BDP Spacehaler; Beclazone; Becloforte; Becodisks; Beconase; Becotide Inhaler; Becotide Rotacaps; Filair Forte; Propaderm; Ventide.

Becodisks

(Allen & Hanburys) is a proprietary, prescription-only preparation of the CORTICOSTEROID and ANTI-ASTHMATIC beclomethasone dipropionate. It can be used to prevent asthmatic attacks, and is available as a powder in discs for inhalation from a *Diskhaler* device.
+▲ Side-effects/warning: See
BECLOMETHASONE DIPROPIONATE.

Beconase

(Allen & Hanburys) is a proprietary, prescription-only preparation of the CORTICOSTEROID and ANTI-INFLAMMATORY beclomethasone dipropionate. It can be used to relieve the symptoms of conditions such as hay fever and rhinitis. It is available as *Beconase nasal spray (aerosol)* and as *Beconase aqueous nasal spray* (some versions for hay fever are available without a prescription).
+▲ Side-effects/warning: See
BECLOMETHASONE DIPROPIONATE.

Becotide Inhaler

(Allen & Hanburys) is a proprietary, prescription-only preparation of the CORTICOSTEROID and ANTI-ASTHMATIC beclomethasone dipropionate. It can be used to prevent asthmatic attacks, and is

B

B

available in an aerosol for inhalation in three forms: *Becotide-50*, *Becotide-100* and *Becotide-200*.

✚▲ Side-effects/warning: See BECLOMETHASONE DIPROPIONATE.

Becotide Rotacaps

(Allen & Hanburys) is a proprietary, prescription-only preparation of the CORTICOSTEROID and ANTI-ASTHMATIC beclomethasone dipropionate. It can be used to prevent asthmatic attacks, and is available as a powder in cartridges, *Becotide Rotacaps*, and for inhalation from the *Becotide Rotahaler*.

✚▲ Side-effects/warning: See BECLOMETHASONE DIPROPIONATE.

Bedranol SR

(Lagap) is a proprietary, prescription-only preparation of the BETA-BLOCKER propranolol hydrochloride. It can be administered as an ANTIHYPERTENSIVE treatment for raised blood pressure, as an ANTI-ANGINA treatment to relieve symptoms and improve a patient's exercise tolerance and as an ANTI-ARRHYTHMIC drug to regularize heartbeat and to treat myocardial infarction. It can also be used as an ANTITHYROID drug for the short-term treatment of thyrotoxicosis, as an ANTIMIGRAINE treatment to prevent attacks, as an ANXIOLYTIC, particularly for symptomatic relief of tremor and palpitations, and, with an ALPHA-ADRENOCEPTOR BLOCKER, in the acute treatment of phaeochromocytoma. It is available as modified-release capsules.

✚▲ Side-effects/warning: See PROPRANOLOL HYDROCHLORIDE.

Beecham Pills

(SmithKline Beecham) is a proprietary, non-prescription preparation of the (*stimulant*) LAXATIVE aloin. It can be used to relieve constipation, and is available as tablets. It is not normally given to children, except on medical advice.

✚▲ Side-effects/warning: See ALOIN.

Beechams 75 mg Aspirin

(SmithKline Beecham) is a proprietary, non-prescription preparation of the (NSAID) NON-NARCOTIC ANALGESIC aspirin (at a lower analgesic dose than is usual). It can be used to treat mild to moderate pain, and is available as tablets. It is not normally given to children under 12 years, except on medical advice.

✚▲ Side-effects/warning: See ASPIRIN.

Beechams All-In-One

(SmithKline Beecham) is a proprietary, non-prescription COMPOUND PREPARATION of the NON-NARCOTIC ANALGESIC and ANTIRHEUMATIC paracetamol, the SYMPATHOMIMETIC and DECONGESTANT phenylephrine hydrochloride and the EXPECTORANT agent GUAIPHENESIN. It can be used for the symptomatic relief of colds, flu, aches and pains and nasal congestion. It is available as a syrup and is not normally given to children under six years, except on medical advice.

✚▲ Side-effects/warning: See PARACETAMOL; PHENYLEPHRINE HYDROCHLORIDE.

Beechams Flu-Plus Hot Lemon

(SmithKline Beecham) is a proprietary, non-prescription COMPOUND PREPARATION of the NON-NARCOTIC ANALGESIC and ANTIRHEUMATIC paracetamol, the SYMPATHOMIMETIC and DECONGESTANT phenylephrine hydrochloride and vitamin C. It can be used for the symptomatic relief of mild to moderate pain, colds, flu, aches and pains and nasal congestion. It is available as a powder and is not normally given to children under 12 years, except on medical advice.

✚▲ Side-effects/warning: See PARACETAMOL; PHENYLEPHRINE HYDROCHLORIDE.

Beechams Hot Blackcurrant

(SmithKline Beecham) is a proprietary, non-prescription COMPOUND PREPARATION of the NON-NARCOTIC ANALGESIC paracetamol, the SYMPATHOMIMETIC and DECONGESTANT

phenylephrine hydrochloride and vitamin C.
It can be used for the symptomatic relief of
mild to moderate pain, colds and flu, aches
and pains and nasal congestion. It is
available as a powder and is not normally
given to children, except on medical advice.
+▲ Side-effects/warning: See PARACETAMOL;
PHENYLEPHRINE HYDROCHLORIDE.

Beechams Hot Lemon
(SmithKline Beecham) is a proprietary,
non-prescription COMPOUND PREPARATION of
the NON-NARCOTIC ANALGESIC and
ANTIRHEUMATIC paracetamol, the
SYMPATHOMIMETIC and DECONGESTANT
phenylephrine hydrochloride and vitamin C.
It can be used for the symptomatic relief of
mild to moderate pain, colds, flu, aches and
pains and nasal congestion. It is available
as a powder and is not normally given to
children under 12 years, except on medical
advice.
+▲ Side-effects/warning: See PARACETAMOL;
PHENYLEPHRINE HYDROCHLORIDE.

Beechams Hot Lemon and Honey
(SmithKline Beecham) is a proprietary,
non-prescription COMPOUND PREPARATION of
the NON-NARCOTIC ANALGESIC and
ANTIRHEUMATIC paracetamol, the
SYMPATHOMIMETIC and DECONGESTANT
phenylephrine hydrochloride and vitamin C.
It can be used for the symptomatic relief of
mild to moderate pain, colds, flu, aches and
pains and nasal congestion. It is available
as a powder and is not normally given to
children under 12 years, except on medical
advice.
+▲ Side-effects/warning: See PARACETAMOL;
PHENYLEPHRINE HYDROCHLORIDE.

Beechams Lemon Tablets
(SmithKline Beecham) is a proprietary,
non-prescription preparation of the (NSAID)
NON-NARCOTIC ANALGESIC and ANTIRHEUMATIC
aspirin with glycine. It can be used for the
symptomatic relief of mild to moderate
pain, colds, flu, aches and pains (including

the pain and inflammation of rheumatic
disease), toothache and period pain. It is
available as tablets and is not normally
given to children under 12 years, except on
medical advice.
+▲ Side-effects/warning: See ASPIRIN.

Beechams Powders
(SmithKline Beecham) is a proprietary,
non-prescription COMPOUND PREPARATION of
the (NSAID) NON-NARCOTIC ANALGESIC and
ANTIRHEUMATIC aspirin and the STIMULANT
caffeine. It can be used for the symptomatic
relief of mild to moderate pain, colds, flu,
aches and pains (including the pain and
inflammation experienced in rheumatic
disease) and period pain. It is available as
tablets and is not normally given to
children, except on medical advice.
+▲ Side-effects/warning: See ASPIRIN;
CAFFEINE.

Beechams Powders Capsules
(SmithKline Beecham) is a proprietary,
non-prescription COMPOUND PREPARATION of
the NON-NARCOTIC ANALGESIC and
ANTIRHEUMATIC paracetamol, the
SYMPATHOMIMETIC and DECONGESTANT
phenylephrine hydrochloride and the
STIMULANT caffeine. It can be used for the
symptomatic relief of mild to moderate
pain, colds, flu, aches and pains and nasal
congestion. It is available as capsules and is
not normally given to children under six
years, except on medical advice.
+▲ Side-effects/warning: See CAFFEINE;
PARACETAMOL; PHENYLEPHRINE HYDROCHLORIDE.

belladonna alkaloids ⚡
are derived from solanaceous plants such
as *Atropa belladonna* (deadly nightshade)
and inlcude the drugs ATROPINE SULPHATE
(hyoscyamine) and HYOSCINE HYDROBROMIDE
(scopolamine). These drugs have
ANTICHOLINERGIC properties and are
administered for a variety of medical
purposes. Poisoning due to eating the
berries of *Atropa belladonna* is not

B

uncommon, particularly in children. Indeed, it has been one of the more popular poisons throughout history, from the time of Imperial Rome to the Borgias in 15th-century Italy. The name *belladonna* literally means 'beautiful lady' and is thought to refer to the use of the plant as a cosmetic in ancient times, when it was used as eye-drops to dilate the pupils.

+▲ Side-effects/warning: See ATROPINE SULPHATE; HYOSCINE BUTYLBROMIDE; HYOSCINE HYDROBROMIDE.

✿ Related entry: Enterosan.

Bendogen

(Lagap) is a proprietary, prescription-only preparation of the ADRENERGIC-NEURONE BLOCKER bethanidine sulphate. It can be used as an ANTIHYPERTENSIVE for moderate to severe high blood pressure, and is available as tablets.

+▲ Side-effects/warning: See BETHANIDINE SULPHATE.

bendrofluazide

(bendroflumethiazide) is a DIURETIC of the THIAZIDE class. It is used as an ANTIHYPERTENSIVE, either alone or in conjunction with other types of diuretic or other drugs. It can also be used in the treatment of oedema associated with congestive heart failure. Administration is oral.

+ Side-effects: There may be mild gastrointestinal upsets, postural hypotension, reversible impotence; low blood potassium, sodium, magnesium and chloride; raised blood urea, glucose and lipids; rarely, gout, photosensitivity, blood disorders, skin reactions and pancreatitis.

▲ Warning: It should not be administered to patients with certain severe kidney or liver disorders. It should be administered with caution to the elderly, or who are pregnant or breast-feeding. It may aggravate diabetes or gout. Blood potassium levels should be monitored in patients taking thiazide diuretics, because they may deplete the body of potassium. It should not be used where

there are abnormal levels of sodium and potassium or in Addison's disease.

✿ Related entries: Aprinox; Berkozide; Corgaretic 40; Corgaretic 80; Inderetic; Inderex; Neo-NaClex; Neo-NaClex-K; Prestim; Prestim Forte.

bendroflumethiazide

see BENDROFLUAZIDE

Benemid

(Merck Sharp & Dohme) is a proprietary, prescription-only preparation of the probenecid. It can be used to prevent gout and to reduce the excretion of certain ANTIBIOTICS by the kidney. It is available as tablets.

+▲ Side-effects/warning: See PROBENECID.

Bengué's Balsam

(Bengué) is a proprietary, non-prescription COMPOUND PREPARATION of MENTHOL and methyl salicylate, which both have COUNTER-IRRITANT, or RUBEFACIENT, actions. It can be applied to the skin for symptomatic relief of underlying muscle or joint pain. It is available as an ointment in a lanolin base.

+▲ Side-effects/warning: See LANOLIN; METHYL SALICYLATE .

Benoral

(Sanofi Winthrop) is a proprietary, non-prescription preparation of the (NSAID) NON-NARCOTIC ANALGESIC and ANTIRHEUMATIC drug benorylate, which is derived from both ASPIRIN and PARACETAMOL. It can be used to treat mild to moderate pain, especially the pain of rheumatic disease and other musculoskeletal disorders. It is available as tablets, as granules in sachets for oral solution and as a sugar-free suspension.

+▲ Side-effects/warning: See BENORYLATE.

benorilate

see BENORYLATE

benorylate

(benorilate) is a (NSAID) NON-NARCOTIC ANALGESIC and ANTIRHEUMATIC drug with

ANTIPYRETIC actions. It is chemically derived from both ASPIRIN and PARACETAMOL, and these two pharmacologically active constituents are released into the bloodstream at different rates. It is used particularly to treat the pain of rheumatic disease and other musculoskeletal disorders and to lower a high temperature in fever. Administration is oral.

+▲ Side-effects/warning: See NSAID; but it is better tolerated and causes less gastrointestinal disturbances than the majority of this class.

✪ **Related entry: Benoral.**

benoxinate

is an alternative name for the LOCAL ANAESTHETIC drug OXYBUPROCAINE HYDROCHLORIDE.

Benoxyl 10 Lotion

(Stiefel) is a proprietary, non-prescription COMPOUND PREPARATION of the ANTIFUNGAL miconazole (as nitrate) and the KERATOLYTIC and ANTIMICROBIAL benzoyl peroxide (10%). It can be used to treat acne, and is available as a cream and a lotion for topical application.

+▲ Side-effects/warning: See BENZOYL PEROXIDE; MICONAZOLE.

Benoxyl 5 Cream

(Stiefel) is a proprietary, non-prescription COMPOUND PREPARATION of the ANTIFUNGAL miconazole (as nitrate) and the KERATOLYTIC and ANTIMICROBIAL benzoyl peroxide (5%). It can be used to treat acne, and is available as a cream and a lotion for topical application.

+▲ Side-effects/warning: See BENZOYL PEROXIDE; MICONAZOLE.

benperidol

is a powerful ANTIPSYCHOTIC and is chemically a butyrophenone. It is used to treat and tranquillize psychotics and is especially suitable for treating antisocial and deviant forms of sexual behaviour. Administration is oral.

+▲ Side-effects/warning: See HALOPERIDOL.

✪ **Related entry: Anquil.**

benserazide hydrochloride

is an ENZYME INHIBITOR which is administered therapeutically in combination with the drug LEVODOPA to treat parkinsonism, but not the parkinsonian symptoms induced by drugs (see ANTIPARKINSONISM). Benserazide prevents levodopa being too rapidly broken down in the body into dopamine and so allowing more levodopa to reach the brain to make up the deficiency of dopamine, which is the major cause of parkinsonian symptoms. The combination of benserazide hydrochloride with levodopa is known in medicine by the simplified name of CO-BENELDOPA. Administration of the combination is oral.

+▲ Side-effects/warning: See LEVODOPA.

✪ **Related entry: Madopar.**

bentonite

is an absorbent powder which is administered therapeutically in emergencies to absorb corrosive substances like paraquat (the toxic horticultural preparation) in cases of accidental poisoning and to reduce further absorption by the body. See ANTIDOTE.

Benylin Chesty Coughs Non-Drowsy

(Warner Wellcome) is a proprietary, non-prescription preparation of the EXPECTORANT agent GUAIPHENESIN and MENTHOL. It can be used for the symptomatic relief of cough, and is available as a syrup. It is not normally given to children under six years, except on medical advice.

Benylin Chesty Coughs Original

(Warner Wellcome) is a proprietary, non-prescription preparation of the ANTIHISTAMINE diphenhydramine hydrochloride. It can be used for the symptomatic relief of cough and associated

B

congestive symptoms, and is available as a syrup. It is not normally given to children under five years, except on medical advice.
+▲ Side-effects/warning: See DIPHENHYDRAMINE HYDROCHLORIDE.

Benylin Children's Coughs Original

(Warner Wellcome) is a proprietary, non-prescription preparation of the ANTIHISTAMINE diphenhydramine hydrochloride. It can be used for the symptomatic relief of cough and its congestive symptoms, and for the treatment of hay fever and other allergic conditions. It is available as a syrup and is not normally given to children under one year, except on medical advice.
+▲ Side-effects/warning: See DIPHENHYDRAMINE HYDROCHLORIDE.

Benylin Children's Coughs Sugar Free/Colour Free

(Warner Wellcome) is a proprietary, non-prescription preparation of the ANTIHISTAMINE diphenhydramine hydrochloride and MENTHOL. It can be used for the symptomatic relief of cough and congestion, and in the treatment of hay fever and other allergic conditions affecting the upper respiratory tract in children. It is available as a syrup and is not normally given to children under one year, except on medical advice.
+▲ Side-effects/warning: See DIPHENHYDRAMINE HYDROCHLORIDE.

Benylin Cough and Congestion

(Warner Wellcome) is a proprietary, non-prescription preparation of the ANTIHISTAMINE diphenhydramine hydrochloride, the ANTITUSSIVE dextromethorphan hydrobromide and the DECONGESTANT pseudoephedrine hydrochloride (with levomenthol). It can be used for the symptomatic relief of cough and congestion associated with colds. It is available as a syrup and is not normally

given to children under six years, except on medical advice.
+▲ Side-effects/warning: See DEXTROMETHORPHAN HYDROBROMIDE; DIPHENHYDRAMINE HYDROCHLORIDE; PSEUDOEPHEDRINE HYDROCHLORIDE.

Benylin Day and Night

(Warner Wellcome) is a proprietary, non-prescription preparation which can be used for the symptomatic relief of colds and flu. It is available in the form of two types of COMPOUND PREPARATIONS in the same pack: a yellow film-coated tablet (taken during the day) contains the NON-NARCOTIC ANALGESIC and ANTIPYRETIC paracetamol and the SYMPATHOMIMETIC phenylpropanolamine hydrochloride; a blue film-coated tablet (taken at night) contains paracetamol and the ANTIHISTAMINE diphenhydramine hydrochloride. It is not normally given to children, except on medical advice.
+▲ Side-effects/warning: See DIPHENHYDRAMINE HYDROCHLORIDE; PARACETAMOL; PHENYLPROPANOLAMINE HYDROCHLORIDE.

Benylin Dry Coughs Non-Drowsy

(Warner Wellcome) is a proprietary, non-prescription preparation of the ANTITUSSIVE dextromethorphan hydrobromide. It can be used for the symptomatic relief of persistent, dry, irritating coughs. It is available as a syrup and is not normally given to children under six years, except on medical advice.
+▲ Side-effects/warning: See DEXTROMETHORPHAN HYDROBROMIDE.

Benylin Dry Coughs Original

(Warner Wellcome) is a proprietary, non-prescription preparation of the ANTIHISTAMINE diphenhydramine hydrochloride, the ANTITUSSIVE dextromethorphan hydrobromide and MENTHOL. It can be used for the symptomatic relief of persistent, dry,

irritating coughs. It is available as a syrup and is not normally given to children under five years, except on medical advice.
+▲ Side-effects/warning: See DEXTROMETHORPHAN HYDROBROMIDE; DIPHENHYDRAMINE HYDROCHLORIDE.

Benylin Four Flu Liquid

(Warner Wellcome) is a proprietary, non-prescription preparation of the NON-NARCOTIC ANALGESIC and ANTIPYRETIC paracetamol, the SYMPATHOMIMETIC pseudoephedrine hydrochloride and the ANTIHISTAMINE diphenhydramine hydrochloride. It can be used for the symptomatic relief of colds and flu and coughs, and is available in the form of an oral liquid. It is not normally given to children under six years, except on medical advice.
+▲ Side-effects/warning: See DIPHENHYDRAMINE HYDROCHLORIDE; PARACETAMOL; PSEUDOEPHEDRINE HYDROCHLORIDE.

Benylin Four Flu Tablets

(Warner Wellcome) is a proprietary, non-prescription preparation of the NON-NARCOTIC ANALGESIC and ANTIPYRETIC paracetamol, the SYMPATHOMIMETIC pseudoephedrine hydrochloride and the ANTIHISTAMINE diphenhydramine hydrochloride. It can be used for the symptomatic relief of colds and flu and coughs, and is available as tablets. It is not normally given to children under six years, except on medical advice.
+▲ Side-effects/warning: See DIPHENHYDRAMINE HYDROCHLORIDE; PARACETAMOL; PSEUDOEPHEDRINE HYDROCHLORIDE.

Benylin with Codeine

(Warner Wellcome) is a proprietary, non-prescription COMPOUND PREPARATION of the ANTITUSSIVE codeine phosphate, the ANTIHISTAMINE diphenhydramine hydrochloride and MENTHOL. It can be used for the symptomatic relief of persistent, dry

cough, and is available as a syrup. It is not normally given to children under six years, except on medical advice.
+▲ Side-effects/warning: See CODEINE PHOSPHATE; DIPHENHYDRAMINE HYDROCHLORIDE.

benzalkonium chloride

is an ANTISEPTIC which has some KERATOLYTIC properties. It can be topically applied to remove hard, dead skin from around wounds or ulcers, or to dissolve warts. It can also be used on minor abrasions and burns and (in the form of lozenges) for mouth ulcers, gum disease and sore throats. For other than oral purposes, administration is topical in the form of a cream or (combined with bromine) as a paint.
+▲ Side-effects/warning: Avoid normal skin when using as a cream.
❂ Related entries: Bradosol Sugar-Free Lozenges; Conotrane; Dermol 500; Drapolene Cream; Emulsiderm; Ionax Scrub; Ionil T; Roccal; Roccal Concentrate 10X.

Benzamycin

(Bioglan) is a proprietary, non-prescription COMPOUND PREPARATION of the ANTIBACTERIAL and (MACROLIDE) ANTIBIOTIC erythromycin and the KERATOLYTIC and ANTIMICROBIAL benzoyl peroxide. It can be used to treat acne, and is available as a gel for topical application.
+▲ Side-effects/warning: See BENZOYL PEROXIDE; ERYTHROMYCIN.

benzatropine mesilate

see BENZTROPINE MESYLATE

benzhexol hydrochloride

(trihexyphenidyl hydrochloride) is an ANTICHOLINERGIC which is used in the treatment of some types of parkinsonism (see ANTIPARKINSONISM). It increases mobility and decreases rigidity and tremor, and the tendency to produce an excess of saliva is also reduced, but it has only a limited effect on bradykinesia. Additionally, the drug has the capacity to treat these symptoms, in some cases, where they are produced by drugs. It is thought to work by correcting the over-effectiveness of the NEUROTRANSMITTER ACETYLCHOLINE (cholinergic excess), which is caused by the deficiency of dopamine that occurs in parkinsonism. Administration, which may be in conjunction with other drugs used to relieve parkinsonism, is oral.

✚ Side-effects: Dry mouth, gastrointestinal disturbances, dizziness, blurred vision; less commonly there is urinary retention, speeding of the heart, sensitivity reactions or nervousness. Rarely, and only in susceptible patients, there may be confusion, excitement and psychological disturbance.

▲ Warning: It should not be used in patients with urinary retention, closed-angle glaucoma, gastrointestinal obstruction. Administer with caution to those with impaired kidney or liver function, or cardiovascular disease. Withdrawal of treatment must be gradual.

✪ Related entries: Artane; Broflex.

benzocaine

is a LOCAL ANAESTHETIC which is used by topical application for the relief of pain in the skin surface or mucous membranes, particularly in or around the mouth and throat, or (in combination with other drugs) in the ears. Administration is topical and in various forms.

▲ Warning: Prolonged use should be avoided and some patients may experience sensitivity reactions.

✪ Related entries: Dequacaine Lozenges; Intralgin; Medilave; Merocaine Lozenges; Solarcaine; Tyrocane Throat Lozenges; Tyrozets; Vicks Ultra Chloraseptic.

benzodiazepines ⚇

are drugs that belong chemically to a large group of agents that have a marked effect upon the central nervous system. The effect varies according to the level of dose, the frequency of dosage and which member of the group is used. They have, to varying degrees, SEDATIVE, ANXIOLYTIC, HYPNOTIC, ANTICONVULSANT, ANTI-EPILEPTIC and SKELETAL MUSCLE RELAXANT actions. They can also cause amnesia and may be used as a postoperative medication in order to allow patients to forget unpleasant procedures. Benzodiazepines that are used as hypnotics have virtually replaced earlier drugs, such as the BARBITURATES and CHLORAL HYDRATE, because they are just as effective but much safer in overdose.

There are now ANTAGONISTS, such as FLUMAZENIL, that can be used to reverse some of the central nervous system effects of benzodiazepines, for instance, at the end of operations. However, it is now realized that dependence may result from prolonged use and there may be a paradoxical increase in hostility and aggression in patients having long-term treatment.

The best-known and most-used benzodiazepines include DIAZEPAM (which can be used for many purposes, including to control anxiety, skeletal muscle relaxation during operations, the convulsions of epilepsy or for drug poisoning), NITRAZEPAM (a widely used hypnotic), CHLORDIAZEPOXIDE and LORAZEPAM (anxiolytic). See also ALPRAZOLAM; BROMAZEPAM; CLONAZEPAM; FLUNITRAZEPAM; FLURAZEPAM; LORMETAZEPAM; NITRAZEPAM; OXAZEPAM; TEMAZEPAM.

✚ Side-effects: Depending on use, dose and type; there may be drowsiness and light-headedness the day after treatment, confusion and impaired gait (particularly in the elderly), dependence, amnesia, aggression; occasionally, vertigo, headache, hypotension, salivation changes, rashes, visual disturbances, changes in libido, urinary retention, blood disorders, jaundice and gastrointestinal disorders.

▲ Warning: Depending on use, dose and type; they should not be given to patients with respiratory depression or acute pulmonary insufficiency, psychosis or phobic or obsessional states. Administer with caution to those with respiratory disease, muscle weakness, history of alcohol or drug abuse, severe personality disorders, liver or kidney impairment; who are elderly or debilitated, or have porphyria, or who are pregnant or breast-feeding. Avoid prolonged use because of the risk of dependence.

benzoic acid

has ANTIFUNGAL and KERATOLYTIC activity and is incorporated into non-proprietary and proprietary ointments and creams.
◑ Related entries: Aserbine; Benzoic Acid Ointment, Compound, BP; Hemocane.

Benzoic Acid Ointment, Compound, BP

is a non-proprietary, non-prescription COMPOUND PREPARATION of the ANTIFUNGAL and KERATOLYTIC agents salicylic acid and benzoic acid. It is commonly used to treat patches of ringworm infection on the limbs, palms, soles of feet and chest. It is available in the form of an ointment, which is also known as *Whitfield's Ointment*.
✚▲ Side-effects/warning: See BENZOIC ACID; SALICYLIC ACID.

Benzoin Tincture, Compound, BP

is a non-proprietary non-prescription COMPOUND PREPARATION of balsam resin and balsamic acid. It is used as a base from which vapours may be inhaled (when added to boiling water) and can be used as a NASAL DECONGESTANT for blocked nose in sinusitis, rhinitis and bronchitis.

benzoyl peroxide

is a KERATOLYTIC and ANTIMICROBIAL drug which is used in combination with other drugs to treat skin conditions and infections such as acne and athlete's foot. Administration is topical.
✚ Side-effects: Some patients experience skin irritation.
▲ Warning: It should not be used to treat the skin disease of the facial blood vessels, rosacea. When applying, avoid the eyes, mouth and mucous membranes. It may bleach fabrics.

◑ Related entries: Acnecide; Acnegel; Acnegel Forte; Acnidazil; Benoxyl 5 Cream; Benoxyl 10 Lotion; Benzamycin; Mediclear 5 Acne Cream; Mediclear 10 Acne Cream; Mediclear Acne Lotion; Nericur; Oxy 5 Lotion; Oxy 10 Lotion; PanOxyl 5 Gel; PanOxyl 10 Gel; PanOxyl Aquagel 5; PanOxyl Aquagel 10; PanOxyl Aquagel 25; PanOxyl Wash; Quinoderm Cream; Quinoderm Cream 5; Quinoderm Lotio-Gel 5%; Quinoped; Ultra Clearasil Maximum Strength; Ultra Clearasil Regular Strength.

benzthiazide

is a DIURETIC of the THIAZIDE class. It is used as an ANTIHYPERTENSIVE, in conjunction with other types of diuretics, and in the treatment of oedema associated with congestive heart failure. Administration is oral.
✚▲ Side-effects/warning: See BENDROFLUAZIDE.
◑ Related entry: Dytide.

benztropine mesylate

(benzatropine mesilate) is an ANTICHOLINERGIC which is used in the treatment of some types of parkinsonism (see ANTIPARKINSONISM). It increases mobility and decreases rigidity and tremor, and the tendency to produce an excess of saliva is also reduced, but it has only a limited effect on bradykinesia. Additionally, it has the capacity to treat these symptoms, in some but not all instances, where they are produced by drugs. It is thought to work by correcting the over-effectiveness of the NEUROTRANSMITTER ACETYLCHOLINE (cholinergic excess), which results from the deficiency of dopamine that occurs in parkinsonism. Because it also has some sedative properties, it is sometimes administered in preference to the similar drug BENZHEXOL HYDROCHLORIDE. Administration, which may be in conjunction with other drugs used to relieve parkinsonism, is either oral or by injection.

✚▲ Side-effects/warning: See BENZHEXOL HYDROCHLORIDE; but it causes sedation rather than stimulation.
⊘ Related entry: Cogentin.

benzydamine hydrochloride

has COUNTER-IRRITANT, or RUBEFACIENT, action and can be used for the symptomatic relief of pain when applied to the skin, mouth ulcers and other sores or inflammation in the mouth and throat. Administration is either oral or by topical application.
✚ Side-effects: Stinging or numbness on initial application.
⊘ Related entry: Difflam.

benzyl benzoate

can be used either as a SCABICIDAL drug to treat infestation of the skin, chest and limbs by itch-mites (scabies) or as a PEDICULICIDAL to treat head lice infestation. Administration is topical.
✚ Side-effects: There may be skin irritation, a burning sensation and occasionally a rash.
▲ Warning: Administer with caution to patients who are pregnant or breast-feeding; avoid contact with the eyes, mucous membranes and broken skin.
⊘ Related entries: Anugesic-HC; Anusol-HC; Ascabiol Emulsion; Sudocrem Antiseptic Cream.

benzylpenicillin

(penicillin G) is the chemical name for the ANTIBACTERIAL drug that was the first of the penicillins to be isolated and used as an ANTIBIOTIC. Despite the many hundreds of antibiotics introduced since, it still remains the drug of choice in treating many severe infections, including those caused by sensitive strains of meningococcus (eg meningitis and septicaemia.), pneumococcus (eg pneumonia and meningitis) and streptococcus (eg bacterial sore throat, scarlet fever and septicaemia), in serious conditions when the micro-organism causing the disease has not be identified for certain (eg endocarditis) and

to prevent bacterial infection following limb amputation. In its long-acting form, PROCAINE PENICILLIN, it has an important role in treating syphilis.

It is usually injected because it is inactivated by digestive acids in the stomach. Its rapid excretion by the kidney also means frequent administration is necessary, unless long-acting preparations are used.
✚ Side-effects: Diarrhoea (after oral administration); more rarely, sensitivity reactions such as rashes, urticaria, angio-oedema and blood changes; high temperature and joint pain. Allergic patients may suffer anaphylactic shock.
▲ Warning: It should not be administered to patients with known allergy to penicillins; use with care in patients with impaired kidney function.
⊘ Related entry: Crystapen.

Berkamil

(Berk) is a proprietary, prescription-only preparation of the (*potassium-sparing*) DIURETIC amiloride hydrochloride. It can be used to treat oedema, ascites in cirrhosis of the liver, congestive heart failure (in conjunction with other diuretics) and as an ANTIHYPERTENSIVE. It is available as tablets.
✚▲ Side-effects/warning: See AMILORIDE HYDROCHLORIDE.

Berkaprine

(Berk) is a proprietary, prescription-only preparation of the IMMUNOSUPPRESSANT azathioprine. It can be used to treat tissue rejection in transplant patients and for a variety of autoimmune diseases. It is available as tablets.
✚▲ Side-effects/warning: See AZATHIOPRINE.

Berkatens

(Berk) is a proprietary, prescription-only preparation of the CALCIUM-CHANNEL BLOCKER verapamil hydrochloride. It can be used as an ANTIHYPERTENSIVE, as an ANTI-ANGINA treatment in the prevention of attacks and

as an ANTI-ARRHYTHMIC to correct heart irregularities. It is available as tablets.
+▲ Side-effects/warning: See VERAPAMIL HYDROCHLORIDE.

Berkmycen

(Berk) is a proprietary, prescription-only preparation of the ANTIBACTERIAL and (TETRACYCLINE) ANTIBIOTIC oxytetracycline. It can be used to treat a wide range of infections, and is available as tablets.
+▲ Side-effects/warning: See OXYTETRACYCLINE.

Berkolol

(Berk) is a proprietary, prescription-only preparation of the BETA-BLOCKER propranolol hydrochloride. It can be used as an ANTIHYPERTENSIVE for raised blood pressure, an ANTI-ANGINA treatment to relieve symptoms and improve exercise tolerance and as an ANTI-ARRHYTHMIC to regularize heartbeat and to treat myocardial infarction. It can also be used as an ANTITHYROID drug for short-term treatment of thyrotoxicosis, as an ANTIMIGRAINE treatment to prevent attacks, as an ANXIOLYTIC, particularly for symptomatic relief of tremor and palpitations, and, with an ALPHA-ADRENOCEPTOR BLOCKER, in the acute treatment of phaeochromocytoma. It is available as tablets.
+▲ Side-effects/warning: See PROPRANOLOL HYDROCHLORIDE.

Berkozide

(Berk) is a proprietary, prescription-only preparation of the (THIAZIDE) DIURETIC bendrofluazide. It can be used, either alone or in conjunction with other drugs, in the treatment of oedema with congestive heart failure and as an ANTIHYPERTENSIVE. It is available as tablets.
+▲ Side-effects/warning: See BENDROFLUAZIDE.

Berotec

(Boehringer Ingelheim) is a proprietary, prescription-only preparation of the BETA-RECEPTOR STIMULANT fenoterol hydrobromide. It can be used as a BRONCHODILATOR in reversible obstructive airways disease, as an ANTI-ASTHMATIC treatment in severe acute asthma and for the alleviation of symptoms of chronic bronchitis and emphysema. It is available as a metered aerosol inhalant.
+▲ Side-effects/warning: See FENOTEROL HYDROBROMIDE.

Beta-Adalat

(Bayer) is a proprietary, prescription-only COMPOUND PREPARATION of the BETA-BLOCKER atenolol and the CALCIUM-CHANNEL BLOCKER nifedipine. It can be used as an ANTIHYPERTENSIVE for raised blood pressure, and is available as tablets.
+▲ Side-effects/warning: See ATENOLOL; NIFEDIPINE.

beta-adrenoceptor stimulants

see BETA-RECEPTOR STIMULANTS

beta-adrenoceptor-blocking drugs

see BETA-BLOCKERS

beta-agonists

see BETA-RECEPTOR STIMULANTS

beta-blockers 🔢

(beta-adrenoceptor-blocking drugs) are drugs that inhibit some actions of the sympathetic nervous system by preventing the actions of ADRENALINE and NORADRENALINE (which are HORMONE and NEUROTRANSMITTER mediators, respectively) by blocking the beta-adrenoceptors on which they act. Correspondingly, alpha-adrenoceptor blockers are drugs used to inhibit the remaining actions by occupying the other main class of adrenoceptor, alpha-adrenoceptors.

These two classes of adrenoceptor are responsible for the very widespread actions of adrenaline and noradrenaline in the body, both in normal physiology and in stress. For example, they speed the heart, constrict or dilate certain blood vessels (thereby increasing blood pressure) and suppress activity in the intestines. In general, they prepare the body for emergency action.

In disease, some of these actions may be inappropriate, exaggerated and detrimental to health, so beta-blockers may be used to restore a more healthy balance. Thus beta-blockers may be used as ANTIHYPERTENSIVES to lower blood pressure when it is abnormally raised in cardiovascular disease; as ANTI-ARRHYTHMICS to correct heartbeat irregularities; as ANTI-ANGINA drugs to prevent the pain of angina pectoris during exercise and to treat myocardial infarction (damage to heart muscle) associated with heart attacks; as ANTIMIGRAINE drugs (prophylaxis; to prevent migraine attacks); as ANXIOLYTICS to reduce anxiety, particularly its manifestations such as tremor; as ANTITHYROID drugs, specifically, shortly before surgery to correct thyrotoxicosis; and, in the form of eye-drops, as a GLAUCOMA TREATMENT to lower raised intraocular pressure.

However, there may be a price to pay, in as much as they will also block beta-receptors elsewhere in the body, thereby reducing the normal, beneficial actions of adrenaline and noradrenaline and these effects may well be undesirable. For instance, they may precipitate asthma attacks and sufferers may require bigger doses of beta-receptor stimulant aerosols for their complaint. Similarly, the blood flow in the extremities will often be reduced, so patients may complain of cold feet or hands. The best-known and most-used beta-blockers include ACEBUTOLOL, OXPRENOLOL HYDROCHLORIDE, PROPRANOLOL HYDROCHLORIDE and SOTALOL HYDROCHLORIDE.

+▲ Side-effects/warning: See PROPRANOLOL HYDROCHLORIDE. Most beta-blockers can cause tiredness, sleep disturbances and coldness in the extremities. They may cause asthma attacks in susceptible patients and, because they slow the heart, heart failure, so

they should only be used in patients where this is not a problem. These side-effects may occur when beta-blockers are used as eye-drops for glaucoma treatment. Some beta-blockers having fewer general side-effects are known as *cardioselective*.

Beta-Cardone

(Evans) is a proprietary, prescription-only preparation of the BETA-BLOCKER sotalol hydrochloride. It can be used as an ANTI-ARRHYTHMIC to regularize heartbeat, and is available as tablets.

+▲ Side-effects/warning: See SOTALOL HYDROCHLORIDE.

beta-lactams 🔲

are chemically the group of ANTIBIOTICS that have a certain chemical structure called a lactam ring. This extensive family includes the PENICILLINS (whose generic names usually end -*cillin*; eg AMOXYCILLIN, AMPICILLIN, METHICILLIN), the CEPHALOSPORINS (whose names often include *cef* or *ceph*; eg cefaclor, ceftazidime), together with newer synthetic classes such as the *carbapenems* (eg IMIPENEM, MEROPENEM) and *monobactams* (eg AZTREONAM). A notable adverse reaction to this family of antibiotics is an allergic drug response, which can be dangerous. Allergy to one class makes reaction to another likely, though not inevitable.

Beta-Prograne

(Tillomed) is a proprietary, prescription-only preparation of the BETA-BLOCKER propranolol hydrochloride. It can be used as an ANTIHYPERTENSIVE for raised blood pressure, as an ANTI-ANGINA treatment to relieve symptoms and improve exercise tolerance and as an ANTI-ARRHYTHMIC to regularize heartbeat and to treat myocardial infarction. It can also be used as an ANTITHYROID drug for the short-term treatment of thyrotoxicosis, as an ANTIMIGRAINE treatment to prevent attacks, as an ANXIOLYTIC, particularly for symptomatic relief of tremor and palpitations, and, with an ALPHA-ADRENOCEPTOR BLOCKER, in the acute treatment of phaeochromocytoma. It is available as modified-release capsules.

+▲ Side-effects/warning: See PROPRANOLOL HYDROCHLORIDE.

beta-receptor stimulants ⧉

(beta-adrenoceptor stimulants; beta-agonists) are a class of drugs that act at beta-receptors, which, along with alpha-adrenoceptors, are the sites that recognize and respond to the natural hormones and neurotransmitters (adrenaline and noradrenaline) of the sympathetic nervous system. Drugs that activate this system, by whatever mechanism, are called SYMPATHOMIMETICS. Notable actions of beta-receptor stimulants include bronchodilation, speeding and strengthening of the heartbeat and relaxation of contraction of the uterus and intestine. Importantly, differences in receptors at different sites allow selectivity of action.

For example, the beta$_2$-receptor stimulant drugs are normally used as BRONCHODILATORS in the treatment of asthma, because they can act within the respiratory tract without significant and potentially dangerous parallel stimulation of the heart (which is a beta$_1$-receptor site). Examples of beta$_2$-stimulant drugs used to cause bronchodilation are SALBUTAMOL and TERBUTALINE SULPHATE. In contrast, beta$_1$-receptor stimulants, for example, XAMOTEROL, may be administered to stimulate a failing heart. Agents that are not selective between the two beta-receptor types (eg ISOPRENALINE SULPHATE; ORCIPRENALINE SULPHATE) are not used that often anymore .

Betacap

(Dermal) is a proprietary, prescription-only, preparation of the CORTICOSTEROID and ANTI-INFLAMMATORY betamethasone (as valerate). It can be used to treat severe, non-infective inflammation of the scalp, and is available in a 'Scalp application' water-miscible form.

+▲ Side-effects/warning: See BETAMETHASONE.

Betadine

(Seton) is a proprietary, non-prescription range of preparations of the ANTISEPTIC povidone-iodine. It is available as a vaginal cleansing kit containing pessaries, a gel and a solution for the treatment of bacterial infections in the vagina and cervix. A more dilute solution may also be used as a mouthwash and gargle for the mouth and throat. For the treatment of skin infections, it is available in solutions of differing concentrations as a paint, a lotion, a scalp and skin cleanser, a shampoo, a skin cleanser solution and a mouthwash or gargle. It is also available as a dry powder and an ointment which can be used to dress minor cuts and abrasions.

+▲ Side-effects/warning: See POVIDONE-IODINE.

Betadur CR

(Monmouth) is a proprietary, prescription-only preparation of the BETA-BLOCKER propranolol hydrochloride. It can be used as an ANTIHYPERTENSIVE for raised blood pressure, as an ANTI-ANGINA treatment to relieve symptoms and improve exercise tolerance and as an ANTI-ARRHYTHMIC to regularize heartbeat and to treat myocardial infarction. It can also be used as an ANTITHYROID drug for short-term treatment of thyrotoxicosis, as an ANTIMIGRAINE treatment to prevent attacks, as an ANXIOLYTIC, particularly for symptomatic relief of tremor and palpitations, and, with an ALPHA-ADRENOCEPTOR BLOCKER, in the acute treatment of phaeochromocytoma. It is available as modified-release capsules.

+▲ Side-effects/warning: See PROPRANOLOL HYDROCHLORIDE.

Betaferon

(Schering Health) is a proprietary, prescription-only preparation of the

B

IMMUNOMODULATOR interferon (in the form of beta-1b). It can be used to treat Relapsing-Remitting Multiple Sclerosis, and is available in a form for injection.

✚▲ Side-effects/warning: See INTERFERON.

Betagan

(Allergan) is a proprietary, prescription-only preparation of the BETA-BLOCKER levobunolol hydrochloride. It can be used for GLAUCOMA TREATMENT, and is available as eye-drops.

✚▲ Side-effects/warning: See LEVOBUNOLOL HYDROCHLORIDE.

betahistine hydrochloride

is an ANTINAUSEANT which is used to treat the vertigo, hearing loss and tinnitus (ringing in the ears) associated with Ménière's disease. Administration is oral.

✚ Side-effects: Gastrointestinal disturbances, headache, rash.

▲ Warning: It is not to be given to patients with phaeochromocytoma; administer with caution to those with peptic ulcer or asthma.

✪ Related entry: Serc.

Betaloc

(Astra) is a proprietary, prescription-only preparation of the BETA-BLOCKER metoprolol tartrate. It can be used as an ANTIHYPERTENSIVE for raised blood pressure, as an ANTI-ANGINA treatment to relieve symptoms and improve exercise tolerance and as an ANTI-ARRHYTHMIC to regularize heartbeat and to treat myocardial infarction. It can also be used as an ANTITHYROID drug for the short-term treatment of thyrotoxicosis and as an ANTIMIGRAINE to prevent attacks. It is available as tablets and in a form for injection.

✚▲ Side-effects/warning: See METOPROLOL TARTRATE.

Betaloc-SA

(Astra) is a proprietary, prescription-only preparation of the BETA-BLOCKER metoprolol

tartrate. It can be used as an ANTIHYPERTENSIVE for raised blood pressure, as an ANTI-ANGINA treatment to relieve symptoms and improve exercise tolerance and as an ANTI-ARRHYTHMIC to regularize heartbeat and to treat myocardial infarction. It can also be used as an ANTIMIGRAINE treatment to prevent attacks. It is available as modified-release tablets.

✚▲ Side-effects/warning: See METOPROLOL TARTRATE.

betamethasone

is a CORTICOSTEROID with ANTI-INFLAMMATORY properties. It is used in the treatment of many kinds of inflammation, particularly inflammation associated with skin conditions, such as eczema and psoriasis, and of the eyes, ears or nose. It is also administered to treat cerebral oedema (fluid retention in the brain) and congenital adrenal hyperplasia (which is the abnormal growth of a part of the adrenal gland called the adrenal cortex). It is administered in several forms by different methods, depending on the form of the drug. Administration as *betamethasone* can be either oral as tablets or by injection; as *betamethasone dipropionate* by topical application as a cream, ointment or a scalp lotion; as *betamethasone sodium phosphate* by topical application as eye-, ear- or nose-drops; and as *betamethasone valerate* also by topical application as a cream, ointment, lotion or a rectal ointment. Additionally, betamethasone is incorporated into several COMPOUND PREPARATIONS with ANTIMICROBIALS and LOCAL ANAESTHETICS.

✚▲ Side-effects/warning: See CORTICOSTEROIDS. Systemic side-effects are unlikely with topical application, but there may be local skin reactions.

✪ Related entries: Betacap; Betnelan; Betnesol; Betnesol-N; Betnovate; Betnovate-C; Betnovate-N; Betnovate-RD; Bettamousse; Diprosalic; Diprosone; Fucibet; Lotriderm; Vista-Methasone; Vista-Methasone-N.

betamethasone dipropionate
see BETAMETHASONE

betamethasone sodium phosphate
see BETAMETHASONE

betamethasone valerate
see BETAMETHASONE

betaxolol hydrochloride
is a BETA-BLOCKER which can be used as an ANTIHYPERTENSIVE for raised blood pressure. Administration can be either oral or by injection. It can also be used, in the form of eye-drops, as a GLAUCOMA TREATMENT for chronic simple glaucoma.

+▲ Side-effect/warning: See PROPRANOLOL HYDROCHLORIDE. When given as eye-drops, it may cause dry eyes and eyelids, and allergic reactions (conjunctivitis). In view of possible absorption, systemic side-effects should be considered, particularly the danger of bronchospasm in asthmatics and interactions with calcium-channel blockers.
○ Related entries: Betoptic; Kerlone.

bethanechol chloride
is a PARASYMPATHOMIMETIC which is used to stimulate motility in the intestines and to treat urinary retention (particularly following surgery). Administration is oral.
+ Side-effects: There may be sweating, blurred vision, nausea and vomiting, intestinal colic and a slow heart rate.
▲ Warning: It should not be administered to patients who suffer from urinary or intestinal obstruction, asthma, epilepsy, parkinsonism, thyroid or certain heart disorders, who have peptic ulceration or are pregnant.
○ Related entry: Myotonine.

bethanidine sulphate
is an ADRENERGIC-NEURONE BLOCKER, which is an ANTISYMPATHETIC class of drug. It prevents the release of noradrenaline from sympathetic nerves, and can be used as an ANTIHYPERTENSIVE for moderate to severe high blood pressure, especially when other forms of treatment have failed and usually with other antihypertensives (eg DIURETICS or BETA-BLOCKERS). Administration is oral.
+▲ Side-effects/warning: See GUANETHIDINE MONOSULPHATE; except it does not cause diarrhoea.
○ Related entry: Bendogen.

Betim
(Leo) is a proprietary, prescription-only preparation of the BETA-BLOCKER timolol maleate. It can be used as an ANTIHYPERTENSIVE for raised blood pressure, as an ANTI-ANGINA treatment to relieve symptoms and improve exercise tolerance and as an ANTI-ARRHYTHMIC to regularize heartbeat and to treat myocardial infarction. It can also be used as an ANTIMIGRAINE treatment to prevent attacks. It is available as tablets.
+▲ Side-effects/warning: See TIMOLOL MALEATE.

Betnelan
(Evans) is a proprietary, prescription-only preparation of the CORTICOSTEROID and ANTI-INFLAMMATORY betamethasone. It can be used to treat inflammation, especially in rheumatic or allergic conditions, cerebral oedema and congenital adrenal hyperplasia. It is available as tablets.
+▲ Side-effects/warning: See BETAMETHASONE.

Betnesol
(Evans) is a proprietary, prescription-only preparation of the CORTICOSTEROID and ANTI-INFLAMMATORY betamethasone (as sodium phosphate). It can be used to treat local inflammations (eg of the ear, eye or nose) as well as more widespread rheumatic or allergic conditions, including severe asthma. It is available as tablets, as ear-, eye- and nose-drops, an eye ointment and in a form for injection.
+▲ Side-effects/warning: See BETAMETHASONE.

B

Betnesol-N

(Evans) is a proprietary, prescription-only
COMPOUND PREPARATION of the ANTI-
INFLAMMATORY and CORTICOSTEROID
betamethasone (as sodium phosphate) and
the ANTIBACTERIAL and ANTIBIOTIC neomycin
sulphate. It can be used to treat local
inflammations, and is available as ear-, eye-
and nose-drops and an eye ointment.
✚▲ Side-effects/warning: See
BETAMETHASONE; NEOMYCIN SULPHATE.

Betnovate

(Glaxo) is a proprietary, prescription-only
preparation of the ANTI-INFLAMMATORY and
CORTICOSTEROID betamethasone (as
valerate). It can be used topically to treat
severe non-infective inflammation of the
skin, rectum and scalp. It is available as a
cream, ointment, lotion and a scalp
preparation. A rectal ointment is also
available as a COMPOUND PREPARATION of
betamethasone (as valerate), the LOCAL
ANAESTHETIC lignocaine hydrochloride and
the SYMPATHOMIMETIC and VASOCONSTRICTOR
phenylephrine hydrochloride.
✚▲ Side-effects/warning: See
BETAMETHASONE; LIGNOCAINE HYDROCHLORIDE;
PHENYLEPHRINE HYDROCHLORIDE.

Betnovate-C

(Glaxo) is a proprietary, prescription-only
COMPOUND PREPARATION of the ANTI-
INFLAMMATORY and CORTICOSTEROID
betamethasone (as valerate) and the
ANTIMICROBIAL clioquinol. It can be used
topically to treat severe, non-infective
inflammation, such as skin eczema, and is
available as a cream.
✚▲ Side-effects/warning: See
BETAMETHASONE; CLIOQUINOL.

Betnovate-N

(Glaxo) is a proprietary, prescription-only
COMPOUND PREPARATION of the ANTI-
INFLAMMATORY and CORTICOSTEROID
betamethasone (as valerate) and the
ANTIBACTERIAL and ANTIBIOTIC neomycin
sulphate. It can be used topically to treat
severe inflammation, such as skin psoriasis
and eczema, and is available as a cream
and an ointment.
✚▲ Side-effects/warning: See
BETAMETHASONE; NEOMYCIN SULPHATE.

Betnovate-RD

(Glaxo) is a proprietary, prescription-only,
preparation of the CORTICOSTEROID and ANTI-
INFLAMMATORY betamethasone (as valerate).
It can be used to treat severe, non-infective
inflammation of the skin and scalp, and is
available as a cream and an ointment.
✚▲ Side-effects/warning: See
BETAMETHASONE.

Betoptic

(Alcon) is a proprietary, prescription-only
preparation of the BETA-BLOCKER betaxolol
hydrochloride, and can be used, in the
form of eye-drops, for GLAUCOMA TREATMENT.
✚▲ Side-effects/warning: See BETAXOLOL
HYDROCHLORIDE.

Bettamousse

(Evans) is a proprietary, prescription-only,
preparation of the CORTICOSTEROID and ANTI-
INFLAMMATORY betamethasone (as valerate).
It can be used to treat severe, non-infective
inflammation of the scalp, and is available
in a form for scalp application.
✚▲ Side-effects/warning: See
BETAMETHASONE.

bezafibrate

is used as a LIPID-LOWERING DRUG in
hyperlipidaemia to reduce the levels, or
change the proportions, of various lipids
(eg cholesterol and LDL) in the
bloodstream. Generally, it is administered
only to patients in whom a strict and
regular dietary regime, alone, is not having
the desired effect. Administration is oral.
✚ Side-effects: There may be nausea,
abdominal pain, loss of appetite; skin
complaints, including rashes and itching;
and impotence. Occasionally, dizziness and
vertigo; fatigue and headache; hair loss;
muscle weakness.

B

▲ Warning: Avoid administering to patients who have severely impaired kidney or liver function, disease of the gall bladder, or who are pregnant or breast-feeding.
◎ Related entries: Bezalip-Mono; Bezalip.

Bezalip

(Boehringer Mannheim) is a proprietary, prescription-only preparation of the LIPID-LOWERING DRUG bezafibrate. It can be used in hyperlipidaemia to reduce the levels, or change the proportions, of various lipids (eg cholesterol and LDL) in the bloodstream. It is available as capsules.
✚▲ Side-effects/warning: See BEZAFIBRATE.

Bezalip-Mono

(Boehringer Mannheim) is a proprietary, prescription-only preparation of the LIPID-LOWERING DRUG bezafibrate. It can be used in hyperlipidaemia to reduce the levels, or change the proportions, of various lipids (eg cholesterol and LDL) in the bloodstream. It is available as tablets.
✚▲ Side-effects/warning: See BEZAFIBRATE.

bicalutamide

is a HORMONE ANTAGONIST (an anti-androgen) which is used as an ANTICANCER drug for the treatment of prostate cancer. Administration is oral.
✚ Side-effects: There may be hot flushes, growth and tenderness of breasts, weakness, pruritus, sleepiness, transient elevation of certain blood enzymes, jaundice and cholestasis, rarely thrombocytopenia, certain cardiovascular disorders (angina, heart failure, arrhythmias); other effects (more common in elderly) include dizziness, insomnia, decreased libido, impotence, anorexia, shortness of breath, gastrointestinal problems (such as flatulence, constipation and dyspepsia), alopecia, rashes, sweating, oedema, dry mouth, chest and abdominal pain.
▲ Warning: Administer with caution to patients suffering certain liver disorders (liver function should be monitored).
◎ Related entry: Casodex.

Bicillin

(Yamanouchi) is a proprietary, prescription-only preparation of the ANTIBACTERIAL and (PENICILLIN) ANTIBIOTIC procaine penicillin. It can be used in long-lasting intramuscular (depot) injections to treat conditions such as syphilis and gonorrhoea. It is released slowly into the blood, therefore avoiding the need for frequent injections.
✚▲ Side-effects/warning: See PROCAINE PENICILLIN.

BiCNU

(Bristol-Myers) is a proprietary, prescription-only preparation of the (CYTOTOXIC) ANTICANCER drug carmustine. It can be used in the treatment of certain myelomas, lymphomas and brain tumours, and is available in a form for injection.
✚▲ Side-effects/warning: See CARMUSTINE.

biguanides 🔋

are a chemical class of orally administered HYPOGLYCAEMIC drugs (of which metformin hydrochloride is the only example currently available in the UK) which are used in DIABETIC TREATMENT for Type II diabetes (non-insulin-dependent diabetes mellitus; NIDDM; maturity-onset diabetes).

BiNovum

(Ortho) is a proprietary, prescription-only COMPOUND PREPARATION which can be used as a (*biphasic*) ORAL CONTRACEPTIVE (and also for certain menstrual problems) of the type that combines an OESTROGEN and a PROGESTOGEN, in this case ethinyloestradiol and norethisterone. It is available as tablets in a calendar pack.
✚▲ Side-effects/warning: See ETHINYLOESTRADIOL; NORETHISTERONE.

Bioplex

(Thames) is a proprietary, prescription-only preparation of the CYTOPROTECTANT drug carbenoxolone sodium. It can be used to treat mouth ulcers, and is available as granules to make up into a mouthwash.

B

+▲ Side-effects/warning: See
CARBENOXOLONE SODIUM.

Bioral Gel

(SmithKline Beecham) is a proprietary,
non-prescription preparation of the ANTI-
INFLAMMATORY carbenoxolone sodium. It can
be used to treat mouth ulcers, and is
available as a gel.
+▲ Side-effects/warning: See
CARBENOXOLONE SODIUM.

Biorphen

(Bioglan) is a proprietary, prescription-
only preparation of the ANTICHOLINERGIC
orphenadrine hydrochloride. It can be used
to relieve some of the symptoms of
parkinsonism, especially muscle rigidity
and the tendency to produce an excess of
saliva (see ANTIPARKINSONISM). The drug also
has the capacity to treat these symptoms, in
some cases, where they are produced by
drugs. It is available as an elixir.
+▲ Side-effects/warning: See
ORPHENADRINE HYDROCHLORIDE.

biosynthetic human growth hormone

see SOMATROPIN

biperiden

is an ANTICHOLINERGIC drug which is used in
the treatment of some types of
parkinsonism (see ANTIPARKINSONISM). It
increases mobility and decreases rigidity
and the tendency to produce an excess of
saliva is also reduced, but it has only a
limited effect on bradykinesia. Additionally,
it has the capacity to treat these symptoms,
in some cases, where they are produced by
drugs. It is thought to work by correcting
the over-effectiveness of the
NEUROTRANSMITTER ACETYLCHOLINE
(cholinergic excess), which results from
the deficiency of dopamine that occurs in
parkinsonism. Because it also has some
sedative properties, it is sometimes used in
preference to the similar drug BENZHEXOL
HYDROCHLORIDE. Administration, which may

be in conjunction with other drugs used to
relieve parkinsonism, is either oral or by
injection.
+▲ Side-effects/warning: See BENZHEXOL
HYDROCHLORIDE; but it may cause sedation;
when administered by injection, it may
cause hypotension.
○ Related entry: Akineton.

biphasic insulin

is a form of purified insulin which is
prepared as a sterile suspension of bovine
insulin crystals in a solution of porcine
insulin. It is used in DIABETIC TREATMENT to
treat and maintain diabetic patients. It is
available in vials for injection and has an
intermediate duration of action.
+▲ Side-effects/warning: See INSULIN.
○ Related entry: Rapitard MC.

biphasic isophane insulin

is a form of purified insulin which is
prepared as a sterile buffered suspension of
porcine insulin complexed with protamine
in a solution of porcine insulin, or human
insulin complex in a solution of human
insulin. It is used in DIABETIC TREATMENT to
maintain diabetic patients. It is available in
vials for injection and has an intermediate
duration of action.
+▲ Side-effects/warning: See INSULIN.
○ Related entries: Human Actraphane
30/70; Human Initard 50/50; Human Mixtard
30/70; Humulin M1; Humulin M2; Humulin
M3; Humulin M4; Humulin M5; Mixtard
30/70; PenMix 10/90; PenMix 20/80; PenMix
30/70; PemMix 40/60; PemMix 50/50; Pur-In
Mix 15/85; Pur-In Mix 25/75; Pur-In Mix
50/50.

bisacodyl

is a (*stimulant*) LAXATIVE which is used to
promote defecation and relieve
constipation. It seems to work by
stimulating motility in the intestine,
however, there are some medical
authorities who do not approve of the
frequent use of *stimulant laxatives* (as
compared to the relatively benign

bulking-agent laxatives, which help establish good bowel habit). Medically, bisacodyl can be administered to evacuate a patient's colon prior to rectal examination or surgery. Administration can be either oral as tablets (when full effects are achieved after several hours) or topical as suppositories (with effects achieved within an hour).

✚ Side-effects: There may be abdominal cramps, griping, nausea or vomiting. Suppositories can sometimes cause local irritation.

▲ Warning: It should not be administered to patients with intestinal obstruction.

✪ Related entries: Dulco-lax Suppositories; Dulco-lax Suppositories for Children; Dulco-lax Tablets; Nylax Tablets.

Bismag Tablets

(Whitehall) is a proprietary, non-prescription COMPOUND PREPARATION of the ANTACIDS sodium bicarbonate, calcium carbonate and mixed magnesium carbonates. It can be used for the symptomatic relief of hyperacidity, indigestion, heartburn, dyspepsia and flatulence. It is available as tablets and is not normally given to children, except on medical advice.

✚▲ Side-effects/warning: See CALCIUM CARBONATE; MAGNESIUM CARBONATE; SODIUM BICARBONATE.

bismuth chelate

see TRIPOTASSIUM DICITRATOBISMUTHATE

bismuth oxide

is a mild ASTRINGENT agent which is used in the treatment of haemorrhoids. Administration is topical as suppositories.

✪ Related entries: Anugesic-HC; Anusol; Anusol HC; Hemocane.

bismuth subgallate

is a mild ASTRINGENT agent which is used in the treatment of haemorrhoids. Administration is topical as suppositories.

✪ Related entry: Anusol-HC.

bismuth subnitrate

is a mild ASTRINGENT agent which is used as a dusting powder in certain skin disorders and as suppositories in the treatment of haemorrhoids.

✪ Related entry: Caved-S.

Bisodol Antacid Powder

(Whitehall) is a proprietary, non-prescription COMPOUND PREPARATION of the ANTACIDS sodium bicarbonate and magnesium carbonate. It can be used for the relief of indigestion, heartburn, dyspepsia, acidity and flatulence. It is available as a powder and is not normally given to children, except on medical advice.

✚▲ Side-effects/warning: See MAGNESIUM CARBONATE; SODIUM BICARBONATE.

Bisodol Antacid Tablets

(Whitehall) is a proprietary, non-prescription COMPOUND PREPARATION of the ANTACIDS sodium bicarbonate, calcium carbonate and mixed magnesium carbonates. It can be used for the relief of indigestion, heartburn, dyspepsia, acidity and flatulence. It is available as tablets and is not normally given to children, except on medical advice.

✚▲ Side-effects/warning: See CALCIUM CARBONATE; MAGNESIUM CARBONATE; SODIUM BICARBONATE.

Bisodol Extra Tablets

(Whitehall) is a proprietary, non-prescription COMPOUND PREPARATION of the ANTACIDS sodium bicarbonate, calcium carbonate and magnesium carbonate and the ANTIFOAMING AGENT dimethicone (as simethicone). It can be used for the relief of indigestion, heartburn, dyspepsia, acidity and flatulence, and is available as tablets.

✚▲ Side-effects/warning: See CALCIUM CARBONATE; DIMETHICONE; MAGNESIUM CARBONATE; SODIUM BICARBONATE.

Bisodol Heartburn

(Whitehall) is a proprietary, non-prescription COMPOUND PREPARATION of the

B

ANTACIDS sodium bicarbonate and magaldrate and the DEMULCENT alginic acid. It can be used for the relief of indigestion, heartburn, dyspepsia, acidity and flatulence. It is available as tablets and is not normally given to children under six years, except on medical advice.

✚▲ Side-effects/warning: See ALGINIC ACID; MAGALDRATE; SODIUM BICARBONATE.

bisoprolol fumarate

is a BETA-BLOCKER which can be used as an ANTIHYPERTENSIVE treatment for raised blood pressure and as an ANTI-ANGINA drug to relieve symptoms and to improve exercise tolerance. It is also available as an antihypertensive in the form of a COMPOUND PREPARATION with a DIURETIC. Administration is oral.

✚▲ Side-effects/warning: See PROPRANOLOL HYDROCHLORIDE.

✪ Related entries: Emcor; Monocor; Monozide 10.

bisphosphonates ⚏

(diphosphonates) are a chemical drug class which are administered as CALCIUM METABOLISM MODIFIERS in the treatment of a number of conditions of disturbed calcium metabolism, including Paget's disease of the bone, malignant hypercalcaemia and osteoporosis, and are also being evaluated for use in treating bone pain associated cancer metastases of the bone.
Bisphosphonate drugs are enzyme-resistant analogues of pyrophosphate, which is a natural inhibitor of bone mineralization, and those used medically are ALENDRONIC ACID, DISODIUM ETIDRONATE, DISODIUM PAMIDRONATE, SODIUM CHLODRONATE and TILUDRONIC ACID .

Blemix

(Ashbourne) is a proprietary, prescription-only preparation of the ANTIBACTERIAL and (TETRACYCLINE) ANTIBIOTIC drug minocycline. It can be used to treat a wide range of infections, and is available as tablets.

✚▲ Side-effects/warning: See MINOCYCLINE.

Bleomycin

(Lundbeck) is a proprietary, prescription-only preparation of the (CYTOTOXIC) ANTICANCER drug bleomycin. It can be used in the treatment of certain cancers, and is available in a form for injection.

✚▲ Side-effects/warning: See BLEOMYCIN.

bleomycin

is a CYTOTOXIC drug (an ANTIBIOTIC in origin) which is used as an ANTICANCER treatment. Administration is by injection.

✚▲ Side-effects/warning: See CYTOTOXICS; but causes little bone marrow depression. Hypersensitivity reactions (chills and fevers) and effects on the lung and skin.

✪ Related entry: Bleomycin.

Blisteze

(DDD) is a proprietary, non-prescription preparation of the ANTISEPTIC phenol (with ammonia solution). It can be used for cold sores and chapped, cracked lips, and is available as a cream.

✚▲ Side-effects/warning: See PHENOL.

Blocadren

(Merck Sharp & Dohme) is a proprietary, prescription-only preparation of the BETA-BLOCKER timolol maleate. It can be used as an ANTIHYPERTENSIVE for raised blood pressure, as an ANTI-ANGINA treatment to relieve symptoms and improve exercise tolerance and as an ANTI-ARRHYTHMIC to regularize heartbeat and to treat myocardial infarction. It may also be used as an ANTIMIGRAINE treatment to prevent attacks. It is available as tablets.

✚▲ Side-effects/warning: See TIMOLOL MALEATE.

BN Liniment

(3M) is a proprietary, non-prescription COMPOUND PREPARATION of TURPENTINE OIL, ammonia and AMMONIUM CHLORIDE, which have COUNTER-IRRITANT, or RUBEFACIENT, actions. It can be applied to the skin for the symptomatic relief of pain associated with rheumatism, neuralgia, fibrosis, sprains and stiffness of joints. It is available as an emulsion for topical application and is not normally used for children under six years, except on medical advice.

Bocasan

(Oral-B Lab) is a proprietary, non-prescription preparation of the ANTISEPTIC sodium perborate. It can be used to cleanse and disinfect the mouth, and is available in a form for making up into a mouthwash.
✚▲ Side-effects/warning: See SODIUM PERBORATE.

Bonefos

(Boehringer Ingelheim) is a recently introduced, proprietary, prescription-only preparation of sodium chlodronate. It is used to treat high calcium levels associated with malignant tumours and bone lesions. It is available in a number of forms (one called *Bonefos Concentrate*), as tablets and in a form for infusion.
✚▲ Side-effects/warning: See SODIUM CHLODRONATE.

Bonjela Antiseptic Pain-Relieving Pastilles

(Reckitt & Colman) is a proprietary, non-prescription COMPOUND PREPARATION of the LOCAL ANAESTHETIC lignocaine hydrochloride and the ANTISEPTIC aminacrine hydrochloride. It can be used to relieve the pain of mouth ulcers.
✚▲ Side-effects/warning: See AMINACRINE HYDROCHLORIDE; LIGNOCAINE HYDROCHLORIDE.

Bonjela Oral Pain-Relieving Gel

(Reckitt & Colman) is a proprietary, non-prescription COMPOUND PREPARATION of the ANTISEPTIC cetalkonium chloride and choline salicylate, which has COUNTER-IRRITANT, or RUBEFACIENT, action. It can be applied to the mouth for symptomatic relief of pain from mouth ulcers, cold sores, denture irritation, inflammation of the tongue and teething in infants. It is available as a gel to be massaged in gently. It should

not be given to babies under four months, except on medical advice.
✚▲ Side-effects/warning: SeeCHOLINE SALICYLATE.

Bonomint

(Intercare) is a proprietary, non-prescription preparation of the (*stimulant*) LAXATIVE phenolphthalein. It can be used to relieve constipation, and is available as a coated tablet with a chewing gum centre. It is not normally given to children under six years, except on medical advice.
✚▲ Side-effects/warning: See PHENOLPHTHALEIN.

Boots Children's Chesty Cough Syrup

(Boots) is a proprietary, non-prescription preparation of the EXPECTORANT agent GUAIPHENESIN. It can be used to relieve chesty coughs, and is available as a sugar-free liquid. It is not normally given to children under one year, except on medical advice.

Boots Covering Cream

(Boots) is a proprietary, non-prescription preparation which is used to mask scars and other skin disfigurements. It is available as a cream and a powder and may be obtained on prescription under certain circumstances.

Boots Travel Calm Tablets

(Boots) is a proprietary, non-prescription preparation of the ANTICHOLINERGIC hyoscine hydrobromide. It can be used as an ANTINAUSEANT in the treatment of motion sickness, and is available as chewable tablets. It is not normally given to children under three years, except on medical advice.
✚▲ Side-effects/warning: See HYOSCINE HYDROBROMIDE.

Botox

(Allergan) is a proprietary, prescription-

B

only preparation of botulinum A toxin-haemagglutin complex. It can be used for treating blepharospasm (a tight contraction of the eyelids) and one-sided facial spasm, and is available in a form for injection.

+▲ Side-effects/warning: See BOTULINUM A TOXIN-HAEMAGGLUTIN COMPLEX.

botulinum A toxin-haemagglutin complex

is a TOXIN used for treating blepharospasm (a tight contraction of the eyelids) and one-sided facial spasm. Administration is by injection.

▲ Warning: Avoid its use in patients who are pregnant, breast-feeding or with certain muscle disorders (eg myasthenia gravis). It may have many effects on the eye such as bruising and swelling.

✪ Related entry: Botox.

botulism antitoxin

is a preparation that neutralizes the TOXINS produced by botulism bacteria (*Clostridium bolulinum* types A, B and E). It can therefore be used in IMMUNIZATION to provide *passive immunity* to people who have been exposed to botulism in order to prevent them from developing the disease. It is also given to an infected patient as a means of treatment. Hypersensitivity reactions are common and it is not effective against some strains of botulism. Administration is by injection.

+▲ Side-effects/warning: See IMMUNIZATION.

✪ Related entry: Botulism Antitoxin.

Botulism Antitoxin

(Department of Health) is a non-proprietary, prescription-only preparation of botulism antitoxin. It can be used to immunize people at risk from the disease following exposure to an infected patient and also as a treatment for those already infected. It is available in a form for injection or intravenous infusion.

+▲ Side-effects/warning: See BOTULISM ANTITOXIN.

bowel-cleansing solutions 🗷

are used prior to colonic surgery, colonoscopy or barium enema to ensure that the bowel is free of solid contents. They are available in sachets for making up with water.

+ Side-effects: Nausea and occasionally vomiting, transient abdominal cramps, bloated feeling, running nose, skin and anal irritations.

▲ Warning: Administer with caution to patients who are pregnant, who have ulcerative colitis or reflux oesophagitis. Bowel-cleansing solutions should not be used for patients suffering from certain gastrointestinal conditions, eg perforated bowel or obstruction.

✪ Related entries: Klean-Prep; Movicol.

Bradosol Plus

(Zyma) is a proprietary, non-prescription COMPOUND PREPARATION of the ANTISEPTIC agent DOMIPHEN BROMIDE and the LOCAL ANAESTHETIC lignocaine hydrochloride. It can be used for the symptomatic relief of a painful sore throat, and is available as lozenges. It is not normally given to children under 12 years, except on medicaladvice.

+▲ Side-effects/warning: See LIGNOCAINE HYDROCHLORIDE.

Bradosol Sugar-Free Lozenges

(Zyma) is a proprietary, non-prescription preparation of the ANTISEPTIC benzalkonium chloride, and can be used for the symptomatic relief of a painful sore throat. (It is also available in a Cherry Menthol form.)

+▲ Side-effects/warning: See BENZALKONIUM CHLORIDE.

bran

is a natural *bulking-agent* LAXATIVE, which is commonly used to keep people 'regular' and to treat constipation. It works by increasing the overall mass of faeces (by retaining a lot of water) and so stimulating bowel movement (the full effect may not be achieved for many hours). As an excellent source of dietary fibre, bran is thought to reduce the risk of diverticular disease while actively assisting digestion. It is useful in managing patients with colostomy, ileostomy, haemorrhoids, chronic diverticular disease, irritable bowel syndrome and ulcerative colitis.

✚ Side-effects: Some patients cannot tolerate bran, particularly those sensitive to the compound gluten.

▲ Warning: It should not be consumed if there is intestinal blockage or coeliac disease. Adequate fluid intake must be maintained to avoid faecal impaction.

✪ Related entry: Trifyba.

Brasivol

(Stiefel) is a proprietary, non-prescription preparation of particles of aluminium oxide, which has abrasive properties that can be used to cleanse skin with acne. It is available as a paste in three grades – fine, medium and coarse – within a soap base.

Bretylate

(Wellcome) is a proprietary, prescription-only preparation of the ADRENERGIC-NEURONE BLOCKER bretylium tosylate. It can be used as an ANTI-ARRHYTHMIC to treat abnormal heart rhythms in resuscitation and where other treatments have not been successful. It is available in a form for injection.

✚▲ Side-effects/warning: See BRETYLIUM TOSYLATE.

bretylium tosilate

see BRETYLIUM TOSYLATE

bretylium tosylate

(bretylium tosilate) is an ADRENERGIC-NEURONE BLOCKER, which is an ANTISYMPATHETIC class of drug that prevents the release of noradrenaline from sympathetic nerves. It can be used in ANTI-ARRHYTHMIC treatment of abnormal heart rhythms in resuscitation, where other therapies have not been successful.

Administration is by injection.

✚ Side-effects: Hypotension; nausea and vomiting; tissue damage at the site of injection.

▲ Warning: It should not be used in patients with phaeochromocytoma.

✪ Related entries: Bretylate; Min-I-Jet Bretylate Tosylate.

Brevibloc

(Du Pont) is a proprietary, prescription-only preparation of the BETA-BLOCKER esmolol hydrochloride. It can be used as an ANTIHYPERTENSIVE for raised blood pressure during operations and as an ANTI-ARRHYTHMIC, in the short term, to regularize heartbeat and to treat myocardial infarction. It is available in a form for injection.

✚▲ Side-effects/warning: See ESMOLOL HYDROCHLORIDE.

Brevinor

(Syntex) is a proprietary, prescription-only COMPOUND PREPARATION which can be used as a (*monophasic*) ORAL CONTRACEPTIVE (and also for certain menstrual problems) of the type that combines an OESTROGEN and a PROGESTOGEN, in this case ethinyloestradiol and norethisterone. It is available as tablets in a calendar pack.

✚▲ Side-effects/warning: See ETHINYLOESTRADIOL; NORETHISTERONE.

Bricanyl

(Astra) is a proprietary, prescription-only preparation of the BETA-RECEPTOR STIMULANT terbutaline sulphate. It can be used as a BRONCHODILATOR in reversible obstructive airways disease, as an ANTI-ASTHMATIC treatment in severe acute asthma or for the alleviation of symptoms of chronic bronchitis and emphysema. It is available as tablets and modified-release tablets (*Bricanyl SA*), in a form for injection or infusion, as a metered aerosol used with a device called a *Spacer inhaler* or a *Nebuhaler*, as a breath-actuated dry powder with an inhaler called a

Turbohaler, in a single-dose nebulization solution called *Respules* and as a respirator solution (for use with a nebulizer or a ventilator). It can also be used as a means of slowing premature labour.

✚▲ Side-effects/warning: See TERBUTALINE SULPHATE.

Brietal Sodium

(Lilly) is a proprietary, prescription-only preparation of the GENERAL ANAESTHETIC methohexitone sodium. It can be used for the induction and maintainance of anaesthesia, and is available in a form for injection.

✚▲ Side-effects/warning: See METHOHEXITONE SODIUM.

Britaject

(Britannia) is a prescription-only preparation of the ANTIPARKINSONISM drug apomorphine hydrochloride. It is available in a form for injection.

✚▲ Side-effects/warning: See APOMORPHINE HYDROCHLORIDE.

Britiazim

(Thames) is a proprietary, prescription-only preparation of the CALCIUM-CHANNEL BLOCKER diltiazem hydrochloride. It can be used as an ANTIHYPERTENSIVE and ANTI-ANGINA treatment, and is available as modified-release tablets.

✚▲ Side-effects/warning: See DILTIAZEM HYDROCHLORIDE.

BritLofex

(Britannia) is a proprietary, prescription-only preparation of the recently introduced drug lofexidine hydrochloride. It can be used to alleviate the symptoms of OPIOID withdrawal, and is available as tablets.

✚▲ Side-effects/warning: See LOFEXIDINE HYDROCHLORIDE.

Broflex

(Bioglan) is a proprietary, prescription-only preparation of the ANTICHOLINERGIC benzhexol hydrochloride. It can be used in the treatment of parkinsonism to control tremors and involuntary movement, and is available as a syrup.

✚▲ Side-effects/warning: See BENZHEXOL HYDROCHLORIDE.

Brol-eze Eye Drops

(Rhône-Poulenc Rorer) is a proprietary, non-prescription preparation of the ANTI-ALLERGIC drug sodium cromoglycate. It can be used to treat allergic conjunctivitis, including when it is associated with hay fever, and is available as eye-drops.

✚▲ Side-effects/warning: See SODIUM CROMOGLYCATE.

Brolene Eye Drops

(Rhône-Poulenc Rorer) is a proprietary, non-prescription preparation of the ANTIBACTERIAL propamidine isethionate. It can be used to treat infections of the eyelids or conjunctiva (including acanthamoeba keratitis), and is available as eye-drops.

✚▲ Side-effects/warning: See PROPAMIDINE ISETHIONATE.

Brolene Eye Ointment

(Rhône-Poulenc Rorer) is a proprietary, non-prescription preparation of the ANTIBACTERIAL dibromopropamidine isethionate. It can be used to treat infections of the eyelids or conjunctiva (including acanthamoeba keratitis), and is available as an eye ointment.

✚▲ Side-effects/warning: See DIBROMOPROPAMIDINE ISETHIONATE.

bromazepam

is a BENZODIAZEPINE which is used as an ANXIOLYTIC in the short-term treatment of anxiety. Administration is oral.

✚▲ Side-effects/warning: See BENZODIAZEPINES.

❍ Related entry: Lexotan.

bromocriptine

is an ERGOT ALKALOID and is used primarily to treat parkinsonism (but not the parkinsonian symptoms caused by certain drug therapies: see ANTIPARKINSONISM). It works by stimulating the DOPAMINE receptors in the brain and so is slightly different from the more commonly used treatment with levodopa, which is converted to dopamine in the body. It is therefore particularly useful in the treatment of patients who, for one reason or another, cannot tolerate levodopa. Occasionally, the two drugs are combined. Bromocriptine has alternative uses (some related to its ability to inhibit prolactin secretion by the pituitary gland): to treat delayed puberty caused by hormonal insufficiency; to relieve certain menstrual disorders, or to reduce or halt lactation (in galactorrhoea), prolactinoma (tumour of the pituitary gland, leading to excess prolactin secretion) and to treat cyclical benign breast disease; and sometimes for treating acromegaly (over-secretion of the anterior pituitary gland due to a tumour). Administration is oral.

✚ Side-effects: There may be nausea, vomiting, headache, dizziness (especially on rising from sitting or lying down – postural hypotension), spasm in the blood vessels of the extremities and drowsiness. High dosage may cause hallucinations, a state of confusion, leg cramps and a variety of rare disorders.

▲ Warning: Do not use in hypertension or in the toxaemia of pregnancy; and in certain liver or kidney disorders. Full, regular monitoring of various body systems is essential during treatment. If the drug fails to stop lactation, women should nevertheless stop breast-feeding.

✪ Related entry: Parlodel.

brompheniramine maleate

is an ANTIHISTAMINE which is used to treat the symptoms of allergic conditions such as hay fever and urticaria, and is also used, in combination with other drugs, in the treatment of coughs. Administration is oral.

✚▲ Side-effects/warning: See ANTIHISTAMINES. Because of its sedative side-effects, the performance of skilled tasks,

such as driving, may be impaired.

✪ Related entries: Dimotane Expectorant; Dimotane Co; Dimotane Co Paediatric; Dimotapp Elixir; Dimotapp Elixir Paediatric; Dimotapp LA Tablets.

Bronalin Decongestant Elixir

(Seton) is a proprietary, non-prescription preparation of the DECONGESTANT pseudoephedrine hydrochloride. It can be used for the symptomatic relief of flu and cold symptoms, catarrh, blocked sinuses, rhinitis and hay fever, and is available as an oral liquid. It is not normally given to children under two years, except on medical advice.

✚▲ Side-effects/warning: See PSEUDOEPHEDRINE HYDROCHLORIDE.

Bronalin Dry Cough Elixir

(Seton) is a proprietary, non-prescription preparation of the ANTITUSSIVE dextromethorphan hydrobromide, the SYMPATHOMIMETIC and DECONGESTANT pseudoephedrine hydrochloride (and alcohol). It can be used for the symptomatic relief of dry, ticklish coughs and colds, and is available as an oral solution. It is not normally given to children under six years, except on medical advice.

✚▲ Side-effects/warning: See DEXTROMETHORPHAN HYDROBROMIDE; PSEUDOEPHEDRINE HYDROCHLORIDE.

Bronalin Expectorant Linctus

(Seton) is a proprietary, non-prescription preparation of the ANTIHISTAMINE diphenhydramine hydrochloride and the EXPECTORANT AMMONIUM CHLORIDE (and sodium citrate). It can be used for the symptomatic relief of dry, ticklish coughs and colds, and is available as an oral solution. It is not normally given to children under six years, except on medical advice.

✚▲ Side-effects/warning: See DIPHENHYDRAMINE HYDROCHLORIDE.

B

Bronalin Junior Linctus

(Seton) is a proprietary, non-prescription preparation of the ANTIHISTAMINE diphenhydramine hydrochloride (and sodium citrate). It can be used for the symptomatic relief of coughs and colds, and is available as an oral solution. It is not normally given to children under one year, except on medical advice.

+▲ Side-effects/warning: See DIPHENHYDRAMINE HYDROCHLORIDE.

Bronchodil

(ASTA Medica) is a proprietary, prescription-only preparation of the BETA-RECEPTOR STIMULANT reproterol hydrochloride. It can be used as a BRONCHODILATOR in reversible obstructive airways disease, as an ANTI-ASTHMATIC treatment in severe acute asthma and for the alleviation of symptoms of chronic bronchitis and emphysema. It is available as a metered aerosol inhalant.

+▲ Side-effects/warning: See REPROTEROL HYDROCHLORIDE.

bronchodilators 🗓

relax the smooth muscle of the bronchioles (air passages in the lungs), so allowing air to flow more easily in or out (the latter being the major problem in obstructive airways disease). There are a number of conditions that cause bronchospasm (spasm in the bronchial muscles) and increased secretion of mucus and hence blockage, but the most common are asthma and bronchitis. The type of drug mainly used to treat bronchospasm is a BETA-RECEPTOR STIMULANT and SYMPATHOMIMETIC drug. These drugs (eg SALBUTAMOL and TERBUTALINE SULPHATE) work by stimulating beta-adrenoceptors on the smooth muscle of the airways, which normally respond to adrenal hormones and sympathetic nerve neurotransmitters (adrenaline and noradrenaline). Other types of bronchodilator, such as the xanthine compounds AMINOPHYLLINE and THEOPHYLLINE, act directly on the smooth

muscle of the bronchioles. All these drugs are best administered directly to the airways (except in emergency situations) in the form of aerosols, ventilator sprays or nebulizing mists, because this minimizes side-effects.

Brooklax

(Intercare) is a proprietary, non-prescription preparation of the *stimulant* LAXATIVE phenolphthalein. It can be used to relieve constipation, and is available as a chocolate bar. It is not normally used for children under six years, except on medical advice.

+▲ Side-effects/warning: See PHENOLPHTHALEIN.

Brufen

(Boots) is a proprietary, prescription-only preparation of the (NSAID) NON-NARCOTIC ANALGESIC and ANTIRHEUMATIC ibuprofen. It can be used to relieve pain, particularly the pain of rheumatic disease and other musculoskeletal disorders. It is available as tablets, a syrup for dilution and effervescent granules.

+▲ Side-effects/warning: See IBUPROFEN.

Brufen Retard

(Boots) is a proprietary, prescription-only preparation of the (NSAID) NON-NARCOTIC ANALGESIC and ANTIRHEUMATIC ibuprofen. It can be used to relieve pain and inflammation, particularly the pain of rheumatic disease and other musculoskeletal disorders, and is available as modified-release tablets.

+▲ Side-effects/warning: See IBUPROFEN.

Brulidine

(Rhône-Poulenc Rorer) is a proprietary, non-prescription preparation of the ANTISEPTIC dibromopropamidine isethionate. It can be used to treat minor burns and abrasions, and is available as a cream for topical application.

+▲ Side-effects/warning: See DIBROMOPROPAMIDINE ISETHIONATE.

Brush Off Cold Sore Lotion

(Seton) is a proprietary, non-prescription preparation of the ANTISEPTIC povidone-iodine. It can be used for the treatment of cold sores, and is available as a quick-drying paint.

+▲ Side-effects/warning: See POVIDONE-IODINE.

Buccastem

(Reckitt & Coleman) is a proprietary, prescription-only preparation of prochlorperazine (as maleate). It can be used as an ANTINAUSEANT to relieve symptoms of nausea caused by the vertigo and loss of balance experienced due to infections of the inner and middle ears, or by cytotoxic drugs in the treatment of cancer. It can also be used as an ANTIPSYCHOTIC to treat schizophrenia and other psychoses and for the short-term treatment of acute anxiety. It is available as buccal tablets (placed between the upper lip and gum and left to dissolve).

+▲ Side-effects/warning: See PROCHLORPERAZINE.

buclizine hydrochloride

is an ANTIHISTAMINE which is included in a proprietary ANTIMIGRAINE treatment.

+▲ Side-effects/warning: See ANTIHISTAMINES.

✪ Related entry: Migraleve.

budesonide

is a CORTICOSTEROID with ANTI-INFLAMMATORY and ANTI-ALLERGIC properties, which is used to treat and prevent attacks of asthma, rhinitis and severe inflammatory skin disorders (eg psoriasis and eczema). Administration is by inhalation or a nasal spray, or topically as a cream or ointment. It is now also used for the induction of remission in mild to moderate Crohn's disease affecting the ileum or ascending colon, when it is administered orally.

+▲ Side-effects/warning: See BECLOMETHASONE DIPROPIONATE.

✪ Related entries: Entocort CR; Preferid; Pulmicort Inhaler; Pulmicort Respules; Pulmicort Turbohaler; Rhinocort; Rhinocort Aqua.

bumetanide

is a powerful DIURETIC, one of the class of *loop diuretics*. It can be used in ther treatment of oedema, particularly pulmonary (lung) oedema in patients with left ventricular or chronic heart failure, and low urine production due to kidney failure (oliguria). Administration is either oral or by injection.

+▲ Side-effects/warning: See FRUSEMIDE; there may also be muscle pain.

✪ Related entries: Burinex; Burinex K.

bupivacaine hydrochloride

is a LOCAL ANAESTHETIC with a long duration of action. It is an amide and chemically related to lignocaine hydrochloride, but is particularly long lasting. It is commonly used for spinal anaesthesia, including epidural injection (especially during labour) and also for nerve block and by local infiltration. Administration is by injection.

+▲ Side-effects/warning: See LIGNOCAINE HYDROCHLORIDE. Heart depression may be more severe.

✪ Related entries: Marcain; Marcain with Adrenaline.

buprenorphine

is a NARCOTIC ANALGESIC, an OPIOID, which is long-acting (its effects last longer than morphine) and used to treat moderate to severe pain, including during surgical operations. Preparations of buprenorphine are on the Controlled Drugs List, because it can cause dependence (addiction). It has some OPIOID ANTAGONIST properties and so may be dangerous to use in combination with other narcotic analgesics, and can precipitate withdrawal symptoms in those habituated to, for instance, morphine or diamorphine. Administration is either oral as tablets placed sublingually (under the tongue) or by injection.

✚▲ Side-effect/warning: See OPIOIDS. It may cause vomiting.
○ Related entry: Temgesic.

Burinex

(Leo) is a proprietary, prescription-only preparation of the (*loop*) DIURETIC bumetanide. It can be used to treat oedema, particularly pulmonary (lung) oedema in patients with left ventricular or chronic heart failure and low urine production due to kidney failure (oliguria). It is available as tablets, an oral liquid and in a form for injection.
✚▲ Side-effects/warning: See BUMETANIDE.

Burinex K

(Leo) is a proprietary, prescription-only COMPOUND PREPARATION of the (*loop*) DIURETIC bumetanide and the potassium supplement POTASSIUM CHLORIDE. It can be used to treat oedema, for instance in congestive heart failure and low urine production due to kidney failure (oliguria). It is available as tablets, which should be swallowed whole with plenty of fluid at mealtimes or when in an upright posture.
✚▲ Side-effects/warning: See BUMETANIDE.

Buscopan

(Boehringer Ingelheim) is a proprietary, prescription-only preparation of the ANTICHOLINERGIC hyoscine butylbromide, which can be used as an ANTISPASMODIC to treat colic and dysmenorrhoea. It is available as tablets and in a form for injection. (The tablets, which are available from Windsor, can also be obtained without a prescription under certain conditions.)
✚▲ Side-effects/warning: See HYOSCINE BUTYLBROMIDE.

buserelin

is an analogue of the hypothalamic HORMONE GONADORELIN (gonadothrophin-releasing hormone; GnRH). It reduces secretion of gonadotrophin by the pituitary gland, which results in reduced secretion of sex hormones by the ovaries or testes.

Buserelin is used to treat endometriosis and as an ANTICANCER drug to treat cancer of the prostate gland. It is also used prior to *in vitro* fertilization. Administration (as buserelin acetate) is by injection or as a nasal spray (because it is absorbed into the systemic circulation from the nasal mucosa).
✚ Side-effects: In women: there may be menstruation-like and breakthrough bleeding and symptoms similar to the menopause (sweating, hot flushes, palpitations, vaginal dryness). There may be mood changes; back, muscle and abdominal pain; changes to breast size and tenderness; acne and dry skin; nervousness, tiredness and sleep disturbances; ovarian cysts; skin disturbances (eg rashes); constipation; blurred vision; vaginal discharge; tingling and sensitivity in fingers and toes; and changes in body hair. In men: there may be bone pain; hot flushes; nausea and diarrhoea; occasional increase in breast size. In men and women: there may be changes in libido; dizziness; vomiting; headache. There may be irritation on using the nasal spray.
▲ Warning: Do not use in pregnancy or when breast-feeding, or where there is vaginal bleeding of unknown origin. Some men initially experience increased tumour growth, to the extent even of compressing the spinal cord and additional drugs may be necessary to counteract this.
○ Related entries: Suprecur; Suprefact.

Buspar

(Bristol-Myers) is a proprietary, prescription-only preparation of the recently introduced ANXIOLYTIC buspirone hydrochloride. It can be used for the short-term treatment of anxiety, and is available as tablets.
✚▲ Side-effects/warning: See BUSPIRONE HYDROCHLORIDE.

buspirone hydrochloride

is a recently introduced ANXIOLYTIC which is thought to work by stimulating SEROTONIN

receptors in the brain. It can be used for
the short-term treatment of anxiety.
Administration is oral.

✚ Side-effects: Nausea, dizziness, headache,
nervousness, excitement, light-headedness;
rarely, increase in heart rate, palpitations,
chest pain, drowsiness, dry mouth,
confusion, fatigue or sweating.

▲ Warning: It should not be given to
patients with epilepsy, severe liver or
kidney impairment; or who are pregnant or
breast-feeding. It may impair the
performance of skilled tasks, such as
driving; avoid alcohol because its effects are
enhanced.

❂ Related entry: Buspar.

busulphan

is a CYTOTOXIC drug which is used as an
ANTICANCER treatment, particularly for
chronic myeloid leukaemia. It works by
direct interference with the DNA.
Administration is oral.

✚▲ Side-effects/warning: See CYTOTOXICS.
However, it should not be administered to
patients with porphyria.

❂ Related entry: Myleran.

Butacote

(Geigy) is a proprietary, prescription-only
preparation of the (NSAID) NON-NARCOTIC
ANALGESIC and ANTIRHEUMATIC
phenylbutazone. Because of its sometimes
severe side-effects, it is used solely in the
treatment of ankylosing spondylitis under
medical supervision in hospitals.
Administration is oral.

✚▲ Side-effects/warning: See
PHENYLBUTAZONE.

butobarbitone

is a BARBITURATE which is used only when
absolutely necessary as a HYPNOTIC to treat
severe and intractable insomnia.
Administration is oral. Preparations
containing butobarbitone are on the
Controlled Drugs List.

✚▲ Side-efects/warning: See BARBITURATES.
❂ Related entry: Soneryl.

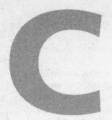

C-Film

(FP) is a proprietary, non-prescription
SPERMICIDAL CONTRACEPTIVE for use in
combination with barrier methods of
contraception (such as a condom). It is
available as a film containing nonoxinol.

✚▲ Side-effects/warning: See NONOXINOL.

cabergoline

is a recently introduced drug with
properties similar to bromocriptine, for
which it may be substituted if one or the
other is not tolerated. There are more
established drugs for ANTIPARKINSONISM, but
for uses in hormonal disorders see
bromocriptine. Administration is oral.

✚▲ Side-effects/warning: See
BROMOCRIPTINE. The side-effects are
somewhat different and there may be
gastrointestinal and epigastric pain and
other side-effects. Do not use in pregnancy.

❂ Related entry: Dostinex.

Cafergot

(Sandoz) is a proprietary, prescription-only
COMPOUND PREPARATION of the
VASOCONSTRICTOR ergotamine tartrate and the
STIMULANT caffeine. It can be used as an
ANTIMIGRAINE treatment for acute attacks,
and is available as tablets and
suppositories.

✚▲ Side-effects/warning: See CAFFEINE;
ERGOTAMINE TARTRATE.

caffeine

is a weak STIMULANT, which is present in tea,
coffee and some soft drinks. It is also

included in many analgesic preparations, partly in the belief that it speeds absorption.

✚ Side-effects: Excessive doses may cause headache, either directly or on withdrawal, and also anxiety.

○ Related entries: Actron; Anadin Analgesic Tablets; Anadin Analgesic Capsules, Maximum Strength; Anadin Extra; Anadin Extra Soluble Tablets; Askit Powders; Beechams Powders; Beechams Powders Capsules; Cafergot; Catarrh-Ex; Cojene Tablets; Cold Relief Capsules; Coldrex Tablets; Do-Do Chesteze; Doloxene Compound; Dristan Decongestant Tablets; Feminax; Flurex Tablets; Hedex Extra Tablets; Lemsip Cold Relief Capsules; Migril; Nurse Sykes Powders; Panadol Extra Soluble Tablets; Panadol Extra Tablets; Phensic; Powerin Analgesic Tablets; Propain Tablets; Solpadeine Capsules; Solpadeine Soluble Tablets; Solpadeine Tablets; Syndol.

Calabren

(Berk) is a proprietary, prescription-only preparation of the SULPHONYLUREA glibenclamide. It can be used in DIABETIC TREATMENT of Type II diabetes (non-insulin-dependent diabetes mellitus; NIDDM; maturity-onset diabetes) and works by augmenting what remains of INSULIN production in the pancreas. It is available as tablets.

✚▲ Side-effects/warning: See GLIBENCLAMIDE.

Caladryl Cream

(Warner Wellcome) is a proprietary, non-prescription COMPOUND PREPARATION of the ANTIHISTAMINE diphenhydramine hydrochloride, CAMPHOR and ZINC OXIDE. It can be used for the relief of skin irritation associated with urticaria, herpes, minor skin afflictions, insect bites, nettle sting and sunburn.

✚▲ Side-effects/warning: See DIPHENHYDRAMINE HYDROCHLORIDE.

Caladryl Lotion

(Warner Wellcome) is a proprietary, non-

prescription COMPOUND PREPARATION of the ANTIHISTAMINE diphenhydramine hydrochloride, CAMPHOR and ZINC OXIDE. It can be used for the relief of skin irritation associated with urticaria, herpes, minor skin afflictions, insect bites, nettle sting and sunburn.

✚▲ Side-effects/warning: See DIPHENHYDRAMINE HYDROCHLORIDE.

calamine

is a suspension containing mainly (basic) zinc carbonate (with added ferric oxide) and has a mild ASTRINGENT action. It is incorporated into several preparations that are used to cool and soothe itching skin in conditions such as pruritus, eczema and psoriasis, and is also used in some EMOLLIENT preparations. Adminsitration is by topical application.

○ Related entries: Calamine and Coal Tar Ointment, BP; Calamine Cream, Aqueous, BP; Calamine Lotion, Aqueous, BP; Hydrocal; Vasogen Cream.

Calamine and Coal Tar Ointment, BP

is a non-proprietary, non-prescription COMPOUND PREPARATION of CALAMINE and coal tar. It can be used by topical application to treat chronic eczema and psoriasis and to relieve itching. It is available as an ointment.

✚▲ Side-effects/warning: See COAL TAR.

Calamine Cream, Aqueous, BP

is a non-proprietary, non-prescription COMPOUND PREPARATION which consists of a suspension of zinc carbonate, zinc oxide, liquid paraffin and other constituents. It is used to cool and soothe itching skin, and is available as a cream.

Calamine Lotion, Aqueous, BP

is a a non-proprietary, non-prescription COMPOUND PREPARATION which consists of a suspension of zinc carbonate, zinc oxide, liquid paraffin and other constituents. It is used to cool and soothe itching skin, and is available as a lotion.

Calcicard CR

(Norton) is a proprietary, prescription-only preparation of the CALCIUM-CHANNEL BLOCKER diltiazem hydrochloride. It can be used as an ANTIHYPERTENSIVE for angina treatment, and is available as tablets.
+▲ Side-effects/warning: See DILTIAZEM HYDROCHLORIDE.

calciferol

see ERGOCALCIFEROL

Calcijex

(Abbott) is a proprietary, prescription-only preparation of calcitriol, which is a VITAMIN D analogue, and can be used in vitamin D deficiency. It is available in a form for injection.
+▲ Side-effects/warning: See CALCITRIOL.

Calcilat

(Eastern) is a proprietary, prescription-only preparation of the CALCIUM-CHANNEL BLOCKER nifedipine. It can be used as an ANTI-ANGINA treatment in the prevention of attacks, as an ANTIHYPERTENSIVE and as a VASODILATOR in peripheral vascular disease (Raynaud's phenomenon). It is available as capsules.
+▲ Side-effects/warning: See NIFEDIPINE.

Calciparine

(Sanofi Winthrop) is a proprietary, prescription-only preparation of the ANTICOAGULANT heparin calcium. It can be used to treat various forms of thrombosis, and is available in a form for injection.
+▲ Side-effects/warning: See HEPARIN.

calcipotriol

is used to treat chronic or milder forms of psoriasis. It is available as a cream ointment and a scalp solution for topical application.
+ Side-effects: Local irritation, various skin irritations (itching, dermatitis, reddening,

photosensitivity); raised blood calcium.
▲ Warning: Do not use in patients with disorders of calcium metabolism. Administer with caution during pregnancy; avoid contact with the face.
✪ Related entry: Dovonex.

Calcisorb

(3M) is a proprietary, non-prescription preparation of sodium cellulose phosphate. It can be used to help reduce high calcium levels in the bloodstream by inhibiting calcium absorption from food. It is available as sachets of powder for solution in water or to sprinkle over food.
+▲ Side-effects/warning: See SODIUM CELLULOSE PHOSPHATE.

Calcitare

(Rhône-Poulenc Rorer) is a proprietary, prescription-only preparation of the THYROID HORMONE calcitonin. It can be used to lower blood levels of calcium when they are abnormally high (hypercalcaemia) and to treat Paget's disease of the bone. It is available in a form for injection.
+▲ Side-effects/warning: See CALCITONIN.

calcitonin

is a THYROID HORMONE produced and secreted by the thyroid gland at the base of the neck. Its function is to lower the levels of calcium and phosphate in the blood and together with the correspondingly opposite action of a parathyroid hormone (parathormone) regulates these levels. Therapeutically, calcitonin is used to lower blood levels of calcium when they are abnormally high (hypercalcaemia), to treat Paget's disease of the bone and when there is cancer. Administration is by injection. It is available in the porcine form and the salmon form (referred to as SALCATONIN).
+ Side-effects: There may be nausea, vomiting and flushing; there may also be a tingling sensation in the hands, a peculiar taste in the mouth and inflammation at the site of injection.
▲ Warning: Prolonged use of calcitonin

C

derived from animals may eventually lead to the body producing antibodies against it and consequent neutralization of its effect. Some patients may become hypersensitive to animal calcitonin. It should be used with caution in pregnant women and not at all by those who are breast-feeding.
○ Related entry: Calcitare.

calcitriol

(1,25-dihydroxycholecalciferol) is a synthesized form of vitamin D which is used to make up vitamin D deficiency in the body, particularly in the treatment of certain forms of hypoparathyroidism and rickets. Administration is oral.
✚▲ Side-effects/warning: See VITAMIN D.
○ Related entries: Calcijex, Rocaltrol.

calcium

is a metallic element essential for normal growth and development, especially (in the form of calcium phosphate) of the bones and teeth. Its level in blood is regulated by the opposing actions of the thyroid hormone CALCITONIN and the parathyroid HORMONE parathormone. Its uptake from food is enhanced by vitamin D (calciferol). Good food sources include most dairy products. Salts of calcium used therapeutically include the ANTACID calcium carbonate, the folinic acid supplement calcium folinate, the MINERAL SUPPLEMENTS calcium gluconate and calcium lactate.
▲ Warning: Deficiency of vitamin D leads to calcium deficiency and corresponding bone, blood and nerve and muscle disorders. Conversely, excess calcium in the body may cause the formation of stones (calculi, generally composed of calcium oxalate), particularly in the kidney or gall bladder.
○ Related entries: Calcium-500; calcium and ergocalciferol tablets; calcium carbonate; calcium folinate; Calcium-Sandoz; Ossopan; Sandocal.

calcium and ergocalciferol tablets

is a non-proprietary, non-prescription COMPOUND PREPARATION of the VITAMIN ergocalciferol (vitamin D_2) and CALCIUM (in the form of calcium lactate and calcium phosphate). It can be used as a MINERAL SUPPLEMENT in the treatment of nutritional or absorptive deficiencies.
✚▲ Side-effects/warning: See CALCIUM; ERGOCALCIFEROL.

calcium antagonists

see CALCIUM-CHANNEL BLOCKERS

calcium carbonate

or chalk, is used therapeutically as an ANTACID. It is incorporated into many proprietary preparations that are used to relieve hyperacidity, dyspepsia and for the symptomatic relief of heartburn and symptoms of peptic ulcer in the treatment of peptic ulcers. It is also used by mouth in the treatment of hyperphosphataemia (abnormally raised levels of phosphates in the blood). Administration is oral.
✚ Side-effects: Treatment with calcium carbonate as an antacid may cause belching (due to carbon dioxide).
▲ Warning: Its prolonged use as an antacid can induce tolerance and eventually cause renewed acid secretion. There may also be abnormally high levels of calcium in the blood. Antacids may impair the absorption of other drugs.
○ Related entries: Andrews Antacid; Bismag Tablets; Bisodol Antacid Tablets; Bisodol Extra Tablets; Calcium-500; Calcium-Sandoz; Didronel PMO; Eno; Fynnon Calcium Aspirin; Gaviscon Liquid; J Collis Browne's Tablets; Maclean Indigestion Tablets; Nulacin Tablets; Original Andrews Salts; Ossopan; Remegel Original; Rennie Rap-Eze; Rennie Tablets, Digestif; Sandocal; Setlers Tablets Peppermint Flavour.

calcium folinate

is the usual form in which folinic acid (a derivative of folic acid, which is a vitamin of the VITAMIN B complex) is administered as a supplement to patients who are susceptible to some of the toxic effects caused by the folate-antagonist activity of certain anticancer drugs, especially METHOTREXATE. Administration is oral.

+▲ Side-effects/warning: See FOLINIC ACID.

Calcium Leucovorin

(Lederle) is a proprietary, prescription-only preparation of folinic acid, which can be used to counteract the toxic effects of certain anticancer drugs, especially METHOTREXATE. It is available as tablets and in a form for injection.

+▲ Side-effects/warning: See FOLINIC ACID.

calcium metabolism modifiers ?

alter the metabolism and therefore the levels of CALCIUM in the body. Calcium has an important role in most body processes and there are many ways in which it can be disrupted in disease. *Parathyroid hormone* (parathormone, see THYROID HORMONES) is a HORMONE secreted by the parathyroid gland, and increases the concentration of calcium in the blood. CALCITONIN is a hormone from the thyroid gland (and is unrelated to THYROXINE). It lowers calcium levels in the blood, and its action is balanced in the body by corresponding opposite action of parathormone from the adjacent parathyroid gland. Calcitonin is used in therapeutics to lower blood levels of calcium when they are abnormally high (hypercalcaemia), to treat Paget's disease of the bone and for some sorts of cancer. It works by reducing calcium uptake by bone. Preparations for clinical use include natural porcine (pig) calcitonin and synthetic SALCATONIN (salmon calcitonin). It is also becoming available in the synthetic human form.

Vitamin D (used as synthetic CALCITRIOL) acts with parathormone to mobilize bone calcium and by increasing calcium absorption from the intestine. Vitamin D occurs in a number of natural forms, including CHOLECALCIFEROL (D_3) and ERGOCALCIFEROL (D_2). It increases the absorption of calcium (and, to a lesser extent, phosphorus) from the intestine, to deposit it in the bones. A deficiency of vitamin D therefore results in bone deficiency disorders, eg rickets in children. Therapeutic replacement of vitamin D in cases of severe deficiency requires quantities of the vitamin best provided by one of the synthetic vitamin D analogues such as ALFACALCIDOL and DIHYDROTACHYSTEROL.

Calcium forms used therapeutically to counter too low levels, include the FOLINIC ACID supplement CALCIUM FOLINATE, and the mineral supplements CALCIUM CARBONATE, CALCIUM GLUCONATE, CALCIUM LACTATE and CALCIUM BICARBONATE.

A drug series that chemically are *bisphosphonates* (diphosphonates) are used to treat a number of conditions of disturbed calcium metabolism, including Paget's disease of the bone, malignant hypercalcaemia, osteoporosis, and are being evaluated for use in treating bone pain associated cancer metastases of the bone. These drugs include DISODIUM ETIDRONATE, DISODIUM PAMIDRONATE and SODIUM CHLODRONATE. Also, OESTROGENS are used in prevention of post-menopausal osteoporosis.

Calcium Resonium

(Sanofi Winthrop) is a proprietary, non-prescription preparation of calcium polystyrene sulphonate, which is a resin that can be used to treat high blood potassium levels, particularly in patients who suffer from fluid retention or undergo kidney dialysis. It is available in the form of a powdered resin for use as a rectal enema or by mouth.

+▲ Side-effects/warning: See POLYSTYRENE SULPHONATE RESINS.

Calcium-500

(Renacare) is a proprietary, non-prescription preparation of calcium carbonate. It can be used as a MINERAL SUPPLEMENT for calcium in cases of deficiency, and is available as tablets.

C

+▲ Side-effects/warning: See CALCIUM CARBONATE.

calcium-channel blockers ⚕

(calcium antagonists; calcium-entry blockers) is a quite a recently introduced class of drugs which are being increasingly used in therapeutics. They work by blocking the entry of calcium through channels (specialized 'pores' in a cell's membrane) that admit calcium ions from the fluid surrounding cells to the interior of the cell. Since calcium has very profound activities within cells (for instance, increasing muscle contraction and electrical excitability), these drugs have powerful effects on cell function. Their main uses include: a direct SMOOTH MUSCLE RELAXANT action causing dilation of blood vessels and effects on heart muscle, which has led to their widespread therapeutic use as ANTIHYPERTENSIVES (eg AMLODIPINE BESYLATE, ISRADIPINE, NICARDIPINE HYDROCHLORIDE, NIFEDIPINE and VERAPAMIL HYDROCHLORIDE); as an ANTI-ANGINA treatment (eg amlodipine besylate, DILTIAZEM HYDROCHLORIDE, nicardipine hydrochloride, nifedipine and verapamil hydrochloride); as ANTI-ARRHYTHMIC agents (eg verapamil hydrochloride); as VASODILATORS to treat peripheral vascular disease – Raynaud's phenomenon (eg nifedipine); in the prevention of damage to the brain due to ischaemia (lack of blood supply) following subarachnoid haemorrhage (bleeding from blood vessels supplying the outer surface of the brain) (eg NIMODIPINE); and as an ANTIMIGRAINE treatment to prevent attacks (eg nifedipine and verapamil hydrochloride).

calcium-entry blockers

see CALCIUM-CHANNEL BLOCKERS

Calcium-Sandoz

(Sandoz) is a proprietary, non-prescription preparation of calcium glubionate and calcium lactobionate. It can be used as a MINERAL SUPPLEMENT for calcium in cases of

calcium deficiency, and is available as a syrup and in a form for injection.
+▲ Side-effects/warning: See CALCIUM CARBONATE.

Calcort

(Hoechst Matior Roussel) is a proprietary, prescription-only preparation of the CORTICOSTEROID deflazacort. It can be used as an ANTI-INFLAMMATORY treatment for the suppression of inflammatory and allergic conditions, and is available as tablets.
+▲ Side-effects/warning: See DEFLAZACORT.

Calfig California Syrup of Figs

(SmithKline Beecham) is a proprietary, non-prescription preparation of the (*stimulant*) LAXATIVE senna. It can be used for the relief of constipation, and is available as a viscous liquid. It is not normally given to children under one year, except on medical advice.
+▲ Side-effects/warning: See SENNA.

Calgel Teething Gel

(Warner Wellcome) is a proprietary, non-prescription COMPOUND PREPARATION of the LOCAL ANAESTHETIC lignocaine hydrochloride and the ANTISEPTIC cetylpyridinium chloride. It can be used for the temporary relief of pain caused by teething in babies, and is available as a gel for topical application.
+▲ Side-effects/warning: See CETYLPYRIDINIUM CHLORIDE; LIGNOCAINE HYDROCHLORIDE.

Calimal

(Sussex) is a proprietary, non-prescription preparation of the ANTIHISTAMINE chlorpheniramine maleate. It can be used to treat allergic conditions such as hay fever, food allergies and urticaria, and is available as tablets. It is not normally given to children under six years, except on medical advice.
+▲ Side-effects/warning: See CHLORPHENIRAMINE MALEATE.

C

Calmurid

(Novex) is a proprietary, non-prescription COMPOUND PREPARATION of lactic acid and the HYDRATING AGENT urea. It can be used for dry, scaly or hard skin, and is available as a cream.

Calmurid HC

(Novex) is a proprietary, prescription-only COMPOUND PREPARATION of the CORTICOSTEROID and ANTI-INFLAMMATORY drug hydrocortisone and the HYDRATING AGENT urea (in combination with lactic acid). It can be administered as a treatment for mild inflammation of the skin caused by conditions such as eczema, and is available as a cream for topical application to the affected area.

✚▲ Side-effects/warning: See HYDROCORTISONE.

Calpol Infant Suspension

(Warner Wellcome) is a proprietary, non-prescription preparation of the NON-NARCOTIC ANALGESIC paracetamol. It can be administered to treat mild to moderate pain (including teething pain) and as an ANTIPYRETIC (for instance, to reduce fever after vaccination, when it can be used in two-month-old babies). It is available as a liquid suspension and is not normally given to infants under three months, except on medical advice.

✚▲ Side-effects/warning: See PARACETAMOL.

Calpol Infant Suspension, Sugar-Free

(Warner Wellcome) is a proprietary, non-prescription preparation of the NON-NARCOTIC ANALGESIC paracetamol. It can be administered to treat mild to moderate pain (including teething pain) and as an ANTIPYRETIC (for instance, to reduce fever after vaccination, when it can be used in two-month-old babies). It is available as a liquid suspension and is not normally given to infants under three months, except on medical advice.

✚▲ Side-effects/warning: See PARACETAMOL.

Calpol Six Plus Suspension

(Warner Wellcome) is a proprietary, non-prescription preparation of the NON-NARCOTIC ANALGESIC and ANTIPYRETIC paracetamol. It can be administered to treat mild to moderate pain and to reduce fever in children. However, it is not normally given to children under six years, except on medical advice. It is available in the form of a liquid suspension; a form called *Calpol Six Plus Sugar Free/Colour Free Suspension* is also available.

✚▲ Side-effects/warning: See PARACETAMOL.

Calsynar

(Rhône-Poulenc Rorer) is a proprietary, prescription-only preparation of the THYROID HORMONE calcitonin, in the form of salcatonin. It can be used to lower blood levels of calcium when they are abnormally high (hypercalcaemia) and to treat Paget's disease of the bone. It is available in a form for injection.

✚▲ Side-effects/warning: See SALCATONIN.

CAM

(Rybar) is a proprietary, prescription-only preparation of the BETA-RECEPTOR STIMULANT ephedrine hydrochloride. It can be used as a BRONCHODILATOR in reversible obstructive airways disease and as an ANTI-ASTHMATIC treatment in severe acute asthma. It is available as a sugar-free mixture.

✚▲ Side-effects/warning: See EPHEDRINE HYDROCHLORIDE.

Camcolit 250

(Norgine) is a proprietary, prescription-only preparation of the ANTIMANIA drug lithium (as lithium carbonate). It can be used to prevent and treat mania and manic-depressive bouts, and is available as tablets.

✚▲ Side-effects/warning: See LITHIUM.

Camcolit 400

(Norgine) is a proprietary, prescription-only preparation of the ANTIMANIA drug lithium (as lithium carbonate). It can be used to prevent and treat mania and manic-

C

depressive bouts, and is available as tablets.
+▲ Side-effects/warning: See LITHIUM.

camphor

is an aromatic substance with mild COUNTER-IRRITANT, or RUBEFACIENT, properties. It is incorporated into a number of topical preparations that are used to help relieve itchiness and also for the symptomatic relief of muscular pains and rheumatism, fibrosis, lumbago, sciatica and skin irritation.

○ Related entries: Aspellin; Balmosa Cream; Caladryl Cream; Caladryl Lotion; Nicobrevin; PR Heat Spray; Radian B Heat Spray; Radian B Muscle Lotion; Radian B Muscle Rub.

Camsilon

(Cambridge) is a proprietary, prescription-only preparation of the ANTICHOLINESTERASE drug edrophonium chloride. It can be used in the diagnosis of myasthenia gravis and at the termination of operations to reverse the actions of neuromuscular blocking agents (when it is often administered with atropine sulphate). It is available in a form for injection. (This preparation was formerly known as *Tensilon*.)
+▲ Side-effects/warning: See EDROPHONIUM CHLORIDE.

Canesten

(Bayer) is the name of several proprietary preparations of the ANTIFUNGAL drug clotrimazole. They can be used to treat fungal infections, particularly vaginal candidiasis (thrush) and skin infections such as nappy rash and balanitis (infection of the glans penis). The preparations are available in several forms and strengths, including a skin cream, a dusting powder, a vaginal cream, vaginal tablets (pessaries) and a *Duopak* that contains vaginal tablets and a cream. Most of these products are now available on a non-prescription basis for stated conditions, though their use will generally follow medical diagnosis, but *Caneston-HC* is available only on

prescription. The various preparations are detailed under separate headings.
+▲ Side-effects/warning: See CLOTRIMAZOLE.

Canesten 1%

(Bayer) is a proprietary, non-prescription preparation of the ANTIFUNGAL drug clotrimazole. It can be used to treat fungal and *Candida* skin infections, including *Candida* nappy rash, vulvitis and balanitis (infection of the glans penis). It is available as a cream for topical application.
+▲ Side-effects/warning: See CLOTRIMAZOLE.

Canesten 1 VT

(Bayer) is a proprietary, non-prescription preparation of the ANTIFUNGAL drug clotrimazole. It can be used particularly to treat vaginal candidiasis (thrush), and is available as vaginal tablets (pessaries). It is not normally given to children, except on medical advice.
+▲ Side-effects/warning: See CLOTRIMAZOLE.

Canesten 10% VC

(Bayer) is a proprietary, non-prescription preparation of the ANTIFUNGAL drug clotrimazole. It can be used particularly to treat vaginal candiasis (thrush), and is available as a vaginal cream to be inserted through a special applicator. It is not normally given to children, except on medical advice.
+▲ Side-effects/warning: See CLOTRIMAZOLE.

Canesten-HC

(Bayer) is a proprietary, prescription-only COMPOUND PREPARATION of the CORTICOSTEROID hydrocortisone and the ANTIFUNGAL drug clotrimazole. It can be used to treat fungal infections, particularly those associated with inflammation, and is available as a cream for topical application.
+▲ Side-effects/warning: See CLOTRIMAZOLE; HYDROCORTISONE.

Cantil

(Boehringer Mannheim) is a proprietary, prescription-only preparation of the ANTICHOLINERGIC mepenzolate bromide. It can be used as an ANTISPASMODIC for the symptomatic relief of smooth muscle spasm in the gastrointestinal tract, and is available as tablets.

✚▲ Side-effects/warning: See MEPENZOLATE BROMIDE.

Capasal

(Dermal) is a proprietary, non-prescription COMPOUND PREPARATION of coal tar and salicylic acid (with coconut oil). It can be used for conditions such as dandruff and psoriasis of the scalp, and is available as a shampoo.

✚▲ Side-effects/warning: See COAL TAR; SALICYLIC ACID.

Capastat

(Dista) is a proprietary, prescription-only preparation of the ANTIBIOTIC and ANTITUBERCULAR drug capreomycin (as capreomycin sulphate). It can be administered to treat tuberculosis that is resistant to other drugs, and is available in a form for injection.

✚▲ Side-effects/warning: See CAPREOMYCIN.

Caplenal

(Berk) is a proprietary, prescription-only preparation of the ENZYME INHIBITOR allopurinol, which is a XANTHINE-OXIDASE INHIBITOR. It can be used to treat excess uric acid in the blood and to prevent renal stones and attacks of gout. It is available as tablets.

✚▲ Side-effects/warning: See ALLOPURINOL.

Capoten

(Squibb) is a proprietary, prescription-only preparation of the ACE INHIBITOR captopril. It can be used as an ANTIHYPERTENSIVE and in HEART FAILURE TREATMENT, usually in conjunction with other classes of drug. It is available as tablets.

✚▲ Side-effects/warning: See CAPTOPRIL.

Capozide

(Squibb) is a proprietary, prescription-only COMPOUND PREPARATION of the ACE INHIBITOR captopril and the DIURETIC hydrochlorothiazide. It can be used as an ANTIHYPERTENSIVE, and is available as tablets.

✚▲ Side-effects/warning: See CAPTOPRIL; HYDROCHLOROTHIAZIDE.

capreomycin

is an ANTIBACTERIAL and ANTIBIOTIC drug. It is used specifically in the treatment of tuberculosis that proves to be resistant to the first-line drugs (see ANTITUBERCULAR), or in cases where those drugs are not tolerated. Administration is by injection in combination with other drugs.

✚ Side-effects: There may be kidney toxicity and impaired hearing with or without tinnitus or vertigo; sometimes there are sensitivity reactions such as rashes or urticaria and blood changes.

▲ Warning: It should not be administered to patients who are pregnant; administer with caution to those who have impaired liver or kidney function or sense of hearing (functions that should be monitored during treatment), or who are already taking other ototoxic antibiotics, or who are breast-feeding.

❂ Related entry: Capastat.

Caprin

(Sinclair) is a proprietary, non-prescription preparation of the (NSAID) NON-NARCOTIC ANALGESIC and ANTIRHEUMATIC aspirin. It can be used to treat headache and rheumatic conditions, and is available as modified-release tablets. It is not normally given to children, except on medical advice.

✚▲ Side-effects/warning: See ASPIRIN.

capsaicin

is the active principle of capsicum, which is often used medically in the form of the resin called CAPSICUM OLEORESIN and is a pungent extract from capsicum peppers. Both capsicum resin and capsaicin are incorporated into medicines with

C

RUBEFACIENT, or COUNTER-IRRITANT, action, and when rubbed in topically to the skin cause a feeling of warmth that offsets the pain from underlying muscles, joints or internal organs.

capsicum oleoresin

or capsicum resin, is a pungent extract from capsicum peppers. The active principle of these 'hot' peppers, which are also used for culinary purposes as chilli and cayenne pepper, is CAPSAICIN. Both capsicum resin and capsaicin are incorporated into medicines with RUBEFACIENT, or COUNTER-IRRITANT, action, and when rubbed in topically to the skin, cause a feeling of warmth that offsets the pain from underlying muscles, joints or internal organs.

✚ Side-effects: There may be local irritation.

▲ Warning: It should not be used on inflamed or broken skin, or on mucous membranes. Keep away from the eyes.

⊙ Related entries: Algipan Rub; Axsain; Balmosa Cream; Cremalgin Balm; Radian B Muscle Rub; Ralgex Cream; Ralgex Stick.

captopril

is an ACE INHIBITOR. It is a powerful VASODILATOR which can be used as an ANTIHYPERTENSIVE and in HEART FAILURE TREATMENT. It is often used in conjunction with other classes of drug, particularly (THIAZIDE) DIURETICS. Additionally, it can be used following myocardial infarction (damage to heart muscle, usually after a heart attack) and in diabetic nephropathy (kidney disease) in insulin-dependent diabetes. Administration is oral.

✚ Side-effects: Hypotension; headache and fatigue; nausea and vomiting; diarrhoea or constipation, abdominal pain and dyspepsia; muscle cramps; dry cough and sore throat with voice changes; loss of taste and body weight; skin rash and itching; impaired kidney function with high blood potassium; blood disorders. A number of other, rarer, side-effects have been reported.

▲ Warning: There may be a rapid initial drop in blood pressure. It should not be given to patients who are breast-feeding, or have porphyria or renovascular disease.

⊙ Related entries: Capoten; Capozide.

Carace

(Du Pont) is a proprietary, prescription-only preparation of the ACE INHIBITOR lisinopril. It can be used as an ANTIHYPERTENSIVE and in HEART FAILURE TREATMENT, and is available as tablets.

✚▲ Side-effects/warning: See LISINOPRIL.

Carace Plus

(Du Pont) is a proprietary, prescription-only COMPOUND PREPARATION of the ACE INHIBITOR lisinopril and the DIURETIC hydrochlorothiazide. It can be used as an ANTIHYPERTENSIVE, and is available as tablets (*Carace 10 Plus* and *Carace 20 Plus*).

✚▲ Side-effects/warning: See HYDROCHLOROTHIAZIDE; LISINOPRIL.

carbachol

is a PARASYMPATHOMIMETIC drug which is used in GLAUCOMA TREATMENT to lower pressure in the eyeball (while constricting the pupil) and to treat urinary retention (particularly following surgery). Administration can be oral, topical or by injection.

✚▲ Side-effects/warning: See BETHANECHOL CHLORIDE.

⊙ Related entry: Isopto Carbachol.

Carbalax

(Pharmax) is a proprietary, non-prescription preparation of the (*osmotic*) LAXATIVE sodium acid phosphate. It can be used to relieve constipation and to evacuate the rectum prior to abdominal procedures, and is available as an effervescent suppository.

✚▲ Side-effects/warning: See SODIUM ACID PHOSPHATE.

carbamazepine

is an ANTICONVULSANT and ANTI-EPILEPTIC drug

which is used in the preventive treatment of most forms of epilepsy (except absence seizures), to relieve the pain of trigeminal neuralgia (a searing pain from the trigeminal nerve in the face), in the management of manic-depressive illness resistant to lithium and in the treatment of diabetes insipidus. Administration is either oral or by suppositories.

✚ Side-effects: There are many and include blood, liver and skin disorders, nausea and vomiting, dizziness, drowsiness, headache, unsteady gait, confusion and agitation (particularly in the elderly), visual disturbances, constipation or diarrhoea, anorexia, kidney failure, hair loss, effect on the heart, growth of breasts in men, impotence, aggression and depression.

▲ Warning: It should not be administered to patients who suffer from certain heart defects, porphyria or bone marrow depression. Use with caution in those with impaired liver, kidney or heart function, a history of blood reactions to other drugs, glaucoma or who are pregnant or breast-feeding. Seek medical advice if fever, bruising, sore throat, rash or mouth ulcers occur.

🟐 Related entries: Epimaz; Tegretol.

carbaryl

is a PEDICULICIDAL drug which is used in the treatment of head lice and crab lice. Administration, as an aqueous or alcohol solution, is either as a lotion or a shampoo.

✚ Side-effects: Skin irritation.

▲ Warning: Avoid contact with the eyes and broken or infected skin. It should not be used by asthmatics.

🟐 Related entries: Carylderm; Clinicide; Derbac-C; Suleo-C .

carbenoxolone sodium

is derived from LIQUORICE and is a synthetic derivative of glycyrrhizinic acid. It can be used as an ULCER-HEALING DRUG for benign gastric ulcers, because it promotes healing of the stomach lining when this has been eroded by acid and enzymes (in a way that

is not well understood) and is used for oesophageal ulceration and inflammation. Oral administration can be in the form of chewable tablets or as a liquid and in both cases with incorporated antacids. It may also be used locally as a gel or mouthwash to soothe mouth ulcers.

✚ Side-effects: There may be oedema, raised blood potassium levels (leading to muscle damage and other problems).

▲ Warning: It should not be administered to patients with cardiac failure, certain liver or kidney disorders, with hyperkalaemia (raised blood potassium) or who are pregnant. Use with caution in patients with hypertension or heart disease.

🟐 Related entries: Bioplex; Bioral Gel; Pyrogastrone.

carbidopa

is a drug that is administered in combination with levodopa to treat parkinsonism, but not the parkinsonian symptoms induced by other drugs (see ANTIPARKINSONISM). It is levodopa that actually has the major effect, but carbidopa inhibits the break down of levodopa to dopamine in the body before it reaches the brain where it carries out its function. The presence of carbidopa allows the dose of levodopa to be at a minimum and so minimizes potentially severe side-effects and speeds the therapeutic response. However, it is also responsible for producing some involuntary body movements. Administration of carbidopa and levodopa is oral as single-compound tablets called CO-CARELDOPA.

✚▲ Side-effects/warning: See LEVODOPA.

🟐 Related entries: Half Sinemet CR; Sinemet; Sinemet CR; Sinemet LS; Sinemet-Plus.

carbimazole

is a drug that acts as an indirect HORMONE ANTAGONIST, by inhibiting the production of the THYROID HORMONES by the thyroid gland, therefore treating an excess in the blood of thyroid hormones and the symptoms that it causes (thyrotoxicosis). Treatment may be on a maintenance basis over a long period (with dosage adjusted to optimum effect) or prior to surgical removal of the thyroid gland. Administration is oral.

✚ Side-effects: There may be rash; nausea and headache; occasionally, jaundice; hair loss; blood disorders; joint pain.

▲ Warning: It should be administered with caution to patients who are pregnant, breast-feeding or who have a large goitre.

⊕ Related entry: Neo-Mercazole.

Carbo-Cort

(Lagap) is a proprietary, prescription-only COMPOUND PREPARATION of the CORTICOSTEROID and ANTI-INFLAMMATORY hydrocortisone and coal tar. It can be used to treat eczema and psoriasis, and is available as a cream for topical application.

✚▲ Side-effects/warning: See COAL TAR; HYDROCORTISONE.

Carbo-Dome

(Lagap) is a proprietary, prescription-only preparation of coal tar. It can be used by topical application to treat eczema and psoriasis, and is available as a cream.

✚▲ Side-effects/warning: See COAL TAR.

carbocisteine

is a MUCOLYTIC drug which is used to reduce the viscosity of sputum and thus acts as an EXPECTORANT in patients with disorders of the upper respiratory tract, such as chronic asthma and bronchitis. Administration is oral.

✚▲ Side-effects/warning: See ACETYLCYSTEINE.

⊕ Related entry: Mucodyne.

carbomer

(CIBA Vision) is a synthetic agent which can be used in artificial tears where there is dryness of the eye due to a disease, such as keratoconjunctivitis. It is available as a liquid gel for application to the eye.

⊕ Related entry: GelTears; Viscotears.

Carbomix

(Penn) is a proprietary, non-prescription preparation of ACTIVATED CHARCOAL. It can be used to treat patients suffering from poisoning or a drug overdose, and is available as a granulated powder.

carbonic anhydrase inhibitors ⚇

are drugs with ENZYME-INHIBITOR actions against the enzyme *carbonic anhydrase*, which is present throughout the body and has an important role in the control of acid-base balance (pH). Medical application of carbonic anhydrase inhibitors include as a weak DIURETIC to treat systemic oedema (accumulation of fluid in the tissues), as a GLAUCOMA TREATMENT in reducing fluid (aqueous humour) and intraocular pressure in the eye (the pressure in the eyeball) and to prevent motion sickness. See ACETAZOLAMIDE and DORZOLAMIDE.

carboplatin

is a CYTOTOXIC drug (derived from cisplatin) which is used as an ANTICANCER treatment specifically for cancer of the ovary. Administration is by injection.

✚▲ Side-effects/warning: See CYTOTOXICS.

⊕ Related entry: Paraplatin.

carboprost

is used to treat haemorrhage following childbirth, which is caused by the muscles of the uterus losing their tone. It is an analogue of PROSTAGLANDIN (a synthetic form related to $PGF_{2\alpha}$), which is a LOCAL HORMONE naturally involved in controlling the muscles of the uterus. It is generally used in patients who are unresponsive to ERGOMETRINE MALEATE and OXYTOCIN. Administration is by injection.

✚ Side-effects: There may be nausea, headache and dizziness, vomiting and diarrhoea; flushing, chills and hyperthermia. There may be raised blood pressure, oedema of the lungs, shortness of breath and sweating. There may be pain at the site of injection.

▲ Warning: Use with caution in patients with a history of glaucoma, anaemia, jaundice, epilepsy, asthma, abnormal blood pressure (high or low) and uterine scars or any other predisposition to uterine rupture. It should not be used in patients with certain acute inflammatory disease; heart, kidney, lung or liver disorders.
✪ Related entry: Hemabate.

Cardene

(Syntex) is a proprietary, prescription-only preparation of the CALCIUM-CHANNEL BLOCKER nicardipine hydrochloride. It can be used as an ANTIHYPERTENSIVE and as an ANTI-ANGINA drug in the prevention and treatment of attacks. It is available as capsules.
✚▲ Side-effects/warning: See NICARDIPINE HYDROCHLORIDE.

Cardene SR

(Syntex) is a proprietary, prescription-only preparation of the CALCIUM-CHANNEL BLOCKER nicardipine hydrochloride. It can be used as an ANTIHYPERTENSIVE and as an ANTI-ANGINA drug in the prevention and treatment of attacks. It is available as modified-release capsules.
✚▲ Side-effects/warning: See NICARDIPINE HYDROCHLORIDE.

cardiac glycosides ▨

are a class of drugs derived from the leaf of the *Digitalis* foxgloves. These drugs have a pronounced effect on the failing heart by increasing the force of contraction and so have been commonly used for their CARDIAC STIMULANT actions to increase the force in congestive HEART FAILURE TREATMENT. They can also correct certain abnormal heart rhythms and are therefore used as an ANTI-ARRHYTHMIC treatment. However, today, these drugs are used much less often, as doses that are useful therapeutically are close to those that are toxic, so dose must be carefully adjusted in the individual. A digitalis antidote for use in overdose, DIGIBIND, is available. Examples of cardiac glycosides include DIGOXIN and DIGITOXIN.

cardiac stimulants ▨

are used in medicine to stimulate the rate or the force of the heartbeat, but only when it is weak as a result of some disease state or in medical emergencies. CARDIAC GLYCOSIDES have a pronounced effect on the failing heart, increasing the force of contraction and so have been widely prescribed in congestive HEART FAILURE TREATMENT. A number of SYMPATHOMIMETICS can be used directly to stimulate the heart through their BETA-RECEPTOR STIMULANT properties; for example DOPEXAMINE HYDROCHLORIDE, DOBUTAMINE HYDROCHLORIDE, ISOPRENALINE and ADRENALINE. Most of these drugs tend to be reserved for acute emergencies, such as cardiogenic shock, septic shock, during heart surgery and in cardiac infarction and cardiac arrest.

Cardilate MR

(Norton) is a proprietary, prescription-only preparation of the CALCIUM-CHANNEL BLOCKER nifedipine. It can be used as an ANTI-ANGINA treatment in the prevention of attacks and as an ANTIHYPERTENSIVE. It is available as tablets.
✚▲ Side-effects/warning: See NIFEDIPINE.

Cardinol

(CP) is a proprietary, prescription-only preparation of the BETA-BLOCKER propranolol hydrochloride. It can be used as an ANTIHYPERTENSIVE for raised blood pressure, as an ANTI-ANGINA treatment to relieve symptoms and improve exercise tolerance and as an ANTI-ARRHYTHMIC to regularize heartbeat and to treat myocardial infarction. It can also be used as an ANTITHYROID drug for short-term treatment of thyrotoxicosis, as an ANTIMIGRAINE treatment to prevent attacks, as an ANXIOLYTIC, particularly for symptomatic relief of tremor and palpitations, and, with an ALPHA-ADRENOCEPTOR BLOCKER, in the acute treatment of phaeochromocytoma. It is available as tablets.
✚▲ Side-effects/warning: See PROPRANOLOL HYDROCHLORIDE.

C

Cardura

(Invicta) is a proprietary, prescription-only preparation of the ALPHA-ADRENOCEPTOR BLOCKER doxazosin. It can be used as an ANTIHYPERTENSIVE, often in conjunction with other antihypertensives, and is available as tablets.

➕▲ Side-effects/warning: See DOXAZOSIN.

Carisoma

(Pharmax) is a proprietary, prescription-only preparation of the SKELETAL MUSCLE RELAXANT carisoprodol. It can be used to treat muscle spasm caused by an injury to or a disease of the central nervous system, and is available as tablets.

➕▲ Side-effects/warning: See CARISOPRODOL.

carisoprodol

is a SKELETAL MUSCLE RELAXANT which can be used for relaxing muscles that are in spasm, particularly when caused by an injury to or a disease of the central nervous system. It works by an action on the central nervous system. Administration is oral.

➕▲ Side-effects/warning: See MEPROBAMATE; but drowsiness is less common. Avoid its use in patients with porphyria.

⊙ Related entry: Carisoma.

carmellose sodium

(sodium carboxymethyl cellulose) is a substance that is used as the basis for a paste or a powder which is spread or sprinkled over lesions in or around the mouth, in order to provide a protective barrier and relieve some of the discomfort while lesions heal.

⊙ Related entries: artificial saliva; Glandosane; Luborant; Orabase; Orahesive; Salivace.

carmustine

is a CYTOTOXIC drug which works by direct interference with DNA and so prevents normal cell replication. It is used as an ANTICANCER drug to treat some myelomas, lymphatic cancer and brain tumours. Administration is by injection.

➕▲ Side-effects/warning: See CYTOTOXICS.

⊙ Related entry: BiCNU.

carteolol hydrochloride

is a BETA-BLOCKER which can be used as a GLAUCOMA TREATMENT for chronic simple glaucoma. It is thought to work by slowing the rate of production of the aqueous humour in the eye. Administration is topical.

➕ Side-effects: There may be some systemic absorption into the body, so some of the side-effects listed under PROPRANOLOL HYDROCHLORIDE may be seen. Dry eyes and some local allergic reactions of the eyelids, including conjunctivitis, may also occur.

▲ Warning: In view of possible systemic absorption, dangerous side-effects should be borne in mind; in particular, the danger of bronchospasm in asthmatics and interactions with calcium-channel blockers.

⊙ Related entry: Teoptic.

Carter's Little Pills

(Carter-Wallace) is a proprietary, non-prescription COMPOUND PREPARATION of the (*stimulant*) LAXATIVES phenolphthalein and aloin. It can be used to relieve constipation, and is available as tablets. It is not normally given to children, except on medical advice.

➕▲ Side-effects/warning: See ALOIN; PHENOLPHTHALEIN.

carvedilol

is a BETA-BLOCKER which can be used as an ANTIHYPERTENSIVE. Administration is oral.

➕▲ Side-effects/warning: See PROPRANOLOL HYDROCHLORIDE. It should not be given to patients with kidney impairment.

⊙ Related entry: Eucardic.

Carylderm

(Napp) is a proprietary, non-prescription preparation of the PEDICULICIDAL carbaryl. It can be used to treat infestations of lice in the scalp and pubic hair, and is available as a lotion and a shampoo.

✚▲ Side-effects/warning: See CARBARYL.

Casodex

(Zeneca) is a proprietary, prescription-only preparation of the anti-androgen, HORMONE ANTAGONIST bicalutamide . It can be used as an ANTICANCER drug to treat cancer of the prostate, and is available as tablets.
✚▲ Side-effects/warning: SeeBICALUTAMIDE.

castor oil

has EMOLLIENT properties and is found in some skin preparations and BARRIER CREAMS. It was once used as a (*stimulant*) LAXATIVE but is now obsolete. It is used in a polyethoxylated form in some drug formulations for injection.
✚▲ Side-effects/warning: It is normally safe and relatively free of side-effects on topical application, but the polyethoxylated form has been associated with anaphylaxis on injection. As a laxative, its irritant properties are powerful, and it can induce labour.
◎ Related entry: Panda Baby Cream & Castor Oil Cream with Lanolin.

Catapres

(Boehringer Ingelheim) is a proprietary, prescription-only preparation of the ANTISYMPATHETIC clonidine hydrochloride. It can be used as an ANTIHYPERTENSIVE and ANTIMIGRAINE treatment, and is available as tablets and in a form for injection.
✚▲ Side-effects/warning: See CLONIDINE HYDROCHLORIDE.

Catapres Perlongets

(Boehringer Ingelheim) is a proprietary, prescription-only preparation of the ANTISYMPATHETIC clonidine hydrochloride. It can be used as an ANTIHYPERTENSIVE, and is available as modified-release capsules.
✚▲ Side-effects/warning: See CLONIDINE HYDROCHLORIDE.

Catarrh-Ex

(Thompson) is a proprietary, non-prescription COMPOUND PREPARATION of the NON-NARCOTIC ANALGESIC paracetamol, the SYMPATHOMIMETIC and DECONGESTANT phenylephrine hydochloride and the STIMULANT caffeine. It can be used for the relief of cold and flu symptoms and sinusitis. It is available as tablets and is not normally given to children, except on medical advice.
✚▲ Side-effects/warning: See CAFFEINE; PARACETAMOL; PHENYLEPHRINE HYDROCHLORIDE.

Caved-S

(Pharmacia) is a proprietary, non-prescription COMPOUND PREPARATION of the ANTACIDS aluminium hydroxide, magnesium carbonate and sodium bicarbonate and the CYTOPROTECTANTS bismuth subnitrate and deglycyrrhizinised liquorice. It can be used to treat peptic ulcers, and is available as tablets.
✚▲ Side-effects/warning: See ALUMINIUM HYDROXIDE; BISMUTH SUBNITRATE; LIQUORICE, DEGLYCYRRHIZINISED; MAGNESIUM CARBONATE; SODIUM BICARBONATE.

Caverject

(Upjohn) is a PROSTAGLANDIN, alprostadil (PGE$_1$). It is a recently introduced, prescription-only treatment for men to manage penile erectile dysfunction. It available in a form for injection and is administered by intracavernosal injection into the penis.
✚▲ Side-effects/warning: See ALPROSTADIL.

CCNU

(Lundbeck) is a proprietary, prescription-only preparation of the (CYTOTOXIC) ANTICANCER drug lomustine. It can be used in the treatment of Hodgkin's disease and some solid tumours, and is available in a form for injection.
✚▲ Side-effects/warning: See LOMUSTINE.

Ceanel Concentrate

(Quinoderm) is a proprietary, non-prescription COMPOUND PREPARATION of the ANTISEPTIC cetrimide and the ANTIFUNGAL undecenoic acid (with phenylethyl

C

alcohol). It can be used to treat psoriasis and other non-infective scalp conditions, and is available as a shampoo.
✚▲ Side-effects/warning: See CETRIMIDE; UNDECENOIC ACID.

Cedax
(Schering-Plough) is a proprietary, prescription-only preparation of the ANTIBACTERIAL and (CEPHALOSPORIN) ANTIBIOTIC ceftibuten. It can be used to treat acute bacterial infections of the urinary and respiratory tracts by Gram-positive and Gram-negative organisms. It is available as capsules and an oral suspension.
✚▲ Side-effects/warning: See CEFTIBUTEN.

Cedocard
(Pharmacia) is a proprietary, non-prescription preparation of the VASODILATOR and ANTI-ANGINA drug isosorbide dinitrate. It can be used to treat and prevent angina pectoris and in HEART FAILURE TREATMENT. It is available as short-acting, sublingual, or oral tablets in three doses: *Cedocard-5*, *Cedocard-10* and *Cedocard-20*.
✚▲ Side-effects/warning: See ISOSORBIDE DINITRATE.

Cedocard-Retard
(Pharmacia) is a proprietary, non-prescription preparation of the VASODILATOR and ANTI-ANGINA drug isosorbide dinitrate. It can be used to prevent angina pectoris, and is available as modified-release tablets.
✚▲ Side-effects/warning: See ISOSORBIDE DINITRATE.

cefaclor
is a broad-spectrum ANTIBACTERIAL and ANTIBIOTIC drug. It is one of the second-generation CEPHALOSPORINS, and is now primarily used to treat Gram-positive and Gram-negative bacterial infections of the respiratory and urinary tracts. It is used particularly for urinary tract infections that do not respond to other drugs, or which occur during pregnancy and pneumonia. Administration is oral.

✚ Side-effects: Nausea, vomiting, diarrhoea, headache, colitis (more likely at high doses); sensitivity reactions that may be serious (from rashes to anaphylaxis); blood and liver disturbances, behavioural and nervous disturbances.
▲ Warning: It should not be administered to patients who are sensitive to penicillins and cephalosporins. Do not use in patients with porphyria and with caution in those who are pregnant or breast-feeding.
○ Related entries: Distaclor; Distaclor MR.

cefadroxil
is a broad-spectrum ANTIBACTERIAL and ANTIBIOTIC drug. It is one of the first-generation CEPHALOSPORINS, and is now primarily used to treat bacterial infections of the urinary tract that do not respond to other drugs, or which occur during pregnancy. Administration is oral.
✚▲ Side-effects/warning: See CEFACLOR.
○ Related entry: Baxan.

cefalexin
see CEPHALEXIN

cefamandole
see CEPHAMANDOLE

cefazolin
see CEPHAZOLIN

cefixime
is a broad-spectrum ANTIBACTERIAL and (CEPHALOSPORIN) ANTIBIOTIC drug. It is used to treat acute bacterial infections by Gram-positive and Gram-negative organisms, particularly of the urinary tract. It has a longer duration of action than any other cephalosporin taken by mouth. Administration is oral.
✚▲ Side-effects/warning: See CEFACLOR.
○ Related entry: Suprax.

cefodizime
is a broad-spectrum ANTIBACTERIAL and ANTIBIOTIC drug. It is one of the third-generation CEPHALOSPORINS, and can be used

to treat infections of the lower respiratory tract, including pneumonia and bronchopneumonia, and of the urinary tract, including cystitis and pyelonephritis. Administration is by injection.
+▲ Side-effects/warning: See CEFACLOR.
۞ Related entry: Timecef.

cefotaxime

is a broad-spectrum ANTIBACTERIAL and ANTIBIOTIC drug. It is one of the third-generation CEPHALOSPORINS, and can be administered to treat a wide range of bacterial infections, particularly of the skin and soft tissues, the urinary tract, the meninges of the brain (in meningitis) and gonorrhoea. It can also be used to prevent infection during surgery. Administration is by injection.
+▲ Side-effects/warning: See CEFACLOR.
۞ Related entry: Claforan.

cefoxitin

is a broad-spectrum ANTIBACTERIAL and ANTIBIOTIC drug. It is one of the second-generation CEPHALOSPORINS, and can be administered to treat a wide range of bacterial infections, particularly Gram-negative infections of the skin and soft tissues, the urinary and respiratory tracts and the peritoneum (in peritonitis). Administration is by injection.
+▲ Side-effects/warning: See CEFACLOR.
۞ Related entry: Mefoxin.

cefpirome

is a broad-spectrum ANTIBACTERIAL and ANTIBIOTIC drug, a recently introduced member of the CEPHALOSPORINS. It is used to treat complicated upper and lower urinary-tract, skin and soft-tissue infections, respiratory tract infections and particularly for severe infections including bacteraemia and septicaemia and infections in neutropenic patients. Administration is by injection.
+▲ Side-effects/warning: See CEFACLOR; also, there may be taste disturbances.
۞ Related entry: Cefrom.

cefpodoxime

is a broad-spectrum ANTIBACTERIAL and (CEPHALOSPORIN) ANTIBIOTIC. It can be used to treat bacterial infections of the respiratory tract, including bronchitis and pneumonia, and tonsillitis infections that are recurrent, chronic or resistant to other drugs. Administration is oral.
+▲ Side-effects/warning: See CEFACLOR.
۞ Related entry: Orelox.

cefradine

see CEPHRADINE

Cefrom

(Roussel) is a proprietary, prescription-only preparation of the ANTIBACTERIAL and (CEPHALOSPORIN) ANTIBIOTIC cefpirome. It can be used to treat serious infections, especially those of the urinary tract, and is available in a form for intravenous injection.
+▲ Side-effects/warning: See CEFPIROME .

ceftazidime

is a broad-spectrum ANTIBACTERIAL and ANTIBIOTIC drug. It is one of the third-generation CEPHALOSPORINS and is among the most effective of the cephalosporins against bacterial infections. It can be used particularly to treat infections of the skin and soft tissues, the urinary and respiratory tracts, the ear, nose and throat (eg *Pseudomonal* lung infections in cystic fibrosis) and to prevent infection following surgery. It can also be used to treat infection in patients whose immune systems are defective. Administration is by injection.
+▲ Side-effects/warning: See CEFACLOR.
۞ Related entries: Fortum; Kefadim.

ceftibuten

is a broad-spectrum ANTIBACTERIAL and (CEPHALOSPORIN) ANTIBIOTIC drug. It can be administered to treat acute bacterial infections caused by Gram-positive and Gram-negative organisms, particularly of the urinary and respiratory tracts. Administration is oral.

C

+▲ Side-effects/warning: See CEFACLOR.
○ **Related entry: Cedax.**

ceftriaxone

is a broad-spectrum ANTIBACTERIAL and
ANTIBIOTIC drug. It is a recently introduced,
third-generation CEPHALOSPORIN, and can be
used to treat a wide range of Gram-negative
bacterial infections, including septicaemia,
pneumonia and gonorrhoea, and to prevent
meningococcal meningitis. It can also be
used to prevent infections during surgery. It
has a much longer duration of action than
others of this class and so only needs to be
taken once a day. Administration is by
injection.
+▲ Side-effects/warning: See CEFACLOR.
Administer with caution to patients with
certain liver disorders; the calcium salt form
of the drug may precipitate or form
gallstones to be passed in the urine.
○ **Related entry: Rocephin.**

cefuroxime

is a broad-spectrum ANTIBACTERIAL and
ANTIBIOTIC drug. It is one of the second-
generation CEPHALOSPORINS, and can be used
to treat a wide range of bacterial infections,
particularly Gram-negative infections of the
urinary, respiratory and genital tracts and
the meninges (in meningitis). It can also be
used to prevent infection during surgery.
Administration is by injection.
+▲ Side-effects/warning: See CEFACLOR.
○ **Related entries: Zinacef; Zinnat.**

Celance

(Lilly) is a proprietary, prescription-only
preparation of pergolide, which can be
used as an ANTIPARKINSONISM drug. It is
available as tablets.
+▲ Side-effects/warning: See PERGOLIDE.

Celectol

(Rhône-Poulenc Rorer) is a proprietary,
prescription-only preparation of the BETA-
BLOCKER celiprolol hydrochloride. It can be
used as an ANTIHYPERTENSIVE for raised
blood pressure, and is available as tablets.

+▲ Side-effects/warning: See CELIPROLOL
HYDROCHLORIDE.

Celevac

(Monmouth) is a proprietary, non-
prescription preparation of the (*bulking-
agent*) LAXATIVE methylcellulose. It can be
used to treat a number of gastrointestinal
disorders, and is available as tablets.
+▲ Side-effects/warning: See
METHYLCELLULOSE.

celiprolol hydrochloride

is a BETA-BLOCKER which can be used as an
ANTIHYPERTENSIVE for raised blood pressure.
Administration is oral.
+▲ Side-effects/warning: See PROPRANOLOL
HYDROCHLORIDE. There may also be
headache, sleepiness, fatigue, nausea,
bronchospasm and slowing of the heart. It
should be prescribed with caution to those
who are breast-feeding or pregnant, or who
have certain liver or kidney disorders.
Withdrawal of treatment should be gradual.
○ **Related entry: Celectol.**

CellCept

(Roche) is a proprietary, prescription-only
preparation of the IMMUNOSUPPRESSANT
mycophenolate mofetil. It can be used to
treat tissue rejection in transplant patients,
and is available as capsules.
+▲ Side-effects/warning: See
MYCOPHENOLATE MOFETIL.

cephalexin

(cefalexin) is a broad-spectrum
ANTIBACTERIAL and ANTIBIOTIC drug. It is one
of the orally active CEPHALOSPORINS, and can
be used to treat a wide range of bacterial
infections, particularly of the urinary tract.
Administration is oral.
+▲ Side-effects/warning: See CEFACLOR.
○ **Related entries: Ceporex; Keflex.**

cephalosporins ▣

are ANTIBIOTICS that are chemically BETA-
LACTAMS. They are broad-spectrum
ANTIBACTERIALS that act against both Gram-

positive and Gram-negative bacteria. Their chemical structure bears a strong resemblance to that of the penicillins as they both contain a beta-lactam ring, hence their classification as *beta-lactam antibiotics*. The similarity in structure extends to their mechanism of action: both classes inhibit the synthesis of the bacterial cell wall, so killing growing bacteria – they are *bactericidal*.

As a group, the cephalosporins are generally active against streptococci, staphylococci and a number of Gram-negative bacteria, including many coliforms. Examples of the original, first-generation cephalosporins are CEPHRADINE and CEFADROXIL. Some second-generation cephalosporins (eg CEFUROXIME and CEPHAMANDOLE) are resistant to inactivation by bacterial PENICILLINASE enzymes, which widens their range of action to include treating sensitive Gram-negative organisms, including *Haemophilus influenzae*.

Some of the latest, third-generation, cephalosporins (eg CEFOTAXIME, CEFTAZIDIME and CEFODIZIME) act as antibacterials against certain Gram-negative bacteria (eg *Haemophilus influenzae*) and pseudomonal infections (eg *Pseudomonas aeruginosa*). Many cephalosporins are actively excreted by the kidney and therefore reach considerably higher concentrations in the urine than in the blood. For this reason, they may be used to treat infections of the urinary tract during their own excretion. In general, cephalosporins are rarely the drug of first choice, but provide a useful alternative, or reserve option, in particular situations. The cephalosporins currently used are relatively non-toxic and only occasional blood-clotting problems, superinfections and hypersensitivity reactions occur (only 10% of patients allergic to penicillin show sensitivity to cephalosporins).

cephamandole
(cefamandole) is a broad-spectrum ANTIBACTERIAL and ANTIBIOTIC drug. It is one of the second-generation CEPHALOSPORINS, and is less susceptible to inactivation by bacterial PENICILLINASES than others in its class and is therefore effective against a greater range of Gram-negative bacteria, for example, penicillin-resistant *Neisseria gonorrhoeae* and *Haemophilus influenzae*. It can be used to treat a wide range of bacterial infections, particularly of the skin and soft tissues, the genito-urinary and upper respiratory tracts and middle ear. It is also used to prevent infection during surgery. Administration is by injection.

+▲ Side-effects/warning: See CEFACLOR.
◐ Related entry: Kefadol.

cephazolin
(cefazolin) is a broad-spectrum ANTIBACTERIAL and ANTIBIOTIC drug. It is one of the first-generation CEPHALOSPORINS, and can be used to treat a wide range of bacterial infections, particularly of the skin and soft tissues, urinary and upper respiratory tracts and middle ear. It can also be used to prevent infection during surgery. Administration is by injection.

+▲ Side-effects/warning: See CEFACLOR.
◐ Related entry: Kefzol.

cephradine
(cefradine) is a broad-spectrum ANTIBACTERIAL and ANTIBIOTIC drug. It is one of the first-generation CEPHALOSPORINS, and can be used to treat a wide range of bacterial infections, particularly streptococcal infections of the skin and soft tissues, the urinary and upper respiratory tracts and middle ear. It is also used to prevent infection during surgery. Administration is either oral or by injection.

+▲ Side-effects/warning: See CEFACLOR.
◐ Related entry: Velosef.

Ceporex
(Glaxo) is a proprietary, prescription-only preparation of the ANTIBACTERIAL and (CEPHALOSPORIN) ANTIBIOTIC cephalexin. It can be used to treat many infections,

C

including of the urinogenital tract, and is available as capsules, tablets, an oral suspension and a syrup.
✚▲ Side-effects/warning: See CEPHALEXIN.

Ceredase

(Genzyme) is a proprietary, prescription-only preparation of the ENZYME alglucerase, which is used as a replacement in the specialist treatment of the enzyme deficiency disease Gaucher's disease. It is available in a form for intravenous infusion.
✚▲ Side-effects/warning: See ALGLUCERASE.

certoparin sodium

is a LOW MOLECULAR WEIGHT HEPARIN and is used as an ANTICOAGULANT. It has some advantages over heparin (longer duration of action), for instance, when used for prophylaxis of deep-vein thrombosis. Administration is by injection.
✚▲ Side-effects/warning: See HEPARIN.
✪ Related entry: Alphaparin.

Cerubidin

(Rhône-Poulenc Rorer) is a proprietary, prescription-only preparation of the (CYTOTOXIC) ANTICANCER drug daunorubicin. It can be used to treat advanced HIV-related Kaposi's sarcoma, and is available in a form for intravenous infusion.
✚▲ Side-effects/warning: See DAUNORUBICIN.

Cerumol Ear Drops

(LAB) is a proprietary, non-prescription COMPOUND PREPARATION of the ANTISEPTIC agent CHLORBUTOL and arachis oil (with paradichlorobenzene). It can be used to remove earwax, and is available as ear-drops.
✚▲ Side-effects/warning: See ARACHIS OIL.

Cesamet

(Lilly) is a proprietary, prescription-only preparation of the ANTINAUSEANT and ANTI-EMETIC nabilone. It can be used to treat nausea in patients undergoing

chemotherapy, and is available as capsules.
✚▲ Side-effects/warning: See NABILONE.

Cetavlex

(Zeneca) is a proprietary, non-prescription COMPOUND PREPARATION of the ANTISEPTIC cetrimide and arachis oil (with paradichlorobenzene). It can be used to treat cuts and abrasions, and is available as a water-based cream.
✚▲ Side-effects/warning: See ARACHIS OIL; CETRIMIDE.

cetirizine

is a recently developed ANTIHISTAMINE with less side-effects (such as sedation) than some of the older members of this class. It can be used for the symptomatic relief of allergic symptoms such as hay fever and urticaria. Administration is oral.
✚▲ Side-effects/warning: See ANTIHISTAMINES. Administer with caution to patients with kidney impairment. The incidence of sedation and anticholinergic effects is low.
✪ Related entry: Zirtek.

cetrimide

is an ANTISEPTIC and DISINFECTANT which is used therapeutically (often in combination with CHLORHEXIDINE) for cleansing the skin and scalp, burns and wounds and, as a cream, as a soap-substitute for conditions such as acne and seborrhoea.
✚ Side-effects: There may be skin irritation.
▲ Warning: Avoid contact with eyes and body cavities.
✪ Related entries: Ceanel Concentrate; Cetavlex; Drapolene Cream; Hibicet Hospital Concentrate; Savlon Antiseptic Cream; Siopel; Tisept; Travasept 100.

cetylpyridinium chloride

is an ANTISEPTIC which is used as a mouthwash or gargle for oral hygiene, and is available as a gel, lozenges and an oral solution.
✪ Related entries: Anbesol Adult Strength Gel; Anbesol Liquid; Anbesol Teething Gel;

Calgel Teething Gel; Dentinox Teething Gel;
Medilave; Meltus Adult Expectorant Linctus;
Meltus Junior Expectorant Linctus;
Merocaine Lozenges; Merocets Lozenges;
Merocets Gargle/Mouthwash; Merothol
Lozenges; Merovit Lozenges; Tyrocane
Junior Antiseptic Lozenges; Rinstead
Teething Gel; Ulc-Aid Gel; Vicks Original
Cough Syrup (Chesty).

chalk
see CALCIUM CARBONATE

chelating agents ?
are drugs that can be used as ANTIDOTES
mainly for metal poisoning. They work by
chemically binding to certain metallic ions
and other substances, making them less
toxic and allowing their excretion. They are
used to reduce unacceptably high levels of
metals of external origin (accidental or
environmental) and due to abnormal
metabolism (eg of copper in Wilson's
disease) and to treat disease states (eg
PENICILLAMINE in rheumatoid arthritis). See
DESFERRIOXAMINE MESYLATE; DICOBALT EDETATE;
DIMERCAPROL; SODIUM CALCIUMEDETATE.

Chemotrim
(RP) is a proprietary, prescription-only
COMPOUND PREPARATION of the
(SULPHONAMIDE) ANTIBACTERIAL
sulphamethoxazole and the antibacterial
trimethoprim, which is a combination
known as co-trimoxazole. It can be used to
treat bacterial infections, particularly
infections of the urinary tract, prostatitis
and bronchitis. It is available as a
paediatric oral suspension.
✚▲ Side-effects/warning: See CO-
TRIMOXAZOLE.

Chendol
(CP) is a proprietary, prescription-only
preparation of chenodeoxycholic acid. It
can be used to dissolve gallstones, and is
available as tablets.
✚▲ Side-effects/warning: See
CHENODEOXYCHOLIC ACID.

chenodeoxycholic acid
(a bile acid) is a drug that can dissolve
gallstones *in situ*. Administration is oral.
✚ Side-effects: There is diarrhoea and
itching, mild liver dysfunction and changes
in blood enzymes.
▲ Warning: It should not be used in
patients with impaired gall bladder, chronic
liver disease, inflammatory disorders of the
intestines or who are pregnant.
❂ Related entries: Chendol; Chenofalk;
Combidol; Lithofalk.

Chenofalk
(Thames) is a proprietary, prescription-
only preparation of chenodeoxycholic acid.
It can be used to dissolve gallstones, and is
available as capsules.
✚▲ Side-effects/warning: See
CHENODEOXYCHOLIC ACID.

Children's Vitamin Drops
(Hough) is a proprietary, non-prescription
MULTIVITAMIN preparation of vitamins A, C
and D. It is recommended by the
Department of Health for routine
supplement to the diet of young children
from 6 months to 2-5 years and in some
cases from as early as 1 month. It is
available direct to families under the
Welfare Food Scheme.
✚▲ Side-effects/warning: See ASCORBIC
ACID; RETINOL; VITAMIN D.

Chloractil
(DDSA Pharmaceuticals) is a proprietary,
prescription-only preparation of the
(PHENOTHIAZINE) ANTIPSYCHOTIC
chlorpromazine hydrochloride. It can be
used in patients undergoing behavioural
disturbances, who are psychotic (especially
schizophrenics) or showing severe anxiety
where sedation is useful. It can also be used
as an ANTINAUSEANT and ANTI-EMETIC to
relieve nausea and vomiting, particularly in
terminal illness and preoperative
medication. It is available as tablets.
✚▲ Side-effects/warning: See
CHLORPROMAZINE HYDROCHLORIDE.

C

Chloral Elixir, Paediatric, BP

is a non-proprietary, prescription-only preparation of the HYPNOTIC drug chloral hydrate, which is used to treat insomnia, and is available as an elixir for children.
✚▲ Side-effects/warning: See CHLORAL HYDRATE.

chloral hydrate

is a short-term SEDATIVE and HYPNOTIC drug. It is considered to be particularly useful in inducing sleep in children or elderly patients. Administration is usually oral.
✚ Side-effects: Stomach irritation, abdominal distension and flatulence; occasionally, rashes, headache, blood changes and excitement. Dependence can occur with prolonged use.
▲ Warning: It should not be administered to patients with severe heart disease, inflammation of the stomach, or severely impaired function of the liver or kidneys. It should be administered with caution to those with respiratory disorders; who are pregnant or breast-feeding, or elderly or debilitated, or who have a history of drug abuse. Avoid contact with the skin or mucous membranes.
✪ Related entries: Chloral Elixir, Paediatric, BP; Chloral Mixture, BP; Welldorm.

Chloral Mixture, BP

is a non-proprietary, prescription-only preparation of the HYPNOTIC drug chloral hydrate, which is used to treat insomnia. It is available as a mixture.
✚▲ Side-effects/warning: See CHLORAL HYDRATE.

chlorambucil

is a CYTOTOXIC drug which is used as an ANTICANCER treatment, particularly for chronic lymphocytic leukaemia, lymphomas and solid tumours. It works by interfering with the DNA and so preventing normal cell replication. It can also be used as an IMMUNOSUPPRESSANT in the treatment of rheumatoid arthritis. Administration is oral.
✚▲ Side-effects/warning: See CYTOTOXICS;

but there may also be haemorrhagic cystitis (though this is rare); avoid its use in patients with porphyria, and administer with care to those with renal impairment.
✪ Related entry: Leukeran.

chloramphenicol

is a broad-spectrum ANTIBACTERIAL and ANTIBIOTIC drug, which can be used to treat many forms of infection. However, the serious side-effects caused by its systemic use mean that it is normally restricted to certain severe infections, such as typhoid fever (*Haemophilus meningitis*) and, in particular, infections caused by *Haemophilus influenzae*. It is useful in treating conditions such as bacterial conjunctivitis, otitis externa or many types of skin infection, because it is applied topically to the eyes, ears or skin and therefore its toxicity is not encountered. Topical administration is by eye-drops, ear-drops or a cream. Systemic administration is oral.
✚ Side-effects: Depending on the route of administration, there may be nausea, vomiting, diarrhoea; certain types of neuritis. Systemic treatment may cause serious damage to the bone marrow, which results in blood disorders.
▲ Warning: It should not be administered to patients who are pregnant, breast-feeding or have porphyria. Administer with caution to those with impaired liver or kidney function. Topical treatment may cause stinging and it should be kept away from open wounds. Prolonged or repeated use should be avoided. Regular blood counts are essential.
✪ Related entries: Actinac; Chloromycetin; Chloromycetin Hydrocortisone; Kemicetine; Minims Chloramphenicol; Sno Phenicol.

Chlorasept 2000

(Baxter) is a proprietary, non-prescription preparation of the ANTISEPTIC chlorhexidine (as acetate). It can be used to cleanse and disinfect skin, wounds and burns, and is available as a solution.

+▲ Side-effects/warning: See
CHLORHEXIDINE.

Chloraseptic

(Procter & Gamble) is a proprietary, non-
prescription preparation of the ANTISEPTIC
phenol. It can be used to treat minor mouth
and gum disorders, sore throats and mouth
ulcers. It is available as a solution for use
as a mouthwash or gargle and is not
normally given to children, except on
medical advice.
+▲ Side-effects/warning: See PHENOL.

Chlorasol

(Seton) is a proprietary, non-prescription
preparation of the ANTISEPTIC sodium
hypochlorite. It can be used as a cleanser to
treat skin infections and particularly for
cleansing wounds and ulcers. It is available
as a solution.
+▲ Side-effects/warning: See SODIUM
HYPOCHLORITE.

chlorbutanol

see CHLORBUTOL

chlorbutol

(chlorbutanol) is used as a preservative in
some drug preparations for removing
earwax.
✪ Related entries: Cerumol Ear Drops;
Eludril Mouthwash; Karvol Decongestant
Capsules; Monphytol.

chlordiazepoxide

is a BENZODIAZEPINE which can be used as an
ANXIOLYTIC in the short-term treatment of
anxiety and, in conjunction with other
drugs, in the treatment of acute alcohol
withdrawal symptoms. Administration is
oral.
+▲ Side-effects/warning: See
BENZODIAZEPINES.
✪ Related entries: Librium; Tropium.

chlorhexidine

is an ANTISEPTIC and DISINFECTANT agent
which is a constituent in many

preparations. It can be used prior to
surgery and in obstetrics, but is
administered mainly (as chlorhexidine
gluconate, chlorhexidine acetate,or
chlorhexidine hydrochloride) either as a
mouthwash for oral hygiene or as a
dressing for minor skin wounds and
infections. It can also be used for
instillation in the bladder to relieve minor
infections.
+ Side-effects: Some patients experience
sensitivity reactions. It may cause irritation,
burning and blood in the urine when used
to irrigate the bladder.
▲ Warning: Avoid contact with the eyes and
delicate body tissues.
✪ Related entries: Chlorohex 2000;
Chlorasept 2000; Corsodyl; CX Antiseptic
Dusting Powder; Dermol 500; Eludril
Mouthwash; Eludril Spray; Germoline
Cream; Hibicet Hospital Concentrate;
Hibisol; Hibitane; Instillagel; Mycil Powder;
Naseptin; Nystaform; Phiso-med; Savlon
Antiseptic Cream; Steripod Chlorhexidine;
Tisept; Travasept 100; Unisept.

chlormethiazole

(clomethiazole) has a number of uses: as a
HYPNOTIC for treating severe insomnia
(especially in elderly patients because it is
relatively free of a 'hangover' effect), as an
ANTICONVULSANT and ANTI-EPILEPTIC to treat
status epilepticus and eclampsia, to reduce
the symptoms of withdrawal from alcohol
(under strict medical supervision), and
also for maintaining unconsciousness
under regional anaesthesia with LOCAL
ANAESTHETICS. Administration is either oral
or by injection.
+ Side-effects: Nasal congestion, sneezing,
irritation of the conjunctiva of the eyes and
nose, headache; when given by injection or
infusion, there is rarely an increase in heart
rate and decrease in blood pressure and
thrombophlebitis excitement, confusion,
gastrointestinal upsets, rashes and urticaria,
anaphylaxis, blood and liver changes, or
dependence.
▲ Warning: It should not be given to

C

patients with acute pulmonary insufficiency, or who are alcoholics who continue to drink. Use with care in patients with heart or respiratory disease, or impaired liver or kidney function, or who have a history of alcohol or drug abuse. Withdrawal of treatment should be gradual. It may cause drowsiness the next day, which can impair the performance of skilled tasks, such as driving. The effects of alcohol may be enhanced.

○ Related entry: Heminevrin.

chlormethine hydrochloride
see MUSTINE HYDROCHLORIDE

chlormezanone
is an ANXIOLYTIC and HYPNOTIC drug which also has SKELETAL MUSCLE RELAXANT properties. It is used in the short-term treatment of anxiety and tension and to induce sleep. It is not of proven value as a muscle relaxant, though it is available as a COMPOUND ANALGESIC preparation with paracetamol (called *Lobak*) intended for the relief of muscle spasm. Administration is oral.

✚ Side-effects: Concentration and speed of thought and movement may be affected; the effects of alcohol may be enhanced. There may be drowsiness, dizziness, nausea, headache, dry mouth and shallow breathing; hypersensitivity reactions or jaundice may occur.

▲ Warning: It should not be administered to patients with certain lung disorders; and only with caution to those who have muscle weakness, a history of drug or alcohol abuse, or with porphyria. Prolonged use or abrupt withdrawal of treatment should be avoided. The sedative effects may persist and impair the performance of skilled tasks, such as driving.

○ Related entry: Lobak.

Chlorohex 2000
(Colgate-Palmolive) is a proprietary, non-prescription preparation of the ANTISEPTIC chlorhexidine (as gluconate). It can be used by topical application to treat inflammations and infections of the mouth, and is available as a mouthwash.

✚▲ Side-effects/warning: See CHLORHEXIDINE.

Chloromycetin
(Parke-Davis) is a proprietary, prescription-only preparation of the broad-spectrum ANTIBACTERIAL and ANTIBIOTIC chloramphenicol. When injected, it can be used to treat potentially dangerous bacterial infections, such as typhoid fever. When applied topically, as creams or drops, it can be used to treat eye infections. It is available as capsules, a suspension for dilution, as an eye ointment (*Redidrops*), eye-drops and in a form for injection.

✚▲ Side-effects/warning: See CHLORAMPHENICOL.

Chloromycetin Hydrocortisone
(Parke-Davis) is a proprietary, prescription-only COMPOUND PREPARATION of the ANTI-INFLAMMATORY and CORTICOSTEROID hydrocortisone (as acetate) and the broad-spectrum ANTIBACTERIAL and ANTIBIOTIC chloramphenicol. It can be used to treat eye infections with inflammation, and is available as an eye ointment.

✚▲ Side-effects/warning: See CHLORAMPHENICOL; HYDROCORTISONE.

chloroquine
is an ANTIMALARIAL drug which is used as an AMOEBICIDAL to treat and to prevent contraction of malaria. In certain areas of the world strains of *Plasmodium falciparum* have recently exhibited resistance to chloroquine, so an alternative therapy is now advised. Chloroquine is also used as an ANTIRHEUMATIC to slow the progress of rheumatic disease (eg rheumatoid arthritis and lupus erythematosus). Administration is either oral or by injection.

✚ Side-effects: There may be nausea and vomiting, headache; gastrointestinal disturbance; some patients itch and break out in a rash. Susceptible patients may suffer psychotic episodes, blood disorders, damage to the eyes and possibly effects to the hair.

▲ Warning: Administer with caution to those with porphyria, G6PD deficiency, psoriasis or who have certain kidney, liver or gastrointestinal disorders, or neurological disorders. Ophthalmic checks should be made for long-term patients.

✪ Related entries: Avloclor; Nivaquine.

chlorothiazide

is a DIURETIC of the THIAZIDE class which is used as an ANTIHYPERTENSIVE, either alone or in conjunction with other drugs, and can also be used in the treatment of oedema associated with congestive heart failure. Administration is oral.

✚▲ Side-effects/warning: See BENDROFLUAZIDE.

✪ Related entries: Co-Betaloc; Co-Betaloc SA; Saluric.

chlorphenamine maleate

see CHLORPHENIRAMINE MALEATE

chlorpheniramine maleate

(chlorphenamine maleate) is an ANTIHISTAMINE used to treat the symptoms of allergic conditions, such as hay fever and urticaria, and also occasionally in emergencies to treat anaphylactic shock. Administration is either oral or by injection.

✚▲ Side-effects/warning: See ANTIHISTAMINES. Because of its sedative side-effects, the performance of skilled tasks, such as driving, may be impaired. Injections may be irritant and cause short-lasting hypotension and stimulation of the central nervous system.

✪ Related entries: Calimal; Contac 400; Dristan Decongestant Tablets; Expulin Children's Cough Linctus – Sugar Free; Expulin Cough Linctus – Sugar Free; Expulin Decongestant For Babies And Children (Linctus); Galpseud Plus; Haymine; Piriton; Tixylix Cough and Cold; Lemsip Night-Time;

Expulin Decongestant for Babies and Children (Linctus).

chlorpromazine hydrochloride

is chemically an important member of the PHENOTHIAZINES and has a number actions and uses. It is used as an ANTIPSYCHOTIC and has marked sedative effects that make it a useful treatment for schizophrenia and other psychoses, particularly during violent behavioural disturbances. It can also be used as an ANXIOLYTIC in the short-term treatment of severe anxiety, to soothe the terminally ill, sometimes as a premedication prior to surgery to induce hypothermia and reduce shivering and to remedy an intractable hiccup. Additionally, it has an important use as an ANTINAUSEANT and ANTI-EMETIC to relieve nausea and vomiting, particularly in terminal illness. Administration can be either oral or by injection.

✚ Side-effects: Extrapyramidal symptoms, drowsiness, apathy, pallor, insomnia, nightmares, depression (or, rarely, agitation), changes in heart rate and rhythm, dry mouth, nasal constriction, difficulty in urination, constipation, blurred vision, changes in hormone function (irregular menstruation, growth of breasts, abnormal milk production, impotence, weight gain), sensitivity reactions, blood changes, photosensitization, contact sensitization, rashes, jaundice and alterations in liver function, lupus-like syndrome and effects on the eye and skin. Intramuscular injection may be painful.

▲ Warning: It should not be given to patients with bone marrow depression, or phaeochromocytoma. Administer with care to those with vascular disease states, respiratory disease, parkinsonism and epilepsy, liver and kidney impairment, a history of jaundice, blood disorders, myasthenia gravis, hypothyroidism, hypertrophy of the prostate gland, closed-angle glaucoma, hypothyroidism; or who are pregnant or breast-feeding. Withdrawal

of treatment should be gradual. Because of its sedative effects, the performance of skilled tasks may be impaired.
⊙ Related entries: Chloractil; Largactil.

chlorpropamide

is a SULPHONYLUREA which is used in DIABETIC TREATMENT of Type II diabetes mellitus (non-insulin-dependent diabetes mellitus; NIDDM; maturity-onset diabetes). It works by augmenting what remains of INSULIN production in the pancreas and its effect lasts longer than that of most similar drugs. Unusually for a sulphonylurea, chlorpropamide can also be used to treat diabetes insipidus, though only mild forms caused by pituitary or thalamic malfunction, because it also reduces frequency of urination. Administration is oral.
✚▲ Side-effects/warning: See GLIBENCLAMIDE; but has more side-effects. The consumption of alcohol may cause flushing.
⊙ Related entry: Diabinese.

chlorquinaldol

is an ANTIMICROBIAL which is included in some preparations that incorporate a CORTICOSTEROID and are used for treatment of inflammatory skin conditions.
⊙ Related entry: Locoid C.

chlortalidone

see CHLORTHALIDONE

chlortetracycline

is a broad-spectrum ANTIBACTERIAL and (TETRACYCLINE) ANTIBIOTIC. It can be used to treat many forms of infection, especially of the eye and skin (such as acne and impetigo). Administration (as chlortetracycline hydrochloride) is topical.
✚▲ Side-effects/warning: See TETRACYCLINE. Although topical application would not usually cause most of these side-effects, but local sensitivity reactions may occur.
⊙ Related entries: Aureocort; Aureomycin; Aureomycin Topical; Deteclo.

chlorthalidone

(chlortalidone) is a DIURETIC related to the THIAZIDES. It is used to treat oedema, hypertension and diabetes insipidus. Administration is oral.
✚▲ Side-effects/warning: See BENDROFLUAZIDE.
⊙ Related entries: AtenixCo; co-tenidone; Hygroton; Kalspare; Tenchlor; Tenoret 50; Tenoretic.

Cho/Vac

is an abbreviation for CHOLERA VACCINE.

Cholera Vaccine

(Evans) (Cho/Vac) is a prescription-only preparation of cholera VACCINE, which is available in a form for injection.

cholera vaccine

is a VACCINE for IMMUNIZATION that contains heat-killed strains of the bacteria that causes cholera, *Vibrio cholerae*, and is effective for about six months. However, it provides only a limited degree of protection and travellers should still take great care over the food and drink they consume. Administration is by injection.
✚▲ Side-effects/warning: See VACCINES.

cholestyramine

(colestyramine) is a resin that binds bile acids in the gut and is used as a LIPID-LOWERING DRUG in hyperlipidaemia to reduce the levels, or change the proportions, of various lipids in the bloodstream. It has various other uses, including as an ANTIDIARRHOEAL and in certain biliary disturbances (including pruritus in biliary obstruction, or biliary cirrhosis). Generally, it is administered only to patients in whom a strict and regular dietary regime, alone, is not having the desired effect. Administration is oral.
✚ Side-effects: Nausea and vomiting; flatulence with abdominal discomfort, constipation or diarrhoea; and heartburn. (Prolonged use may lead to vitamin K deficiency with increased bleeding.)

▲ Warning: It should not be administered to patients who suffer from complete blockage of the bile ducts; use with caution in those who are pregnant or breast-feeding. High dosage may require simultaneous administration of fat-soluble vitamins and folic acid.

○ Related entries: Questran; Questran A.

choline salicylate

is a drug with mild, local pain-relieving properties, which are principally due to a COUNTER-IRRITANT, or RUBEFACIENT, action. It can be used by topical application in the mouth or ears to relieve, for example, the pain of teething, ulcers or of minor scratches. Administration is oral.

✚▲ Side-effects/warning: See METHYL SALICYLATE.

○ Related entries: Audax Ear Drops; Bonjela Oral Pain-Relieving Gel; Teejel Gel.

chorionic gonadotrophin

(human chorionic gonadotrophin; HCG) is secreted by the placenta and so is obtained from the urine of pregnant women. Its main actions are the same as those of LUTEINISING HORMONE (LH). It can be used as an infertility treatment and also to correct deficiencies in prepubertal males, including aiding decent of testicles and to treat delayed puberty (though use of testosterone for this purpose may be preferred). Administration is by injection.

✚ Side-effects: Oedema, tiredness and mood changes, headache; breast enlargement in males; sexual precocity, over-stimulation of the ovary; reactions at site of injection.

▲ Warning: It should be given with caution to patients with certain heart or kidney disorders, asthma, epilepsy or migraine.

○ Related entries: Gonadotraphon LH; Pregnyl; Profasi.

chymotrypsin

is an enzyme that can be administered to dissolve a suspensory ligament of the lens of the eye (zonulysin) to aid surgical removal of the lens because of cataract.

Administration is by injection.

○ Related entry: Zonulysin.

Cicatrin

(Wellcome) is a proprietary, prescription-only preparation of the (AMINOGLYCOSIDE) ANTIBIOTICS neomycin sulphate and bacitracin zinc. It can be used to treat skin infections, and is available as a cream, a dusting-powder and an aerosol powder-spray.

✚▲ Side-effects/warning: See BACITRACIN ZINC; NEOMYCIN SULPHATE.

ciclosporin

see CYCLOSPORIN

Cidomycin

(Roussel) is a proprietary, prescription-only preparation of the ANTIBACTERIAL and (AMINOGLYCOSIDE) ANTIBIOTIC gentamicin (as sulphate). It can be used to treat many forms of infection, particularly serious infections by Gram-negative bacteria. It is available in various forms for intravenous and intramuscular injection, as ear- or eye-drops and as an eye ointment.

✚▲ Side-effects/warning: See GENTAMICIN.

Cidomycin Topical

(Roussel) is a proprietary, prescription-only preparation of the ANTIBACTERIAL and (AMINOGLYCOSIDE) ANTIBIOTIC gentamicin (as sulphate). It can be used to treat skin infections, particularly by Gram-negative bacteria, and is available as a cream and an ointment for topical application.

✚▲ Side-effects/warning: See GENTAMICIN.

cilastin

is an ENZYME INHIBITOR that inhibits an enzyme in the kidney which breaks down the ANTIBACTERIAL and (BETA-LACTAM) ANTIBIOTIC imipenem and so prolongs and enhances the antibiotic's effects. Cilastin and imipenem are are administered together in a preparation called impenem with cilastin. Administration is by injection.

✚▲ Side-effects/warning: See IMIPENEM

WITH CILASTIN.
○ Related entry: Primaxin.

cilazapril

is an ACE INHIBITOR. It is a powerful VASODILATOR that can be used as an ANTIHYPERTENSIVE, often in conjunction with other classes of drug, particularly (THIAZIDE) DIURETICS. Administration is oral.
✚▲ Side-effects/warning: See CAPTOPRIL.
○ Related entry: Vascace.

Cilest

(Cilag) is a proprietary, prescription-only COMPOUND PREPARATION which can be used as a (*monophasic*) ORAL CONTRACEPTIVE (and also for certain menstrual problems) of the type that combines an OESTROGEN and PROGESTOGEN, in this case ethinyloestradiol and norgestimate. It is available as tablets in a calendar pack.
✚▲ Side-effects/warning: See ETHINYLOESTRADIOL; NORGESTIMATE.

Ciloxan

(Alcon) is a proprietary, prescription-only preparation of the ANTIBACTERIAL and (QUINOLONE) ANTIBIOTIC ciprofloxacin. It can be used to treat a variety of infections, especially ones that are resistant to more conventional drugs, and also corneal ulcers. It is available as eye-drops.
✚▲ Side-effects/warning: See CIPROFLOXACIN.

cimetidine

is an effective and much-prescribed H_2-ANTAGONIST and ULCER-HEALING DRUG. It is used to assist in the treatment of benign peptic (gastric and duodenal) ulcers, to relieve heartburn in cases of reflux oesophagitis, Zollinger-Ellison syndrome and a variety of conditions where reduction of acidity is beneficial. It is now also available without prescription – in a limited amount and for short-term uses only – for the relief of heartburn, dyspepsia and hyperacidity. It works by reducing the secretion of gastric acid (by acting as a histamine receptor H_2-receptor antagonist), so reducing erosion and bleeding from peptic ulcers and allowing them a chance to heal. However, treatment with cimetidine should not be given before full diagnosis of gastric bleeding or serious pain has been carried out, because its action in restricting gastric secretions may possibly mask the presence of other serious disorders such as stomach cancer. Cimetidine can also be used to treat ulceration induced by NSAID treatment. Administration can be either oral or by injection.
✚ Side-effects: There are effects on bowel function, tiredness, rash, dizziness, headache or confusion (especially in the elderly) and reversible liver damage. Rarely, there may be blood disorders, muscle or joint pain, changes in heart, kidney and pancreas function. In men, high doses may cause reversible and temporary feminization (growth of breasts) and impotence.
▲ Warning: It should be administered with caution to patients with impaired liver or kidney function, who are pregnant or breast-feeding. Treatment of undiagnosed dyspepsia may potentially mask the onset of stomach or duodenal cancer and is therefore undesirable. Cimetidine (but not the other available H_2-antagonists) inhibits microsomal metabolic enzymes (such as the microsomal oxidative system of the liver), so it interacts with a number of other drugs: this is of special importance in patients stabilized on the drugs warfarin, theophylline, aminophylline and phenytoin.
○ Related entries: Algitec; Dyspamet; Galenamet; Peptimax; Phimetin; Tagamet; Tagamet Dual Action Liquid; Ultec; Zita.

cinchocaine

is a LOCAL ANAESTHETIC which is used to relieve pain, particularly in dental surgery but also in the skin or mucous membranes. Administration is by topical application.
✚▲ Side-effects/warning: See LIGNOCAINE HYDROCHLORIDE.
○ Related entries: Proctosedyl; Scheriproct; Ultraproct; Uniroid-HC.

cinchona alkaloids ▣

are chemically complex substances extracted from the bark of the cinchona tree (it is also known as Peruvian, Jesuit's or Cardinal's bark). The best-known and most-used cinchona alkaloid is QUININE, which has been used for many centuries to treat fevers and is still an important drug in the treatment of malaria. It has a bitter taste and is incorporated into non-medicinal drinks to mask its flavour. People who are sensitive to it or who consume large quantities of 'tonic water' may experience one of its more marked side-effects, which is tinnitus (a ringing in the ears). The other main cinchona alkaloid is QUINDIDINE (which is chemically similar to quinine, but is its isomer) which is used as an ANTI-ARRHYTHMIC to treat heartbeat irregularities.

cineole

is a TERPENE which is included, as a NASAL DECONGESTANT, in a number of preparations used for the relief of cold symptoms.
◎ Related entries: Copholco; Merothol Lozenges; Vicks Sinex Decongestant Nasal Spray.

cinnarizine

has ANTIHISTAMINE properties and is used for a number of purposes. It is mainly used as an ANTINAUSEANT (and thus an ANTI-EMETIC), for example, in the treatment of vestibular balance disorders (especially vertigo, tinnitus, nausea and vomiting in Ménière's diseases) and motion sickness. Quite separately, it has VASODILATOR properties that affect the blood vessels of the hands and feet and so may be used to improve the circulation in peripheral vascular disease (Raynaud's phenomenon). Administration is oral.
✚▲ Side-effects/warning: See CYCLIZINE. It may also cause fatigue and skin reactions. Rarely, there may be extrapyramidal symptoms in the elderly and hypotension at high doses. Do not administer to those with porphyria.
◎ Related entry: Stugeron.

Cinobac

(Lilly) is a proprietary, prescription-only preparation of the ANTIBACTERIAL and (QUINOLONE) ANTIBIOTIC cinoxacin. It can be used to treat various infections, particularly of the urinary tract, and is available as capsules.
✚▲ Side-effects/warning: See CINOXACIN.

cinoxacin

is an ANTIBACTERIAL and (QUINOLONE) ANTIBIOTIC which is used primarily to treat infections of the urinary tract. Administration is oral.
✚▲ Side-effects/warning: See QUINOLONES. Avoid its use in patients with severe kidney impairment. Other side-effects include oedema and tinnitus.
◎ Related entry: Cinobac.

Cipramil

(Lundbeck, Du Pont) is a proprietary, prescription-only preparation of the (SSRI) ANTIDEPRESSANT citalopram, which has less sedative effects than some other antidepressants. It is available as tablets.
✚▲ Side-effects/warning: See CITALOPRAM.

ciprofibrate

is used as a LIPID-LOWERING DRUG in hyperlipidaemia to reduce the levels, or change the proportions, of various lipids in the bloodstream. It is usually administered only to patients in whom a strict and regular dietary regime, alone, is not having the desired effect. Administration is oral.
✚▲ Side-effects/warning: See BEZAFIBRATE.
◎ Related entry: Modalim.

ciprofloxacin

is a ANTIBACTERIAL and ANTIBIOTIC drug which is a member of the QUINOLONE family. It can be used to treat infections in patients who are allergic to penicillin or whose strain of bacterium is resistant to standard antibiotics. It is active against Gram-negative bacteria including Salmonella, Shigella, Campylobacter, Neisseria and Pseudomonas; and to a lesser extent against

C

Gram-positive bacteria of the Streptococcal family. It is used to treat infections of the urinary, gastrointestinal and respiratory tracts, gonorrhoea and septicaemia. But usually only when these cases are resistant to more conventional agents. It can also be used to prevent meningococcal meningitis and infection during surgical procedures. Administration can be oral, topical or by injection.

+▲ Side-effects/warning: See QUINOLONES. Other side-effects include dyspepsia, flatulence, liver and kidney impairment, difficulty in swallowing. An adequate fluid intake should be maintained. Use with caution in patients with G6PD deficiency.
۞ Related entries: Ciloxan; Ciproxin.

Ciproxin

(Baypharm) is a proprietary, prescription-only preparation of the ANTIBACTERIAL and (QUINOLONE) ANTIBIOTIC ciprofloxacin. It can be used to treat a variety of infections, for example, of the urinary tract and gonorrhoea. It is available as tablets and in a form for intravenous infusion.
+▲ Side-effects/warning: See CIPROFLOXACIN.

cisapride

is a recently introduced MOTILITY STIMULANT. It acts within the stomach and small intestine and can be used to treat oesophageal reflux, for short-term management of non-ulcer dyspepsia, for symptomatic relief of delayed gastric emptying associated with diabetes and systemic sclerosis and autonomic neuropathy. It is thought to act, though it is not known for certain, by releasing the NEUROTRANSMITTER acetylcholine from the nerves of the stomach and intestine. Administration is oral.
+ Side-effects: There may be abdominal cramps, diarrhoea; sometimes headache and light-headedness. Extrapyramidal symptoms have been reported.
▲ Warning: It should not be administered to patients who are pregnant, or where

stimulation of the intestine may be dangerous. Use with care in those with impaired liver or kidney function.
۞ Related entries: Alimix; Prepulsid.

cisatracurium

is a *non-depolarizing* SKELETAL MUSCLE RELAXANT which can be used to induce muscle paralysis (of medium duration) during surgery. Administration is by injection.
+▲ Side-effects/warning: See TUBOCURARINE CHLORIDE.
۞ Related entry: Nimbex.

cisplatin

is a CYTOTOXIC drug (an organic complex of platinum) that works by damaging the DNA of replicating cells and so can be used as an ANTICANCER drug in the treatment of certain solid tumours, including ovarian cancer and testicular teratoma. Administration is by injection.
+▲ Side-effects/warning: See CYTOTOXICS; but also severe nausea and vomiting, kidney damage, ototoxicity and peripheral nerve effects.

citalopram

is a recently introduced (SSRI) ANTIDEPRESSANT which is used to treat depressive illness and has the advantage over some other antidepressants because it has relatively less SEDATIVE and ANTICHOLINERGIC side-effects. The onset of action may take some weeks to reach full effect and offset on discontinuation is also slow. Administration is oral.
+▲ Side-effects/warning: See FLUOXETINE.
۞ Related entry: Cipramil.

Citanest

(Astra) is a proprietary, prescription-only preparation of the LOCAL ANAESTHETIC prilocaine hydrochloride. It can be used for various types of anaesthesia, and is available in a form for injection.
+▲ Side-effects/warning: See PRILOCAINE HYDROCHLORIDE.

Citanest with Octapressin

(Astra) is a proprietary, prescription-only COMPOUND PREPARATION of the LOCAL ANAESTHETIC prilocaine hydrochloride and the VASOCONSTRICTOR felypressin. It can be used in dental surgery, and is available in a form for injection.

+▲ Side-effects/warning: See FELYPRESSIN; PRILOCAINE HYDROCHLORIDE.

Citramag

(Bioglan) is a proprietary, non-prescription preparation of the (*osmotic*) LAXATIVE magnesium citrate. It can be used to relieve constipation, and is available as an effervescent powder.

cladribine

is a CYTOTOXIC drug which is administered as an ANTICANCER treatment for hairy cell leukaemia. Administration is by injection.

+▲ Side-effects/warning: See CYTOTOXICS.
✪ Related entry: Leustat.

Claforan

(Roussel) is a proprietary, prescription-only preparation of the ANTIBACTERIAL and (CEPHALOSPORIN) ANTIBIOTIC cefotaxime. It can be used to treat many infections, including meningitis, and is available in a form for injection.

+▲ Side-effects/warning: See CEFOTAXIME.

clarithromycin

is an ANTIBACTERIAL and (MACROLIDE) ANTIBIOTIC which is a derivative of erythromycin, and is usually given to patients who are allergic to penicillin. It can be administered to treat various skin, soft tissue and respiratory tract infections. Administration can be either oral or by injection.

+▲ Side-effects/warning: See ERYTHROMYCIN. Adminster with caution to patients who are pregnant or breast-feeding. Blood disorders have been reported. There may be headache, effects on taste and inflammation of the tongue and mouth.
✪ Related entry: Klaricid.

Clarityn

(Schering-Plough) is a proprietary, prescription-only preparation of the ANTIHISTAMINE loratadine. It can be used to treat the symptoms of allergic disorders, such as hay fever and urticaria, and is available as tablets and a syrup.

+▲ Side-effects/warning: See LORATADINE.

clavulanic acid

is chemically an ANTIBIOTIC but is only weakly ANTIBACTERIAL and is used instead as a PENICILLINASE INHIBITOR to combat bacterial resistance. It works as an ENZYME INHIBITOR by inhibiting the penicillinase enzymes ('beta-lactamases') that are produced by some bacteria. These enzymes can inactivate many antibiotics of the penicillin family, such as amoxycillin and ticarcillin, and so prevent the antibiotics from working. Clavulanic acid is therefore used in combination with amoxycillin or ticarcillin.

✪ Related entries: Augmentin; Timentin.

Clearine Eye Drops

(Crookes) is a non-prescription preparation of the SYMPATHOMIMETIC and VASOCONSTRICTOR naphazoline hydrochloride. It can be used to treat redness in the eyes due to minor infections, and is available as eye-drops. It is not normally given to children, except on medical advice.

+▲ Side-effects/warning: See NAPHAZOLINE HYDROCHLORIDE.

clemastine

is an ANTIHISTAMINE which can be used for the symptomatic relief of allergic symptoms, such as hay fever and urticaria. Administration is oral.

+▲ Side-effects/warning: See ANTIHISTAMINES. Because of its sedative side-effects, the performance of skilled tasks, such as driving and operating machinery, may be impaired.
✪ Related entries: Aller-eze; Aller-eze Plus; Tavegil.

C

Clexane
(Rhône-Poulenc Rorer) is a proprietary, prescription-only preparation of the ANTICOAGULANT enoxaparin, which is a low molecular weight version of heparin. It can be used for long-duration prevention of venous thrombo-embolism, particularly in orthopaedic use. It is available in a form for injection.
➕▲ Side-effects/warning: See ENOXAPARIN.

Climagest
(Sandoz) is a proprietary, prescription-only COMPOUND PREPARATION of the female SEX HORMONES oestradiol (as valerate; an OESTROGEN) and norethisterone (a PROGESTOGEN). It can be used to treat menopausal problems, including in HRT (hormone replacement therapy), and is available as tablets.
➕▲ Side-effects/warning: See NORETHISTERONE; OESTRADIOL.

Climaval
(Sandoz) is a proprietary, prescription-only preparation of the OESTROGEN oestradiol (as valerate). It can be used in HRT (hormone replacement therapy), and is available as tablets in a calendar pack.
➕▲ Side-effects/warning: See OESTRADIOL.

Climesse
(Sandoz) is a proprietary, prescription-only COMPOUND PREPARATION of the female SEX HORMONES oestradiol (an OESTROGEN) and norethisterone (as acetate; a progestogen). It can be used as HRT, and is available as tablets.
➕▲ Side-effects/warning: See NORETHISTERONE; OESTRADIOL.

clindamycin
is an ANTIBACTERIAL and ANTIBIOTIC drug which is used to treat infections of bones and joints, peritonitis (inflammation of the peritoneal lining of the abdominal cavity) and to assist in the prevention of endocarditis. It is active against many anaerobic bacteria (including *Bacteroides*

fragilis and Gram-positive cocci (including penicillin-resistant *Staphylococci*). It can also be used topically to treat acne and vaginal infections. However, it is not widely used because of its serious side-effects. Administration can be oral, by topical application or by injection.
➕ Side-effects: If diarrhoea or colitis appear during treatment, administration must be halted (see below). There may be nausea and vomiting; abdominal discomfort; jaundice, liver dysfunction; blood disorders.
▲ Warning: It should not be administered to patients suffering from diarrhoea; and if diarrhoea or other symptoms of colitis appear during treatment, administration must be stopped. This is because clindamycin greatly alters the normal balance of bacteria in the gut and in a few cases this allows a superinfection by the anaerobe *Clostridium difficile*, which causes a form of colitis that can be serious. It should be administered with caution to those with certain liver or kidney disorders, or who are pregnant or breast-feeding.
✪ Related entries: Dalacin; Dalacin C; Dalacin T.

Clinicide
(De Witt) is a proprietary, non-prescription preparation of the PEDICULICIDAL drug carbaryl. It can be used to treat infestations of the scalp and pubic hair by lice. It is available as a lotion and a shampoo and is not normally given to infants under six months, except on medical advice.
➕▲ Side-effects/warning: See CARBARYL.

Clinitar
(Shire) is a proprietary, prescription-only preparation of coal tar. It can be used to treat eczema and psoriasis, and is available as a cream and a shampoo.
➕▲ Side-effects/warning: See COAL TAR.

Clinoril
(Merck Sharp & Dohme) is a proprietary, prescription-only preparation of the (NSAID) NON-NARCOTIC ANALGESIC and ANTIRHEUMATIC

sulindac. It can be used to treat rheumatic conditions and other musculoskeletal disorders and acute gout. It is available as tablets.

+▲ Side-effects/warning: See SULINDAC.

clioquinol

is an ANTIMICROBIAL drug which is chemically an iodine-containing member of the 8-hydroxyquinoline group. It can be used as an ANTIFUNGAL and AMOEBICIDAL, and its primary use is to treat *Candida* fungal infections of the skin and outer ear. Administration is topical as drops, creams, ointments and anal suppositories.

+ Side-effects: Some patients experience sensitivity reactions.

✪ Related entries: Betnovate-C; Locorten-Vioform; Oralcer; Synalar C; Vioform-Hydrocortisone.

clobazam

is a BENZODIAZEPINE which is used as an ANXIOLYTIC in the short-term treatment of anxiety. It can also be used, in conjunction with other drugs, as an ANTI-EPILEPTIC treatment. Administration is oral.

+▲ Side-effects/warning: See BENZODIAZEPINES.

✪ Related entry: Frisium.

clobetasol propionate

is an extremely powerful CORTICOSTEROID with ANTI-INFLAMMATORY properties. It is used to treat severe, non-infective inflammation of the skin caused by conditions such as eczema and psoriasis, especially in cases where less powerful steroid treatments have failed. Administration is by topical application.

+▲ Side-effects/warning: See CORTICOSTEROIDS; though systemic side-effects are unlikely with topical application, but there may be local skin reactions. The amount applied to the skin each week should be below a certain maximum amount.

✪ Related entries: Dermovate; Dermovate-NN.

clobetasone butyrate

is a CORTICOSTEROID with ANTI-INFLAMMATORY properties. It is administered in the treatment of severe inflammation of the skin caused by conditions such as eczema and certain types of dermatitis, especially as a maintenance treatment between courses of more potent corticosteroids. Administration is by topical application.

+▲ Side-effects/warning: See CORTICOSTEROIDS; though systemic effects are unlikely with topical application, but there may be local skin reactions.

✪ Related entries: Eumovate; Eumovate-N; Trimovate.

clofazimine

is an ANTIBACTERIAL which is administered, in combination with the drugs dapsone and rifampicin, in the treatment of the major form of leprosy. The fact that the treatment of leprosy now requires the use of no fewer than three drugs is because of the increasing resistance exhibited by the leprosy bacterium. Administration is oral.

+ Side-effects: There may be nausea and giddiness, diarrhoea and headache. The skin and urine may have a reddish tinge and skin lesions may be discoloured.

▲ Warning: It should be administered with caution to patients with impaired kidney or liver function. Regular tests on both functions are essential.

✪ Related entry: Lamprene.

clofibrate

is used as a LIPID-LOWERING DRUG in hyperlipidaemia to reduce the levels, or change the proportions, of various lipids in the bloodstream. It is usually administered only to patients in whom a strict and regular dietary regime, alone, is not having the desired effect. Administration is oral.

+▲ Side-effects/warning: see BEZAFIBRATE.

✪ Related entry: Atromid-S.

clomethiazole

see CHLORMETHIAZOLE

C

Clomid

(Merrell) is a proprietary, prescription-only preparation of the HORMONE ANTAGONIST clomiphene citrate, which is an ANTI-OESTROGEN. It can be used to treat infertility due to ovulatory failure, and is available as tablets.

✚▲ Side-effects/warning: See CLOMIPHENE CITRATE.

clomiphene citrate

is a sex HORMONE ANTAGONIST (an ANTI-OESTROGEN) which is used as a fertility treatment in women whose condition is linked to the persistent presence of oestrogens and a consequent failure to ovulate (characterized by sparse or infrequent periods). Clomiphene prevents the action of oestrogens and this therefore increases the secretion of GONADOTROPHINS, which cause ovulation. Administration is oral.

✚ Side-effects: Multiple births may result. Hot flushes; nausea; vomiting; visual disturbances; dizziness and insomnia; breast tenderness; weight gain; rashes; and hair loss may occur.

▲ Warning: It should not be administered to patients with ovarian cysts; cancer of the womb lining; certain liver disorders; abnormal uterine bleeding; or who are pregnant.

✪ Related entries: Clomid; Serophene.

clomipramine hydrochloride

is a (TRICYCLIC) ANTIDEPRESSANT that also has SEDATIVE properties. It is administered primarily to treat depressive illness, but can also be used to assist in treating phobic or obsessional states and to try to reduce the incidence of catalepsy in narcoleptic patients (those who fall asleep in quiet or monotonous periods). Administration can be either oral or by injection.

✚▲ Side-effects/warning: See AMITRIPTYLINE HYDROCHLORIDE.

✪ Related entry: Anafranil.

clonazepam

is a BENZODIAZEPINE which is used as an ANTICONVULSANT and ANTI-EPILEPTIC for all forms of epilepsy, especially myoclonus and status epilepticus. Administration can be either oral or by injection.

✚▲ Side-effects/warning: See BENZODIAZEPINES; but it is not to be administered to patients with certain lung disorders.

✪ Related entry: Rivotril.

clonidine hydrochloride

is an ANTISYMPATHETIC drug which decreases the release of NORADRENALINE from sympathetic nerves. It can be used as an ANTIHYPERTENSIVE, an ANTIMIGRAINE treatment (for reducing the incidence of attacks) and for vascular headaches and menopausal flushing (however, authorities are not convinced of its efficacy for this purpose). Additionally, there is some use for it in treating the symptoms (tics) of Gilles de la Tourette syndrome. Administration is either oral or by injection.

✚ Side-effects: Sedation, drowsiness, headache, depression or euphoria; dry mouth; fluid retention; rashes; nausea and constipation; blood disorders; slow heart rate, poor circulation in the extremities; rarely, there may be a failure to ejaculate and sleep disturbances.

▲ Warning: It should not be administered to patients who have a history of depression. It must be given with caution to those with porphyria or peripheral vascular disease. The drug may cause drowsiness and impair the ability to drive or operate machinery. Withdrawal of treatment should be gradual.

✪ Related entries: Catapres; Catapres Perlongets; Dixarit.

clopamide

is a (THIAZIDE) DIURETIC which can be used as an ANTIHYPERTENSIVE in conjunction with BETA-BLOCKERS. Administration is oral.

✚▲ Side-effects/warning: See BENDROFLUAZIDE.

✪ Related entry: Viskaldix.

Clopixol

(Lundbeck) is a proprietary, prescription-only preparation of the ANTIPSYCHOTIC zuclopenthixol dihydrochloride, and can be used for the long-term maintenance of schizophrenia and other psychoses. It is available as tablets (as zuclopenthixol dihydrochloride) and a depot deep intramuscular injection called (as zuclopenthixol decanoate). There is a range of *Clopixol* preparations which differ in their duration of action and may be used according to the length of treatment intended.

✚▲ Side-effects/warning: See ZUCLOPENTHIXOL DECANOATE; ZUCLOPENTHIXOL DIHYDROCHLORIDE.

Clopixol Acuphase

(Lundbeck) is a proprietary, prescription-only preparation of the ANTIPSYCHOTIC zuclopenthixol acetate. It can be administered for the short-term management of acute psychosis and mania or exacerbation of a chronic psychotic disorder. It is available in a form for depot deep intramuscular injection.

✚▲ Side-effects/warning: See ZUCLOPENTHIXOL ACETATE.

Clopixol Conc.

(Lundbeck) is a proprietary, prescription-only preparation of the ANTIPSYCHOTIC zuclopenthixol decanoate, and can be used for long-term maintenance of schizophrenia and other psychoses. It is available in a form for depot deep intramuscular injection.

✚▲ Side-effects/warning: See ZUCLOPENTHIXOL DECANOATE.

clorazepate dipotassium

(dipotassium clorazepate) is a BENZODIAZEPINE which is used as an ANXIOLYTIC in the short-term treatment of anxiety. Administration is oral.

✚▲ Side-effects/warning: See BENZODIAZEPINES.

✿ Related entry: Tranxene.

Clostet

(Evans) is a proprietary, prescription-only VACCINE preparation of adsorbed tetanus vaccine. It can be used for active IMMUNIZATION against tetanus, and is available in a form for injection.

clotrimazole

is an (AZOLE) ANTIMICROBIAL and ANTIFUNGAL drug. It can be used in topical application to treat fungal infections of the skin and mucous membranes (especially the vagina, outer ear and toes). Administration is by topical application.

✚ Side-effects: Rarely, there may be a burning sensation or irritation; a very few patients experience sensitivity reactions.

✿ Related entries: Canesten; Canesten 1 VT; Canesten 1%; Canesten 10% VC; Canesten-HC; Lotriderm; Masnoderm.

cloxacillin

is an ANTIBACTERIAL and ANTIBIOTIC drug of the PENICILLIN family. It is *penicillinase-resistant* which means that it is not inactivated by the penicillinase enzymes produced by bacteria such as *Staphylococci*, and is therefore primarily used to treat infections that other penicillins are incapable of countering due to the presence of this enzyme. Administration is either oral or by injection.

✚▲ Side-effects/warning: See BENZYLPENICILLIN.

✿ Related entries: Ampiclox; Ampiclox Neonatal; Orbenin.

clozapine

is an ANTIPSYCHOTIC drug which can be used for the treatment of schizophrenia in patients who do not respond to, or who can not tolerate, conventional antipsychotic drugs. Because clozapine can cause serious blood disorders, its use is restricted to patients registered with the Sandoz Clozaril Patient Monitoring Service. Administration is oral.

✚ Side-effects: See CHLORPROMAZINE HYDROCHLORIDE. But it is less sedating and

C

with a higher incidence of anticholinergic symptoms. Extrapyramidal symptoms are less frequent. There are potentially very serious effects on the blood (agranulocytosis and neutropenia). Headache and dizziness, salivation, urinary incontinence, persistent erection, heart dysfunction, delirium, nausea and vomiting.

▲ Warning: Because of its effects on the blood (especially to depress the white cell count), this drug can only be used on registration with and concurrent monitoring by the special patient monitoring service. It should not be given to patients who are pregnant or breast-feeding.
✪ Related entry: Clozaril.

Clozaril

(Sandoz) is a proprietary, prescription-only preparation of the ANTIPSYCHOTIC clozapine. It can be used to treat schizophrenics who are unresponsive to other drugs, and is subject to special monitoring because of its potentially severe effects on the blood. It is available as tablets.
✚▲ Side-effects/warning: See CLOZAPINE.

coal tar

is a black, viscous liquid obtained by the distillation of coal. It is used on the skin to reduce inflammation and itching and also has some KERATOLYTIC properties. Therapeutically, it is used to treat psoriasis and eczema, where it is used in solution at a concentration determined by a patient's condition and response. It is a constituent in many non-proprietary and proprietary preparations, especially pastes.
✚ Side-effects: Skin irritation, an acne-like rash and sensitivity to light.
▲ Warning: Avoid contact with broken or inflamed skin and the eyes. Coal tar stains skin, hair and fabric.
✪ Related entries: Alphosyl; Alphosyl 2 in 1 Shampoo; Alphosyl HC; Balneum with Tar; Baltar; Calamine and Coal tar Ointment, BP; Capasal; Carbo-Cort; Carbo-Dome; Clinitar; Coal Tar and Salicylic Acid Ointment, BP; Cocois; Gelcosal; Gelcotar; Ionil T; Pentrax;

Polytar Emollient; Pragmatar; Psoriderm; PsoriGel; Psorin; T/Gel; Tarcortin.

Coal Tar and Salicylic Acid Ointment, BP

is a non-proprietary, non-prescription preparation of coal tar and salicylic acid. It can be used by topical application to treat chronic eczema and psoriasis, and is available as an ointment.
✚▲ Side-effects/warning: See COAL TAR; SALICYLIC ACID.

co-amilofruse 10/80

is a simplified name for the COMPOUND PREPARATION of the (*potassium-sparing*) DIURETIC amiloride hydrochloride and the (*loop*) diuretic frusemide; in the ratio of 10:80 (mg).
✚▲ Side-effects/warning: See AMILORIDE HYDROCHLORIDE; FRUSEMIDE.
✪ Related entry: Frumil Forte.

co-amilofruse 5/40

is a simplified name for the COMPOUND PREPARATION of the (*potassium-sparing*) DIURETIC amiloride hydrochloride and the (*loop*) diuretic frusemide; in the ratio of 5:40 (mg).
✚▲ Side-effects/warning: See AMILORIDE HYDROCHLORIDE; FRUSEMIDE.
✪ Related entries: Fru-Co; Frumil; Lasoride.

co-amilozide 2.5/25

is a simplified name for the COMPOUND PREPARATION of the (*potassium-sparing*) DIURETIC amiloride hydrochloride and the THIAZIDE diuretic hydrochlorothiazide; in the ratio 2.5:25 (mg).
✚▲ Side-effects/warning: See AMILORIDE HYDROCHLORIDE; HYDROCHLORITHIAZIDE.
✪ Related entry: Moduret-25.

co-amilozide 5/50

is a simplified name for the COMPOUND PREPARATION of the (*potassium-sparing*) DIURETIC amiloride hydrochloride and the THIAZIDE diuretic hydrochlorothiazide; in the ratio 5:50 (mg).

+▲ Side-effects/warning: See AMILORIDE HYDROCHLORIDE; HYDROCHLOROTHIAZIDE.
✪ Related entries: Amil-Co; Delvas; Moduretic.

co-amoxclav

is a simplified name for the COMPOUND PREPARATION of the broad-spectrum ANTIBACTERIAL and (PENICILLIN) ANTIBIOTIC amoxycillin and the ENZYME INHIBITOR clavulanic acid (in the form of its potassium salt). Clavulanic acid interferes with the action of beta-lactamase and so makes amoxycillin *penicillinase-resistant* when it is used against *Staphylococcus aureus*, *Haemophilus influenzae* and certain other bacteria that would otherwise inactivate the antibiotic. Co-amoxclav can be used to treat many infections including those of the upper respiratory tract, of the ear, nose and throat and of the urinogenital tracts. Administration is either oral or by injection.
+▲ Side-effects/warning: See AMOXYCILLIN. Administer with caution to patients with liver impairment, jaundice, certain blood disorders; or who are pregnant or breast-feeding.
✪ Related entry: Augmentin.

Cobadex

(Cox) is a proprietary, prescription-only COMPOUND PREPARATION of the CORTICOSTEROID and ANTI-INFLAMMATORY hydrocortisone and the ANTIFOAMING AGENT dimethicone. It can be used to treat mild inflammatory skin conditions, such as eczema, and is available as a cream.
+▲ Side-effects/warning: See DIMETHICONE; HYDROCORTISONE.

Cobalin-H

(Link) is a proprietary, prescription-only preparation of the VITAMIN hydroxocobalamin. It can be used to correct deficiency of vitamin B_{12}, including pernicious anaemia, and is available in a form for injection.
+▲ Side-effects/warning: See HYDROXOCOBALAMIN.

co-beneldopa

is a simplified name for the COMPOUND PREPARATION of the ANTIPARKINSONISM drug levodopa and the ENZYME INHIBITOR benserazide hydrochloride (in a ratio of benzeride/levodopa 1:4). It is used to treat parkinsonism, but not drug-induced parkinsonian symptoms. Benserazide prevents levodopa from being broken down too rapidly in the body (into dopamine), so allowing more of it to reach the brain to make up the deficiency of dopamine, which is the cause of parkinsonian symptoms. Administration is oral.
+▲ Side-effects/warning: See LEVODOPA.
✪ Related entry: Madopar.

Co-Betaloc

(Astra) is a proprietary, prescription-only COMPOUND PREPARATION of the BETA-BLOCKER metoprolol tartrate and the (THIAZIDE) DIURETIC chlorothiazide. It can be used as an ANTIHYPERTENSIVE for raised blood pressure, and is available as tablets.
+▲ Side-effects/warning: See CHLOROTHIAZIDE; METOPROLOL TARTRATE.

Co-Betaloc SA

(Astra) is a proprietary, prescription-only COMPOUND PREPARATION of the BETA-BLOCKER metoprolol tartrate and the (THIAZIDE) DIURETIC chlorothiazide. It can be used as an ANTIHYPERTENSIVE for raised blood pressure, and is available as modified-release tablets.
+▲ Side-effects/warning: See CHLOROTHIAZIDE; METOPROLOL TARTRATE.

cocaine

is a central nervous system STIMULANT which rapidly causes dependence (addiction). Therapeutically, it is used as a LOCAL ANAESTHETIC for topical application to the throat, nose or eyes.
+ Side-effects: Stimulation of the central nervous system, sympathomimetic effects and heart arrhythmias.
▲ Warning: Avoid its use in patients with porphyria.

C

C

co-careldopa

is a simplified name for the COMPOUND PREPARATION of the ANTIPARKINSONISM drug levodopa and the ENZYME INHIBITOR carbidopa (the proportion of carbidopa to levodopa varies). It is used to treat parkinsonism, but not the parkinsonian symptoms induced by drugs. Carbidopa prevents levodopa from being broken down too rapidly in the body (into dopamine) and so allowing more of it to reach the brain to make up the deficiency of dopamine, which is the cause of parkinsonian symptoms. Administration is oral.

+▲ Side-effects/warning: See LEVODOPA.

✪ Related entries: Half Sinemet CR; Sinemet; Sinemet CR; Sinemet LS; Sinemet-Plus.

co-codamol

is a COMPOUND ANALGESIC preparation of the (OPIOID) NARCOTIC ANALGESIC codeine phosphate and the NON-NARCOTIC ANALGESIC paracetamol; in either a ratio of 8:500 (mg) – *co-codamol 8/500*, or the stronger and more recently introduced 30:500 (mg) – *co-codamol 30/500*. The 8/500 preparation is available on a non-prescription basis (as it has a lower codeine content) either as one of an extensive range of generic preparations or in proprietary forms that cannot be prescribed under the National Health Service. The 30/500 preparation is available only on prescription and should be used with caution, especially in the elderly.

+▲ Side-effects/warning: See CODEINE PHOSPHATE; PARACETAMOL.

✪ Related entries: Kapake; Panadeine Tablets; Paracodol Capsules; Paracodol Tablets; Parake; Solpadol; Tylex.

co-codaprin

(8/400) is a COMPOUND ANALGESIC preparation of the (OPIOID) NARCOTIC ANALGESIC codeine phosphate and the (NSAID) NON-NARCOTIC ANALGESIC and ANTIRHEUMATIC aspirin; in a ratio of 8:400 (mg). Administration is oral.

+▲ Side-effects/warning: See ASPIRIN; CODEINE PHOSPHATE.

Cocois

(Bioglan) is a proprietary, non-prescription COMPOUND PREPARATION of salicylic acid, coal tar and sulphur (in coconut oil). It is used to treat eczema and psoriasis, and is available as a scalp ointment.

+▲ Side-effects/warning: See COAL TAR; SALICYLIC ACID; SULPHUR.

cod-liver oil

has EMOLLIENT properties and is one of the constituents of a proprietary COMPOUND PREPARATION that is administered by topical application to the skin in the form of a cream. At one time cod-liver oil was commonly used as a source of VITAMIN A and VITAMIN D, but now HALIBUT-LIVER OIL is preferred.

✪ Related entry: Morhulin Ointment.

Codafen Continus

(Napp) is a proprietary, prescription-only COMPOUND ANALGESIC preparation of the (NSAID) NON-NARCOTIC ANALGESIC and ANTIRHEUMATIC ibuprofen and the (OPIOID) NARCOTIC ANALGESIC codeine phosphate (in higher amounts than in proprietary, non-prescription, over-the-counter compound analgesics). It can be used in particular for treating the pain of musculoskeletal disorders, and is available as tablets.

+▲ Side-effects/warning: See CODEINE PHOSPHATE; IBUPROFEN.

Codalax

(Napp) is a proprietary, prescription-only preparation of co-danthramer 25/200, which is a (*stimulant*) LAXATIVE based on danthron. It can be used to treat constipation and to prepare patients for abdominal procedures, and is available as an oral suspension.

+▲ Side-effects/warning: See DANTHRON.

Codalax Forte

(Napp) is a proprietary, prescription-only preparation of co-danthramer 75/1000, which is a (*stimulant*) LAXATIVE based on danthron. It can be used to treat constipation and to prepare patients for abdominal procedures, and is available as an oral suspension.

+▲ Side-effects/warning: See DANTHRON.

Codanin Tablets

(Whitehall) is a proprietary, non-prescription COMPOUND ANALGESIC preparation of the NON-NARCOTIC ANALGESIC and ANTIPYRETIC paracetamol and the (OPIOID) NARCOTIC ANALGESIC codeine phosphate. It can be used for the symptomatic relief of mild to moderate pain and raised body temperature. It is available as tablets and is not normally given to children under six years, except on medical advice.

+▲ Side-effects/warning: See CODEINE PHOSPHATE; PARACETAMOL.

co-danthramer 25/200

is a non-proprietary, prescription-only COMPOUND PREPARATION of the (*stimulant*) LAXATIVE danthron and poloxamer '188'. Administration is oral.

+▲ Side-effects/warning: See DANTHRON.
☯ Related entry: Codalax.

co-danthramer 75/1000

is a non-proprietary, prescription-only COMPOUND PREPARATION of the (*stimulant*) LAXATIVE danthron and poloxamer '188'. Administration is oral.

+▲ Side-effects/warning: See DANTHRON.
☯ Related entry: Codalax Forte.

co-danthrusate 50/60

is a non-proprietary, prescription-only COMPOUND PREPARATION of the (*stimulant*) LAXATIVES danthron and docusate sodium. Administration is oral.

+▲ Side-effects/warning: See DANTHRON; DOCUSATE SODIUM.
☯ Related entry: Normax.

codeine phosphate

is an (OPIOID) NARCOTIC ANALGESIC that also has the properties of an ANTITUSSIVE. As an analgesic, codeine is a common but often minor constituent of non-proprietary and proprietary preparations for the relief of mild to moderate pain. The drug also has the capacity to reduce intestinal motility and so can be used as an ANTIDIARRHOEAL and antimotility treatment. Administration is either oral or by injection.

+▲ Side-effects/warning: See OPIOIDS. Tolerance occurs readily, though dependence (addiction) is relatively unusual.

☯ Related entries: Aspav; Benylin with Codeine; co-codamol; co-codaprin; Codafen Continus; Codanin Tablets; Codis 500; Cojene Tablets; Diarrest; Dimotane Co; Dimotane with Codiene Pediatric; Famel Original Cough Syrup; Feminax; Galcodine; Galcodine Paediatric; Kapake; Migraleve; Nurofen Plus; Panadeine Tablets; Panadol Ultra; Paracodol Capsules; Paracodol Tablets; Parake; Propain Tablets; Solpadeine Capsules; Solpadeine Soluble Tablets; Solpadeine Tablets; Solpadol; Syndol; Tylex; Veganin Tablets.

co-dergocrine mesylate

is a VASODILATOR drug which affects the blood vessels of the brain. It consists of a mixture of dihydroergocornine mesylate, dihydroergocristine mesylate and alpha- and beta-dihydroergocryptine mesylates, which have ALPHA-ADRENOCEPTOR BLOCKING actions. It has on occasion been claimed to be a NOOTROPIC AGENT, improving brain function; but clinical results of psychological tests during and following treatment have neither proved nor disproved such a claim. It is for the treatment of senile dementia that the drug is most frequently used. Administration is oral.

+ Side-effects: There may be gastrointestinal disturbances, flushing, a blocked nose, headache and a rash. Postural hypotension (low blood pressure on standing up from a lying or sitting position, causing dizziness).

▲ Warning: It should be administered with caution to patients who have a particularly slow heart rate.

✪ Related entry: Hydergine.

Codis 500

(Reckitt & Colman) is a proprietary, non-prescription COMPOUND ANALGESIC preparation of the (NSAID) NON-NARCOTIC ANALGESIC and ANTIRHEUMATIC aspirin and the (OPIOID) NARCOTIC ANALGESIC codeine phosphate. It can be used to relieve mild to moderate pain and high body temperature. It is available as soluble tablets and is not normally given to children under12 years, except on medical advice.

✚▲ Side-effects/warning: See ASPIRIN; CODEINE PHOSPHATE.

co-dydramol

is a prescription-only COMPOUND ANALGESIC preparation of the (OPIOID) NARCOTIC ANALGESIC dihydrocodeine tartrate and the NON-NARCOTIC ANALGESIC paracetamol; in a ratio of 10:500 (mg) – though some non-prescription preparations have different ratios. It is available in many generic and some proprietary preparations. There are further prescription-only versions that are similar, but have a higher proportion of dihydrocodeine (SEE REMEDEINE). This compound analgesic has the advantages and disadvantages of both drugs. It is particularly dangerous in overdose because of the opioid dihydrocodeine tartrate component. It is available as tablets.

✚▲ Side-effects/warning: See DIHYDROCODEINE TARTRATE; PARACETAMOL.

✪ Related entries: Galake; Paramol Tablets.

co-fluampicil

is a simplified name for the COMPOUND PREPARATION of the broad-spectrum, penicillin-like ANTIBACTERIAL and ANTIBIOTIC ampicillin and the *penicillinase-resistant*, penicillin-like antibacterial and antibiotic flucloxacillin. It can be used to treat severe

infection where the causative organism has not been identified, but Gram-positive staphylococcal infection is suspected or where penicillin-resistant bacterial infection is probable. Administration is either oral or by injection.

✚▲ Side-effects/warning: See AMPICILLIN; FLUCLOXACILLIN.

✪ Related entries: Flu-Amp; Magnapen.

co-flumactone 25/25

is a simplified name for the COMPOUND PREPARATION of the (*aldosterone-antagonist* and *potassium-sparing*) DIURETIC spironolactone and the (*potassium-depleting* THIAZIDE) diuretic hydroflumethiazide; in the ratio 25:25 (mg).

✚▲ Side-effects/warning: See HYDROFLUMETHIAZIDE; SPIRONOLACTONE.

✪ Related entries: Aldactide 25; Spiro-Co.

co-flumactone 50/50

is a simplified name for the COMPOUND PREPARATION of the (*aldosterone-antagonist* and *potassium-sparing*) DIURETIC spironolactone and the (*potassium-depleting* THIAZIDE) diuretic hydroflumethiazide; in the ratio of 50:50 (mg).

✚▲ Side-effects/warning: See HYDROFLUMETHIAZIDE; SPIRONOLACTONE.

✪ Related entries: Aldactide 50; Spiro-Co 50.

Cogentin

(Merck Sharp & Dohme) is a proprietary, prescription-only preparation of the ANTICHOLINERGIC benztropine mesylate. It can be used in the treatment of parkinsonism, and is available as tablets and in a form for injection.

✚▲ Side-effects/warning: See BENZTROPINE MESYLATE.

Cojene Tablets

(Roche) is a proprietary, non-prescription COMPOUND PREPARATION of the (NSAID) NON-NARCOTIC ANALGESIC and ANTIRHEUMATIC

aspirin, the (OPIOID) NARCOTIC ANALGESIC codeine phosphate and the STIMULANT caffeine. It can be used to relieve pain (especially rheumatic pain), fever and flu and cold symptoms. It is available as tablets and is not normally given to children under 12 years, except on medical advice.
✚▲ Side-effects/warning: See ASPIRIN; CAFFEINE; CODEINE PHOSPHATE.

colchicine

is a drug derived from the autumn crocus *Colchicum autnale*. It is used in the treatment of gout, particularly as a short-term, introductory measure to prevent acute attacks during initial treatment with other drugs that reduce uric acid levels in the blood. Administration is oral.
✚ Side-effects: Nausea, vomiting and abdominal pain. High or excessive dosage may lead to gastrointestinal bleeding and diarrhoea, rashes and even kidney damage. Rarely, peripheral nerve disorders, loss of hair or blood disorders.
▲ Warning: Administer with caution to patients with gastrointestinal disease, impaired kidney function; or who are pregnant or breast-feeding.

Cold Relief Capsules

(Sussex) is a proprietary, non-prescription COMPOUND PREPARATION of the NON-NARCOTIC ANALGESIC paracetamol, the DECONGESTANT phenylephrine hydrochloride and the STIMULANT caffeine. It can be used to relieve cold and flu symptoms, and is available as capsules. It is not normally given to children, except on medical advice.
✚▲ Side-effects/warning: See CAFFEINE; PARACETAMOL; PHENYLEPHRINE HYDROCHLORIDE.

Coldrex Tablets

(Sterling) is a proprietary, non-prescription COMPOUND PREPARATION of the NON-NARCOTIC ANALGESIC paracetamol, the SYMPATHOMIMETIC and DECONGESTANT phenylephrine hydochloride and the STIMULANT caffeine (with terpin and vitamin C). It can be used to relieve cold and flu symptoms, and is

available as tablets. It is not normally given to children, except on medical advice.
✚▲ Side-effects/warning: See CAFFEINE; PARACETAMOL; PHENYLEPHRINE HYDROCHLORIDE.

Colestid

(Upjohn) is a proprietary, prescription-only preparation of the LIPID-LOWERING DRUG colestipol hydrochloride. It can be used in hyperlipidaemia to reduce the levels, or change the proportions, of lipids in the bloodstream. It is available as granules to be taken with liquids.
✚▲ Side-effects/warning: See COLESTIPOL HYDROCHLORIDE.

colestipol hydrochloride

is a resin that binds bile acids and lowers LDL-cholesterol. It is used as a LIPID-LOWERING DRUG in hyperlipidaemia to reduce the levels, or change the proportions, of various lipids in the bloodstream. It is usually administered only to patients in whom a strict and regular dietary regime, alone, is not having the desired effect. Administration is oral.
✚▲ Side-effects/warning: See CHOLESTYRAMINE.
✪ Related entry: Colestid.

colestyramine

see CHOLESTYRAMINE

Colifoam

(Stafford-Miller) is a proprietary prescription-only preparation of the CORTICOSTEROID hydrocortisone (as acetate). It can be used to treat inflammation with colitis and proctitis, and is available as a foam and applied with an aerosol.
✚▲ Side-effects/warning: See HYDROCORTISONE.

colistin

is an ANTIBACTERIAL and ANTIBIOTIC drug which is a comparatively toxic member of the POLYMIXIN family. It is active against Gram-negative bacteria, including *Pseudomonas aeruginosa*, and can be

C

used in topical application (as colistin sulphate) to treat infections of the skin. However, in certain conditions and under strict supervision, the drug may be administered orally (primarily to sterilize the bowel and is not absorbed) or by injection, infusion or inhalation (as an adjunct to standard antibiotic treatment).

✚ Side-effects: There may be breathlessness, vertigo, numbness round the mouth and muscular weakness and a tingling sensation. Rarely, slurred speech, confusion and visual disturbances.

▲ Warning: It should not be administered to patients who suffer from the neuromuscular disease myasthenia gravis, or who are pregnant or breast-feeding. It should be administered with caution to those who suffer from impaired kidney function or porphyria.

◖ Related entry: Colomycin.

Colofac

(Duphar) is a proprietary, prescription-only preparation of the ANTISPASMODIC mebeverine hydrochloride. It can be used to treat gastrointestinal spasm, and is available as tablets and an oral suspension.

✚▲ Side-effects/warning: See MEBEVERINE HYDROCHLORIDE.

Colomycin

(Pharmax) is a proprietary, prescription-only preparation of the ANTIBACTERIAL and (POLYMIXIN) ANTIBIOTIC colistin. It can be used by topical application to treat skin infections, burns and wounds; and also by mouth and by injection. It is available as a sterile powder (to make up into a topical solution), tablets, as a syrup and in a form for injection (as colistin sulphomethate sodium).

✚▲ Side-effects/warning: See COLISTIN.

Colpermin

(Pharmacia) is a proprietary, non-prescription preparation of the ANTISPASMODIC peppermint oil. It can be used to relieve the discomfort of abdominal colic and distension, particularly in irritable bowel syndrome, and is available as capsules.

✚▲ Side-effects/warning: See PEPPERMINT OIL.

Combidol

(CP) is a proprietary, prescription-only COMPOUND PREPARATION of chenodeoxycholic acid and ursodeoxycholic acid. It can be used to dissolve gallstones, and is available as tablets.

✚▲ Side-effects/warning: See CHENODEOXYCHOLIC ACID; URSODEOXYCHOLIC ACID.

Comixco

(Ashbourne) is a proprietary, prescription-only COMPOUND PREPARATION of the (SULPHONAMIDE) ANTIBACTERIAL sulphamethoxazole and the antibacterial trimethoprim, which is a combination called co-trimoxazole. It can be used to treat bacterial infections, particularly infections of the urinary tract, prostatitis and bronchitis, and is available as soluble tablets.

✚▲ Side-effects/warning: See CO-TRIMOXAZOLE.

Comox

(Norton) is a proprietary, prescription-only COMPOUND PREPARATION of the (SULPHONAMIDE) ANTIBACTERIAL sulphamethoxazole and the antibacterial trimethoprim, which is a combination called co-trimoxazole. It can be used to treat bacterial infections, particularly infections of the urinary tract, prostatitis and bronchitis, and is available as soluble tablets.

✚▲ Side-effects/warning: See CO-TRIMOXAZOLE.

compound analgesics ▣

are drug preparations that combine two or more ANALGESICS in one preparation. There are a number of proprietary preparations with some combination of the NON-NARCOTIC

ANALGESIC PARACETAMOL, the NSAID analgesics ASPIRIN and IBUPROFEN and the (OPIOID) NARCOTIC ANALGESICS CODEINE PHOSPHATE, DEXTROPROPOXYPHENE HYDROCHLORIDE and DIHYDROCODEINE TARTRATE. There are also several 'official', non-proprietary compound analgesics that contain specified amounts of various analgesics: see CO-CODAMOL, CO-CODAPRIN, CO-DYDRAMOL and CO-PRAXAMOL.

compound preparations ▣

are drug formulations that are a combination of two or more pharmacologically active constituents in a single preparation. Many proprietary preparations contain a number of active constituents with differing actions (especially in cough and cold remedies). However, medical attitudes to compound preparations are mixed. The main criticism is that in certain circumstances it may be necessary to adjust the dose of one or all of the constituents independently, in order to achieve a reliable and safe response, but this is impossible in a compound preparation. For instance, POTASSIUM CHLORIDE is now rarely included in preparations containing DIURETICS that cause potassium loss from the body, because the amount of potassium required is very variable and best controlled independently of the (critical) dose of the diuretic. On the other hand, certain combinations of drugs (in a standard ratio of doses) have gained an established place in both prescription-only and non-prescription applications. Most examples of these compound preparations have a *co-*prefix, which means compound. For example, CO-CODAMOL 8/500 is a compound preparation of CODEINE PHOSPHATE and PARACETAMOL, in a ratio of 8 mg of codeine phosphate to 500 mg of paracetamol.

Compound Thymol Glycerin, BP

is a non-proprietary non-prescription preparation of GLYCEROL and THYMOL (with colour and flavouring). It can be used as a mouthwash for oral hygiene.

Concordin

(Merck Sharp & Dohme) is a proprietary, prescription-only preparation of the (TRICYCLIC) ANTIDEPRESSANT protriptyline hydrochloride. It can be used to treat depressive illness, especially in apathetic or withdrawn patients, and is available as tablets.
+▲ Side-effects/warning: See PROTRIPTYLINE HYDROCHLORIDE.

Condyline

(Yamanouchi) is a proprietary, prescription-only COMPOUND PREPARATION of the KERATOLYTIC agent podophyllum. It can be used in men to treat and remove penile warts, or in women on the external genitalia. It is available as a solution for topical application.
+▲ Side-effects/warning: See POPOPHYLLIN.

conjugated oestrogens

are naturally obtained OESTROGENS obtained from the urine of pregnant mares, which are used in HRT (hormone replacement therapy). Administration is oral.
+▲ Side-effects/warning: See OESTROGEN.
✪ Related entries: Premarin; Premique; Prempak-C.

Conotrane

(Yamanouchi) is a proprietary, non-prescription preparation of the ANTISEPTIC benzalkonium chloride (with dimethicone '350'). It can be used for the relief of nappy rash and skin sores, and is available as a cream.
+▲ Side-effects/warning: See BENZALKONIUM CHLORIDE.

Contac 400

(SmithKline Beecham) is a proprietary, non-prescription COMPOUND PREPARATION of the SYMPATHOMIMETIC and DECONGESTANT phenylpropanolamine hydrochloride and the ANTIHISTAMINE chlorpheniramine maleate. It can be used for symptomatic relief of nasal over-secretion, and is available as capsules.

➕▲ Side-effects/warning: See CHLORPHENIRAMINE MALEATE; PHENYLPROPANOLAMINE HYDROCHLORIDE.

Contac Coughcaps

(SmithKline Beecham) is a proprietary, non-prescription preparation of the ANTITUSSIVE and (OPIOID) NARCOTIC ANALGESIC dextromethorphan hydrobromide. It can be used for the symptomatic relief of unproductive coughs, and is available as controlled-release beads in capsules. It is not normally given to children, except on medical advice.

➕▲ Side-effects/warning: See DEXTROMETHORPHAN HYDROBROMIDE.

contraceptives ⧄

are drugs, methods or devices that prevent conception. Contraceptive drugs include ORAL CONTRACEPTIVES (most notably the Pill), which contain either a hormonal combination of PROGESTOGENS plus an OESTROGEN (combined oral contraceptive pill; COC) just a progestogen (progesterone-only contraceptive pill; POP) or parenteral contraceptives (progesterone-only preparations given by injection or implantation and renewable every three months). SPERMICIDAL preparations contain drugs that kill sperm and/or prevent sperm motility within the vagina or cervix, and should only be used in combination with barrier methods of contraception (such as a condom or diaphragm). Post-coital emergency contraception consists of a high dose of a combined preparation of oestrogen and progestogen (known as the *morning-after pill*). Intra-uterine contraceptive devices are not normally regarded as drugs (and are not within the scope of this book), but have a copper wire or ring incorporated which is thought to be pharmacologically active in changing production of local mediators (especially PROSTAGLANDINS), which effect implantation.

All contraceptives that involve the use of drugs produce side-effects and expert advice is required to identify the form ideally suited to an individual's circumstances.

Contraflam

(Berk) is a proprietary, prescription-only preparation of the (NSAID) NON-NARCOTIC ANALGESIC and ANTIRHEUMATIC mefenamic acid. It can be used to treat pain in rheumatoid arthritis, osteoarthritis and other musculoskeletal disorders and also period pain. It is available as capsules.

➕▲ Side-effects/warning: See MEFENAMIC ACID.

Convulex

(Pharmacia) is a proprietary, prescription-only preparation of the ANTICONVULSANT and ANTI-EPILEPTIC valproic acid. It is a valuable drug in the treatment of all forms of epilepsy, and is available as capsules.

➕▲ Side-effects/warning: See SODIUM VALPROATE.

Cool Lemon Lemsip

(Reckitt & Colman) is a proprietary, non-prescription preparation of the NON-NARCOTIC ANALGESIC and ANTIPYRETIC paracetamol and the DECONGESTANT phenylephrine hydrochloride (with vitamin C). It can be used for the relief of flu and cold symptoms, and is available as sachets for making up in water. It is not to be given to children under six years, except on medical advice.

➕▲ Side-effects/warning: See PARACETAMOL; PHENYLEPHRINE HYDROCHLORIDE.

co-phenotrope

is an ANTIDIARRHOEAL COMPOUND PREPARATION of the OPIOID diphenoxylate hydrochloride and the ANTICHOLINERGIC atropine sulphate. It can be administered to treat chronic diarrhoea (eg in mild chronic ulcerative colitis), but dependency may occur with prolonged use. It is available as tablets and a sugar-free liquid.

+▲ Side-effects/warning: See ATROPINE
SULPHATE; DIPHENOXYLATE HYDROCHLORIDE.
✪ Related entries: Diarphen: Lomotil.

Copholco

(Roche) is a proprietary, non-prescription
preparation of the ANTITUSSIVE and
EXPECTORANT pholcodine, along with terpin,
CINEOLE and MENTHOL. It can be used for the
symptomatic relief of ticklish cough, and is
available as a linctus.
+▲ Side-effects/warning: See PHOLCODINE.

Copholcoids Cough Pastilles

(Roche) is a proprietary, non-prescription
preparation of the ANTITUSSIVE and
EXPECTORANT pholcodine, along with
MENTHOL and terpin hydrate. It can be used
for the symptomatic relief of ticklish
coughs.
+▲ Side-effects/warning: See PHOLCODINE.

Coppertone Ultrashade 23 Lotion

(Scholl) is a proprietary, non-prescription
SUNSCREEN preparation, which protects
against UVA and UVB ultraviolet radiation
(UVB-SPF 23). It contains several agents
used to help protect the skin, such as
ethylhexyl-methoxycinnamate, oxybenzone
and padimate-O. A patient whose skin
condition requires this sort of protection
may be prescribed it at the discretion of his
or her doctor.

co-praxamol

is a COMPOUND ANALGESIC preparation of the
(OPIOID) NARCOTIC ANALGESIC
dextropropoxyphene hydrochloride and the
NON-NARCOTIC ANALGESIC paracetamol; in a
ratio of 32.5:325 (mg). It is available in
many generic and some proprietary
preparations, and has the advantages and
disadvantages of both drugs. It is
particularly dangerous to overdose because
of the opioid dextropropoxyphene
component. Administration is oral.
+▲ Side-effects/warning: See
DEXTROPROPOXYPHENE HYDROCHLORIDE;

PARACETAMOL.
✪ Related entries: Cosalgesic; Distagesic.

Coracten

(Evans) is a proprietary, prescription-only
preparation of the CALCIUM-CHANNEL BLOCKER
nifedipine. It can be used as an ANTI-ANGINA
treatment in the prevention of attacks and
as an ANTIHYPERTENSIVE. It is available as
capsules.
+▲ Side-effects/warning: See NIFEDIPINE.

Cordarone X

(Sanofi Winthrop) is a proprietary,
prescription-only preparation of the ANTI-
ARRHYTHMIC amiodarone hydrochloride. It
can be used to treat heartbeat irregularities,
and is available as tablets and in a form for
injection.
+▲ Side-effects/warning: See AMIODARONE
HYDROCHLORIDE.

Cordilox

(Baker Norton) is a proprietary,
prescription-only preparation of the
CALCIUM-CHANNEL BLOCKER verapamil
hydrochloride. It can be used as an
ANTIHYPERTENSIVE, as an ANTI-ANGINA
treatment in the prevention of attacks and
as an ANTI-ARRHYTHMIC to correct heart
irregularities. It is available as tablets and
in a form for injection.
+▲ Side-effects/warning: See VERAPAMIL
HYDROCHLORIDE.

Corgard

(Sanofi Winthrop) is a proprietary,
prescription-only preparation of the BETA-
BLOCKER nadolol. It can be used as an
ANTIHYPERTENSIVE for raised blood pressure,
as an ANTI-ANGINA treatment to relieve
symptoms and improve exercise tolerance
and as an ANTI-ARRHYTHMIC to regularize
heartbeat and to treat myocardial
infarction. It can also be used as a
preventive ANTIMIGRAINE treatment and as an
ANTITHYROID for short-term treatment of
thyrotoxicosis. It is available as tablets.
+▲ Side-effects/warning: See NADOLOL.

Corgaretic 40

(Sanofi Winthrop) is a proprietary, prescription-only COMPOUND PREPARATION of the BETA-BLOCKER nadolol and the DIURETIC bendrofluazide. It can be used as an ANTIHYPERTENSIVE for raised blood pressure, and is available as tablets.

+▲ Side-effects/warning: See BENDROFLUAZIDE; NADOLOL.

Corgaretic 80

(Sanofi Winthrop) is a proprietary, prescription-only COMPOUND PREPARATION of the BETA-BLOCKER nadolol and the DIURETIC bendrofluazide. It can be used as an ANTIHYPERTENSIVE for raised blood pressure, and is available as tablets.

+▲ Side-effects/warning: See BENDROFLUAZIDE; NADOLOL.

Corlan

(Evans) is a proprietary, non-prescription preparation of the CORTICOSTEROID and ANTI-INFLAMMATORY hydrocortisone (as sodium succinate). It can be used to treat ulcers and sores in the mouth, and is available as lozenges.

+▲ Side-effects/warning: See HYDROCORTISONE.

Coro-nitro Spray

(Boehringer Mannheim) is a proprietary, non-prescription preparation of the VASODILATOR and ANTI-ANGINA drug glyceryl trinitrate. It can be used to treat and prevent angina pectoris and in HEART FAILURE TREATMENT. It is available in the form of a sublingual (beneath the tongue) aerosol spray in metered doses.

+▲ Side-effects/warning: See GLYCERYL TRINITRATE.

Correctol

(Schering-Plough) is a proprietary, non-prescription COMPOUND PREPARATION of the (*stimulant*) LAXATIVES docusate sodium and phenolphthalein. It can be used to relieve constipation, and is available as tablets. It is not normally given to children, except on medical advice.

+▲ Side-effects/warning: See DOCUSATE SODIUM; PHENOLPHTHALEIN.

Corsodyl

(SmithKline Beecham) is a proprietary, non-prescription preparation of the ANTISEPTIC chlorhexidine (as gluconate). It can be used by topical application to treat inflammations and infections of the mouth. It is available as a dental gel, a mouthwash and an oral spray.

+▲ Side-effects/warning: See CHLORHEXIDINE.

corticosteroids ⚡

are steroid hormones secreted by the cortex (outer part) of the adrenal glands, or are synthetic substances that closely resemble the natural forms. There are two main types, *glucocorticoids* and *mineralocorticoids*. The latter assist in maintaining the salt-and-water balance of the body. Corticosteroids such as the glucocorticoid HYDROCORTISONE and the mineralocorticoid FLUDROCORTISONE ACETATE can be given to patients for replacement therapy where there is a deficiency, in Addison's disease or following adrenalectomy or hypopituitarism. The glucocorticoids are potent ANTI-INFLAMMATORY and ANTI-ALLERGIC drugs and are frequently used to treat inflammatory and/or allergic reactions of the skin, airways and elsewhere. COMPOUND PREPARATIONS are available that contain both an ANTIBACTERIAL or ANTIFUNGAL with an anti-inflammatory corticosteroid, and can be used in conditions where an infection is also present. However, these preparations must be used with caution because the corticosteroid component diminishes the patient's natural immune response to the infective agent. Absorption of a high dose of corticosteroid over a period of time may also cause undesirable, systemic side-effects.

+ Side-effects: *Mineralocorticoid* adverse effects include hypertension, sodium and water retention and potassium loss. *Glucocorticoid* adverse effects include diabetes, osteoporosis, avascular necrosis, mental disturbances, euphoria, muscle wasting and possibly peptic ulceration. Corticosteroids may also cause Cushing's syndrome, suppressed growth in children and adrenal atrophy. If administered during pregnancy, they may affect adrenal gland development in the child. Suppression of the symptoms of infection may occur.

▲ Warning: Withdrawal of treatment must be gradual (patients are given a *steroid card* with general advice).

corticotrophin

or adrenocorticotrophic hormone (ACTH), is a HORMONE produced and secreted by the pituitary gland in order to control the production and secretion of other hormones – CORTICOSTEROIDS – in the adrenal glands, generally as a response to stress. Therapeutically, synthetic corticotrophin analogues (eg TETRACOSACTRIN) can be administered in order to make up for hormonal deficiency in the pituitary gland, to cause the production of extra corticosteroids in the treatment of certain inflammatory conditions, such as rheumatoid arthritis and Crohn's disease, or to test the function of the adrenal glands.

cortisol

is another name for HYDROCORTISONE.

cortisone acetate

is a CORTICOSTEROID hormone with ANTI-INFLAMMATORY properties and has both *glucocorticoid* and *mineralocorticoid* activity. It can therefore be used to make up for hormonal deficiency (especially in relation to the salt-and-water balance in the body), for instance, following the surgical removal of the adrenal glands. Administration is oral.

➕▲ Side-effects/warning: See CORTICOSTEROIDS.

⚙ Related entry: Cortisyl.

Cortisyl

(Roussel) is a proprietary, prescription-only preparation of the CORTICOSTEROID and ANTI-INFLAMMATORY cortisone acetate. It can be used in replacement therapy to make up hormonal deficiency, for instance, following surgical removal of one or both of the adrenal glands. It is available as tablets.x

➕▲ Side-effects/warning: See CORTISONE ACETATE.

Corwin

(Stuart) is a proprietary, prescription-only preparation of the SYMPATHOMIMETIC and CARDIAC STIMULANT xamoterol (as xamoterol fumarate). It can be used for the treatment of heart conditions where moderate stimulation of the force of heartbeat is required, such as chronic moderate heart failure. It is available as tablets.

➕▲ Side-effects/warning: See XAMOTEROL.

Cosalgesic

(Cox) is a proprietary, prescription-only COMPOUND ANALGESIC preparation of the (OPIOID) NARCOTIC ANALGESIC dextropropoxyphene hydrochloride and the NON-NARCOTIC ANALGESIC paracetamol (a combination called co-proxamol). It can be used to treat many types of pain, and is available as tablets. It is not normally given to children, except on medical advice.

➕▲ Side-effects/warning: See DEXTROPROPOXYPHENE HYDROCHLORIDE; PARACETAMOL.

Cosmegen Lyovac

(Merck Sharp & Dohme) is a proprietary, prescription-only preparation of the (CYTOTOXIC) ANTICANCER drug dactinomycin. It is used particularly to treat cancer in children, and is available in form for injection.

➕▲ Side-effects/warning: See DACTINOMYCIN.

Cosuric

(DDSA Pharmaceuticals) is a proprietary, prescription-only preparation of the ENZY.ME

C

INHIBITOR allopurinol, which is a XANTHINE-OXIDASE INHIBITOR. It can be used to treat excess uric acid in the blood and to prevent renal stones and attacks of gout. It is available as tablets.

✚▲ Side-effects/warning: See ALLOPURINOL.

co-tenidone

is a COMPOUND PREPARATION of the BETA-BLOCKER atenolol and the DIURETIC chlorthalidone. It can be used as an ANTIHYPERTENSIVE for raised blood pressure, and is available as tablets.

✚▲ Side-effects/warning: See ATENOLOL; CHLORTHALIDONE.

✪ Related entries: AtenixCo; Tenchlor.

co-triamterzide 50/25

is a simplified name for the COMPOUND PREPARATION of the (*potassium-sparing*) DIURETIC triamterine and the (THIAZIDE) diuretic hydrochlorothiazide; in the ratio 50:25 (mg).

✚▲ Side-effects/warning: See HYDROCHLOROTHIAZIDE; TRIAMTERINE.

✪ Related entries: Dyazide; Triam-Co; TrimazCo.

co-trimoxazole

is a simplified name for the COMPOUND PREPARATION of the (SULPHONAMIDE) ANTIBACTERIAL sulphamethoxazole and the similar, but not related, antibacterial trimethoprim (a folic acid inhibitor); in the ratio of 5:1. It is thought that each drug enhances the action of the other, giving a combined effect greater than the sum of the two. Although there is little evidence to support this, the combination remains a useful antibacterial preparation, though because of adverse reactions its use now restricted to certain specific situations. These include treatment of *Pneumocystis carinii* pneumonia toxoplasmosis and nocardiasis, and only where other treatments are not effective for exacerbations of chronic bronchitis, infections of the urinary tract and in acute otitis media in children. Administration is either oral or by injection.

✚ Side-effects: These are thought to be largely caused by the sulphonamide and may include nausea and vomiting; diarrhoea and rashes. Blood disorders and generalized skin disorders may occur.

▲ Warning: It should not be administered to patients who are pregnant; who have certain blood, liver or kidney disorders, or jaundice. Administer with caution to patients who are elderly or breast-feeding. Adequate fluid intake must be maintained. Prolonged treatment requires regular blood counts. Restrictions on the use of this combination and its constituents has been recommended by the CSM.

✪ Related entries: Bactrim; Chemotrim; Comixco; Comox; Fectrim; Laratrim; Septrim.

counter-irritants

also called RUBEFACIENTS, are preparations that cause a feeling of warmth and offset the pain from underlying muscle and joints or viscera when rubbed in topically to the skin. A number of them are aromatic or volatile oils. How these agents act is uncertain, but the reddening of the skin (denoted by the name *rube*facient) indicates a dilatation of the blood vessels which gives a soothing feeling of warmth. The term counter-irritant refers to the idea that irritation of the sensory nerve endings alters or offsets pain in the underlying muscle or joints that are served by the same nerves. See CAPSAICIN; CAPSICUM OLEORESIN; CHOLINE SALICYLATE; ETHYL SALICYLATE; GLYCOL SALICYLATE; METHYL SALICYLATE; MENTHOL; SALICYLIC ACID; TURPENTINE OIL.

Coversyl

(Servier) is a proprietary, prescription-only preparation of the ACE INHIBITOR perindopril. It can be used as an ANTIHYPERTENSIVE and in HEART FAILURE TREATMENT, and is available as tablets.

✚▲ Side-effects/warning: See PERINDOPRIL.

Covonia Bronchial Balsam

(Thornton & Ross) is a proprietary,

non-prescription COMPOUND PREPARATION of the ANTITUSSIVE and (OPIOID) NARCOTIC ANALGESIC dextromethorphan hydrobromide and the EXPECTORANT agent GUAIPHENESIN along with menthol. It can be used for the symptomatic relief of non-productive coughs, such as those associated with colds and bronchitis. It is available as a linctus and is not normally given to children under six years, except on medical advice.

✚▲ Side-effects/warning: See DEXTROMETHORPHAN HYDROBROMIDE.

Covonia for Children

(Thornton & Ross) is a proprietary, non-prescription preparation of the ANTITUSSIVE and (OPIOID) NARCOTIC ANALGESIC dextromethorphan hydrobromide. It can be used for the symptomatic relief of non-productive coughs, including those associated with the common cold. It is available as a sugar-free linctus and is not normally given to children under two years, except on medical advice.

✚▲ Side-effects/warning: See DEXTROMETHORPHAN HYDROBROMIDE.

Cozaar

(Merck Sharp & Dohme) is a proprietary prescription-only preparation of losartan potassium, which is a recently introduced member of the ANGIOTENSIN-RECEPTOR BLOCKERS. It can be used as an ANTIHYPERTENSIVE, and is available as tablets.

✚▲ Side-effects/warning: See LOSARTAN POTASSIUM.

Cremalgin Balm

(Rhône-Poulenc Rorer) is a proprietary, non-prescription COMPOUND PREPARATION of capsicum oleoresin, METHYL NICOTINATE and GLYCOL SALICYLATE, which all have COUNTER-IRRITANT, or RUBEFACIENT, actions. It can be applied to the skin for symptomatic relief of underlying muscle or joint pain, and is available as a balm.

✚▲ Side-effects/warning: See CAPSICUM OLEORESIN.

Creon

(Duphar) is a proprietary, non-prescription preparation of the digestive ENZYME pancreatin. It can be used to treat deficiencies of digestive juices that are normally supplied by the pancreas, and is available as capsules and granules (a higher strength version, *Creon 25 000*, is also available).

✚▲ Side-effects/warning: See PANCREATIN.

Creon 25 000

(Duphar) is a proprietary, non-prescription preparation of the digestive ENZYME pancreatin. It can be used to treat deficiencies of digestive juices that are normally supplied by the pancreas, and is available as capsules (this is a higher strength version of *Creon*).

✚▲ Side-effects/warning: See PANCREATIN.

cristantaspase

is an ENZYME called asparaginase which is used as a ANTICANCER treatment almost exclusively for acute lymphoblastic leukaemia. Administration is by injection.

✚ Side-effects: There may be nausea, vomiting, central nervous system depression; changes in liver function and blood lipids (requiring monitoring, including of the urine for glucose); and anaphylaxis.

✪ Related entry: Erwinase.

Crixivan

(Merck Sharp & Dohme) is a proprietary, prescription-only preparation of the ANTIVIRAL indinavir. It can be used in AIDS, and is available as capsules.

✚▲ Side-effects/warning: See INDINAVIR.

crotamiton

is used to relieve pruritus (itching) of the skin, for example, with scabies. Administration is topical.

▲ Warning: It should not be used on broken skin or near the eyes.

✪ Related entries: Eurax; Eurax-Hydrocortisone.

C

crystal violet

(gentian violet; methyl violet; methylrosanilium chloride) is a dye with both astringent and oxidizing properties which is used as an ANTISEPTIC. It is occasionally administered to treat certain bacterial and fungal skin infections or abrasions and minor wounds. Administration is usually by topical application. As a non-proprietary, antiseptic paint preparation, it is used specifically to prepare skin for surgery.

✚ Side-effects: It may cause mucosal ulcerations.

▲ Warning: It should not be applied to mucous membranes or broken skin. It stains clothes as well as skin.

Crystapen

(Britannia) is a proprietary, prescription-only preparation of the ANTIBACTERIAL and (PENICILLIN) ANTIBIOTIC benzylpenicillin (as sodium). It can be used to treat infections of the skin, middle ear, throat, respiratory tract (such as tonsillitis) and certain severe systemic infections (such as meningitis). It is available in a form for injection or infusion.

✚▲ Side-effects/warning: See BENZYLPENICILLIN.

Cultivate

(Glaxo) is a proprietary, prescription-only preparation of the CORTICOSTEROID and ANTI-INFLAMMATORY fluticasone propionate. It can be used to treat inflammatory skin disorders, such as dermatitis, eczema and psoriasis, and is available as a cream for topical application.

✚▲ Side-effects/warning: See FLUTICASONE PROPIONATE.

Cupanol Over 6 Paracetamol Oral Suspension

(Seton) is a proprietary, non-prescription preparation of the NON-NARCOTIC ANALGESIC and ANTIPYRETIC paracetamol. It can be used to treat mild to moderate pain, migraine, toothache, headache and feverish conditions. It is available as a liquid suspension and is not normally given to children under six years, except on medical advice.

✚▲ Side-effects/warning: See PARACETAMOL.

Cupanol Under 6 Paracetamol Oral Suspension

(Seton) is a proprietary, non-prescription preparation of the NON-NARCOTIC ANALGESIC and ANTIPYRETIC paracetamol. It can be used to treat mild to moderate pain, such as teething and feverish conditions (including after vaccination, when it may be given to two-month-old babies). It is available as a liquid suspension and is not normally given to infants under three months, except on medical advice.

✚▲ Side-effects/warning: See PARACETAMOL,

Cuplex

(Smith & Nephew) is a proprietary, non-prescription preparation of the KERATOLYTIC agent salicylic acid (together with lactic acid and copper acetate). It can be used to remove warts and hard skin, and is available as a gel.

✚▲ Side-effects/warning: See SALICYLIC ACID.

Cuprofen Ibuprofen Tablets

(Seton) is a proprietary, non-prescription preparation of the (NSAID) NON-NARCOTIC ANALGESIC and ANTIRHEUMATIC ibuprofen. It can be used for the relief of headache, period pain, muscular pain, dental pain, feverishness and cold and flu symptoms. It is available as tablets and is not normally given to children under 12 years, except on medical advice.

✚▲ Side-effects/warning: See IBUPROFEN.

Cuprofen Tablets Maximum Strength

(Seton) is a proprietary, non-prescription preparation of the (NSAID) NON-NARCOTIC ANALGESIC and ANTIRHEUMATIC drug ibuprofen. It can be used for the relief of headache, period pain, muscular pain, dental pain, feverishness and cold and flu symptoms. It is available as tablets and is not normally given to children under 12 years, except on medical advice.

+▲ Side-effects/warning: See IBUPROFEN.

Curatoderm

(Merck) is a is a proprietary, prescription-only preparation of derivative tacalcitol, a VITAMIN D analogue which can be used as a skin treatment for plaque psoriasis. It is available as an ointment.

+▲ Side-effects/warning: See TACALCITOL.

CX Antiseptic Dusting Powder

(Bio-Medical) is a proprietary, non-prescription preparation of the ANTISEPTIC chlorhexidine (as acetate). It can be used by topical application for disinfection and antisepsis.

+▲ Side-effects/warning: See CHLORHEXIDINE.

cyanocobalamin

is a form of vitamin B_{12} which is readily found in most normal, well-balanced diets (for example, in fish, eggs, liver and red meat). Vegans, who eat no animal products at all, may eventually suffer from deficiency of this vitamin. A deficiency of vitamin B_{12} eventually causes megaloblastic anaemia, degeneration of nerves in the central and peripheral nervous systems and abnormalities of epithelia (particularly the lining of the mouth and gut). Apart from poor diet, deficiency can also be caused by the lack of an *intrinsic factor* necessary for absorption in the stomach (pernicious anaemia) and by various malabsorption syndromes in the gut (sometimes due to drugs). Deficiency may be rectified by giving HYDROXOCOBALAMIN (a form of vitamin B_{12}), and supplements of vitamin B_{12} are administered by injection. There is no real beneficial effect from the inclusion of vitamin B_{12} (as cyanocobalamin) in proprietary multivitamin 'tonics'.

Cyclimorph

(Wellcome) is a proprietary, prescription-only preparation of the (OPIOID) NARCOTIC ANALGESIC morphine tartrate and the ANTI-EMETIC cyclizine tartrate. It can be used to treat moderate to severe pain, especially in serious conditions of fluid within the lungs. It is available, in two strengths (*Cyclimorph-10* and *Cyclimorph-15*) for injection and is on the Controlled Drugs List.

+▲ Side-effects/warning: See MORPHINE SUPLHATE; CYCLIZINE TARTRATE.

cyclizine

is an ANTIHISTAMINE and ANTINAUSEANT which can be used to treat nausea, vomiting, vertigo, motion sickness and disorders of the balance function of the inner ear. Administration is either oral or by injection.

+ Side-effects: See ANTIHISTAMINES; there may also be drowsiness, occasional dry mouth and blurred vision.

▲ Warning: It may aggravate severe heart failure. Drowsiness may impair the performance of skilled tasks, such as driving; avoid alcohol because its effects may be enhanced.

✪ Related entries: Cyclimorph; Diconal; Femigraine; Migril; Valoid.

Cyclo-Progynova

(Schering) is a proprietary, prescription-only COMPOUND PREPARATION of female SEX HORMONES oestradiol (as valerate; an OESTROGEN) and norgestrel (a PROGESTOGEN). It can be used in HRT, and is available as tablets.

+▲ Side-effects/warning: See NORGESTREL; OESTRADIOL.

Cyclodox

(Berk) is a proprietary, prescription-only preparation of the ANTIBACTERIAL and (TETRACYCLINE) ANTIBIOTIC doxycycline. It can be administered to treat quite an extensive range of infections, and is available as capsules.

+▲ Side-effects/warning: See DOXYCYCLINE.

C

Cyclogest

(Hoechst) is a proprietary, prescription-only preparation of the PROGESTOGEN progesterone. It can be used to treat many conditions of hormonal deficiency in women, including menstrual difficulty and premenstrual syndrome, and is available as (vaginal or anal) pessaries.

+▲ Side-effects/warning: See PROGESTERONE.

cyclopenthiazide

is a (THIAZIDE) DIURETIC which can be used as an ANTIHYPERTENSIVE (either alone or in conjunction with different types of diuretic or other drugs) and in the treatment of oedema. Administration is oral.

+▲ Side-effects/warning: See BENDROFLUAZIDE.

✪ Related entries: Navidrex; Navispare; Trasidrex.

cyclopentolate hydrochloride

is an ANTICHOLINERGIC drug which can be used to dilate the pupil and paralyse the focusing of the eye for ophthalmic examination. Administration is topical as eye-drops.

+▲ Side-effects/warning: See ATROPINE SULPHATE. Although when applied locally it has few side-effects, but it should not be used in patients with raised intraocular pressure (it may precipitate glaucoma).

✪ Related entries: Minims Cyclopentolate; Mydrilate.

cyclophosphamide

is a CYTOTOXIC drug which is used as an ANTICANCER treatment of chronic lymphatic leukaemia, lymphomas and some solid tumours. It works by interfering with DNA and so preventing normal cell replication. It can also be used as an IMMUNOSUPPRESSANT in the treatment of complicated rheumatoid arthritis (unlicensed use). Administration is either oral or by injection.

+▲ Side-effects/warning: See CYTOTOXICS. Avoid its use in patients with porphyria;

rarely, it may cause haemorrhagic cystitis.

✪ Related entry: Endoxana.

cyclopropane

is a gas that is used as an inhalant GENERAL ANAESTHETIC for rapid induction and maintenance of general anaesthesia. Administration is by inhalation.

Cycloserine

(Lilly) is a proprietary, prescription-only preparation of the ANTIBACTERIAL cycloserine. It can be used specifically as an ANTITUBERCULAR treatment for tuberculosis that is resistant to the powerful drugs ordinarily used first, or in cases where those drugs are not tolerated. It is available as capsules.

+▲ Side-effects/warning: See CYCLOSERINE.

cycloserine

is an ANTIBACTERIAL drug which is used specifically as an ANTITUBERCULAR treatment for tuberculosis that is resistant to the powerful drugs ordinarily used first, or in cases where those drugs are not tolerated. Administration is oral.

+ Side-effects: There may be headache, dizziness, drowsiness, depression, convulsions, tremor and allergic dermatitis.

▲ Warning: It should not be administered to patients with epilepsy, alcoholism, depressive illness, anxiety or psychosis, porphyria or severe kidney impairment; it should be administered with caution to those with impaired kidney function, or who are pregnant or breast-feeding. Blood, kidney and liver function should be monitored.

✪ Related entry: Cycloserine.

cyclosporin

(ciclosporin) is an IMMUNOSUPPRESSANT drug which is used particularly to limit tissue rejection during and following organ transplant surgery. It can also be used to treat severe, active rheumatoid arthritis and some skin conditions such as severe, resistant atopic dermatitis and (under special supervision) psoriasis. It has very little effect on the blood-cell producing capacity of the bone marrow, but does have liver toxicity. Administration can be either oral or by injection.

✚ Side-effects: These include changes in blood enzymes, disturbances in liver, kidney and cardiovascular function, excessive hair growth, gastrointestinal disturbances, tremor, gum growth, oedema, fatigue and also burning sensations in both the hands and feet.

▲ Warning: Treatment with cyclosporin inevitably leaves the body vulnerable to infection. Administer with caution to patients who are pregnant or breast-feeding, or with porphyria. Body functions (liver, kidney and cardiovascular system) should be monitored. When used for rheumatoid arthritis; it should not be given to patients with abnormal kidney function, uncontrolled hypertension, infections or malignancy.

✪ Related entries: Neoral; Sandimmun.

Cyklokapron

(Pharmacia) is a proprietary, prescription-only preparation of the antifibrinolytic drug tranexamic acid. It can be used to stop bleeding in circumstances such as dental extraction in a haemophiliac patient or menorrhagia (excessive period bleeding). It may also be administered in the treatment of hereditary angioedema and in streptokinase overdose. It is available as tablets, a dilute syrup and in a form for injection.

✚▲ Side-effects/warning: See TRANEXAMIC ACID.

Cymevene

(Syntex) is a proprietary, prescription-only preparation of the ANTIVIRAL ganciclovir. It can be used to treat life-threatening or sight-threatening viral infections and in immunocompromised patients. It is available as capsules and in a form for intravenous infusion.

✚▲ Side-effects/warning: See GANCICLOVIR.

cyproheptadine hydrochloride

is an ANTIHISTAMINE which can be used for the symptomatic relief of allergic symptoms such as hay fever and urticaria. It differs from other antihistamines in having additional actions as an antagonist of SEROTONIN and as a CALCIUM-CHANNEL BLOCKER, and is useful in a wider range of conditions, such as the prevention of migraine attacks. Administration is oral.

✚▲ Side-effects/warning: See ANTIHISTAMINES. It may cause weight gain. Because of its sedative side-effects, the performance of skilled tasks, such as driving, may be impaired.

✪ Related entry: Periactin.

Cyprostat

(Schering) is a proprietary, prescription-only preparation of the sex HORMONE ANTAGONIST cyproterone acetate, which is an ANTI-ANDROGEN. It can be used as an ANTICANCER treatment for cancer of the prostate gland. It works by neutralizing the effects of the male sex hormones (androgens) that contribute to the cancer, and is available as tablets.

✚▲ Side-effects/warning: See CYPROTERONE ACETATE.

cyproterone acetate

is a sex HORMONE ANTAGONIST, an ANTI-ANDROGEN, which reduces the effects of male sex hormones (androgens) in the body. It is used as an ANTICANCER treatment for cancer of the prostate gland. It can also be used for the treatment of hypersexuality or sexual deviation in men; in whom the drug causes a condition of reversible sterility through a reduction in the production of sperm. Additionally, it can be used (in a preparation containing oestrogen) to treat acne and excess body hair (hirsutism) in women. Administration is oral.

✚ Side-effects: Concentration and speed of thought and movement may be affected; breathlessness; weight gain; fatigue and lethargy. Hormonal effects include changes

C

in hair-growth patterns and enlargement of the breasts and inhibition of sperm production in men. Rarely, there is osteoporosis, and liver abnormalities.

▲ Warning: Except for use in prostate cancer, it should not be administered to patients who have sickle-cell anaemia, severe diabetes, liver disease or severe depression; who have a history of thrombosis; who are pregnant; or who are adolescent boys (in whom bone growth and testicular development may be arrested). It should be administered with caution to those with diabetes or insufficient secretion of adrenal hormones, or who are breast-feeding. Regular checks on liver function, adrenal gland function, blood counts and determination of levels of glucose are needed.

✿ Related entries: Androcur; Cyprostat; Dianette.

Cystrin

(Pharmacia Upjohn) is a proprietary, prescription-only preparation of the ANTICHOLINERGIC oxybutynin hydrochloride. It can be used as an ANTISPASMODIC in the treatment of urinary frequency and incontinence. It is available as tablets.

✚▲ Side-effects/warning: See OXYBUTYNIN HYDROCHLORIDE.

cytarabine

is a CYTOTOXIC drug which is used as an ANTICANCER treatment primarily of acute leukaemia. It works by by interfering with pyrimidine synthesis (a chemical needed for cell replication/DNA) and so prevents normal cell replication. Administration is by injection.

✚▲ Side-effects/warning: See CYTOTOXICS.

✿ Related entry: Cytosar.

cytoprotectants 🔋

are drugs with the capacity to protect the gastric mucosa (the lining of the stomach) from the normal stomach contents of acid and enzymes, which can cause erosion and pain in peptic ulcers (gastric and duodenal

ulcers). They may be used as long-term ULCER-HEALING DRUGS, as well as affording short-term relief from discomfort. Examples of cytoprotectants include: *liquorice extracts*, LIQUORICE, DEGLYCYRRHIZINISED and CARBENOXOLONE SODIUM; *bismuth salts*; and TRIPOTASSIUM DICITRATOBISMUTHATE (bismuth chelate) and SUCRALFATE.

Cytosar

(Upjohn) is a proprietary, prescription-only preparation of the (CYTOTOXIC) ANTICANCER drug cytarabine. It can be used to treat acute leukaemia, and is available in a form for injection.

✚▲ Side-effects/warning: See CYTARABINE.

Cytotec

(Searle) is a proprietary, prescription-only preparation of the synthetic PROSTAGLANDIN analogue misoprostol. It can be used to treat gastric and duodenal ulcers, and is available as tablets.

✚▲ Side-effects/warning: See MISOPROSTOL.

cytotoxics 🔋

are agents are used mainly in the treatment of cancer and are an important group of ANTICANCER drugs. They have the essential property of preventing normal cell replication and so inhibiting the growth of tumours or of excess cells in body fluids.

There are several mechanisms by which they do this, but in every case they inevitably also affect the growth of normal healthy cells and cause toxic side-effects, generally nausea and vomiting with hair loss. The most-used cytotoxics are the *alkylating agents*, which work by interfering with the action of DNA in cell replication (eg BUSULPHAN, CHLORAMBUCIL, CISPLATIN, CYCLOPHOSPHAMIDE, LOMUSTINE, MELPHALANM, THIOTEPA). The VINCA ALKALOIDS are also effective cytotoxic drugs and work by damaging part of the metabolic features of new-forming cells, however, they have severe side-effects (such as damage to peripheral nerves) which limits their use. A number of cytotoxics are ANTIBIOTICS in origin, but ANTIMICROBIAL actions do not contribute an important part of their action (eg BLEOMYCIN, DACTINOMYCIN, DOXORUBICIN HYDROCHLORIDE, EPIRUBICIN HYDROCHLORIDE). A new development has been the development of the *taxane* drugs based on a principle found in the yew tree (eg PACLITAXEL, DOCETAXEL). There are some cytotoxics that are not primarily administered in anticancer treatment, but are used as IMMUNOSUPPRESSANTS to limit tissue rejection during and following transplant surgery and in the treatment of autoimmune diseases, such as rheumatoid arthritis and lupus erythematosus (eg AZATHIOPRINE, chlorambucil, cyclophosphamide, CYCLOSPORIN, METHOTREXATE).

✚ Side-effects: Vomiting and nausea, bone-marrow suppression, hair loss and teratogenetic damage to the foetus are seen with many drugs of this class. Specialist advice is required about likely frequencies of adverse action experienced with each of the fifty (approximately) drugs in use, according to dosage and use.

▲ Warning: Under no circumstances are they to be administered in the period before conception or during pregnancy.

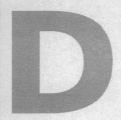

D

dacarbazine

is a CYTOTOXIC which is used comparatively rarely because of its high toxicity. It may be administered to treat the skin (mole) cancer melanoma and, in combination with other ANTICANCER drugs, in some soft-tissue sarcomas and the lymphatic cancer Hodgkin's disease. Administration is by injection.

✚▲ Side-effects/warning: See CYTOTOXICS. There is also intense nausea and vomiting; myelosuppression.

○ Related entry: DTIC-Dome.

dactinomycin

(actinomycin D) is a CYTOTOXIC (in fact, an ANTIBIOTIC in origin) which is used as an ANTICANCER treatment, particularly to treat cancer in children. Administration is by injection.

✚▲ Side-effects/warning: See CYTOTOXICS; similar side-effects to DOXORUBICIN, but with less heart toxicity.

○ Related entry: Cosmegen Lyovac.

Daktacort

(Janssen) is a proprietary, prescription-only COMPOUND PREPARATION of the CORTICOSTEROID hydrocortisone and the (IMIDAZOLE) ANTIFUNGAL drug miconazole (as nitrate). It can be used to treat various skin infections with accompanying inflammation, and is available as a cream and an ointment for topical application to the affected area.

✚▲ Side-effects/warning: See HYDROCORTISONE; MICONAZOLE.

Daktarin

(Janssen) is a proprietary, prescription-only preparation of the (IMIDAZOLE) ANTIFUNGAL miconazole. It can be used to treat both systemic and skin-surface fungal infections, and is available as tablets, an oral gel and as a solution for infusion. (There are other forms for topical application that are available without prescription.)

✚▲ Side-effects/warning: See MICONAZOLE.

Daktarin Cream

(Janssen) is a proprietary, non-prescription preparation of the (IMIDAZOLE) ANTIFUNGAL miconazole (as nitrate). It can be used for the prevention and treatment of fungal (and associated bacterial) infections of the skin, such as athlete's foot, intertrigo and infected nappy rash. It is available as a cream for topical application.

✚▲ Side-effects/warning: See MICONAZOLE.

Daktarin Oral Gel

(Janssen) is a proprietary, non-prescription preparation of the (IMIDAZOLE) ANTIFUNGAL miconazole (as base). It can be used for the prevention and treatment of fungal infections of the mouth, and is available as an oral gel for use by adults and children.

✚▲ Side-effects/warning: See MICONAZOLE.

Daktarin Powder

(Janssen) is a proprietary, non-prescription preparation of the (IMIDAZOLE) ANTIFUNGAL miconazole (as nitrate). It can be used for the prevention and treatment of fungal (and associated bacterial) infections of the skin, such as athlete's foot, intertrigo and infected nappy rash. It is available as a powder for application to the skin and clothes.

✚▲ Side-effects/warning: See MICONAZOLE.

Daktarin Spray Powder

(Janssen) is a proprietary, non-prescription preparation of the (IMIDAZOLE) ANTIFUNGAL miconazole (as nitrate). It can be used for the prevention and treatment of fungal

D

infections of the mouth, and is available as a powder spray for application to the skin, clothes and shoes.
✚▲ Side-effects/warning: See MICONAZOLE.

Dalacin

(Upjohn) is a proprietary, prescription-only preparation of the ANTIBACTERIAL and ANTIBIOTIC clindamycin. It can be used to treat vaginal infections, and is available as a cream.
✚▲ Side-effects/warning: See CLINDAMYCIN; the vaginal cream may damage latex condoms and diaphragms.

Dalacin C

(Upjohn) is a proprietary, prescription-only, preparation of the ANTIBACTERIAL and ANTIBIOTIC clindamycin. It can be used to treat infections of the bones and joints, and peritonitis (inflammation of the peritoneal lining of the abdominal cavity). It is available as capsules, a paediatric suspension and in a form for injection.
✚▲ Side-effects/warning: See CLINDAMYCIN.

Dalacin T

(Upjohn) is a proprietary, prescription-only preparation of the ANTIBACTERIAL and ANTIBIOTIC clindamycin. It can be used to treat acne, and is available as a lotion and a solution for topical application.
✚▲ Side-effects/warning: See CLINDAMYCIN.

Dalmane

(Roche) is a proprietary, prescription-only preparation of the BENZODIAZEPINE flurazepam. It can be used as a relatively long-acting HYPNOTIC for the short-term treatment of insomnia, where a degree of sedation during the daytime is acceptable. It is available as capsules.
✚▲ Side-effects/warning: See FLURAZEPAM.

dalteparin

is a LOW MOLECULAR WEIGHT HEPARIN which is used as an ANTICOAGULANT. It has some advantages over heparin when used in the long-duration prevention of venous

thrombo-embolism, particularly in orthopaedic use. Administration is by injection.
✚▲ Side-effects/warning: See HEPARIN.
✪ Related entry: Fragmin.

danaparoid sodium

is a version of heparin, called a HEPARINOID, that is used as an ANTICOAGULANT. It has some advantages over heparin when used for prevention of deep-vein thrombosis, particularly in orthopaedic surgery. It may be used in some patients who are hypersensitive to heparin itself. Administration is by injection.
✚▲ Side-effects/warning: See HEPARIN. There may also be thrombocytopenia, liver changes, hypersensitivity, osteoporosis and pain or tissue damage at injection site. Administer with care to pateints who are pregnant, breast-feeding, or have certain liver or kidney disorders.
✪ Related entry: Organ.

danazol

is a drug with weak androgen activity, plus HORMONE ANTAGONIST actions as an ANTI-OESTROGEN and antiprogesterone. It inhibits the release of pituitary hormones, GONADOTROPHINS. It can be used to treat endometriosis (the presence of areas of uterus-lining, endometrium, outside the uterus); gynaecomastia (the development of breasts on a male); menorrhagia (excessive menstrual flow) and other menstrual disorders; benign breast cysts and breast pain. It can also be used to treat hereditary angio-oedema. Administration is oral.
✚ Side-effects: Backache, dizziness, flushing, weight gain, menstrual disorders, nervousness, rash, flushing, smaller breasts, muscle spasm, hair loss, masculinization in women (oily skin, acne, hair growth, voice changes, enlarged clitoris), blood disorders, visual disturbances, jaundice and insulin resistance.
▲ Warning: It should not be administered to patients who are pregnant or breast-feeding; non-hormonal contraceptive

177

D

methods should be used where applicable. Use with caution in patients with certain heart, liver or kidney disorders; diabetes, epilepsy, migraine, hypertension, thrombosis, blood disorders, have thrombo-embolitic diseases, androgen-dependent tumours, or porphyria.
✪ Related entry: Danol.

Daneral SA

(Hoechst) is a proprietary, prescription-only preparation of the ANTIHISTAMINE pheniramine maleate. It can be used to treat the symptoms of allergic disorders, such as hay fever and urticaria, and is available as tablets.
✚▲ Side-effects/warning: See PHENIRAMINE MALEATE.

Danol

(Sanofi Winthrop) is a proprietary, prescription-only preparation of danazol, which acts as an indirect HORMONE ANTAGONIST by inhibiting the release of the pituitary HORMONES gonadotrophins, which in turn prevents the release of sex hormones. It is used to treat inflammation of the endometrial lining of the uterus, gynaecomastia and menstrual disorders. It is available as capsules.
✚▲ Side-effects/warning: See DANAZOL.

danthron

(dantron) is a (*stimulant*) LAXATIVE. It is used to promote defecation and so relieve constipation, and seems to work by stimulating motility in the intestine. Therapeutically, it is used for constipation in geriatric practice (particularly analgesic-induced constipation in the terminally ill) and in cardiac failure and coronary thrombosis (to avoid strain). It is also available in COMPOUND PREPARATIONS with DOCUSATE SODIUM (CO-DANTHRUSATE 50/60) or poloxamer '188'.
✚ Side-effects: There may be abdominal pain, griping, nausea or vomiting. The urine may be coloured red. Prolonged contact with the skin may cause irritation.

▲ Warning: It should not be taken when pregnant or breast-feeding.
✪ Related entries: co-danthramer 25/200; co-danthramer 75/1000; Codalax; Codalax Forte; Normax.

Dantrium

(Procter & Gamble) is a proprietary, prescription-only preparation of the SKELETAL MUSCLE RELAXANT dantrolene sodium. It can be used for relieving severe spasticity of muscles in spasm, and is available as capsules and in a form for injection.
✚▲ Side-effects/warning: See DANTROLENE SODIUM.

dantrolene sodium

is a SKELETAL MUSCLE RELAXANT which acts directly on skeletal muscle and can be used for relieving severe spasticity of muscles in spasm. Administration is either oral or by injection.
✚ Side-effects: Transient drowsiness, dizziness, weakness, general malaise, diarrhoea (stop treatment if severe), nausea, anorexia, headache, rash; sometimes constipation, difficulty in swallowing, visual and speech disturbances, confusion, nervousness, depression, insomnia, seizures, chills, urinary frequency; rarely, speeding of the heart, irregular blood pressure, breathing difficulty, various urinary problems, liver toxicity.
▲ Warning: Do not administer to patients with liver impairment or acute muscle spasm. Administer with caution to those with impaired heart and liver function (liver function should be checked regularly); effect is slow to develop. Drowsiness may impair the performance of skilled tasks, such as driving.
✪ Related entry: Dantrium.

dantron

see DANTHRON

Daonil

(Hoechst) is a proprietary, prescription-

D

only preparation of the SULPHONYLUREA glibenclamide. It can be used in DIABETIC TREATMENT of Type II diabetes (non-insulin-dependent diabetes mellitus; NIDDM; maturity-onset diabetes), and is available as tablets at twice the strength of *Semi-Daonil* tablets.

✚▲ Side-effects/warning: See GLIBENCLAMIDE.

dapsone
is a (SULPHONE) ANTIBACTERIAL drug which is used as an ANTITUBERCULAR treatment against leprosy in both lepromatous and tuberculoid forms. It is also sometimes used to treat severe forms of dermatitis (dermatitis herpetiformis) or, in combination with the ENZYME INHIBITOR pyrimethamine (as *Maloprim*), to prevent travellers in tropical regions from contracting malaria. Administration is either oral or by injection.

✚ Side-effects: These are rare at low doses (when used for leprosy), but with higher dosage there may be nausea, vomiting and headache, insomnia and increased heart rate, severe weight loss, anaemia, hepatitis, peripheral nerve disease and blood changes.

▲ Warning: It should be administered with caution to patients with anaemia, porphyria, G6PH deficiency, certain heart or lung diseases; or who are pregnant or breast-feeding.

✪ Related entry: Maloprim.

Daraprim
(Wellcome) is a proprietary, non-prescription preparation of the ANTIMALARIAL drug pyrimethamine. It can be used to prevent or treat malaria in combination with other drugs, but is not administered as the sole agent of prevention. It is available as tablets.

✚▲ Side-effects/warning: See PYRIMETHAMINE.

daunorubicin
is a recently introduced CYTOTOXIC drug (of ANTIBIOTIC origin) with properties similar to

doxorubicin. It is used as an ANTICANCER treatment particularly for advanced HIV-related Kaposi's sarcoma. Administration is as a liposomal formulation for intravenous infusion.

✚▲ Side-effects/warning: See CYTOTOXICS.

✪ Related entries: Cerubidin; DaunoXome.

DaunoXome
(NeXstar) is a proprietary, prescription-only preparation of the (CYTOTOXIC) ANTICANCER drug daunorubicin. It can be used to treat advanced HIV-related Kaposi's sarcoma, and is available in a liposomal form for intravenous infusion.

✚▲ Side-effects/warning: See DAUNORUBICIN.

Day Cold Comfort Capsules
(Boots) is a proprietary, non-prescription COMPOUND PREPARATION of the NON-NARCOTIC ANALGESIC paracetamol, the SYMPATHOMIMETIC and DECONGESTANT pseudoephedrine hydrochloride and the ANTITUSSIVE pholcodine. It can be used for the relief of cold and flu symptoms, and is available as capsules. It is not normally given to children under six years, except on medical advice.

✚▲ Side-effects/warning: See PARACETAMOL; PHOLCODINE; PSEUDOEPHEDRINE HYDROCHLORIDE.

Day Nurse Capsules
(SmithKline Beecham) is a proprietary, non-prescription COMPOUND PREPARATION of the NON-NARCOTIC ANALGESIC paracetamol, the SYMPATHOMIMETIC and DECONGESTANT phenylpropanolamine hydrochloride and the ANTITUSSIVE dextromethorphan hydrobromide. It can be used for the relief of cold and flu symptoms, and is available as capsules. It is not normally given to children under six years, except on medical advice.

✚▲ Side-effects/warning: See DEXTROMETHORPHAN HYDROBROMIDE; PARACETAMOL; PHENYLPROPANOLAMINE HYDROCHLORIDE.

D

Day Nurse Liquid

(SmithKline Beecham) is a proprietary, non-prescription COMPOUND PREPARATION of the NON-NARCOTIC ANALGESIC paracetamol, the SYMPATHOMIMETIC and DECONGESTANT phenylpropanolamine hydrochloride and the ANTITUSSIVE dextromethorphan hydrobromide. It can be used for the relief of cold and flu symptoms, and is available as a liquid. It is not normally given to children under six years, except on medical advice.

+▲ Side-effects/warning: See DEXTROMETHORPHAN HYDROBROMIDE; PARACETAMOL; PHENYLPROPANOLAMINE HYDROCHLORIDE.

DDAVP

(Ferring) is a proprietary, prescription-only preparation of desmopressin, which is an analogue of the pituitary HORMONE vasopressin (ADH). It is administered primarily to diagnose or to treat pituitary-originated diabetes insipidus. It can be used for some other diagnostic tests, to boost the blood concentration of blood-clotting factors in haemophiliac patients and to treat bed-wetting. It is available as tablets (as the acetate), as nose-drops (it is absorbed into the systemic circulation from the nasal mucosa) and in a form for injection.

+▲ Side-effects/warning: See DESMOPRESSIN.

DDC

see ZALCITABINE

DDI

see DIDANOSINE

De Witt's Worm Syrup

(De Witt) is a proprietary, non-prescription preparation of the ANTHELMINTIC drug piperazine (as citrate). It can be used to treat infections by threadworm and roundworm, and is available as an oral powder. It is not normally given to children under four years, except on medical advice.

+▲ Side-effects/warning: See PIPERAZINE.

De-capeptyl sr

(Speywood) is a proprietary, prescription-only preparation of the HORMONE triptorelin, which is an analogue of gonadorelin (gonadotrophin-releasing hormone). It can be used as an ANTICANCER treatment for cancer of the prostate gland, and is available in a form for injection.

+▲ Side-effects/warning: See TRIPTORELIN.

De-Nol

(Yamanouchi) is a proprietary, non-prescription preparation of the CYTOPROTECTANT tripotassium dicitratobismuthate. It can be used as an ULCER-HEALING DRUG for benign peptic ulcers in the stomach and duodenum, and is available as an oral liquid.

+▲ Side-effects/warning: See TRIPOTASSIUM DICITRATOBISMUTHATE.

De-Noltab

(Yamanouchi) is a proprietary, non-prescription preparation of the CYTOPROTECTANT tripotassium dicitratobismuthate. It can be used as an ULCER-HEALING DRUG for benign peptic ulcers in the stomach and duodenum, and is available as tablets.

+▲ Side-effects/warning: See TRIPOTASSIUM DICITRATOBISMUTHATE.

debrisoquine

is an ADRENERGIC-NEURONE BLOCKER, which is an ANTISYMPATHETIC class of drug that prevents the release of the hormone noradrenaline from sympathetic nerves. It can be administered, usually in combination with other drugs (such as a DIURETIC or BETA-BLOCKER), as an ANTIHYPERTENSIVE treatment for moderate to severe high blood pressure, especially in cases where alternative forms of treatment have not been successful. Administration is oral.

+▲ Side-effects/warning: See GUANETHIDINE MONOSULPHATE; except it does not cause diarrhoea.

✪ Related entry: Declinax.

Deca-Durabolin

(Organon) is a proprietary, prescription-only preparation of the (*anabolic*) STEROID nandrolone (as decanoate). It can be used to treat osteoporosis in postmenopausal women and aplastic anaemia. It is available in a form for injection and also in a higher-dose preparation under the name of *Deca-Durabolin 100*.

+▲ Side-effects/warning: See NANDROLONE.

Decadron

(Merck Sharp & Dohme) is a proprietary, prescription-only preparation of the CORTICOSTEROID and ANTI-INFLAMMATORY dexamethasone. It can be used in the suppression of allergic and inflammatory conditions in shock, diagnosis of Cushing's disease, congenital adrenal hyperplasia and cerebral oedema. It is available as tablets and in a form for injection.

+▲ Side-effects/warning: See DEXAMETHASONE.

Decadron Shock-Pak

(Merck Sharp & Dohme) is a proprietary, prescription-only preparation of the CORTICOSTEROID and ANTI-INFLAMMATORY dexamethasone (as sodium phosphate). It can be used in the treatment of shock, and is available in a form for intravenous injection.

+▲ Side-effects/warning: See DEXAMETHASONE.

Decazate

(Berk) is a proprietary, prescription-only preparation of the ANTIPSYCHOTIC fluphenazine decanoate. It can be used in the long-term maintenance of the tranquillization of patients suffering from psychotic disorders (including schizophrenia). It is available in forms for depot deep intramuscular injection.

+▲ Side-effects/warning: See FLUPHENAZINE DECANOATE.

Declinax

(Roche) is a proprietary, prescription-only preparation of the ADRENERGIC-NEURONE BLOCKER debrisoquine. It can be used as an ANTIHYPERTENSIVE for moderate to severe high blood pressure, and is available as tablets.

+▲ Side-effects/warning: See DEBRISOQUINE.

decongestants ▣

are administered to relieve or reduce the symptoms of congestion of the airways and/or nose. NASAL DECONGESTANTS are generally applied in the form of nose-drops or as a nasal spray. This particular route of administration avoids the tendency of such drugs to have side-effects, for example, raising the blood pressure, though some are administered orally.

Most decongestants are SYMPATHOMIMETICS which work by constricting blood vessels in the mucous membranes of the airways and nasal cavity, so reducing the membranes' thickness, improving drainage and possibly decreasing mucous and fluid secretions. However, rhinitis, especially when caused by an allergy (such as hay fever), is usually dealt with by using ANTIHISTAMINES, which inhibit the detrimental and congestive effects of histamine released by an allergic response, or by drugs, and so inhibit the allergic response itself and therefore effectively reduce inflammation (eg CORTICOSTEROIDS or SODIUM CROMOGLYCATE).

Decongestants are often included in COMPOUND PREPARATIONS that are used to treat colds and which may contain a number of other constituents. However, most people are unaware that there are several constituents, but it is important to realize that the vasoconstriction, speeding of the heart and hypertension often caused by sympathomimetic drugs are detrimental and potentially dangerous in a number of cardiovascular disorders. It should also be borne in mind that sympathomimetics can have serious interactions with a number of other drug classes, especially (MAOI) ANTIDEPRESSANTS.

D

Deep Heat Massage Liniment

(Mentholatum) is a proprietary, non-prescription COMPOUND PREPARATION of MENTHOL and methyl salicylate, which both have COUNTER-IRRITANT, or RUBEFACIENT, actions. It can be applied to the skin for symptomatic relief of underlying muscle or joint pain. It is available as a liquid emulsion for topical application and is not normally used for children under five years, except on medical advice.

+▲ Side-effects/warning: See METHYL SALICYLATE.

Deep Heat Maximum Strength

(Mentholatum) is a proprietary, non-prescription COMPOUND PREPARATION of MENTHOL and methyl salicylate, which all have COUNTER-IRRITANT, or RUBEFACIENT, actions. It can be applied to the skin for symptomatic relief of underlying muscle or joint pain. It is available as an emulsion cream for topical application and is not normally used for children under five years, except on medical advice.

+▲ Side-effects/warning: See METHYL SALICYLATE.

Deep Heat Spray

(Mentholatum) is a proprietary, non-prescription COMPOUND PREPARATION of methyl salicylate, methyl nicotinate, ethyl salicylate; which all have COUNTER-IRRITANT, or RUBEFACIENT, actions. It can be applied to the skin for symptomatic relief of underlying muscle or joint pain. It is available as a spray for topical application and is not normally used for children under five years, except on medical advice.

+▲ Side-effects/warning: See METHYL SALICYLATE; ETHYL SALICYLATE.

deflazacort

is a recently introduced CORTICOSTEROID which has predominantly *glucocorticoid* activity. It can be used as an ANTI-INFLAMMATORY for a variety of inflammatory and allergic disorders. Administration is oral.

+▲ Side-effects/warning: See CORTICOSTEROIDS.

✪ Related entry: Calcort.

Delfen

(Ortho) is a proprietary, non-prescription SPERMICIDAL CONTRACEPTIVE for use in combination with barrier methods of contraception (such as a condom). It is available as a foam containing nonoxinol.

+▲ Side-effects/warning: See NONOXINOL.

Deltacortril Enteric

(Pfizer) is a proprietary, prescription-only preparation of the CORTICOSTEROID and ANTI-INFLAMMATORY prednisolone. It can be used to treat allergic and rheumatic conditions, particularly those affecting the joints and soft tissues. It is available as tablets.

+▲ Side-effects/warning: See PREDNISOLONE.

Deltastab

(Boots) is a proprietary, prescription-only preparation of the CORTICOSTEROID and ANTI-INFLAMMATORY prednisolone. It can be used to treat allergic and rheumatic conditions, particularly those affecting the joints and soft tissues. It is available in a form for injection.

+▲ Side-effects/warning: See PREDNISOLONE.

Delvas

(Berk) is a proprietary, prescription-only COMPOUND PREPARATION of the (*potassium-sparing*) DIURETIC amiloride hydrochloride and the (THIAZIDE) diuretic hydrochlorothiazide (a combination called co-amilozide 5/50). It can be used to treat oedema, congestive heart failure and as an ANTIHYPERTENSIVE. It is available as tablets.

+▲ Side-effects/warning: See AMILORIDE HYDROCHLORIDE; HYDROCHLOROTHIAZIDE.

demeclocycline hydrochloride

is a broad-spectrum ANTIBACTERIAL and ANTIBIOTIC drug, which is one of the TETRACYCLINES. It can be used to treat many kinds of infection, but particularly those of the respiratory tract, the ear, nose and throat, the gastrointestinal and genitourinary tracts and a wide variety of soft-tissue infections. Administration is oral. It is also used, quite separately to its use as an antibiotic, as a HORMONE ANTAGONIST to treat over-secretion of antidiuretic hormone (ADH) through an action on the kidney.
+▲ Side-effects/warning: See TETRACYCLINE; but the incidence of photosensitivity is greater.
✪ Related entries: Detecto; Ledermycin.

Demix
(Ashbourne) is a proprietary, prescription-only preparation of the ANTIBACTERIAL and (TETRACYCLINE) ANTIBIOTIC doxycycline. It can be used to treat infections of many kinds, and is available as capsules.
+▲ Side-effects/warning: See DOXYCYCLINE.

Demser
(Merck Sharp & Dohme) is a proprietary, prescription-only preparation of the ANTISYMPATHETIC metirosine. It can be used in the preoperative treatment of phaeochromocytoma, and is available as capsules.
+▲ Side-effects/warning: See METIROSINE.

demulcents 🗎
are agents or preparations that protect the mucous membranes and relieve pain and irritation. They work by forming a protective film and are incorporated into ANTACID preparations for protecting the gastric mucosa (stomach lining) and into mouthwashes, gargles, etc., to soothe the membranes of the mouth. The most commonly used demulcent agent is ALGINIC ACID or one of its alginate salts.

Dentinox Infant Colic Drops
(DDD) is a proprietary, non-prescription preparation of the ANTIFOAMING AGENT

dimethicone. It can be used for the relief of wind and griping pain in infants (from birth onwards), and is available as an oral suspension.
+▲ Side-effects/warning: See DIMETHICONE.

Dentinox Teething Gel
(DDD) is a proprietary, non-prescription COMPOUND PREPARATION of the LOCAL ANAESTHETIC lignocaine hydrochloride and the ANTISEPTIC cetylpyridinium chloride. It can be used for the temporary relief of pain caused by teething in babies, and is available as a gel for topical application.
+▲ Side-effects/warning: See CETYLPYRIDINIUM CHLORIDE; LIGNOCAINE HYDROCHLORIDE.

Dentomycin
(Lederle) is a proprietary, prescription-only preparation of the ANTIMICROBIAL metronidazole, which has ANTIBACTERIAL and ANTIPROTOZOAL actions. It can be used for the treatment of local infections in dental surgery, and is available as a gel.
+▲ Side-effects/warning: See METRONIDAZOLE.

Depixol
(Lundbeck) is a proprietary, prescription-only preparation of the ANTIPSYCHOTIC flupenthixol. It can be used to treat patients suffering from psychotic disorders (including schizophrenia), especially those with a type of psychosis that renders them apathetic and withdrawn. It can also be used for short-term treatment of depressive illness. It is available as tablets (as flupenthixol) and in a forms for depot deep intramuscular injection (as flupenthixol decanoate).
+▲ Side-effects/warning: See FLUPENTHIXOL; FLUPENTHIXOL DECANOATE.

Depixol Conc.
(Lundbeck) is a proprietary, prescription-only preparation of the ANTIPSYCHOTIC flupenthixol decanoate. It can be used in the maintenance of patients suffering from

D

schizophrenia and other psychotic disorders. It is available in a form for depot deep intramuscular injection.

+▲ Side-effects/warning: See FLUPENTHIXOL DECANOATE.

Depixol Low Volume

(Lundbeck) is a proprietary, prescription-only preparation of the ANTIPSYCHOTIC flupenthixol decanoate. It can be used in the maintenance of patients suffering from schizophrenia and other psychotic disorders. It is available in a form for depot deep intramuscular injection.

+▲ Side-effects/warning: See FLUPENTHIXOL DECANOATE.

Depo-Medrone

(Upjohn) is a proprietary, prescription-only preparation of the CORTICOSTEROID and ANTI-INFLAMMATORY methylprednisolone (as acetate). It can be used to relieve allergic and inflammatory disorders, particularly of the joints and soft tissues, and also to treat shock and cerebral oedema. It is available in a form for injection.

+▲ Side-effects/warning: See METHYLPREDNISOLONE.

Depo-Medrone with Lidocaine

(Upjohn) is a proprietary, prescription-only COMPOUND PREPARATION of the CORTICOSTEROID and ANTI-INFLAMMATORY methylprednisolone (as acetate) and the LOCAL ANAESTHETIC lignocaine hydrochloride. It can be used to treat inflammation in the joints (for example, in rheumatic disease) or soft tissue, and is available in a form for injection.

+▲ Side-effects/warning: See LIGNOCAINE HYDROCHLORIDE; METHYLPREDNISOLONE.

Depo-Provera

(Upjohn) is a proprietary, prescription-only preparation of the SEX HORMONE medroxyprogesterone acetate (a PROGESTOGEN). It can be used as an ANTICANCER treatment for cancer of the uterus, breast or prostate, as a hormonal supplement in women whose progestogen level requires boosting (eg in endometriosis or dysfunctional uterine bleeding) and as a long-lasting *progesterone-only* CONTRACEPTIVE preparation (administered by intramuscular injection every three months). It is available as tablets and in a form for injection.

+▲ Side-effects/warning: See MEDROXYPROGESTERONE ACETATE.

Deponit

(Schwarz) is a proprietary, non-prescription preparation of the VASODILATOR and ANTI-ANGINA drug glyceryl trinitrate. It can be used to treat and prevent angina pectoris. It is available as a self-adhesive dressing (patch) and so when placed on the chest the drug is absorbed through the skin and helps to give lasting relief.

+▲ Side-effects/warning: See GLYCERYL TRINITRATE.

Depostat

(Schering) is a proprietary, prescription-only preparation of gestronol hexanoate, which is a synthetic SEX HORMONE (PROGESTOGEN). It is used in women to treat cancer of the endometrium, and in men to treat benign enlargement of the prostate gland and malignant enlargement of the kidneys. It is available in a form for injection.

+▲ Side-effects/warning: See GESTRONOL HEXANOATE.

Dequacaine Lozenges

(Crookes) is a proprietary, non-prescription COMPOUND PREPARATION of the ANTISEPTIC dequalinium chloride and the LOCAL ANAESTHETIC benzocaine. It can be used to relieve the discomfort of a severe sore throat. It is not normally given to children under 12 years, except on medical advice.

+▲ Side-effects/warning: See BENZOCAINE; DEQUALINIUM CHLORIDE.

Dequadin Lozenge

(Crookes) is a proprietary, non-prescription preparation of the ANTISEPTIC dequalinium chloride. It can be used to treat common infections of the mouth and throat. It is not normally given to children under ten years, except on medical advice.

+▲ Side-effects/warning: See DEQUALINIUM CHLORIDE.

dequalinium chloride

is a mild ANTISEPTIC agent with some weak ANTIFUNGAL properties. It can be used to treat infections of the mouth and throat, and administration is oral. It is also available in some COMPOUND PREPARATIONS combined with LOCAL ANAESTHETICS.

✪ Related entries: Dequacaine Lozenges; Dequadin Lozenge; Labosept Pastilles.

Derbac-C

(Napp) is a proprietary, non-prescription preparation of the PEDICULICIDAL drug carbaryl. It can be used to treat infestations of the scalp and pubic hair by lice (pediculosis). It is available as a liquid and a shampoo, and is not normally used for infants under six months, except on medical advice.

+▲ Side-effects/warning: See CARBARYL.

Derbac-M

(Napp) is a proprietary, non-prescription preparation of the SCABICIDAL and PEDICULICIDAL drug malathion. It can be used to treat infestations of the scalp and pubic hair by lice (pediculosis) or of the skin by the itch-mite (scabies). It is available as a liquid and is not normally used for infants under six months, except on medical advice.

+▲ Side-effects/warning: See MALATHION.

Dermalex

(Sanofi Winthrop) is a proprietary, non-prescription preparation of the ANTISEPTIC hexachlorophane. It can be used to treat urinary rash and to prevent bedsores, and is available as a skin lotion. It is not normally used for children under two years, except on medical advice.

+▲ Side-effects/warning: See HEXACHLOROPHANE.

Dermol 500

(Dermal) is a proprietary, non-prescription preparation of the ANTISEPTICS benzalkonium chloride and chlorhexidine hydrochloride (with liquid paraffin and isopropyl myristate). It can be used in the treatment of acne, and is available as a lotion.

+▲ Side-effects/warning: See BENZALKONIUM CHLORIDE; CHLORHEXIDINE HYDROCHLORIDE.

Dermovate

(Glaxo) is a proprietary, prescription-only preparation of the CORTICOSTEROID and ANTI-INFLAMMATORY clobetasol propionate. It can be used for the short-term treatment of severe, inflammatory skin disorders, such as eczema and psoriasis, that are resistant to weaker corticosteroids. It is available as a cream, an ointment and a scalp application for topical application.

+▲ Side-effects/warning: See CLOBETASOL PROPIONATE.

Dermovate-NN

(Glaxo) is a proprietary, prescription-only COMPOUND PREPARATION of the CORTICOSTEROID clobetasol propionate, the ANTIBACTERIAL and (AMINOGLYCOSIDE) ANTIBIOTIC neomycin sulphate and the ANTIFUNGAL and antibiotic nystatin. It can be used, in the short term, to treat inflammation of the skin in which infection is also present. It is available as an ointment and a cream for topical application.

+▲ Side-effects/warning: See CLOBETASOL PROPIONATE; NEOMYCIN SULPHATE; NYSTATIN.

desensitizing vaccines ▣

are preparations of particular allergens (substances to which a patient has an allergic reaction) which are administered, in progressive doses, to reduce the degree of allergic reaction the patient suffers when

D

exposed to the allergen. For example, preparations of grass pollens are administered for the treatment of hay fever, or bee venom or wasp venom to protect against the effects of subsequent stings. The mechanism by which they work is not clear.
✚ Side-effects: Allergic reactions, especially in small children.
▲ Warning: They are not to be used in patients who are pregnant, who have acute asthma or febrile conditions. A heavy meal must not be eaten before treatment. Injections should be administered under close medical supervision and in locations where emergency facilities for full cardio-respiratory resuscitation are immediately available.
○ Related entry: Pharmalgen.

Deseril

(Sandoz) is a proprietary, prescription-only preparation of methysergide. It can be used as an ANTIMIGRAINE treatment to prevent severe, recurrent migraine and similar headaches in patients for whom other forms of treatment have failed. It is available as tablets.
✚▲ Side-effects/warning: See METHYSERGIDE.

Desferal

(Ciba) is a proprietary, prescription-only preparation of the CHELATING AGENT desferrioxamine mesylate. It can be used as an ANTIDOTE to treat iron poisoning and iron overload. It is available as an oral solution or in a form for injection.
✚▲ Side-effects/warning: See DESFERRIOXAMINE MESYLATE.

desferrioxamine mesylate

is a CHELATING AGENT which is used as an ANTIDOTE to treat IRON poisoning or an overload of iron in the tissues (eg in aplastic anaemia due to repeated blood transfusion). Administration is either oral or by injection.
✚ Side-effects: There may be pain at the site of injection, gastrointestinal disturbances,

hypotension, heart rate changes, anaphylaxis, convulsions, dizziness, disturbances in vision and hearing and skin disorders.
▲ Warning: Avoid its use in patients with kidney impairment; or who are pregnant or breast-feeding.
○ Related entry: Desferal.

desflurane

is a recently introduced inhalant GENERAL ANAESTHETIC which can be used along with nitrous oxide-oxygen mixtures for the induction and maintenance of anaesthesia during surgery. Administration is by inhalation.
✚ Side-effects: Coughing, laryngospasm and increased airways secretions and breath-holding.
○ Related entry: Suprane.

desipramine hydrochloride

is a (TRICYCLIC) ANTIDEPRESSANT which can be used to treat depressive illness and has less sedative properties than many tricyclics, which makes it more suitable for the treatment of withdrawn and apathetic patients. Administration is oral.
✚▲ Side-effects/warning: See AMITRYPTYLINE HYDROCHLORIDE; but with a less sedative effect.
○ Related entry: Pertofran.

desmopressin

is one of two major analogues of the antidiuretic HORMONE vasopressin (ADH), which naturally reduces urine production. It is used to diagnose or to treat certain (pituitary-originated) types of diabetes insipidus, to test renal function and to prevent bed-wetting. It is also used to boost blood concentrations of some blood-clotting factors in haemophiliac patients. Administration can be oral, or topical as nose-drops or a nasal spray (it is absorbed into the systemic circulation from the nasal mucosa).
✚▲ Side-effects/warning: See VASOPRESSIN. There is less rise in blood pressure, but

nevertheless care is needed in patients with certain cardiovascular or kidney disorders, or hypertension. Fluid retention and raised sodium levels may occur unless fluid intake is restricted. There may be vomiting, headache and nosebleeds.
○ Related entries: DDAVP; Desmospray; Desmotabs.

Desmospray

(Ferring) is a proprietary, prescription-only preparation of desmopressin, which is an analogue of the pituitary HORMONE vasopressin (ADH). It is administered primarily to diagnose or to treat pituitary-originated diabetes insipidus. It can be used for some other diagnostic tests, to boost the blood concentration of blood-clotting factors in haemophiliac patients and to prevent bed-wetting. It is available as a nasal spray (it is absorbed into the systemic circulation from the nasal mucosa).
+▲ Side-effects/warning: See DESMOPRESSIN.

Desmotabs

(Ferring) is a proprietary, prescription-only preparation of desmopressin, which is an analogue of the pituitary HORMONE vasopressin (ADH). It is used primarily to diagnose or to treat pituitary-originated diabetes insipidus. It can also be used for some other diagnostic tests, to boost the blood concentration of blood-clotting factors in haemophiliac patients and to prevent bed-wetting. It is available (as desmopressin acetate) as tablets.
+▲ Side-effects/warning: See DESMOPRESSIN.

desogestrel

is a PROGESTOGEN which is used as a constituent of the *combined* ORAL CONTRACEPTIVES that contain an OESTROGEN and a PROGESTOGEN. Administration is oral.
+▲ Side-effects/warning: See PROGESTOGEN.
○ Related entries: Marvelon; Mercilon.

desoximetasone
see DESOXYMETHASONE

desoxymethasone

(desoximetasone) is a CORTICOSTEROID with ANTI-INFLAMMATORY properties. It is used in the treatment of severe, acute inflammation of the skin and chronic skin disorders, such as psoriasis. Administration is by topical application.
+▲ Side-effects/warning: See CORTICOSTEROIDS; though systemic effects are unlikely with topical application, but there may be local skin reactions.
○ Related entry: Stiedex.

desquamating agents
see KERATOLYTIC

Destolit

(Merrell) is a proprietary, prescription-only preparation of ursodeoxycholic acid. It is used to dissolve gallstones, and is available as tablets.
+▲ Side-effects/warning: See URSODEOXYCHOLIC ACID.

Deteclo

(Lederle) is a proprietary, prescription-only COMPOUND PREPARATION of the ANTIBACTERIAL and (TETRACYCLINE) ANTIBIOTICS chlortetracycline (as hydrochloride), tetracycline (as hydrochloride) and demeclocycline hydrochloride. It can be used to treat many kinds of infection, and is available as tablets.
+▲ Side-effects/warning: See CHLORTETRACYCLINE; DEMECLOCYCLINE HYDROCHLORIDE; TETRACYCLINE.

Dexa-Rhinaspray

(Boehringer Ingelheim) is a proprietary, prescription-only COMPOUND PREPARATION of the ANTI-INFLAMMATORY and CORTICOSTEROID dexamethasone (as isonicotinate), the (AMINOGLYCOSIDE) ANTIBIOTIC neomycin sulphate and the SYMPATHOMIMETIC and VASOCONSTRICTOR tramazoline hydrochloride. It can be used to treat allergic rhinitis, and

D

is available as an aerosol for nasal inhalation.

✚▲ Side-effects/warning: See
DEXAMETHASONE; NEOMYCIN SULPHATE;
TRAMAZOLINE HYDROCHLORIDE.

dexamethasone

is a CORTICOSTEROID with ANTI-INFLAMMATORY properties. It is used for a variety of purposes, including the suppression of inflammatory and allergic disorders, in the treatment of shock, in the diagnosis of Cushing's disease, to treat congenital adrenal hyperplasia, cerebral oedema and in rheumatic disease to relieve pain and to increase mobility and decrease deformity of joints. It is used in several forms: dexamethasone, dexamethasone sodium phosphate and dexamethasone isonicotinate. Administration can be oral, topical or by injection.

✚▲ Side-effects/warning: See
CORTICOSTEROIDS; though systemic effects are unlikely with topical application, but there may be local skin reactions.

○ Related entries: Decadron; Decadron Shock-Pak; Dexa-Rhinaspray; Dexamethasone; Maxidex; Maxitrol; Otomize; Sofradex.

Dexamethasone

(Organon) is a proprietary, prescription-only preparation of the CORTICOSTEROID and ANTI-INFLAMMATORY dexamethasone. It can be used in the suppression of allergic and inflammatory conditions, in the treatment of shock, congenital adrenal hyperplasia, cerebral oedema and in the diagnosis of Cushing's disease. It is available as tablets and in a form for injection.

✚▲ Side-effects/warning: See
DEXAMETHASONE.

dexamphetamine sulphate

is a drug that, in adults, works directly on the brain as a STIMULANT and can be used to treat narcolepsy (a condition involving irresistible attacks of sleep during the daytime). Paradoxically, in children it has

more of a sedative action and can be used in the treatment of hyperactivity. It is on the Controlled Drugs List because of its addictive potential. Administration is oral.

✚ Side-effects: Insomnia, irritability, restlessness, night terrors, euphoria, tremor, dizziness, headache, dependence, tolerance, psychosis, gastrointestinal symptoms, anorexia, growth retardation in children, dry mouth, sweating and effects on the cardiovascular system.

▲ Warning: It should not be administered to patients with heart disease, hypertension, hyperexcitability states, hyperthyroidism, history of drug abuse, glaucoma, extrapyramidal disorders, or who are pregnant or breast-feeding. Avoid its use in those with porphyria; and avoid alcohol because of the potential of unpredictable reactions. It may impair the performance of skilled tasks, such as driving. Withdrawal of treatment should be gradual.

○ Related entry: Dexedrine.

Dexedrine

(Evans) is a proprietary, prescription-only preparation of the powerful STIMULANT dexamphetamine sulphate, and is on the Controlled Drugs List. It can be used to treat narcolepsy in adults and medically diagnosed hyperactivity in children. It is available as tablets.

✚▲ Side-effects/warning: See
DEXAMPHETAMINE SULPHATE.

dexfenfluramine hydrochloride

is an APPETITE SUPPRESSANT which is used therapeutically for the treatment of medically diagnosed obesity. It is the dextro-isomer of the powerful appetite-suppressant drug fenfluramine hydrochloride. Dexfenfluramine is a sedative rather than a stimulant, which is the case with most other appetite suppressants, and may affect a patient's thought and movement and is potentially addictive (though this is rare). Administration is oral.

+▲ Side-effects/warning: See FENFLURAMINE HYDROCHLORIDE. It should not be used in patients with certain liver or kidney disorders.

◎ Related entry: Adifax.

dextromethorphan hydrobromide

is an (OPIOID) ANTITUSSIVE which is used alone or in combination with other drugs in linctuses, syrups and lozenges to relieve dry or painful coughs.

+▲ Side-effects/warning: See OPIOIDS; but side-effects are rare.

◎ Related entries: Actifed Compound Linctus; Actifed Junior Cough Relief; Benylin Cough and Congestion; Benylin Dry Coughs Non-Drowsy; Benylin Dry Coughs Original; Bronalin Dry Cough Elixir; Benylin Coughs and Congestion; Contac Coughcaps; Covonia Bronchial Balsam; Covonia for Children; Day Nurse Capsules; Day Nurse Liquid; Flurex Cold/Flu Capsules with Cough Suppressant; Franolyn for Dry Cough; Lemsip Night-time; Meltus Dry Cough Elixir, Adult; Meltus Junior Dry Cough Elixir; Night Nurse Capsules; Night Nurse Liquid; Nirolex Lozenges; Owbridge's for Dry Tickly and Allergy Coughs; Robitussin Dry Cough; Robitussin Junior Persistent Cough Medicine; Sudafed Linctus; Tancolin; Vicks Mednite; Vicks Vaposyrup for Dry Coughs; Vicks Vaposyrup for Dry Coughs and Nasal Congestion.

dextromoramide

is an (OPIOID) NARCOTIC ANALGESIC drug that is a synthetic derivative of morphine. It can be administered to treat severe and intractable pain, particularly in the final stages of terminal illness, and is less sedating and shorter acting than morphine. Its proprietary forms are on the Controlled Drugs List because, as with morphine, it is potentially addictive. Administration can be either oral or topical.

+▲ Side-effects/warning: See OPIOIDS. It is not used in obstetrics because it may affect the unborn child.

◎ Related entry: Palfium.

dextropropoxyphene hydrochloride

is an (OPIOID) NARCOTIC ANALGESIC which is used to treat pain anywhere in the body. It is usually combined with other analgesics (especially paracetamol or aspirin) as a COMPOUND ANALGESIC. Administration of the drug on its own is oral.

+▲ Side-effects/warning: See OPIOIDS. There may be occasional liver toxicity, porphyria in susceptible individuals and convulsions in overdose. It is not to be used in patients with suicidal tendencies or with a history of addiction.

◎ Related entries: co-proxamol; Cosalgesic; Distalgesic; Doloxene; Doloxene Compound.

dextrose

or dextrose monohydrate, is another term for glucose.

DF118

(Napp) is a proprietary, prescription-only preparation of the (OPIOID) NARCOTIC ANALGESIC dihydrocodeine tartrate, which is on the Controlled Drugs List. It can be used to treat moderate to severe pain, and is available in a form for injection (this brand name was formerly used for a tablet form).

+▲ Side-effects/warning: See DIHYDROCODEINE TARTRATE.

DF118 Forte

(Napp) is a proprietary, prescription-only preparation of the (OPIOID) NARCOTIC ANALGESIC dihydrocodeine tartrate. It can be used to treat acute and chronic severe pain, and is available as tablets.

+▲ Side-effects/warning: See DIHYDROCODEINE TARTRATE.

DHC Continus

(Napp) is a proprietary, prescription-only preparation of the (OPIOID) NARCOTIC ANALGESIC dihydrocodeine tartrate. It can be used to treat moderate to severe pain, and is available as modified-release tablets.

+▲ Side-effects/warning: See DIHYDROCODEINE TARTRATE.

D

Diabetamide

(Ashbourne) is a proprietary, prescription-only preparation of the SULPHONYLUREA glibenclamide. It is used in DIABETIC TREATMENT of Type II diabetes (non-insulin-dependent diabetes mellitus; NIDDM; maturity-onset diabetes), and is available as tablets.

✚▲ Side-effects/warning: See GLIBENCLAMIDE.

diabetes insipidus treatment ⊡

involves the administration of drugs to counteract the under-production of ANTIDIURETIC HORMONE (ADH; also called VASOPRESSIN) by the pituitary gland, which is a characteristic of diabetes insipidus. Vasopressin itself may be used, but must be given by injection (it is a peptide that is broken down in the gastrointestinal tract). The analogues LYPRESSIN and DESMOPRESSIN can both be administered in the form of a nasal spray (they are absorbed into the systemic circulation from the nasal mucosa) and desmopressin (a synthetic peptide) can also be given by mouth. Diabetes insipidus is a rare disease and has no connection at all with diabetes mellitus, which is also a HORMONE disorder, but due to the under-production of INSULIN by the pancreas. However, in both conditions there is thirst and a production of large quantities of dilute urine.

diabetic treatment ⊡

(*diabetes mellitus* treatment) uses two types of drugs. The first treatment involves the use of ORAL HYPOGLYCAEMICS. These are synthetic agents taken by mouth to reduce the levels of glucose (sugar) in the bloodstream and are used primarily in the treatment of Type II diabetes (non-insulin-dependent diabetes mellitus; NIDDM; maturity-onset diabetes) when there is still some residual capacity in the pancreas for the production of the HORMONE insulin. The main oral hypoglycaemics used are the SULPHONYLUREAS and BIGUANIDES. The second

treatment involves the administration of INSULIN, which is mainly used in Type I diabetes (insulin-dependent diabetes mellitus; IDDM; juvenile-onset diabetes) and must be injected. There are many insulin preparations available and the difference between them is mainly their duration of action.

Diabinese

(Pfizer) is a proprietary, prescription-only preparation of the SULPHONYLUREA chlorpropamide. It is used in DIABETIC TREATMENT of Type II diabetes (non-insulin-dependent diabetes mellitus; NIDDM; maturity-onset diabetes), and is available as tablets.

✚▲ Side-effects/warning: See CHLORPROPAMIDE.

Diagesil

(Berk) is a proprietary, prescription-only preparation of the (OPIOID) NARCOTIC ANALGESIC and ANTITUSSIVE diamorphine hydrochloride (heroin hydrochloride), and is on the Controlled Drugs List. It can be used primarily to relieve intractable pain, especially during the final stages of terminal malignant disease, and is available in a form for injection.

✚▲ Side-effects/warning: See DIAMORPHINE HYDROCHLORIDE.

Dialar

(Lagap) is a proprietary, prescription-only preparation of the BENZODIAZEPINE diazepam. It can be used as an ANXIOLYTIC in the short-term treatment of anxiety, as a HYPNOTIC to relieve insomnia, as an ANTICONVULSANT and ANTI-EPILEPTIC for status epilepticus, as a SEDATIVE in preoperative medication, as a SKELETAL MUSCLE RELAXANT and to assist in the treatment of alcohol withdrawal symptoms. It is available as an oral solution.

✚▲ Side-effects/warning: See DIAZEPAM.

Diamicron

(Servier) is a proprietary, prescription-only

preparation of the SULPHONYLUREA drug gliclazide. It can be used in DIABETIC TREATMENT of Type II diabetes (non-insulin-dependent diabetes mellitus; NIDDM; maturity-onset diabetes), and is available as tablets.

✚▲ Side-effects/warning: See GLICLAZIDE.

diamorphine hydrochloride

is the chemical name of heroin hydrochloride (which is a chemical derivative of morphine) and is a powerful (OPIOID) NARCOTIC ANALGESIC. It can be used in the treatment of moderate to severe pain (though it has a shorter duration of action than morphine). It is also occasionally used as an ANTITUSSIVE to treat severe and painful cough and for acute airways oedema (especially in the treatment of terminal lung cancer). However, its use quickly tends to tolerance and then dependence (addiction). Administration can be either oral or by injection. All proprietray preparations of this drug are on the Controlled Drugs List.

✚▲ Side-effects/warning: See OPIOIDS; but it may cause less nausea and hypotension.

✪ Related entries: Diagesil; Diaphine.

Diamox

(Storz) is a proprietary, prescription-only preparation of the CARBONIC ANHYDRASE INHIBITOR acetazolamide. It is mainly used in GLAUCOMA TREATMENT, but also has DIURETIC properties. It is available as tablets and as a modified-release capsules (*Diamox SR*).

✚▲ Side-effects/warning: See ACETAZOLAMIDE.

Dianette

(Schering) is a proprietary, prescription-only COMPOUND PREPARATION of the OESTROGEN HORMONE ethinyloestradiol and the ANTI-ANDROGEN cyproterone acetate. It can be used in women, in certain circumstances, to treat acne, and is available as tablets.

✚▲ Side-effects/warning: See CYPROTERONE ACETATE; ETHINYLOESTRADIOL.

Diaphine

(Napp) is a proprietary, prescription-only preparation of the (OPIOID) NARCOTIC ANALGESIC and ANTITUSSIVE diamorphine hydrochloride (heroin hydrochloride), and is on the Controlled Drugs List. It is used mainly to relieve intractable pain, especially in terminal malignant disease. It is available in a form for injection.

✚▲ Side-effects/warning: See DIAMORPHINE HYDROCHLORIDE.

Diareze

(Boots) is a proprietary, non-prescription preparation of the (OPIOID) ANTIDIARRHOEAL loperamide hydrochloride. It can be used for the symptomatic relief of acute diarrhoea and its associated pain and discomfort, and is available as capsules.

✚▲ Side-effects/warning: See LOPERAMIDE HYDROCHLORIDE.

Diarphen

(Mepra-pharm) is a proprietary, prescription-only COMPOUND PREPARATION of the (OPIOID) ANTIDIARRHOEAL diphenoxylate hydrochloride and the ANTICHOLINERGIC atropine sulphate (a combination called CO-PHENOTROPE). It can be used to treat chronic diarrhoea, for example, in mild chronic ulcerative colitis. Dependence may occur with prolonged use. It is available as tablets and is not normally given to young children, except on medical advice.

✚▲ Side-effects/warning: See ATROPINE SULPHATE; DIPHENOXYLATE HYDROCHLORIDE.

Diarrest

(Galen) is a proprietary, prescription-only preparation of the (OPIOID) ANTIDIARRHOEAL codeine phosphate with sodium and potassium salts. It can be used to supplement or replace minerals lost through vomiting or diarrhoea. It should be used only for short-term treatment of diarrhoea and cramps, and is available as an oral liquid.

✚▲ Side-effects/warning: See CODEINE PHOSPHATE.

D

Diazemuls

(Dumex) is a proprietary, prescription-only preparation of the BENZODIAZEPINE diazepam. It has quite a range of uses: it can be administered as an ANXIOLYTIC (but only in the short-term treatment of anxiety), as a HYPNOTIC to relieve insomnia, as an ANTICONVULSANT and ANTI-EPILEPTIC for status epilepticus, as a SEDATIVE in preoperative medication, as a SKELETAL MUSCLE RELAXANT and to assist in the treatment of alcohol withdrawal symptoms. It is available in a form for injection.

✚▲ Side-effects/warning: See DIAZEPAM.

diazepam

is chemically a BENZODIAZEPINE. It has quite a range of uses: it can be administered as an ANXIOLYTIC (but only in the short-term treatment of anxiety), as a HYPNOTIC to relieve insomnia, as an ANTICONVULSANT and ANTI-EPILEPTIC for status epilepticus and convulsions due to poisoning, as a SEDATIVE in preoperative medication, as a SKELETAL MUSCLE RELAXANT and to assist in the treatment of alcohol withdrawal symptoms. Administration can be oral, topical or by injection.

✚▲ Side-effects/warning See BENZODIAZEPINES. When injected, there may be pain, inflammation and swelling at the injection site.

◐ Related entries: Atensine; Dialar; Diazemuls; Diazepam Rectubes; Rimapam; Stesolid; Tensium; Valclair; Valium.

Diazepam Rectubes

(CP) is a proprietary, prescription-only preparation of the BENZODIAZEPINE diazepam. It can be used as an ANXIOLYTIC in the short-term treatment of anxiety, as a HYPNOTIC to relieve insomnia, as an ANTICONVULSANT and ANTI-EPILEPTIC for status epilepticus, as a SEDATIVE in preoperative medication, as a SKELETAL MUSCLE RELAXANT and to assist in the treatment of alcohol withdrawal symptoms. It is available as a rectal solution.

✚▲ Side-effects/warning: See DIAZEPAM.

diazoxide

has two separate actions and uses. First, it can lower blood pressure rapidly on injection and can therefore be used as an ANTIHYPERTENSIVE in treating acute hypertensive crisis. Second, it is a hyperglycaemic drug and can be used by mouth to treat chronic hypoglycaemia (abnormally low levels of glucose in the bloostream), for example, where a pancreatic tumour causes excessive secretion of INSULIN. Administration is either oral or by injection.

✚ Side-effects: There may be nausea and vomiting, an increased heart rate with hypotension, loss of appetite, oedema, heart arrhythmias and increased heart rate and hyperglycaemia; excessive growth of hair with chronic treatment.

▲ Warning: Administer with caution to those patients who have a reduced blood supply to the heart, certain kidney disorders, who are pregnant or in labour. During prolonged treatment, regular monitoring of blood constituents and blood pressure is required.

◐ Related entries: Eudemine (injection); Eudemine (tablets).

Dibenyline

(Forley) is a proprietary, prescription-only preparation of the ALPHA-ADRENOCEPTOR BLOCKER phenoxybenzamine hydrochloride. It can be used, in conjunction with a BETA-BLOCKER, as an ANTIHYPERTENSIVE in hypertensive crises in phaeochromocytoma and severe shock. It is available as capsules and in a form for injection.

✚▲ Side-effects/warning: See PHENOXYBENZAMINE HYDROCHLORIDE.

dibromopropamidine isethionate

is an ANTIBACTERIAL which is used specifically to treat infections of the eyelids or conjunctiva, including the amoebic infection acanthamoeba keratitis (sometimes with additional drugs). Administration is topical.

○ Related entries: Brolene Eye Ointment; Brulidine; Golden Eye Ointment.

diclofenac sodium

is a (NSAID) NON-NARCOTIC ANALGESIC and ANTIRHEUMATIC drug. It is used to treat pain and inflammation in rheumatic disease and other musculoskeletal disorders (such as juvenile arthritis and gout). It is being increasing used to treat pain immediately after certain surgical procedures, and for renal colic, usually by injection (or suppositories). Administration can be oral, topical or by injection.
✚▲ Side-effects/warning: See NSAID. Avoid its use in patients with porphyria. There may be local irritation if using suppositories, or pain at the site of injection.
○ Related entries: Arthrotec; Diclomax Retard; Diclozip; Flamrase SR; Isclofen; Motifene 75 mg; Rhumalgan; Valenac; Volraman; Voltarol; Voltarol Emulgel; Voltarol Optha.

Diclomax Retard

(Parke-Davis) is a proprietary, prescription-only preparation of the (NSAID) NON-NARCOTIC ANALGESIC and ANTIRHEUMATIC diclofenac sodium. It can be used to treat arthritic and rheumatic pain and inflammation and other musculoskeletal disorders. It is available as modified-release capsules.
✚▲ Side-effects/warning: See DICLOFENAC SODIUM.

Diclozip

(Ashbourne) is a prescription-only, non-proprietary version of the (NSAID) NON-NARCOTIC ANALGESIC and ANTIRHEUMATIC diclofenac sodium. It can be used to treat arthritic and rheumatic pain and inflammation and other musculoskeletal disorders. It is available as tablets.
✚▲ Side-effects/warning: See DICLOFENAC SODIUM.

dicobalt edetate

is used as an ANTIDOTE to acute cyanide

poisoning. It acts as a CHELATING AGENT by binding to cyanide to form a compound that can be excreted from the body. Administration is by injection.
✚ Side-effects: Vomiting, transient hypotension and tachycardia.
▲ Warning: Because of its toxicity, it is normally used only when the patient is losing, or has lost, consciousness.
○ Related entry: Kelocyanor.

Diconal

(Wellcome) is a proprietary, prescription-only COMPOUND PREPARATION of the (OPIOID) NARCOTIC ANALGESIC dipipanone hydrochloride and the ANTIHISTAMINE and ANTINAUSEANT cyclizine hydrochloride. It can be used to treat moderate to severe pain, and is available as tablets. It is on the Controlled Drugs List and is not normally given to children, except on medical advice.
✚▲ Side-effects/warning: See CYCLIZINE; DIPIPANONE.

dicyclomine hydrochloride

(dicyloverine hydrochloride) is an ANTICHOLINERGIC drug which can be used as an ANTISPASMODIC for the symptomatic relief of muscle spasm in the gastrointestinal tract. Administration is oral.
✚▲ Side-effects/warning: See ATROPINE SULPHATE.
○ Related entries: Kolanticon Gel; Merbentyl; Merbentyl 20.

dicyloverine hydrochloride

see DICYCLOMINE HYDROCHLORIDE

Dicynene

(Delandale) is a proprietary, prescription-only preparation of ethamsylate, which is a HAEOMOSTATIC drug that can be used in certain situations where antifibrinolytic drugs might be administered. It can be used for a variety of purposes, including bleeding in premature infants and in menorrhagia. It is available as tablets and in a form for injection.
✚▲ Side-effects/warning: See ETHAMSYLATE.

D

didanosine

(ddI; DDI) is a (*reverse transcriptase*) ANTIVIRAL which can be used in the treatment of AIDS. It is mainly administered in combination with other antivirals to patients who are intolerant to, or have not benefited from, other antivirals. Administration is oral.

✚ Side-effects: Pancreatitis, peripheral neuropathy or raised uric acid levels in the blood (monitoring is necessary). Other possible side-effects include nausea, headache, vomiting, confusion, fever and headache.

▲ Warning: It should not be given to patients with peripheral neuropathy or diabetes, or who are breast-feeding. Administer with caution where there is a history of pancreatitis, in peripheral neuropathy, where there is raised blood uric acid and in those who have impaired liver or kidney function; and to patients who are pregnant.

✪ Related entry: Videx.

Didronel

(Procter & Gamble) is a proprietary, prescription-only preparation of disodium etidronate. It can be used to reduce the rate of bone turnover in treating the condition known as Paget's disease of the bone, and also to treat high calcium levels associated with malignant tumours. It is available as tablets.

✚▲ Side-effects/warning: See DISODIUM ETIDRONATE.

Didronel PMO

(Procter & Gamble) is a proprietary, prescription-only COMPOUND PREPARATION of the CALCIUM METABOLISM MODIFIER disodium etidronate and calcium carbonate. It can be used to reduce the rate of bone turnover in treating the condition known as Paget's disease of the bone, and also to treat high calcium levels associated with malignant tumours. It is available as tablets.

✚▲ Side-effects/warning: See CALCIUM CARBONATE; DISODIUM ETIDRONATE.

dienoestrol

is a synthetic OESTROGEN, a SEX HORMONE, which can be used as part of HRT (hormone replacement therapy). Administration is by topical application.

✚▲ Side-effects/warning: See OESTROGENS.

✪ Related entry: Ortho Dienoestrol.

diethyl ether

is an inhalant GENERAL ANAESTHETIC which is more familiarly known as ether. It is now rarely administered in developed countries, but is still used elsewhere in the world because it is cheap, requires only simple apparatus to administer and is suitable for single-handed use.

✚ Side-effects: It is irritant to the upper airways and tends to cause nausea and vomiting.

diethylamine salicylate

is a constituent with a COUNTER-IRRITANT, or RUBEFACIENT, action. It can be applied to the skin for symptomatic relief of underlying muscle or joint pain.

✚▲ Side-effects/warning: On topical administration there may be local irritation. It should not be used on broken skin or mucous membranes.

✪ Related entries: Algesal; Lloyd's Cream.

diethylstilbestrol

see STILBOESTROL

Difflam

(3M) is a proprietary, non-prescription preparation of benzydamine hydrochloride, which has a COUNTER-IRRITANT, or RUBEFACIENT, action. It can be used for symptomatic relief of pain on the skin, mouth ulcers and other sores or inflammation in the mouth and throat. It is available as a cream for topical application and as a liquid mouthwash or spray.

✚▲ Side-effects/warning: See BENZYDAMINE HYDROCHLORIDE.

Diflucan

(Pfizer) is a proprietary, prescription-only

preparation of the ANTIFUNGAL fluconazole. It can be used to treat candidiasis (thrush) of the vagina, mouth and other tissue areas. It is available as capsules and in a form for intravenous infusion.

+▲ Side-effects/warning: See FLUCONAZOLE.

diflucortolone valerate

is a CORTICOSTEROID with ANTI-INFLAMMATORY properties. It is used in the treatment of severe, acute inflammatory skin disorders, such as eczema and psoriasis, that are unresponsive to less potent corticosteroids. Administration is by topical application.

+▲ Side-effects/warning: See CORTICOSTEROIDS; though systemic effects are unlikely with topical application, but there may be local skin reactions.

❂ Related entry: Nerisone.

diflunisal

is a (NSAID) NON-NARCOTIC ANALGESIC and ANTIRHEUMATIC drug derived from aspirin, but is quite powerful and with a longer duration of action. It can be used in the treatment of pain and inflammation (especially in rheumatic disease and other musculoskeletal disorders) and for period pain. Administration is oral.

+▲ Side-effects/warning: See NSAID. Administer with care to patients who are breast-feeding.

❂ Related entry: Dolobid.

Diftavax

(Mérieux) is a proprietary, prescription-only VACCINE preparation of adsorbed diphtheria and tetanus vaccine for adults (DT/Vac/Ads for Adults), which combines (toxoid) vaccines for diphtheria and tetanus vaccine adsorbed onto a mineral carrier. It is available in a form for injection.

+▲ Side-effects/warning: See DIPHTHERIA VACCINES; TETANUS VACCINE.

Digibind

(Wellcome) is a proprietary, prescription-only preparation which can be used as an ANTIDOTE to overdosage by the CARDIAC GLYCOSIDES digoxin and digitoxin. It comprises antibody fragments that react with the glycosides, and is administered for emergency use by injection.

digitoxin

is a CARDIAC GLYCOSIDE derived from the leaves of *Digitalis* foxgloves. It can be used as a CARDIAC STIMULANT, because it increases the force of contraction in congestive HEART FAILURE TREATMENT and as an ANTI-ARRHYTHMIC to treat certain heartbeat irregularities. Administration is oral.

+▲ Side-effects/warning: See DIGOXIN.

digoxin

is a CARDIAC GLYCOSIDE derived from the leaves of *Digitalis* foxgloves. It can be used as a CARDIAC STIMULANT, because it increases the force of contraction in congestive HEART FAILURE TREATMENT, and as an ANTI-ARRHYTHMIC to treat certain heartbeat irregularities. Administration is either oral or by injection.

+ Side-effects: There are serious and common side-effects (the minimization of which depends on finding a suitable dosage schedule in each patient and regular monitoring): loss of appetite, nausea and vomiting, with a consequent weight loss; diarrhoea and abdominal pain; visual disturbances; fatigue, confusion, delirium and hallucinations. Overdosage may lead to arrhythmias or heart block.

▲ Warning: It should be administered with caution to patients who have had a recent heart attack, certain arrhythmias and heart conditions, hypothyroidism, who are elderly, have impaired kidney function and where there is raised blood potassium. Regular monitoring of the blood potassium level is also recommended.

❂ Related entries: Lanoxin; Lanoxin-PG.

dihydrocodeine tartrate

is an (OPIOID) NARCOTIC ANALGESIC which is similar to CODEINE PHOSPHATE but more powerful. It is also available in some

D

COMPOUND ANALGESIC preparations (eg in co-dydramol, where it is combined with paracetamol). Administration is either oral or by injection.

+▲ Side-effects/warning: See OPIOIDS.
✪ Related entries: DF118; DF118 Forte; DHC Continus; Galake; Paramol Tablets; Remedeine.

dihydrotachysterol
is a synthetic form of vitamin D (related to D_2 and D_3) which is used to make up body deficiencies of this vitamin. Administration is oral.

+▲ Side-effects/warning: See VITAMIN D.
✪ Related entry: AT 10.

Dijex Suspension
(Seton) is a proprietary, non-prescription COMPOUND PREPARATION of the ANTACIDS aluminium hydroxide and magnesium hydroxide. It can be used to relieve acid indigestion and dyspepsia, and is available as a liquid suspension. It is not normally given to children under six years, except on medical advice.

+▲ Side-effects/warning: See ALUMINIUM HYDROXIDE; MAGNESIUM HYDROXIDE.

Dijex Tablets
(Seton) is a proprietary, non-prescription COMPOUND PREPARATION of the ANTACIDS aluminium hydroxide and magnesium carbonate. It can be used to relieve acid indigestion and dyspepsia, and is available as tablets. It is not normally given to children under five years, except on medical advice.

+▲ Side-effects/warning: See ALUMINIUM HYDROXIDE; MAGNESIUM CARBONATE.

diloxanide furoate
is an ANTIPROTOZOAL and AMOEBICIDAL drug. It can be used to treat chronic infection of the intestine by amoebae (*Entamoeba histolytica*) that cause amoebic dysentery. Administration is oral.

+ Side-effects: Flatulence; vomiting, pruritus (skin itching) and/or urticaria.

✪ Related entry: Furamide.

diltiazem hydrochloride
is a CALCIUM-CHANNEL BLOCKER which is used as an ANTIHYPERTENSIVE and as an ANTI-ANGINA drug in the prevention of attacks. Administration is oral in the form of tablets and capsules (several in long-acting formulations).

+ Side-effects: Slowing of the heart and altered heart function, hypotension, flushing; fatigue and malaise, headache; depression, swelling of the ankles; gastrointestinal disturbances; rashes; and altered liver function.

▲ Warning: Administer with caution and reduce dose to patients with certain liver, kidney or heart disorders; and with abnormal blood states. It should not be given to patients who are pregnant.

✪ Related entries: Adizem-60; Adizem-SR; Adizem-XL; Adizem-XL Plus; Angiozem; Britiazim; Calcicard CR; Dilzem SR; Dilzem XL; Slozem; Tildiem; Tildiem LA; Tildiem Retard.

Dilzem SR
(Elan) is a proprietary, prescription-only preparation of the CALCIUM-CHANNEL BLOCKER diltiazem hydrochloride. It can be used as an ANTIHYPERTENSIVE and as an ANTI-ANGINA treatment, and is available as modified-release capsules.

+▲ Side-effects/warning: See DILTIAZEM HYDROCHLORIDE.

Dilzem XL
(Elan) is a proprietary, prescription-only preparation of the CALCIUM-CHANNEL BLOCKER diltiazem hydrochloride. It can be used as an ANTIHYPERTENSIVE and as an ANTI-ANGINA treatment, and is available as modified-release capsules.

+▲ Side-effects/warning: See DILTIAZEM HYDROCHLORIDE.

dimenhydrinate
is an ANTIHISTAMINE which is principally used as an ANTINAUSEANT, particularly for treating

nausea and vomiting associated with motion sickness, disorders of the balance function of the inner ear and vertigo. Administration is oral.

✚▲ Side-effects/warning: See CYCLIZINE; ANTIHISTAMINES. It should not be given to patients with porphyria.

○ Related entry: Dramamine.

dimercaprol

(BAL) is a CHELATING AGENT which is used as an ANTIDOTE to poisoning with antimony, arsenic, bismuth, gold, mercury, thallium and (with sodium calciumedetate) lead. Administration is by injection.

✚ Side-effects: Hypertension, increase in heart rate, sweating, malaise, nausea and vomiting, excessive tears, constriction of the throat and chest, burning sensation (eyes and mouth), headache, muscle spasms, pain in the abdomen, tingling in extremities, raised temperature in children, pain and abscess at injection site.

▲ Warning: It should not be given to patients with severe liver impairment; administer with care to those with hypertension.

○ Related entry: Dimercaprol Injection.

Dimercaprol Injection

(Boots) is a proprietary, prescription-only preparation of the CHELATING AGENT dimercaprol. It can be used as an ANTIDOTE to poisoning by a number of toxic metals, and is available in a form for injection.

✚▲ Side-effects/warning: See DIMERCAPROL.

dimethicone

is a water-repellent silicone which is used as an ANTIFOAMING AGENT and, when taken orally, is thought to reduce flatulence while protecting mucous membranes. It is also a constituent in many BARRIER CREAMS that can be used to protect against irritation or chapping (eg nappy rash). *Dimethicone activated* is also known as *simethicone*.

▲ Warning: Do not use topically on acutely inflamed or weeping skin.

○ Related entries: Altacite Plus; Asilone Liquid; Asilone Suspension; Asilone Tablets; Bisodol Extra Tablets; Cobadex; Dentinox Infant Colic Drops; Diovol; Infacol; Kolanticon Gel; Maalox Plus Suspension; Maalox Plus Tablets; Piptalin; Siopel; Sprilon; Vaseline Dermacare; Vasogen Cream; Windcheaters Capsules.

Dimotane Co

(Whitehall) is a proprietary, non-prescription COMPOUND PREPARATION of the ANTITUSSIVE codeine phosphate, the ANTIHISTAMINE brompheniramine maleate and the SYMPATHOMIMETIC and VASOCONSTRICTOR pseudoephedrine hydrochloride. It can be used for the symptomatic relief of coughs associated with colds. It is available as a liquid and is not normally given to children under two years, except on medical advice.

✚▲ Side-effects/warning: See BROMPHENIRAMINE MALEATE; CODEINE PHOSPHATE; PSEUDOEPHEDRINE HYDROCHLORIDE.

Dimotane Co Paediatric

(Whitehall) is a proprietary, non-prescription COMPOUND PREPARATION of the ANTITUSSIVE codeine phosphate, the ANTIHISTAMINE brompheniramine maleate and the SYMPATHOMIMETIC and VASOCONSTRICTOR pseudoephedrine hydrochloride. It can be used for the symptomatic relief of coughs associated with colds and other respiratory disorders in children. It is available as a liquid and is not normally given to children under two years, except on medical advice.

✚▲ Side-effects/warning: See BROMPHENIRAMINE MALEATE; CODEINE PHOSPHATE; PSEUDOEPHEDRINE HYDROCHLORIDE.

Dimotane Expectorant

(Whitehall) is a proprietary, non-prescription COMPOUND PREPARATION of the EXPECTORANT agent GUAIPHENESIN, the ANTIHISTAMINE brompheniramine maleate

D

and the SYMPATHOMIMETIC and DECONGESTANT pseudoephedrine hydrochloride. It can be used for the symptomatic relief of upper respiratory tract disorders, and is available as a liquid. It is not normally given to children under two years, except on medical advice.

✚▲ Side-effects/warning: See BROMPHENIRAMINE MALEATE; PSEUDOEPHEDRINE HYDROCHLORIDE.

Dimotapp Elixir

(Whitehall) is a proprietary, non-prescription COMPOUND PREPARATION of the SYMPATHOMIMETIC and DECONGESTANT drugs phenylpropanolamine hydrochloride and phenylephrine hydrochloride and the ANTIHISTAMINE brompheniramine maleate. It can be used for the relief of upper respiratory tract disorders, including congestion, hypersecretion sinusitis and rhinitis. It is available as an elixir and is not normally given to children under two years, except on medical advice.

✚▲ Side-effects/warning: See BROMPHENIRAMINE MALEATE; PHENYLEPHRINE HYDROCHLORIDE; PHENYLPROPANOLAMINE HYDROCHLORIDE.

Dimotapp Elixir Paediatric

(Whitehall) is a proprietary, non-prescription COMPOUND PREPARATION of the SYMPATHOMIMETIC and DECONGESTANT drugs phenylpropanolamine hydrochloride and phenylephrine hydrochloride and the ANTIHISTAMINE brompheniramine maleate. It can be used for the relief of upper respiratory tract disorders, including congestion, hypersecretion sinusitis and rhinitis. It is available as an elixir and is not normally given to children under two years, except on medical advice.

✚▲ Side-effects/warning: See BROMPHENIRAMINE MALEATE; PHENYLEPHRINE HYDROCHLORIDE; PHENYLPROPANOLAMINE HYDROCHLORIDE.

Dimotapp LA Tablets

(Whitehall) is a proprietary, non-

prescription COMPOUND PREPARATION of the SYMPATHOMIMETIC and DECONGESTANT drugs phenylpropanolamine hydrochloride and phenylephrine hydrochloride and the ANTIHISTAMINE brompheniramine maleate. It can be used for the relief of upper respiratory tract disorders, including congestion, hypersecretion sinusitis and rhinitis. It is available as modified-release tablets and is not normally given to children, except on medical advice.

✚▲ Side-effects/warning: See BROMPHENIRAMINE MALEATE; PHENYLEPHRINE HYDROCHLORIDE; PHENYLPROPANOLAMINE HYDROCHLORIDE.

Dindevan

(Goldshield) is a proprietary, prescription-only preparation of the ANTICOAGULANT phenindione. It can be used to treat and prevent thrombosis, and is available as tablets.

✚▲ Side-effects/warning: See PHENINDIONE.

dinoprost

is the PROSTAGLANDIN $F_{2\alpha}$, which has the effect of causing contractions in the muscular walls of the uterus. It is used almost solely to induce termination of pregnancy (abortion). Administration is by injection, usually into the amniotic sac that surrounds the foetus.

✚▲ Side-effects/warning: See DINOPROSTONE.

❂ Related entry: Prostin F2 alpha.

dinoprostone

is the PROSTAGLANDIN E_2, which has the effect of causing contractions in the muscular walls of the uterus. It can be used to induce labour and as an ABORTIFACIENT. Administration can be oral, topical or by injection.

✚ Side-effects: There may be nausea, vomiting, flushing and shivering, headache and dizziness, a raised temperature and diarrhoea, severe contractions of the uterus and increased white blood cell count. There will be uterine pain.

▲ Warning: When administered by infusion, there may be redness at the injection site. It should be used with caution to those with certain gynaecological or obstetric disorders.

✪ Related entries: Prepidil; Propess-RS; Prostin E2.

Diocalm

(Seton) is a proprietary, non-prescription preparation of the (OPIOID) ANTIDIARRHOEAL morphine (as hydrochloride), along with attapulgite (magnesium aluminium silicate) and activated attapulgite. It can be used for the relief of occasional diarrhoea and its associated pain and discomfort, and is available as tablets.

✚▲ Side-effects/warning: See MORPHINE SULPHATE.

Diocalm Replenisher

(SmithKline Beecham) is a proprietary, non-prescription preparation of sodium chloride, sodium citrate, potassium chloride and glucose. It can be used as an electrolyte replacement in ANTIDIARRHOEAL treatment (usually in conjunction with another preparation that reduces diarrhoea, eg *Diocalm* or *Diocalm Ultra*). It is available as a powder for the relief of occasional diarrhoea and its associated pain and discomfort.

✚▲ Side-effects/warning: See SODIUM CITRATE; SODIUM CHLORIDE.

Diocalm Ultra

(SmithKline Beecham) is a proprietary, non-prescription preparation of the (OPIOID) ANTIDIARRHOEAL loperamide hydrochloride. It can be used for the symptomatic relief of acute diarrhoea and its associated pain and discomfort. It is available as capsules and is not normally given to children, except on medical advice.

✚▲ Side-effects/warning: See LOPERAMIDE HYDROCHLORIDE.

Diocaps

(Berk) is a non-proprietary, prescription-

only preparation of the (OPIOID) ANTIDIARRHOEAL loperamide hydrochloride. It can be used for the symptomatic relief of acute diarrhoea and its associated pain and discomfort, and is available as capsules.

✚▲ Side-effects/warning: See LOPERAMIDE HYDROCHLORIDE.

Dioctyl

(Schwarz) is a proprietary, non-prescription preparation of the (*stimulant*) LAXATIVE docusate sodium. It can be used to relieve constipation and also to evacuate the rectum prior to abdominal procedures. It is available as capsules and a syrup (in two strengths, the weaker one is a *Paediatric Oral Solution*).

✚▲ Side-effects/warning: See DOCUSATE SODIUM.

dioctyl sodium sulphosuccinate

see DOCUSATE SODIUM

Dioderm

(Dermal) is a proprietary, prescription-only preparation of the CORTICOSTEROID and ANTI-INFLAMMATORY hydrocortisone. It can be used to treat mild, inflammatory skin conditions, such as eczema, and is available as a cream for topical application.

✚▲ Side-effects/warning: See HYDROCORTISONE.

Dioralyte

(Rhône-Poulenc Rorer) is a proprietary, non-prescription, preparation of sodium chloride, sodium bicarbonate, potassium chloride, citric acid and glucose. It can be used as an electrolyte and water replacement in dehydration or kidney disease, and is available as soluble tablets and an oral powder.

✚▲ Side-effects/warning: See SODIUM CHLORIDE.

Diovan

(Ciba) is a proprietary prescription-only preparation of the ANGIOTENSIN-RECEPTOR

D

BLOCKER valsartan. It can be used as an ANTIHYPERTENSIVE, and is available as capsules.
+▲ Side-effects/warning: See LOSARTAN POTASSIUM.

Diovol

(Pharmax) is a proprietary, non-prescription COMPOUND PREPARATION of the ANTACIDS aluminium hydroxide and magnesium hydroxide and the ANTIFOAMING AGENT dimethicone. It can be used for the symptomatic relief of hyperacidity, hiatus hernia, flatulence and peptic ulcers. It is available as a liquid and is not normally given to children, except on medical advice.
+▲ Side-effects/warning: See ALUMINIUM HYDROXIDE; DIMETHICONE; MAGNESIUM HYDROXIDE.

Dip/Ser

is an abbreviation for DIPHTHERIA ANTITOXIN.

Dipentum

(Pharmacia) is a proprietary, prescription-only preparation of the AMINOSALICYLATE olsalazine sodium. It can be used to treat patients who suffer from ulcerative colitis, and is available as tablets and capsules.
+▲ Side-effects/warning: See OLSALAZINE SODIUM.

diphenhydramine hydrochloride

is an ANTIHISTAMINE which can be used for the symptomatic relief of allergic symptoms, such as hay fever and urticaria, and is incorporated into a number of proprietary cough and cold preparations. It has marked SEDATIVE properties and can be used for the relief of occasional insomnia. It is administered in several ways, including orally.
+▲ Side-effects/warning: See ANTIHISTAMINES. Because of its sedative side-effects, the performance of skilled tasks, such as driving, may be impaired.
✪ Related entries: Benylin Chesty Coughs Original; Benylin Children's Coughs Original;

Benylin Children's Coughs Sugar Free/Colour Free; Benylin Cough and Congestion; Benylin Day and Night; Benylin Dry Coughs Original; Benylin Four Flu Liquid; Benylin Four Flu Tablets; Benylin with Codeine; Bronalin Expectorant Linctus; Bronalin Junior Linctus; Caladryl Cream; Caladryl Lotion; Night Cold Comfort Capsules; Nytol; Nytol One-a-Night; Propain Tablets; Tixylix Catarrh Syrup.

diphenoxylate hydrochloride

is an (OPIOID) ANTIDIARRHOEAL drug which is used to treat chronic diarrhoea. It is commonly used in combination with atropine sulphate to form a preparation known as co-phenotrope.
+ Side-effects: See CODEINE PHOSPHATE; overdosage causes sedation. Prolonged use may lead to impaired gastrointestinal function and eventual dependence.
▲ Warning: Overdosage is uncommon but does occur, particularly in young children. However, the symptoms of overdose (chiefly sedation) do not appear until some 48 hours after treatment, so monitoring of patients for at least this period is necessary. Fluid intake must be maintained during treatment. In elderly patients, monitoring is essential to detect possible faecal impaction. The drug should not be used in patients with gastrointestinal obstruction or jaundice. Care should be taken in patients with severe ulcerative colitis.
✪ Related entries: Diarphen; Lomotil.

diphenylpyraline hydrochloride

is an ANTIHISTAMINE which is used for the symptomatic relief of allergy, such as hay fever and urticaria. It is also incorporated into some proprietary cold treatment preparations. Administration is oral.
+▲ Side-effects/warning: See ANTIHISTAMINES. Because of its sedative side-effects, the performance of skilled tasks, such as driving, may be impaired.
✪ Related entry: Eskornade Capsules.

D

diphosphonates
see bisphosphonates

diphtheria antitoxin
(Dip/Ser) is a preparation that neutralizes the toxins which are produced by diphtheria bacteria (*Corynebacerium diphtheriae*), because of IMMUNIZATION it is not used for prevention but only to provide *passive immunity* to those who have been exposed to people suspected of having diphtheria. Because the antitoxin is produced in horses, hypersensitivity reactions are common. Administration is by injection.
+▲ Side-effects/warning: See IMMUNIZATION.
✪ Related entry: Diphtheria Antitoxin.

Diphtheria Antitoxin
(Mérieux) is a proprietary, prescription-only preparation of diphtheria antitoxin. It can be used to treat suspected cases of diphtheria, and is available in a form for injection.
+▲ Side-effects/warning: See IMMUNIZATION.

diphtheria vaccines
for IMMUNIZATION are VACCINE preparations of inactivated, but still antigenic, toxins (toxoid) of the diphtheria bacteria *Corynebacterium diphtheriae* that provide active immunity to diphtheria. In most instances, they are not administered alone but as a constituent in the *triple vaccine* ADSORBED DIPHTHERIA, TETANUS AND PERTUSSIS VACCINE (DTPer/Vac/Ads), or as a *double vaccine* ADSORBED DIPHTHERIA AND TETANUS VACCINE (DT/Vac/Ads). Diphtheria vaccines are used for the primary immunization of children. Administration is by injection.
+▲ Side-effects/warning: See VACCINES.
✪ Related entries: Adsorbed Diphtheria Vaccine; Adsorbed Diphtheria and Tetanus Vaccine for Adults and Adolescents; Adsorbed Diphtheria Vaccine for Adults; Diftavax; Trivac-AD.

dipipanone
is a rapidly acting and powerful (OPIOID) NARCOTIC ANALGESIC. It is used in combination with an ANTI-EMETIC (the antihistamine cyclizine) for the relief of acute, moderate and severe pain. Its proprietary form is on the Controlled Drugs List. Administration (in the form of dipipanone hydrochloride) is oral.
+▲ Side-effects/warning: See OPIOIDS. It is less sedating than morphine, but in combination with an anti-emetic it is unsuitable for use in chronic pain therapy.
✪ Related entry: Diconal.

dipivefrine hydrochloride
is a derivative of the SYMPATHOMIMETIC adrenaline and is converted in the body to adrenaline. It is often used in GLAUCOMA TREATMENT to reduce intraocular pressure (pressure in the eyeball) and is administered instead of adrenaline because it is thought to pass more rapidly through the cornea. Administration is topical.
+▲ Side-effects/warning: See ADRENALINE.
✪ Related entry: Propine.

dipotassium clorazepate
see CLORAZEPATE DIPOTASSIUM

Diprivan
(Zeneca) is a proprietary, prescription-only preparation of the GENERAL ANAESTHETIC propofol. It can be used for the induction and maintenance of anaesthesia, and is available in a form for injection or infusion.
+▲ Side-effects/warning: See PROPOFOL.

Diprobase
(Schering-Plough) is a proprietary, non-prescription preparation of liquid paraffin (and other paraffins). It can be used as an EMOLLIENT, and is available as an ointment and a cream.
+▲ Side-effects/warning: See LIQUID PARAFFIN.

Diprobath
(Schering-Plough) is a proprietary, non-

D

prescription preparation of liquid paraffin (and isopropyl myristate). It can be used as an EMOLLIENT for dry skin, and is available as a bath oil.

+▲ Side-effects/warning: See LIQUID PARAFFIN.

Diprosalic

(Schering-Plough) is a proprietary, prescription-only COMPOUND PREPARATION of the CORTICOSTEROID and ANTI-INFLAMMATORY betamethasone (as dipropionate) and the KERATOLYTIC salicylic acid. It can be used to treat severe inflammatory skin disorders, such as eczema and psoriasis. It is available as an ointment and a scalp lotion for topical application.

+▲ Side-effects/warning: See BETAMETHASONE; SALICYLIC ACID.

Diprosone

(Schering-Plough) is a proprietary, prescription-only preparation of the CORTICOSTEROID and ANTI-INFLAMMATORY betamethasone (as dipropionate). It can be used to treat severe inflammatory skin disorders, such as eczema and psoriasis. It is available as a cream, an ointment and a lotion for topical application.

+▲ Side-effects/warning: See BETAMETHASONE.

dipyridamole

is an ANTIPLATELET (antithrombotic) drug which is used to prevent thrombosis (blood-clot formation), but does not have an ANTICOAGULANT action. It seems to work by stopping platelets sticking to one another or to surgically inserted tubes and valves (particularly artificial heart valves). Administration is either oral or by injection.

+ Side-effects: There may be nausea and diarrhoea, headache and low blood pressure.

▲ Warning: It may cause hypotension or worsen migraine. There may be dangerous interactions with adenosine (which is used in heart conditions as an anti-arrhythmic). Administer with caution to patients with

certain heart disorders.

✪ Related entry: Persantin.

Dirythmin SA

(Astra) is a proprietary, prescription-only preparation of the ANTI-ARRHYTHMIC disopyramide (as disopyramide phosphate), and is available as modified-release tablets (*Durules*).

+▲ Side-effects/warning: See DISOPYRAMIDE.

disinfectants ▨

are agents used to destroy micro-organisms, or inhibit their activity to such extent that they are less or no longer harmful to health. It can be applied to agents used on inanimate objects (including surgical equipment, catheters, etc.) as well as to preparations that are used to treat the skin and living tissue (although in the latter case the name ANTISEPTIC is often used instead).

Disipal

(Yamanouchi) is a proprietary, prescription-only preparation of the ANTICHOLINERGIC orphenadrine hydrochloride. It can be used to relieve some of the symptoms of parkinsonism, especially muscle rigidity and the tendency to produce an excess of saliva (see ANTIPARKINSONISM). It also has the capacity to treat these conditions, in some cases, where they are produced by drugs. It is available as tablets.

+▲ Side-effects/warning: See ORPHENADRINE HYDROCHLORIDE.

disodium etidronate

(a biphosphonate) is a CALCIUM METABOLISM MODIFIER used to treat disorders of bone metabolism due to HORMONE disorders, tumour-induced high blood calcium levels (hypercalcaemia) and specifically to treat Paget's disease of the bone. It is also available in a COMPOUND PREPARATION with calcium carbonate to treat established osteoporosis of the vertebrae.

Administration is either oral or by injection.

✚ Side-effects: There may be nausea and diarrhoea. With high dosage, increased bone pain and the risk of fractures. Rarely, a short-lived loss of the sense of taste, skin reactions, abdominal pain and constipation.

▲ Warning: Administer with caution to patients with certain kidney disorders. It is not for use in pregnancy or breast-feeding.

○ Related entries: Didronel; Didronel PMO.

disodium pamidronate

(a biphosphonate) is a CALCIUM METABOLISM MODIFIER used to treat disorders of bone metabolism due to HORMONE disorders and malignant tumour-induced high blood calcium levels (hypercalcaemia). Administration is by injection.

✚ Side-effects: There may be nausea and diarrhoea, low blood calcium, blood upsets and transient fever.

▲ Warning: Administer with caution to patients with certain kidney disorders. It is not for use in pregnancy or breast-feeding.

○ Related entry: Aredia.

disopyramide

is an ANTI-ARRHYTHMIC drug which is used to regularize the heartbeat, especially following a heart attack (myocardial infarction). Administration, as disopyramide or disopyramide phosphate, is oral or by slow intravenous injection.

✚ Side-effects: There may be hypotension, gastrointestinal disturbances, dry mouth, blurred vision, urinary retention and effects on the heart.

▲ Warning: It should be administered with caution to patients with depressed heart function (eg heart failure), certain kidney or liver disorders, glaucoma or who are pregnant or breast-feeding. It should not be given to patients with certain heart disorders.

○ Related entries: Dirythmin SA; Isomide CR; Rythmodan; Rythmodan Retard.

Disprin

(Reckitt & Colman) is a proprietary, non-prescription preparation of the (NSAID) NON-NARCOTIC ANALGESIC and ANTIRHEUMATIC aspirin. It can be used to treat mild to moderate pain and to relieve flu and cold symptoms, rheumatism and lumbago. It is available as soluble tablets and is not normally given to children under 12 years, except on medical advice.

✚▲ Side-effects/warning: See ASPIRIN.

Disprin CV

(Reckitt & Colman) is a proprietary, non-prescription preparation of the ANTIPLATELET aggregation drug aspirin. It can be used to help prevent certain cardiovascular diseases, including heart attack.

✚▲ Side-effects/warning: See ASPIRIN.

Disprin Direct

(Reckitt & Colman) is a proprietary, non-prescription preparation of the (NSAID) NON-NARCOTIC ANALGESIC and ANTIRHEUMATIC aspirin. It can be used to treat mild to moderate pain, to relieve flu and cold symptoms and feverishness. It is available as chewable tablets and is not normally given to children under 12 years, except on medical advice.

✚▲ Side-effects/warning: See ASPIRIN.

Disprin Extra

(Reckitt & Colman) is a proprietary, non-prescription COMPOUND ANALGESIC preparation of the (NSAID) NON-NARCOTIC ANALGESIC and ANTIRHEUMATIC aspirin and the non-narcotic analgesic paracetamol. It can be used to treat mild to moderate pain, relieve rheumatic aches and pains and flu and cold symptoms. It is available as tablets and is not normally given to children under 12 years, except on medical advice.

✚▲ Side-effects/warning: See ASPIRIN; PARACETAMOL.

Disprol

(Reckitt & Colman) is a proprietary, non-prescription preparation of the NON-NARCOTIC ANALGESIC paracetamol. It can be used to treat mild to moderate pain, relieve

D

flu and cold symptoms, feverishness and rheumatic aches and pains. It is available as tablets and is not normally given to children under six years, except on medical advice.
✚▲ Side-effects/warning: See PARACETAMOL.

Disprol Junior

(Reckitt & Colman) is a proprietary, non-prescription preparation of the NON-NARCOTIC ANALGESIC and ANTIPYRETIC paracetamol (for children). It can be used to treat mild to moderate pain (including teething), relieve flu and cold symptoms, feverishness and to reduce high body temperature. It is available as effervescent tablets. Even as a paediatric preparation, however, it is not normally given to infants under three months, except on medical advice.
✚▲ Side-effects/warning: See PARACETAMOL.

Disprol Paracetamol Suspension

(Reckitt & Colman) is a proprietary, non-prescription preparation of the NON-NARCOTIC ANALGESIC and ANTIPYRETIC paracetamol. It can be used to treat mild to moderate pain, including period pain, teething and to reduce high body temperature. It is available as a sugar-free suspension and is not normally given to infants under three months, except on medical advice.
✚▲ Side-effects/warning: See PARACETAMOL.

Distaclor

(Dista) is a proprietary, prescription-only preparation of the ANTIBACTERIAL and (CEPHALOSPORIN) ANTIBIOTIC cefaclor (as monohydrate). It can be used to treat a wide range of bacterial infections, particularly of the urinary tract. It is available as capsules and an oral suspension.
✚▲ Side-effects/warning: See CEFACLOR.

Distaclor MR

(Lilly) is a proprietary, prescription-only preparation of the ANTIBACTERIAL and (CEPHALOSPORIN) ANTIBIOTIC cefaclor (as monohydrate). It can be used to treat a wide range of bacterial infections, particularly of the urinary tract, and is available as tablets.
✚▲ Side-effects/warning: See CEFACLOR.

Distalgesic

(Dista) is a proprietary, prescription-only COMPOUND ANALGESIC preparation of the (OPIOID) NARCOTIC ANALGESIC dextropropoxyphene hydrochloride and the NON-NARCOTIC ANALGESIC paracetamol (a combination known as CO-PRAXAMOL). It can be used to relieve pain, and is available as tablets. It is not not normally given to children, except on medical advice.
✚▲ Side-effects/warning: See DEXTROPROPOXYPHENE HYDROCHLORIDE; PARACETAMOL.

Distamine

(Dista) is a proprietary, prescription-only preparation of the CHELATING AGENT penicillamine. It can be used as an ANTIDOTE to copper or lead poisoning, to reduce copper levels in Wilson's disease and in the long-term treatment of rheumatoid arthritis. It is available as tablets.
✚▲ Side-effects/warning: See PENICILLAMINE.

distigmine bromide

is an ANTICHOLINESTERASE drug which enhances the effects of the NEUROTRANSMITTER acetylcholine (and certain cholinergic drugs). Because of this, it has PARASYMPATHOMIMETIC actions and can be used to stimulate the bladder to treat urinary retention and the intestine to treat paralytic ileus. It can also be used to treat the neuromuscular transmission disorder myasthenia gravis. Administration is oral.
✚ Side-effects: There may be nausea and vomiting, sweating and blurred vision, slow heart rate and colic.
▲ Warning: It should not be administered to patients who suffer from urinary or intestinal blockage, or where increased

activity of the intestine or bladder could be harmful. It should be administered with caution to patients with asthma, hyperthyroidism, parkinsonism, epilepsy, peptic ulcer, who have recently had a heart attack or are pregnant.
✪ Related entry: Ubretid.

disulfiram

is an ENZYME INHIBITOR, which blocks a stage in the break down of alcohol (ethanol) in the body with a resultant accumulation in a metabolite (acetaldehyde). If even only a very small amount of alcohol is taken, disulfiram causes very unpleasant, potentially dangerous, reactions – such as flushing, headache, palpitations, nausea and vomiting. Therefore, if an alcoholic takes disulfiram on a regular basis there is a powerful disincentive to drink alcoholic beverages. Administration is oral.
✚ Side-effects: Initial drowsiness and fatigue; nausea and vomiting; halitosis, reduced libido; rarely, there may be psychotic reactions, skin reactions, peripheral nerve and liver damage.
▲ Warning: It should not be administered to patients with certain heart disorders or who are pregnant. Simultaneous use of medications or toiletries containing forms of alcohol should also be avoided.
✪ Related entry: Antabuse 200.

dithranol

is the most powerful drug presently used to treat chronic or milder forms of psoriasis in topical application and is incorporated in a number of preparations. Lesions are covered for a period with a dressing on which there is a preparation of dithranol in weak solution; the concentration is adjusted to suit individual response and tolerance of the associated skin irritation. It is thought to work by inhibiting cell division (antimitotic) and may be used in combination with KERATOLYTICS or with agents that have a moisturizing effect (such as UREA). It may also be used in some preparations as dithranol triacetate.

✚ Side-effects: Irritation and a local sensation of burning.
▲ Warning: It is not suitable for the treatment of acute forms of psoriasis. It stains skin, hair and fabrics. Avoid contact with healthy skin and the eyes.
✪ Related entries: Anthranol; Dithranol Ointment, BP; Dithrocream; Dithrolan; Micanol; Psorin.

Dithranol Ointment, BP

is a non-proprietary, prescription-only preparation of dithranol. It can be used for subacute and chronic psoriasis, and is available as an ointment.
✚▲ Side-effects/warning: See DITHRANOL.

dithranol triacetate

see DITHRANOL

Dithrocream

(Dermal) is a proprietary, non-prescription preparation of dithranol. It can be used to treat subacute and chronic psoriasis, and is available as an ointment in four strengths: 0.1% , 0.25%, 0.5% and 1%. A stronger version, 2%, is available only on prescription.
✚▲ Side-effects/warning: See DITHRANOL.

Dithrolan

(Dermal) is a proprietary, non-prescription COMPOUND PREPARATION of dithranol and salicylic acid. It can be used for subacute and chronic psoriasis, and is available as an ointment.
✚▲ Side-effects/warning: See DITHRANOL; SALICYLIC ACID.

Ditropan

(Smith & Nephew) is a proprietary, prescription-only preparation of the ANTICHOLINERGIC oxybutynin hydrochloride. It can be used as an ANTISPASMODIC in the treatment of urinary frequency and incontinence, and is available as tablets and an elixir.
✚▲ Side-effects/warning: See OXYBUTYNIN HYDROCHLORIDE.

D

Diumide-K Continus

(ASTA Medica) is a proprietary, prescription-only COMPOUND PREPARATION of the (*loop*) DIURETIC frusemide and the potassium supplement POTASSIUM CHLORIDE. It can be used to treat oedema, and is available as tablets, which should be swallowed whole with plenty of fluid at mealtimes or when in an upright posture.

+▲ Side-effects/warning: See FRUSEMIDE.

diuretics ▣

are drugs used to reduce fluid in the body by increasing the excretion of water and mineral salts by the kidney, so increasing urine production (hence 'water tablets'). They have a wide range of uses, because oedema in sites such as the lungs, ankles and eyeball is symptomatic of a number of disorders. Reducing oedema is, in itself, of benefit in some of these disorders; and diuretic drugs may be used in acute pulmonary (lung) oedema, congestive heart failure, some liver and kidney disorders, glaucoma and in certain electrolyte disturbances such as hypercalcaemia (raised calcium levels) and hyperkalaemia (raised potassium levels). Their most common use is as ANTIHYPERTENSIVES, where their action of reducing oedema is of value in relieving the load on the heart, which then (over some days or weeks) gives way to a beneficial reduction in blood pressure (which seems to be associated with VASODILATOR action).

In relation to their specific actions and uses, the diuretics are divided into a number of distinct classes. *Osmotic diuretics* (eg MANNITOL) are inert compounds secreted into the kidney proximal tubules and are not resorbed and therefore carry water and salts with them into the urine. *Loop diuretics* (eg ETHACRYNIC ACID, FRUSEMIDE and BUMETANIDE) have a very vigorous action on the ascending tubules of the loop of Henlé (inhibiting resorption of sodium and water and also some potassium) and are used for short periods, especially in heart failure.

Thiazide and *thiazide-like* diuretics (eg CHLOROTHIAZIDE, HYDROCHLOROTHIAZIDE and XIPAMIDE) are the most commonly used and have a moderate action in inhibiting sodium reabsorption at the distal tubule of the kidney, allowing their prolonged use as antihypertensives. But they may cause potassium loss from the blood to the urine, which needs correction (sometimes through using preparations that combine the diuretic and a potassium salt in tablets). *Potassium-sparing* diuretics (eg AMILORIDE HYDROCHLORIDE, TRIAMTERENE and SPIRONOLACTONE) have a weak action on the distal tubule of the kidney and – as the name suggests – cause retention of potassium, making them suitable for combination with some of the other diuretic classes and for some specific conditions. *Aldosterone antagonists* (eg POTASSIUM CANRENOATE and spironolactone) work by blocking the action of the normal mineralocorticoid hormone aldosterone, and this makes them suitable for treating oedema associated with aldosteronism, liver failure and certain heart conditions. *Carbonic anhydrase inhibitors* (eg ACETAZOLAMIDE) are weak diuretics and are now rarely used to treat systemic oedema, though they are useful in reducing fluid in the anterior chamber of the eye which causes glaucoma. In the treatment of hypertension, diuretics are commonly used in combination with other classes of drugs, particularly BETA-BLOCKERS.

Diurexan

(ASTA Medica) is a proprietary, prescription-only preparation of the (THIAZIDE-like) DIURETIC xipamide. It can be used, either alone or in conjunction with other drugs, in the treatment of oedema and as an ANTIHYPERTENSIVE. It is available as tablets.

+▲ Side-effects/warning: See XIPAMIDE.

Dixarit

(Boehringer Ingelheim) is a proprietary, prescription-only preparation of the

ANTISYMPATHETIC clonidine hydrochloride. It can be used in ANTIMIGRAINE treatment for reducing the frequency of attacks, and is available as tablets.

✚▲ Side-effects/warning: See CLONIDINE HYDROCHLORIDE.

Do-Do Chesteze

(Zyma) is a proprietary, non-prescription COMPOUND PREPARATION of the SYMPATHOMIMETIC and DECONGESTANT ephedrine hydrochloride, the BRONCHODILATOR theophylline (anhydrous) and the STIMULANT caffeine. It can be used for the relief of bronchial cough, wheezing and breathlessness and to help clear the chest after infections. It is available as tablets and is not normally given to children under 12 years, except on medical advice.

✚▲ Side-effects/warning: See CAFFEINE; EPHEDRINE HYDROCHLORIDE; THEOPHYLLINE.

Do-Do Expectorant Linctus

(Zyma) is a proprietary, non-prescription preparation of the EXPECTORANT agent GUAIPHENESIN. It can be used for the relief of productive and non-productive cough associated with irritation due to infection of the upper airways. It is not normally given to children under six years, except on medical advice.

Doan's Backache Pills

(Zyma) is a proprietary, non-prescription COMPOUND ANALGESIC preparation of the (NSAID) NON-NARCOTIC ANALGESIC and ANTIRHEUMATIC paracetamol and the non-narcotic analgesic sodium salicylate. It can be used for the symptomatic relief of rheumatic aches and pains, including lumbago, backache, sprains and other muscle pains, and is available as tablets.

✚▲ Side-effects/warning: See PARACETAMOL; SODIUM SALICYLATE.

dobutamine hydrochloride

is a CARDIAC STIMULANT with SYMPATHOMIMETIC and BETA-RECEPTOR STIMULANT properties. It is used to treat serious heart disorders,

including cardiogenic shock, septic shock, during heart surgery and in cardiac infarction. It works by increasing the heart's force of contraction. Administration is by intravenous infusion.

✚ Side-effects: The heart rate following treatment may increase too much and result in hypertension.

▲ Warning: Administer with caution to patients with severe hypotension (low blood pressure).

✪ Related entries: Dobutrex; Posiject.

Dobutrex

(Lilly) is a proprietary, prescription-only preparation of the CARDIAC STIMULANT dobutamine hydrochloride, which has SYMPATHOMIMETIC and BETA-RECEPTOR STIMULANT properties. It can be used to treat serious heart disorders, including cardiogenic shock, septic shock, during heart surgery and in cardiac infarction. It works by increasing the heart's force of contraction. It is available in a form for intravenous infusion.

✚▲ Side-effects/warning: See DOBUTAMINE HYDROCHLORIDE.

docetaxel

is a CYTOTOXIC drug, the first of a new group of drugs termed the *taxanes*, which is used as an ANTICANCER treatment of (anthracycline-resistant) breast cancer. Administration is by intravenous infusion.

✚▲ Side-effects/warning: See CYTOTOXICS.

✪ Related entry: Taxotere.

docusate sodium

(dioctyl sodium sulphosuccinate) is a LAXATIVE with both *stimulant* and *faecal softener* properties. It is used to relieve constipation and also to evacuate the rectum prior to abdominal X-rays. It is a constituent of many proprietary compound laxatives because it seems to have few adverse side-effects. It works like a surfactant, by applying a very thin film of low surface tension (similar to a detergent) over the surface of the intestinal wall. It can

D

also be used to dissolve and remove earwax and is a constituent of proprietary ear-drop preparations. Administration is either oral or topical.

✚ Side-effects: It may cause abdominal cramps.

▲ Warning: Rectal preparations should not be used in patients with haemorrhoids or an anal fissure.

✪ Related entries: co-danthrusate 50/60; Correctol; Dioctyl; Fletchers' Enemette; Molcer; Norgalex Micro-enema; Normax; Waxsol Ear Drops.

Dolmatil

(Delandale) is a proprietary, prescription-only preparation of the ANTIPSYCHOTIC sulpiride. It can be used to treat schizophrenia and also other conditions that may cause tremor, tics, involuntary movements or utterances (such as in Gilles de la Tourette syndrome). It is available as tablets.

✚▲ Side-effects/warning: See SULPIRIDE.

Dolobid

(Morson) is a proprietary, prescription-only preparation of the (NSAID) NON-NARCOTIC ANALGESIC and ANTIRHEUMATIC drug diflunisal. It can be used to treat various types of moderate to mild pain, in particular the pain of rheumatic disease and other musculoskeletal disorders and also period pain. It is available as tablets and is not normally given to children, except on medical advice.

✚▲ Side-effects/warning: See DIFLUNISAL.

Doloxene

(Lilly) is a proprietary, prescription-only preparation of the (OPIOID) NARCOTIC ANALGESIC dextropropoxyphene hydrochloride. It can be used to treat mild to moderate pain anywhere in the body, and is available as capsules. It is not normally given to children, except on medical advice.

✚▲ Side-effects/warning: See DEXTROPROPOXYPHENE HYDROCHLORIDE.

Doloxene Compound

(Lilly) is a proprietary, prescription-only COMPOUND ANALGESIC preparation of the (NSAID) NON-NARCOTIC ANALGESIC and ANTIRHEUMATIC aspirin, the (OPIOID) NARCOTIC ANALGESIC dextropropoxyphene (as napsylate) and the STIMULANT caffeine. It can be used to treat mild to moderate pain, and is available as capsules.

✚▲ Side-effects/warning: See ASPIRIN; CAFFEINE; DEXTROPROPOXYPHENE HYDROCHLORIDE.

Domical

(Berk) is a proprietary, prescription-only preparation of the (TRICYCLIC) ANTIDEPRESSANT amitriptyline hydrochloride. It can be used to treat depressive illness, especially in cases where some degree of sedation is required, and also bed-wetting by children at night. It is available as tablets.

✚▲ Side-effects/warning: See AMITRIPTYLINE HYDROCHLORIDE.

domiphen bromide

is an ANTISEPTIC which is used in throat lozenges.

✪ Related entry: Bradosol Plus.

domperidone

is an ANTI-EMETIC and ANTINAUSEANT which is thought to work, in part, as a DOPAMINE antagonist, and is used particularly for the relief of nausea and vomiting in patients undergoing treatment with CYTOTOXIC drugs. It is also used to prevent vomiting in patients treated for parkinsonism with the drugs levodopa or bromocriptine. Administration is either oral or topical.

✚ Side-effects: Occasionally, spontaneous lactation in women or the development of feminine breasts in men may occur; rashes and changes in libido.

▲ Warning: It should be administered with caution to those who suffer from impaired kidney function, or who are pregnant or breast-feeding.

✪ Related entry: Motilium.

Dopacard

(Porton) is a proprietary, prescription-only preparation of the CARDIAC STIMULANT and SYMPATHOMIMETIC dopexamine hydrochloride. It can be used for the treatment of heart conditions where moderate stimulation of the force of heartbeat with vasodilatation is required in heart failure associated with heart surgery. It is available in a form for intravenous infusion.

✚▲ Side-effects/warning: See DOPEXAMINE HYDROCHLORIDE.

Dopamet

(Berk) is a proprietary, prescription-only preparation of the ANTISYMPATHETIC methyldopa. It can be used as an ANTIHYPERTENSIVE, and is available as tablets.

✚▲ Side-effects/warning: See METHYLDOPA.

dopamine

is a NEUROTRANSMITTER and is chemically a catecholamine (like ADRENALINE and NORADRENALINE). It is both an intermediate product in the biosynthetic pathway in the brain and sympathetic nervous system that manufactures and stores noradrenaline and adrenaline, and a neurotransmitter in its own right in relaying nerve messages. It is particularly concentrated in the brain and in the adrenal glands. It is quite possible that certain psychoses may, in some way, be caused by abnormalities in the metabolism of dopamine, because drugs that prevent some of its actions (dopamine-receptor antagonists; eg CHLORPROMAZINE HYDROCHLORIDE, HALOPERIDOL, PIMOZIDE) can be administered as ANTIPSYCHOTICS to relieve some schizophrenic symptoms. Conversely, drugs that lead to increased dopamine production or concentrations in the brain (for example, LEVODOPA) play an important part in the therapy of parkinsonism and drugs that mimic some aspects of the action of dopamine in the brain (for example, BROMOCRIPTINE) can be used both for ANTIPARKINSONISM treatment and to relieve a number of hormone

disorders. In the periphery (that is, in the body rather than the brain), dopamine hydrochloride may be administered therapeutically as a CARDIAC STIMULANT in the treatment of the cardiogenic shock associated with a heart attack or heart surgery, when its beneficial actions are thought to result partly through actions at beta-receptors in the heart and partly at dopamine receptors in blood vessels. Administration of dopamine is by injection or infusion.

✚ Side-effects: There may be nausea and vomiting, changes in heart rate and blood pressure, the fingertips and toes may become cold due to constriction of blood vessels.

▲ Warning: Dopamine hydrochloride should not be administered to patients who suffer from phaeochromocytoma or heartbeat irregularities.

⊙ Related entries: Dopamine Hydrochloride in Dextrose (Glucose) Injection; Intropin; Select-A-Jet Dopamine.

dopamine hydrochloride

is the chemical form of the naturally occurring DOPAMINE that is used in medicine.

Dopamine Hydrochloride in Dextrose (Glucose) Injection

(Abbott) is a proprietary, prescription-only preparation of the SYMPATHOMIMETIC and CARDIAC STIMULANT dopamine (as dopamine hydrochloride). It is used to treat cardiogenic shock following a heart attack or during heart surgery, and is available in a form for infusion.

✚▲ Side-effects/warning: See DOPAMINE.

dopexamine hydrochloride

is a SYMPATHOMIMETIC and CARDIAC STIMULANT drug which is used for the treatment of heart conditions where moderate stimulation of the force of heartbeat with vasodilatation is required in heart failure associated with heart surgery. Its beneficial

D

actions are thought partly to result from stimulation of beta-receptors in the heart and partly of dopamine receptors in the kidney. It is available in a form for intravenous infusion.

✚ Side-effects: There may be stimulation of the rate of heartbeat, irregular heartbeats; also, angina pain, nausea, vomiting and muscle tremor.

▲ Warning: It should not be used in patients with certain heart outlet obstructions (eg aortic stenosis), with low blood platelet counts and with certain endocrine disorders (phaeochromocytoma). Administer with care to those with myocardial infarction and recent angina, who have low blood potassium or are hyperglycaemic. Various blood parameters should be monitored (eg blood pressure, potassium and glucose levels and pulse). Withdrawal of treatment should be gradual.
○ Related entry: Dopacard.

Dopram

(Wyeth) is a proprietary, prescription-only preparation of the respiratory stimulant doxapram hydrochloride. It can be used to relieve severe respiratory difficulties in patients with chronic obstructive airways disease or who undergo respiratory depression following major surgery, particularly where ventilatory support is not possible. It is available in a form for intravnous infusion or injection.

✚▲ Side-effects/warning: See DOXAPRAM HYDROCHLORIDE.

Doralese

(Bencard) is a proprietary, prescription-only preparation of the ALPHA-ADRENOCEPTOR BLOCKER indoramin. It can be used to treat urinary retention, for example, in benign prostatic hyperplasia, and is available as tablets.

✚▲ Side-effects/warning: See INDORAMIN.

Dormonoct

(Roussel) is a proprietary, prescription-only preparation of the BENZODIAZEPINE

flurazepam. It can be used as a relatively long-acting HYPNOTIC for the short-term treatment of insomnia, where a degree of sedation during the daytime is acceptable. It is available as capsules.

✚▲ Side-effects/warning: See FLURAZEPAM.

dorzolamide

is a CARBONIC ANHYDRASE INHIBITOR which is used in GLAUCOMA TREATMENT because it reduces the formation of aqueous humour in the eye. It can be used in patients resistant to beta-blockers or those in whom beta-blockers are contraindicated. Administration is topical.

✚ Side-effects: Blurred vision, stinging, burning and itching of the eye, tear formation; eyelid inflammation and conjunctivitis; headache and nausea; rarely rash and certain other disorders reported; bitter taste from drug travelling down the lacrimal duct.

▲ Warning: It should not be administered to patients who are pregnant or breast-feeding. There may be systemic absorption after using as eye-drops. It should not be used in liver or severe kidney impairment, or in certain disorders where there is raised levels of chloride in the blood. Administer with care to those with liver impairment.
○ Related entry: Trusopt.

Dostinex

(Farmitalia Carlo Erba) is a proprietary, prescription-only preparation of cabergoline. It is used primarily to treat parkinsonism, but not the parkinsonian symptoms caused by certain drug therapies (see ANTIPARKINSONISM), and may also be used to treat a number of other hormonal disorders. It is available as tablets and capsules.

✚▲ Side-effects/warning: See CABERGOLINE.

Dothapax

(Ashbourne) is a proprietary, prescription-only preparation of the (TRICYCLIC) ANTIDEPRESSANT dothiepin hydrochloride. It can be used to treat depressive illness,

especially in cases where some degree of sedation is considered appropriate, and is available as tablets and capsules.
+▲ Side-effects/warning: See DOTHIEPIN HYDROCHLORIDE.

dothiepin hydrochloride

is an ANTIDEPRESSANT of the TRICYCLIC group. It can be used to treat depressive illness, especially in cases where some degree of sedation is considered appropriate. Administration is oral.
+▲ Side-effects/warning: See AMITRIPTYLINE HYDROCHLORIDE.
○ Related entries: Dothapax; Prepadine; Prothiaden.

Double Check

(FP) is a proprietary, non-prescription SPERMICIDAL CONTRACEPTIVE, which is used in combination with barrier methods of contraception (for example, a condom). It is available as pessaries containing nonoxinol.
+▲ Side-effects/warning: See NONOXINOL.

Dovonex

(Leo) is a proprietary, prescription-only preparation of calcipotriol. It can be used for psoriasis, and is available as an ointment, a cream and a scalp solution.
+▲ Side-effects/warning: See CALCIPOTRIOL.

doxapram hydrochloride

is a RESPIRATORY STIMULANT which is used to relieve severe respiratory difficulties in patients who suffer from chronic obstructive airways disease, or who undergo respiratory depression following major surgery, particularly in cases where ventilatory support is not possible. Administration is by injection or intravenous infusion.
+ Side-effects: Increase in blood pressure and heart rate; dizziness.
▲ Warning: It should not be administered to patients with severe hypertension, coronary artery disease or thyrotoxicosis.

Administer with care to those with epilepsy or liver impairment.
○ Related entry: Dopram.

doxazosin

is a selective ALPHA-ADRENOCEPTOR BLOCKER which is used as an ANTIHYPERTENSIVE, often in conjunction with other antihypertensives (eg BETA-BLOCKERS or (THIAZIDE) diuretics). It can also be used to treat urinary retention in benign prostatic hypertrophy. Administration is oral.
+▲ Side-effects/warning: See PRAZOSIN HYDROCHLORIDE.
○ Related entry: Cardura.

doxepin

is an ANTIDEPRESSANT of the TRICYCLIC group. It can be used, as doxepin hydrochloride, to treat depressive illness, especially in cases where some degree of sedation is required. Administration is oral.
+▲ Side-effects/warning: See AMITRIPTYLINE HYDROCHLORIDE. It should not be used if breast-feeding.
○ Related entry: Sinequan.

doxorubicin hydrochloride

is a CYTOTOXIC drug (an ANTIBIOTIC in origin) which is used as an ANTICANCER treatment particularly for acute leukaemia, lymphomas and solid tumours (eg some bladder tumours). Administration is by intravenous infusion or bladder instillation.
+▲ Side-effects/warning: See CYTOTOXICS. Administer with care to patients with cardiovascular disease because it has effects on the heart.
○ Related entries: Doxorubicin Rapid Dissolution; Doxorubicin Solution for Injection.

Doxorubicin Rapid Dissolution

(Pharmacia) is a proprietary, prescription-only preparation of the (CYTOTOXIC) ANTICANCER drug doxorubicin hydrochloride. It is used particularly in the treatment of acute leukaemias, Lymphomas and some

D

solid tumours, and is available in a form for infusion.

+▲ Side-effects/warning: See DOXORUBICIN HYDROCHLORIDE.

Doxorubicin Solution for Injection

(Pharmacia) is a proprietary, prescription-only preparation of the (CYTOTOXIC) ANTICANCER drug doxorubicin hydrochloride. It is used particularly in the treatment of acute leukaemias, lymphomas and some solid tumours, and is available in a form for intravenous infusion.

+▲ Side-effects/warning: See DOXORUBICIN HYDROCHLORIDE.

doxycycline

is a broad-spectrum ANTIBACTERIAL and ANTIBIOTIC drug which is one of the TETRACYCLINES. It can be used to treat many kinds of infection, for example, of the respiratory and genital tracts, acne, chronic sinusitis and prostatitis. It can also be administered, in combination with other drugs, to treat brucellosis and pelvic inflammatory disease. Administration is oral.

+▲ Side-effects/warning: See TETRACYCLINE; it can be administered in patients with kidney impairment, but not with porphyria.

○ Related entries: Cyclodox; Demix; Doxylar; Ramysis; Vibramycin; Vibramycin D.

doxylamine succinate

is an ANTIHISTAMINE which is incorporated into a proprietary ANALGESIC preparation.

+▲ Side-effects/warning: See ANTIHISTAMINES.

○ Related entry: Syndol.

Doxylar

(Lagap) is a proprietary, prescription-only preparation of the ANTIBACTERIAL and (TETRACYCLINE) ANTIBIOTIC drug doxycycline. It can be administered to treat a wide range of infections, and is available as capsules.

+▲ Side-effects/warning: See DOXYCYCLINE.

Dozic

(RP) is a proprietary, prescription-only preparation of the ANTIPSYCHOTIC haloperidol. It can be used to treat psychoses, especially patients with schizophrenia and the hyperactive, euphoric condition mania, and to tranquillize patients undergoing behavioural disturbance. It can also be administered in the short-term treatment of severe anxiety and to treat some involuntary motor disturbances (and also intractable hiccup). It is available as an oral liquid.

+▲ Side-effects/warning: See HALOPERIDOL.

Dramamine

(Searle) is a proprietary, non-prescription preparation of the ANTIHISTAMINE and ANTINAUSEANT dimenhydrinate. It can be used to treat nausea and vomiting, particularly when it is associated with motion sickness, disorders of the balance function of the inner ear and vertigo. It is available as tablets and is not normally given to children under one year, except on medical advice.

+▲ Side-effects/warning: See DIMENHYDRINATE.

Drapolene Cream

(Wellcome) is a proprietary, non-prescription COMPOUND PREPARATION of the ANTISEPTIC agents benzalkonium chloride and cetrimide. It can be used for the relief of nappy rash and to dress minor burns and wounds, and is available as a cream.

+▲ Side-effects/warning: See BENZALKONIUM CHLORIDE; CETRIMIDE.

Driclor

(Stiefel) is a proprietary, non-prescription preparation of aluminium chloride (as hexahydrate). It can be used as an antiperspirant to treat hyperhidrosis (excessive sweating), and is available in a roll-on applicator.

+▲ Side-effects/warning: See ALUMINIUM CHLORIDE.

Dried Tub/Vac/BCG
see BACILLUS CALMETTE-GUÉRIN VACCINE, DRIED

Dristan Decongestant Tablets
(Whitehall) is a proprietary, non-prescription COMPOUND PREPARATION of the (NSAID) NON-NARCOTIC ANALGESIC and ANTIRHEUMATIC aspirin, the SYMPATHOMIMETIC and DECONGESTANT phenylephrine hydrochloride, the ANTIHISTAMINE chlorpheniramine maleate and the STIMULANT caffeine. It can be used to relieve cold and flu symptoms, and is available as tablets. It is not normally given to children under six years, except on medical advice.
+▲ Side-effects/warning: See ASPIRIN; CAFFEINE; CHLORPHENIRAMINE MALEATE; PHENYLEPHRINE HYDROCHLORIDE.

Dristan Nasal Spray
(Whitehall) is a proprietary, non-prescription preparation of the SYMPATHOMIMETIC oxymetazoline hydrochloride. It can be used as a NASAL DECONGESTANT for the relief of rhinitis in a head cold, and is available as a nasal spray. It is not normally given to children under six years, except on medical advice.
+▲ Side-effects/warning: See OXYMETAZOLINE HYDROCHLORIDE.

Drogenil
(Schering-Plough) is a proprietary, prescription-only preparation of the anti-androgen, HORMONE ANTAGONIST flutamide. It can be used as an ANTICANCER drug to treat cancer of the prostate, and is available as tablets.
+▲ Side-effects/warning: See FLUTAMIDE.

Droleptan
(Janssen) is a proprietary, prescription-only preparation of the ANTIPSYCHOTIC droperidol. It can be used primarily in emergencies to subdue or soothe psychotic (particularly manic) patients during behavioural disturbances. It can also be used in patients about to undergo certain

diagnostic procedures that may be difficult or painful, because it promotes a sensation of detachment, and to treat nausea and vomiting caused by chemotherapy. It is available as tablets, a liquid and in a form for injection.
+▲ Side-effects/warning: See DROPERIDOL.

droperidol
is an ANTIPSYCHOTIC drug which is used primarily in emergencies to subdue or soothe psychotic (particularly manic) patients during behavioural disturbances. It is also used in patients about to undergo certain diagnostic procedures that may be difficult or painful, because it promotes a sensation of detachment, and to treat nausea and vomiting caused by chemotherapy. Administration is either oral or by injection.
+▲ Side-effects/warning: See HALOPERIDOL.
✪ Related entry: Droleptan.

Dryptal
(Berk) is a proprietary, prescription-only preparation of the (*loop*) DIURETIC frusemide. It can be used to treat oedema, particularly pulmonary (lung) oedema in patients with chronic heart failure and low urine production due to kidney failure (oliguria). It is available as tablets.
+▲ Side-effects/warning: See FRUSEMIDE.

DT/Vac/Ads
see ADSORBED DIPHTHERIA AND TETANUS VACCINE

DTIC-Dome
(Bayer) is a proprietary, prescription-only preparation of the (CYTOTOXIC) ANTICANCER drug dacarbazine. It can be used in the treatment of melanoma, some soft-tissue sarcomas and the lymphatic cancer Hodgkin's disease. It is available in a form for injection.
+▲ Side-effects/warning: See DACARBAZINE.

DTPer/Vac/Ads
see ADSORBED DIPHTHERIA, TETANUS AND PERTUSSIS VACCINE

D

D

Dubam

(Norma) is a proprietary, non-prescription COMPOUND PREPARATION of methyl salicylate, ethyl salicylate, glycol salicylate and methyl nicotinate, which all have COUNTER-IRRITANT, or RUBEFACIENT, actions. It can be used for the symptomatic relief of underlying muscle or joint pain, and is available as an aerosol spray for application to the skin.

+▲ Side-effects/warning: See ETHYL SALICYLATE; GLYCOL SALICYLATE; METHYL NICOTINATE; METHYL SALICYLATE.

Dulco-lax Suppositories

(Windsor) is a proprietary, non-prescription preparation of the (*stimulant*) LAXATIVE bisacodyl. It can be used to relieve constipation, and is available as suppositories. It is not normally given to children under ten years, except on medical advice.

+▲ Side-effects/warning: See BISACODYL.

Dulco-lax Suppositories for Children

(Windsor) is a proprietary, non-prescription preparation of the (*stimulant*) LAXATIVE bisacodyl. It can be used to relieve constipation, and is available as suppositories.

+▲ Side-effects/warning: See BISACODYL.

Dulco-lax Tablets

(Windsor) is a proprietary, non-prescription preparation of the (*stimulant*) LAXATIVE bisacodyl. It can be used to relieve constipation. It is not normally given to children under ten, except on medical advice.

+▲ Side-effects/warning: See BISACODYL.

Duofilm

(Stiefel) is a proprietary, non-prescription preparation of the KERATOLYTIC salicylic acid (with lactic acid). It can be used to remove warts and hard skin, and is available as a liquid paint.

+▲ Side-effects/warning: See SALICYLIC ACID.

Duovent

(Boehringer Ingelheim) is a proprietary, prescription-only COMPOUND PREPARATION of the SYMPATHOMIMETIC and BETA-RECEPTOR STIMULANT fenoterol hydrobromide and the ANTICHOLINERGIC ipratropium bromide, which both have bronchodilator properties. It can be used as an ANTI-ASTHMATIC and chronic bronchitis treatment, and is available in a metered-dose *Autoinhaler*, as an aerosol and a nebulizer solution.

+▲ Side-effects/warning: See FENOTEROL HYDROBROMIDE; IPRATROPIUM BROMIDE.

Duphalac

(Solvay) is a proprietary, non-prescription preparation of the (*osmotic*) LAXATIVE lactulose. It can be used to relieve constipation, and is available as an oral solution.

+▲ Side-effects/warning: See LACTULOSE.

Duphaston

(Duphar) is a proprietary, prescription-only preparation of the PROGESTOGEN dydrogesterone. It can be used to treat many conditions of hormonal deficiency in women, including menstrual problems, premenstrual syndrome, endometriosis, recurrent miscarriage and infertility, and as part of HRT. It is available (also in a packaging called *Duphaston HRT*) as tablets.

+▲ Side-effects/warning: See DYDROGESTERONE.

Duracreme

(LRC) is a proprietary, non-prescription SPERMICIDAL CONTRACEPTIVE which is used in combination with barrier methods of contraception (such as a condom). It is available as a cream containing nonoxinol.

+▲ Side-effects/warning: See NONOXINOL.

Duragel

(LRC) is a proprietary, non-prescription SPERMICIDAL CONTRACEPTIVE which is used in combination with barrier methods of contraception (such as a condom). It is available as a gel containing nonoxinol.

+▲ Side-effects/warning: See NONOXINOL.

Durogesic

(Janssen) is a proprietary, prescription-only preparation of the (OPIOID) NARCOTIC ANALGESIC fentanyl and is on the Controlled Drugs List. It can be used to treat moderate to severe pain, and is available as skin patches.

+▲ Side-effects/warning: See FENTANYL.

Duromine

(3M) is a proprietary, prescription-only preparation of the APPETITE SUPPRESSANT phentermine, which is a strong STIMULANT and on the Controlled Drugs List. It can be used in the treatment of obesity, and is available as modified-release tablets.

+▲ Side-effects/warning: See PHENTERMINE.

Dutonin

(Bristol-Myers) is a proprietary, prescription-only preparation of the (SSRI) ANTIDEPRESSANT nefazodone hydrochloride, which has less sedative effects than some other antidepressants. It is available as tablets.

+▲ Side-effects/warning: See NEFAZODONE HYDROCHLORIDE.

Dyazide

(SK&F) is a proprietary, prescription-only COMPOUND PREPARATION of the (THIAZIDE) DIURETIC hydrochlorothiazide and the (*potassium-sparing*) diuretic triamterene (a combination called co-triamterzide 50/25). It can be used in the treatment of oedema and as an ANTIHYPERTENSIVE, and is available as tablets.

+▲ Side-effects/warning: See HYDROCHLOROTHIAZIDE; TRIAMTERENE; also, the urine may be coloured blue.

dydrogesterone

is a PROGESTOGEN, an analogue of the sex hormone PROGESTERONE, which is used to treat many conditions of hormonal

deficiency in women, including menstrual problems, premenstrual syndrome, displacement of uterus-lining tissue (endometriosis), recurrent miscarriage and infertility and as part of HRT. Administration is oral.

+▲ Side-effects/warning: See PROGESTOGEN. May cause breakthrough bleeding.

◒ Related entries: Duphaston; Femapak 80; Femoston.

Dynese

(Galen) is a proprietary, non-prescription preparation of the ANTACID magaldrate. It can be used for the symptomatic relief of dyspepsia, and is available as a sugar-free oral suspension.

+▲ Side-effects/warning: See MAGALDRATE.

Dysman 250

(Ashbourne) is a proprietary, prescription-only preparation of the (NSAID) NON-NARCOTIC ANALGESIC and ANTIRHEUMATIC mefenamic acid. It can be used to treat pain and inflammation in rheumatoid arthritis, osteoarthritis and other musculoskeletal disorders and period pain. It is available as capsules.

+▲ Side-effects/warning: See MEFENAMIC ACID.

Dysman 500

(Ashbourne) is a proprietary, prescription-only preparation of the (NSAID) NON-NARCOTIC ANALGESIC and ANTIRHEUMATIC mefenamic acid. It can be used to treat pain and inflammation in rheumatoid arthritis, osteoarthritis and other musculoskeletal disorders and period pain. It is available as capsules.

+▲ Side-effects/warning: See MEFENAMIC ACID.

Dyspamet

(SK&F) is a proprietary preparation of the H$_2$-ANTAGONIST cimetidine. It is available on prescription or without a prescription in a limited amount and for short-term uses

D

only. It can be used as an ULCER-HEALING DRUG for benign peptic ulcers (in the stomach or duodenum), gastro-oesophageal reflux, dyspepsia and associated conditions. It is available as chewable tablets (*Chewtab*) and an oral suspension.

+▲ Side-effects/warning: See CIMETIDINE.

Dysport

(Porton) is a proprietary, prescription-only preparation of botulinum A toxin-haemagglutin complex. It can be used for treating blepharospasm (a tight contraction of the eyelids) and one-sided facial spasm, and is available in a form for injection.

Dytac

(Pharmark) is a proprietary, prescription-only preparation of the (*potassium-sparing*) DIURETIC triamterene. It can be used to treat oedema, and is available as capsules.

+▲ Side-effects/warning: See TRIAMTERENE.

Dytide

(Pharmark) is a proprietary, prescription-only COMPOUND PREPARATION of the (THIAZIDE) DIURETIC benzthiazide and the (*potassium-sparing*) diuretic triamterene. It can be used to treat oedema and as an ANTIHYPERTENSIVE, and is available as capsules.

+▲ Side-effects/warning: See BENZTHIAZIDE; TRIAMTERENE.

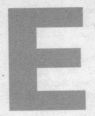

E45 Cream

(Crookes) is a proprietary, non-prescription COMPOUND PREPARATION of liquid paraffin, WHITE SOFT PARAFFIN and wool fat. It can be used as an EMOLLIENT for dry skin and minor abrasions and burns, and is available as a cream, a wash and a bath oil.

+▲ Side-effects/warning: See LIQUID PARAFFIN; WOOL FAT.

Ebufac

(DDSA) is a proprietary, prescription-only preparation of the (NSAID) NON-NARCOTIC ANALGESIC and ANTIRHEUMATIC ibuprofen. It can be used to relieve pain, particularly the pain of rheumatic disease and other musculoskeletal disorders, and is available as tablets.

+▲ Side-effects/warning: See IBUPROFEN.

Econacort

(Squibb) is a proprietary, prescription-only COMPOUND PREPARATION of the CORTICOSTEROID hydrocortisone and the ANTIFUNGAL econazole nitrate. It can be used to treat inflammation in which there is fungal infection, and is available as a cream for topical application.

+▲ Side-effects/warning: See ECONAZOLE NITRATE; HYDROCORTISONE.

econazole nitrate

is a broad-spectrum (IMIDAZOLE) ANTIFUNGAL which can be used to treat fungal infections of the skin, nails or mucous membranes (eg vaginal candidiasis). Administration is by topical application.

+▲ Side-effects/warning: See
CLOTRIMAZOLE.
☉ Related entries: Econacort; Ecostatin;
Gyno-Pevaryl; Pevaryl; Pevaryl TC.

Ecostatin

(Squibb) is a proprietary, prescription-only
preparation of the ANTIFUNGAL econazole
nitrate. It can be used primarily to treat
fungal infections of the skin and mucous
membranes, especially of the vagina and
vulva. It is available as a cream, vaginal
pessaries (the stronger form is called
Ecostatin 1) and a *Twinpack* with
pessaries and cream (the cream is available
without prescription).
+▲ Side-effects/warning: See ECONAZOLE
NITRATE.

Edecrin

(Merck Sharp & Dohme) is a proprietary,
prescription-only preparation of the (*loop*)
DIURETIC ethacrynic acid. It can be used to
treat oedema, particularly pulmonary
(lung) oedema in patients with left
ventricular and chronic heart failure and
low urine production due to kidney failure
(oliguria). It is available in a form for
injection or infusion.
+▲ Side-effects/warning: See ETHACRYNIC
ACID.

edrophonium chloride

is an ANTICHOLINESTERASE drug which
enhances the effects of the
NEUROTRANSMITTER acetylcholine (and of
certain cholinergic drugs). It has a short
duration of action and can be used in the
diagnosis of myasthenia gravis and at the
termination of operations to reverse the
actions of neuromuscular blocking agents
(when it is often administered with atropine
sulphate). Administration is by injection.
+▲ Side-effects/warning: See NEOSTIGMINE.
☉ Related entry: Camsilon.

Efalith

(Searle) is a proprietary, prescription-only
COMPOUND PREPARATION of lithium succinate

and zinc sulphate. It can be used for
seborrhoeic dermatitis, and is available as
an ointment.
+▲ Side-effects/warning: See LITHIUM
SUCCINATE; ZINC SULPHATE.

Efamast

(Searle) is a proprietary, prescription-only
preparation of gamolenic acid (in evening
primrose oil). It can be used for the relief
of breast pain (mastalgia), and is available
as capsules.
+▲ Side-effects/warning: See GAMOLENIC
ACID.

Efcortelan

(Glaxo) is a proprietary, prescription-only
preparation of the CORTICOSTEROID and ANTI-
INFLAMMATORY drug hydrocortisone. It can
be used to treat mild inflammatory skin
conditions, such as eczema, and is available
as a cream and an ointment.
+▲ Side-effects/warning: See
HYDROCORTISONE.

Efcortesol

(Glaxo) is a proprietary, prescription-only
preparation of the CORTICOSTEROID and ANTI-
INFLAMMATORY hydrocortisone (as sodium
phosphate). It can be used to treat
inflammation, especially inflammation
caused by allergy, to treat shock or to make
up a deficiency of steroid hormones. It is
available in a form for injection.
+▲ Side-effects/warning: See
HYDROCORTISONE.

Efexor

(Wyeth) is a proprietary, prescription-only
preparation of the (SSRI) ANTIDEPRESSANT
venlafaxine. It can be used to treat
depressive illness, and is available as
tablets.
+▲ Side-effects/warning: See VENLAFAXINE.

Effercitrate

(Typharm) is a proprietary, non-
prescription preparation of potassium
citrate. It can be used as an alkalizing agent

for the relief of discomfort of mild urinary tract infection and to make the urine alkaline. It is available as effervescent tablets for solution.

+▲ Side-effects/warning: See POTASSIUM CITRATE.

eformoterol

is a recently introduced SYMPATHOMIMETIC and BETA-RECEPTOR STIMULANT with β_2-receptor selectivity. It is mainly used as a BRONCHODILATOR in reversible obstructive airways disease and as an ANTI-ASTHMATIC treatment, for example, for nocturnal asthma and to prevent exercise-induced bronchospasm, in patients who require long-term therapy. It is similar to SALMETEROL but has a more rapid onset of action. Patients should also be cautioned not to exceed the stated dose, and if a previously effective dose fails to relieve symptoms they should consult their doctor. Administration is as a powder for inhalation.

+▲ Side-effects/warning: See SALBUTAMOL; but the effects are more prolonged. Avoid its use with patients who are pregnant or breast-feeding.

✪ Related entry: Foradil.

Efudix

(Roche) is a proprietary, prescription-only preparation of the (CYTOTOXIC) ANTICANCER drug fluorouracil. It can be used to treat malignant skin lesions, and is available as a cream for topical application.

+▲ Side-effects/warning: See CYTOTOXICS.

Elantan

(Schwarz) is a proprietary preparation of the VASODILATOR and ANTI-ANGINA drug isosorbide mononitrate. It can be used to treat and prevent angina pectoris and for heart failure. It is available as tablets in a non-prescription preparation, *Elantan 10* and two prescription-only preparations, *Elantan 20* and *Elantan 40*.

+▲ Side-effects/warning: See ISOSORBIDE MONONITRATE.

Elantan LA

(Schwarz) is a proprietary, non-prescription preparation of the VASODILATOR and ANTI-ANGINA drug isosorbide mononitrate. It can be used to treat and prevent angina pectoris, and is available as modified-release capsules in two forms, *Elantan LA 25* and *Elantan LA 50*.

+▲ Side-effects/warning: See ISOSORBIDE MONONITRATE.

Elavil

(DDSA Pharmaceuticals) is a proprietary, prescription-only preparation of the (TRICYCLIC) ANTIDEPRESSANT amitriptyline hydrochloride. It can be used to treat depressive illness, especially in cases where some degree of sedation is required, and has also been used to treat bed-wetting by children at night. It is available as tablets.

+▲ Side-effects/warning: See AMITRIPTYLINE HYDROCHLORIDE.

Eldepryl

(Britannia) is a proprietary, prescription-only preparation of the ANTIPARKINSONISM drug selegiline. It can be used to assist in the treatment of the symptoms of parkinsonism, and is available as tablets and a liquid.

+▲ Side-effects/warning: See SELEGILINE.

Eldisine

(Lilly) is a proprietary, prescription-only preparation of the (CYTOTOXIC) ANTICANCER drug vindesine sulphate. It can be used to treat acute leukaemia, lymphomas and some solid tumours, and is available in a form for injection.

+▲ Side-effects/warning: See VINDESINE SULPHATE.

Elleste-Duet

(Searle) is a proprietary, prescription-only COMPOUND PREPARATION of the female SEX HORMONES oestradiol (an OESTROGEN) and norethisterone (as acetate; a progestogen). It can be used in HRT, and is available as tablets.

+▲ Side-effects/warning: See
NORETHISTERONE; OESTRADIOL.

Elleste-Solo

(Searle) is a proprietary, prescription-only preparation of the female SEX HORMONE oestradiol (an OESTROGEN). It can be used in HRT, and is available as tablets.
+▲ Side-effects/warning: See OESTRADIOL.

Ellimans Universal Embrocation

(Seton) is a proprietary, non-prescription preparation of TURPENTINE OIL (along with acetic acid). It has a COUNTER-IRRITANT, or RUBEFACIENT, properties and can be applied to the skin for symptomatic relief of underlying muscle or joint pain. It is available as an embrocation for topical application and is not normally used for children under 12 years, except on medical advice.

Eltroxin

(Goldshield) is a proprietary, prescription-only preparation of thyroxine sodium, which is a form of thyroid hormone. It can be used to make up a hormonal deficiency and to treat associated symptoms, and is available as tablets.
+▲ Side-effects/warning: See THYROXINE SODIUM.

Eludril Mouthwash

(Chefaro) is a proprietary, non-prescription COMPOUND PREPARATION of the ANTISEPTICS chlorhexidine (as gluconate) and CHLORBUTOL. It can be used in the treatment and prevention of gingivitis, for oral hygiene and minor throat infections. It is not normally given to children, except on medical advice.
+▲ Side-effects/warning: See CHLORHEXIDINE.

Eludril Spray

(Chefaro) is a proprietary, non-prescription COMPOUND PREPARATION of the ANTISEPTIC chlorhexidine (as gluconate) and the LOCAL ANAESTHETIC amethocaine hydrochloride. It can be administered in the local treatment of mouth and throat conditions, such as gingivitis and ulcers, minor infections of the throat and mouth and for oral hygiene. It is available as a pressurized spray and is not normally given to children, except on medical advice.
+▲ Side-effects/warning: See AMETHOCAINE HYDROCHLORIDE; CHLORHEXIDINE.

Elyzol

(Dumex) is a proprietary, prescription-only preparation of the ANTIMICROBIAL metronidazole, which has both ANTIBACTERIAL and ANTIPROTOZOAL actions. It can be used for the treatment of local infections in dental surgery, and is available as a gel.
+▲ Side-effects/warning: See METRONIDAZOLE.

Emblon

(Berk) is a proprietary, prescription-only preparation of the sex HORMONE ANTAGONIST tamoxifen, which, because it inhibits the effect of OESTROGENS, is used primarily as an ANTICANCER treatment for cancers that depend on the presence of oestrogen in women, particularly breast cancer. It can also be used to treat certain conditions of infertility, and is available as tablets.
+▲ Side-effects/warning: See TAMOXIFEN.

Emcor

(Merck) is a proprietary, prescription-only preparation of the BETA-BLOCKER bisoprolol fumarate. It can be used as an ANTIHYPERTENSIVE for raised blood pressure and as an ANTI-ANGINA treatment to relieve symptoms and improve exercise tolerance. It is available as tablets.
+▲ Side-effects/warning: See BISOPROLOL FUMARATE.

Emeside

(LAB) is a proprietary, prescription-only preparation of the ANTICONVULSANT and ANTI-EPILEPTIC ethosuximide. It can be used to treat absence (petit mal), myoclonic and some other types of seizure, and is available as capsules and a syrup.

➕▲ Side-effects/warning: See ETHOSUXIMIDE.

emetics 🗷

are drugs or other agents that cause vomiting (emesis). Emetics are used primarily to treat poisoning by non-corrosive substances when the patient is conscious, especially drugs taken in overdose. Some affect the vomiting centre in the brain and/or irritate the gastrointestinal tract. Among the best-known and most-used emetics is IPECACUANHA, but several drugs used as EXPECTORANTS can, in higher concentrations, also cause emesis.

Emflex

(Merck) is a proprietary, prescription-only preparation of the (NSAID) NON-NARCOTIC ANALGESIC and ANTIRHEUMATIC acemetacin. It can be used to treat the pain of rheumatic and other musculoskeletal disorders and for postoperative pain. It is available as capsules.

➕▲ Side-effects/warning: See ACEMETACIN.

Eminase

(Beecham) is a proprietary, prescription-only preparation of the FIBRINOLYTIC anistreplase. It can be used to treat myocardial infarction, and is available in a form for injection.

➕▲ Side-effects/warning: See ANISTREPLASE.

Emla

(Astra) is a proprietary, prescription-only COMPOUND PREPARATION of the LOCAL ANAESTHETICS lignocaine hydrochloride and prilocaine hydrochloride. It can be used for surface anaesthesia, including in the preparation for injections, and is available as a cream.

➕▲ Side-effects/warning: See LIGNOCAINE HYDROCHLORIDE; PRILOCAINE HYDROCHLORIDE.

Emmolate

(Bio-Medical) is a proprietary, non-prescription preparation of liquid paraffin, along with acetylated wool alcohol. It has an EMOLLIENT action and can be used for dry skin. It is available as a bath oil.

➕▲ Side-effects/warning: See LIQUID PARAFFIN.

emollients 🗷

are agents that soothe, soften and moisturize the skin, particularly when it is dry and scaling. They are usually emulsions of water, fats, waxes and oils (eg LANOLIN and LIQUID PARAFFIN). They can be used alone to help hydrate the skin, or combined with HYDRATING AGENTS such as UREA. A notable example of a skin condition that may be treated with emollients is atopic eczema, when the skin is very dry. Emollients can be applied as creams, ointments, lotions or added to bath water. Such preparations contain preservatives (eg parabens) which in some patients may worsen the condition by causing contact allergic dermatitis, and similarly some patients are allergic to some of the major constituents (particularly lanolin or WOOL FAT). There are a number of additives that may help itchiness (eg MENTHOL, CAMPHOR and PHENOL) and some preparations have a beneficial ASTRINGENT action (eg ZINC OXIDE or CALAMINE). In conditions that also involve a skin infection, emollients may have an ANTIMICROBIAL or ANTIFUNGAL drug added to them, or, in cases of severe inflammation, ANTI-INFLAMMATORY and CORTICOSTEROID drugs may be incorporated.

Emulsiderm

(Dermal) is a proprietary, non-prescription preparation of the ANTISEPTIC benzalkonium chloride and the skin EMOLLIENT liquid paraffin (with isopropyl myristate). It is available as a liquid emulsion that can be added to a bath.

➕▲ Side-effects/warning: See BENZALKONIUM CHLORIDE; LIQUID PARAFFIN.

Emulsifying Ointment, BP

is a non-proprietary, non-prescription COMPOUND PREPARATION formulation comprising a combination of wax, white soft paraffin and liquid paraffin. It can be used as a base for medications that require topical application.

enalapril maleate

is an ACE INHIBITOR and acts as a VASODILATOR. It can be used as an ANTIHYPERTENSIVE, in HEART FAILURE TREATMENT and to prevent ischaemia (lack of blood supply) in patients with left ventricular failure. It is often used in conjunction with other classes of drug, particularly (THIAZIDE) DIURETICS. Administration is oral.

✚▲ Side-effects/warning: See CAPTOPRIL.

✪ Related entries: Innovace; Innozide.

Endoxana

(ASTA Medica) is a proprietary, prescription-only preparation of the (CYTOTOXIC) ANTICANCER drug cyclophosphamide. It can be used to treat chronic lymphatic leukaemia, lymphomas and some solid tumours. It is available as tablets and a form for injection.

✚▲ Side-effects/warning: See CYCLOPHOSPHAMIDE.

enflurane

is an inhalant GENERAL ANAESTHETIC which is similar to HALOTHANE. It is often used along with nitrous oxide-oxygen mixtures for the induction and maintenance of anaesthesia during major surgery. Administration is by inhalation.

✚ Side-effects: It depresses heart function (lowers blood pressure) and respiration.

▲ Warning: It is not to be used in patients with porphyria.

✪ Related entry: Enflurane.

Enflurane

(Abbott) is a proprietary preparation of the inhalant GENERAL ANAESTHETIC enflurane. It can be used for the induction and maintenance of anaesthesia during major surgery, and is available in a form for inhalation.

✚▲ Side-effects/warning: See ENFLURANE.

Engerix B

(SmithKline Beecham) is a proprietary, prescription-only VACCINE preparation of hepatitis B vaccine (rby), prepared from yeast cells by recombinant DNA technique. It can be used to protect people at risk from infection with hepatitis B, and is available in a form for injection.

✚▲ Side-effects/warning: See HEPATITIS B VACCINE.

Eno

(SmithKline Beecham) is a proprietary, non-prescription COMPOUND PREPARATION of the ANTACIDS calcium carbonate and sodium bicarbonate together with citric acid. It can be used for the symptomatic relief of indigestion, flatulence and nausea. It is available as a powder for making up as a sparkling drink (also available in a form called *Lemon Eno*). It is not normally given to children, except on medical advice.

✚▲ Side-effects/warning: See CALCIUM CARBONATE; SODIUM BICARBONATE.

enoxaparin

is a LOW MOLECULAR WEIGHT HEPARIN. It has some advantages as an ANTICOAGULANT when used for long-duration prevention of venous thrombo-embolism, particularly in orthopaedic use. Administration is by injection.

✚▲ Side-effects/warning: See HEPARIN.

✪ Related entry: Clexane.

enoximone

is a PHOSPHODIESTERASE INHIBITOR and is used in congestive HEART FAILURE TREATMENT, especially where other drugs have been unsuccessful. Administration is by intravenous injection or infusion.

✚ Side-effects: There may be irregular heartbeats, hypotension, headache, nausea and vomiting, insomnia, chills and fever,

E

diarrhoea, retention of urine and pain in the limbs.

▲ Warning: It should be given with caution to patients with certain forms of heart failure and vascular disease. The blood pressure and electrocardiogram should be monitored.

✪ Related entry: Perfan.

Enterosan

(Monmouth) is a proprietary, non-prescription preparation of the (OPIOID) ANTIDIARRHOEAL morphine (as hydrochloride), kaolin and the ANTICHOLINERGIC Belladonna extract. It can be used for the symptomatic relief of occasional diarrhoea and its associated pain and discomfort, and is available as tablets. It is not normally given to children, except on medical advice.

✚▲ Side-effects/warning: See BELLADONNA ALKALOIDS; KAOLIN; MORPHINE SULPHATE.

Entocort CR

(Astra) is a proprietary, prescription-only preparation of the CORTICOSTEROID budesonide. It can be used for the induction of remission in mild to moderate Crohn's disease affecting the ileum or ascending colon. It is available as capsules and an enema.

✚▲ Side-effects/warning: See BUDESONIDE.

enzyme inhibitors ⓘ

are drugs that work by inhibiting enzymes, which are proteins that play an essential part in the metabolism by acting as catalysts in specific, necessary biochemical reactions. Certain drugs have been developed that act only on certain enzymes and so can be used to manipulate the biochemistry of the body. For example, ANTICHOLINESTERASE drugs (eg NEOSTIGMINE, PYRIDOSTIGMINE and PHYSOSTIGMINE) inhibit enzymes called cholinesterases, which are normally involved in the rapid breakdown of ACETYLCHOLINE (an important NEUROTRANSMITTER). Acetylcholine is released from cholinergic nerves and has

many actions throughout the body. Consequently, since anticholinesterase drugs enhance the effects of acetylcholine on its release from these nerves, they can have a wide range of actions. Their actions at the junction of nerves with skeletal (voluntary) muscles are used in the diagnosis and treatment of the muscle weakness disease myasthenia gravis; also, at the end of surgical operations in which SKELETAL MUSCLE RELAXANTS have been used, the anaesthetist is able to reverse the muscle paralysis by injecting an anticholinesterase. In organs innervated by parasympathetic division of the autonomic nervous system, anticholinesterases cause an exaggeration of the nerves' actions, known as PARASYMPATHOMIMETIC actions and can be used for a number of purposes, such as stimulation of the bladder (in cases of urinary retention), the intestine (in paralytic ileus) and the pupil of the eye (on local application in glaucoma treatment). However, anticholinesterases have a number of undesirable side-effects, including slowing of the heart, constriction of the airways with excessive production of secretions and actions in the brain. In anticholinesterase poisoning, their diverse actions can be life-threatening. Chemicals with anticholinesterase properties are used as insecticides and in chemical warfare. ANTIDOTES are available to treat cases of poisoning, for example, due to a farming accident.

MONOAMINE-OXIDASE INHIBITORS, or MAOIs, (eg ISOCARBOXAZID, PHENELZINE and TRANYLCYPROMINE) are one of the three major classes of ANTIDEPRESSANTS. They work by inhibiting an enzyme in the brain that metabolizes monoamines (including NORADRENALINE and SEROTONIN), which results in a change of mood. However, this same enzyme detoxifies other amines, so if certain foods are eaten or medicines taken that contain amines (eg sympathomimetic amines in cough and cold treatments), then dangerous side-effects could occur. MOCLOBEMIDE is a newly introduced MAOI which is an inhibitor of only one type of monoamine oxidase (type A) and is claimed to show less potentiation of the amine in foodstuffs.

ACE INHIBITORS (angiotensin-converting enzyme inhibitors), such as CAPTOPRIL, ENALAPRIL MALEATE and RAMIPRIL, are drugs that are used as ANTIHYPERTENSIVES and in HEART FAILURE TREATMENT. They work by inhibiting the conversion of the natural circulating HORMONE angiotensin I to angiotensin II and because the latter form is a potent VASOCONSTRICTOR, the overall effect is VASODILATION with a HYPOTENSIVE action.

Further examples of enzyme inhibitors include the CARBONIC ANHYDRASE INHIBITORS (which are used for their DIURETIC actions and in GLAUCOMA TREATMENT), the PHOSPHODIESTERASE INHIBITORS (for congestive heart failure treatment), CARBIDOPA (in ANTIPARKINSONISM treatment), CLAVULANIC ACID (to prolong and enhance the effects of certain ANTIBIOTICS) and DISULFIRAM (which is used in the treatment of alcoholism).

enzymes 🔊

are proteins that play an essential part in the metabolism of the body by acting as catalysts in specific, necessary biochemical reactions. Their physiological functions range from digestion of food within the digestive tract through to elaborations of proteins and other structural elements of the body.

Impaired function of enzymes underlies many (particularly familial) diseases, and may cause some food intolerances that require special diets (eg phenylkenonuria and favism). Specialized enzymes are involved in the metabolism and detoxification of chemicals, including drugs, that are foreign to the body. Impaired capacity of these enzymes (which again is often familial) may make persons hypersensitive to these chemicals, and is a prominent cause of adverse drug reactions (eg G6PD deficiency, porphyria) and metabolism by liver enzymes is often slower

in the young, the elderly and in liver disease (including cirrhosis).

Many drugs (see ENZYME INHIBITORS) have been developed that in exerting their beneficial effects, achieve selectivity of action through affecting only certain enzymes and so can be used to manipulate the biochemistry of the body (eg MONOAMINE-OXIDASE INHIBITORS, ANTICHOLINESTERASES and PHOSPHODIESTERASE INHIBITORS). In a few instances enzymes, themselves, are used as drugs, but their chemical nature makes it difficult to deliver them to their proposed sites of action. Also, because they are proteins, in most cases derived from animals, there are commonly serious allergic side-effects.

Some FIBRINOLYTICS are enzymes and are administered by injection or infusion to dissolve blood clots in the treatment of life-threatening conditions, such as acute myocardial infarction, venous thrombi, pulmonary embolism and clots in the eye (eg ALTEPLASE, ANISTREPLASE, STREPTOKINASE and UROKINASE).

A number of enzymes have been given by mouth with food to supplement defiencies in production of proteolytic (protein-digesting) enzymes. This approach, however, is not generally very successful and such agents tend to erode the upper gastrointestinal tract (eg PANCREATIN, which is isolated from the pancreas of a cow or pig). Other proteolytic enzymes have diverse uses, for example, dissolving wound debris, by inhalation into the lungs to liquefy visous sputum (TRYPSIN) or to aid cataract surgery (CHYMOTRYPSIN). Other enzymes that dissolve connective tissue are used in the treatment of skin extravastion injuries such as burns and inflammatory injuries (to promote reabsorption of excess fluids and blood), to increase the permeability of soft tissues to injected drugs and in ophthalmological practice (eg HYALURONIDASE). The ANTICOAGULANT agent ANCROD is a protease enzyme obtained from the venom of the Malaysian pit viper.

ALGLUCERASE is an enzyme that is used as a replacement in the specialist treatment of Gaucher's disease, which is a genetically determined enzyme-deficiency disease that affects the spleen, liver, bone marrow and lymph nodes. Enzymes also can be used in ANTICANCER therapy (eg ASPARAGINASE; an enzyme isolated from the *E. coli* bacterium).

Epanutin

(Parke-Davis) is a proprietary, prescription-only preparation of the ANTICONVULSANT and ANTI-EPILEPTIC phenytoin. It can be used to treat and prevent most forms of seizure and also the pain of trigeminal (facial) neuralgia. It is available as capsules, chewable tablets (*Epanutin Infatabs*) and as a liquid suspension.

✚▲ Side-effects/warning: See PHENYTOIN.

Epanutin Ready Mixed Parenteral

(Parke-Davis) is a proprietary, prescription-only preparation of the ANTICONVULSANT and ANTI-EPILEPTIC phenytoin. It can be used in the emergency treatment of status epilepticus and convulsive seizures during neurosurgical operations. It is available in a form for injection.

✚▲ Side-effects/warning: See PHENYTOIN.

ephedrine hydrochloride

is an ALKALOID that is a SYMPATHOMIMETIC drug (also called an *indirect sympathetic*, because it works indirectly through the release of NORADRENALINE from sympathetic nerve endings). It is occasionally used as a BRONCHODILATOR and VASOCONSTRICTOR, but is primarily used as an ANTI-ASTHMATIC and for chronic bronchitis and similar conditions, especially allergy-based ones (this is also the major use of the closely related PSEUDOEPHEDRINE HYDROCHLORIDE). Overall, its effects are similar to those of ADRENALINE, except that in adults it is a quite powerful central nervous STIMULANT, though it has

SEDATIVE properties in children. It is also used to treat bed-wetting in children and as a NASAL DECONGESTANT. Administration can be either oral or topical.

✚ Side-effects: There may be changes in heart rate and blood pressure, anxiety, restlessness, tremor, insomnia, dry mouth, cold fingertips and toes and changes in the prostate gland. When used as a nasal decongestant, it may cause irritation in the nose.

▲ Warning: Administer with caution to patients with certain heart, kidney and thyroid disorders, diabetes and hypertension; care should be taken to avoid interaction with other drugs.

✪ Related entries: Anestan Bronchial Tablets; CAM; Do-Do Tablets; Expulin Decongestant for Babies and Children (Linctus); Franol; Franol Plus; Franolyn for Chesty Coughs; Haymine; Nirolex for Chesty Coughs.

Epifen

(ALK) is a proprietary prescription-only preparation of the natural HORMONE adrenaline. It is used as a SYMPATHOMIMETIC and BRONCHODILATOR drug in emergency treatment of acute and severe bronchoconstriction and other symptoms of acute anaphylaxis (allergic reaction; eg an insect sting). It is available as an auto-injector, which delivers a single intramuscular dose, and also as a version for children, *Epipen Jr Auto-injector*.

✚▲ Side-effects/warning: See ADRENALINE.

Epilim

(Sanofi Winthrop) is a proprietary, prescription-only preparation of the ANTICONVULSANT and ANTI-EPILEPTIC sodium valproate. It can be used to treat all forms of epilepsy, and is available as tablets, a liquid and a syrup.

✚▲ Side-effects/warning: See SODIUM VALPROATE.

Epilim Chrono

(Sanofi Winthrop) is a proprietary,

prescription-only preparation of the ANTICONVULSANT and ANTI-EPILEPTIC sodium valproate. It can be used to treat all forms of epilepsy, and is available as modified-release tablets.

✚▲ Side-effects/warning: See SODIUM VALPROATE.

Epilim Intravenous

(Sanofi Winthrop) is a proprietary, prescription-only preparation of the ANTICONVULSANT and ANTI-EPILEPTIC sodium valproate. It can be used to treat all forms of epilepsy, and is available in a form for injection.

✚▲ Side-effects/warning: See SODIUM VALPROATE.

Epimaz

(Norton) is a proprietary, prescription-only preparation of the ANTICONVULSANT and ANTI-EPILEPTIC carbamazepine. It can be used to treat most forms of epilepsy (except absence seizures), diabetes insipidus, trigeminal neuralgia and in the management of manic-depressive illness. It is available as tablets.

✚▲ Side-effects/warning: See CARBAMAZEPINE.

epinephrine

see ADRENALINE

epirubicin hydrochloride

is a CYTOTOXIC drug (an ANTIBIOTIC in origin) which is used as an ANTICANCER treatment of severe breast and kidney tumours. Administration is by injection or bladder instillation.

✚▲ Side-effects/warning: See CYTOTOXICS; but it also has cardiac toxicity.

◐ Related entries: Pharmorubicin Rapid Dissolution; Pharmorubicin Solution for Injection.

Epivir

(GlaxoWellcome) is a proprietary, prescription-only preparation of the ANTIVIRAL lamivudine. It can be used in the treatment of AIDS, and is available as tablets and as an oral solution.

✚▲ Side-effects/warning: See LAMIVUDINE.

epoetin

is a synthesized form of human erythropoitetin. It is used as an ANAEMIA TREATMENT for the type of anaemia known to be associated with erythropoetic deficiency in chronic renal failure in dialysis patients. It is available as epoetin alpha and beta and is administered intravenously.

✚ Side-effects: Cardiovascular symptoms including high blood pressure (hypertension) and cardiac complications; anaphylactic reactions, flu-like symptoms, skin reactions; oedema and effects on the blood.

▲ Warning: It should be not be administered to patients with uncontrolled hypertension. Administer with care to patients with poorly controlled blood pressure, a history of convulsions, vascular disease, liver failure or a malignant disease; or who are pregnant or breast-feeding.

◐ Related entries: Eprex; Recormon.

Epogam

(Searle) is a proprietary, prescription-only preparation of gamolenic acid (in evening primrose oil). It can be used for the symptomatic relief of atopic eczema, and is available as capsules and paediatric capsules.

✚▲ Side-effects/warning: See GAMOLENIC ACID.

epoprostenol

(prostacyclin) is a PROSTAGLANDIN present naturally in the walls of blood vessels. When administered therapeutically by intravenous infusion it has ANTITHROMBOTIC or antithrombotic activity and so inhibits blood coagulation by preventing the aggregation of platelets. It is also a potent VASODILATOR. Its main use is to act as an ANTICOAGULANT during procedures such as kidney dialysis (though it has a very short lifetime in the body).

E

✚ Side-effects: Flushing, hypotension and headache.

▲ Warning: It must be administered in continuous intravenous infusion because it is rapidly removed from the blood. Blood monitoring is essential, especially when there is simultaneous administration of heparin.

✪ Related entry: Flolan.

Eppy

(Smith & Nephew) is a proprietary, prescription-only preparation of the SYMPATHOMIMETIC adrenaline. It is used to treat glaucoma, and is available as eye-drops.

✚▲ Side-effects/warning: See ADRENALINE.

Eprex

(Cilag) is a proprietary, prescription-only preparation of epoetin alpha (which is synthesized human erythropoitetin alpha). It can be administered as an ANAEMIA TREATMENT in conditions known to be associated with chronic renal failure in dialysis patients. It is available in a form for injection.

✚▲ Side-effects/warning: See EPOETIN.

Epsom salt(s)

see MAGNESIUM SULPHATE

Equagesic

(Wyeth) is a proprietary COMPOUND PREPARATION of the potentially habituating (addictive) ANXIOLYTIC and SEDATIVE drug meprobamate, the (NSAID) NON-NARCOTIC ANALGESIC and ANTIRHEUMATIC aspirin and ethoheptazine citrate, and is on the Controlled Drugs List. It can be used primarily for the short-term treatment of rheumatic pain and for the relief of the symptoms of other musculoskeletal disorders, and is available as tablets.

✚▲ Side-effects/warning: See ASPIRIN; MEPROBAMATE. It should also be noted that there are interactions with a wide variety of drugs, including alcohol and depressants of the nervous system.

Equanil

(Wyeth) is a proprietary, prescription-only preparation of the ANXIOLYTIC meprobamate and is on the Controlled Drugs List. It can be used in the short-term treatment of anxiety, and is available as tablets.

✚▲ Side-effects/warning: See MEPROBAMATE.

ergocalciferol

is one of the natural forms of calciferol (vitamin D) which are formed in plants by the action of sunlight. It is vitamin D_2 but in medicine it is usually referred to as ergocalciferol or simply calciferol, and is used to make up deficiencies. Administration can be either oral or by injection.

✚▲ Side-effects/warning: See VITAMIN D.

✪ Related entry: calcium and ergocalciferol tablets.

ergometrine maleate

is an alkaloid VASOCONSTRICTOR and uterine stimulant which is used routinely in obstetric practice. It is administered to women in childbirth to speed up the third stage of labour (the delivery of the placenta), as a measure to prevent excessive postnatal bleeding and also bleeding due to incomplete abortion (when it may be combined with OXYTOCIN). Administration is either oral or by injection.

✚ Side-effects: There may be nausea and vomiting; palpitations, breathlessness, slowing of the heart, temporary high blood pressure; headache, dizziness; abdominal and chest pain; rarely, cardiovascular complications.

▲ Warning: It is not administered to patients for induction or in the first and second stages of labour; it should not be administered to those with vascular disease, certain kidney, liver or lung disorders, sepsis, severe hypertension or eclampsia. Administer with caution to those with heart disease, hypertension, blood disorders, multiple pregnancy or porphyria.

✪ Related entry: Syntometrine.

ergot alkaloids 🔟

are ALKALOIDS derived, directly or indirectly,
from a mould or fungus called *Claviceps
purpurea*, which grows on infected damp
rye. These alkaloids are powerful
VASOCONSTRICTOR substances that narrow the
blood vessels in the extremities, in
particular, and cause a tingling sensation
that progressively develops into pain then
gangrene. Ergot poisoning was known as St.
Anthony's Fire and was caused by eating
bread made from rye contaminated with
ergot. In medicine, the dose of individual
alkaloids is adjusted carefully to avoid the
development of the more serious side-
effects. ERGOTAMINE TARTRATE is the principle
vasoconstrictor used in medicine and is
mainly given as an ANTIMIGRAINE treatment.
ERGOMETRINE MALEATE is used to contract the
uterus in the last stages of labour and to
minimize post-partum haemorrhage (it is
the drug of choice because its effects on
blood vessels are less pronounced). Some
notable examples of semi-synthetic ergot
derivatives, which are used for a variety of
purposes, include BROMOCRIPTINE, CO-
DERGORINE MESYLATE, LYSURIDE MALEATE,
METHYSERGIDE and PERGOLIDE. All the ergot
alkaloids are chemically derivatives of
lysergide acid, and lysuride (lysergic acid
diethylamide) is the medical name for LSD.

ergotamine tartrate

is a vegetable ALKALOID which is given to
patients who suffer from migraine that is
not relieved by the ordinary forms of
painkilling drug. It is most effective if
administered during the aura – the initial
symptoms – of an attack and probably
works by constricting the cranial arteries.
However, although the pain may be relieved
other symptoms, such as the visual
disturbances and nausea, may not (but
other drugs may be used to treat these
symptoms separately). Repeated
administration of high doses can, in some
patients, cause ergot poisoning, which can
cause gangrene of the fingers and toes and
also confusion.

Administration is oral in the form of
tablets that are either swallowed or held
under the tongue until they dissolve, or as
an aerosol inhalant. One proprietary
compound preparation is available as
suppositories.

✚ Side-effects: Vomiting, nausea, vertigo,
abdominal pain and diarrhoea, cramps,
myocardial ischaemia and heart pain.
Repeated high doses may cause confusion,
gangrene and peritoneal fibrosis.

▲ Warning: It is not to be used in
prophylaxis of migraine attacks. If there is
numbness or tingling in the extremities,
stop treatment and seek medical advice. It is
not to be used in patients who are pregnant
or breast-feeding, who have vascular disease
(eg Raynaud's disease), certain kidney or
liver disorders, severe hypertension, sepsis or
hyperthyroidism.

⊘ Related entries: Cafergot; Lingraine;
Medihaler-Ergotamine; Migril.

Erwinase

(Porton) is a proprietary, prescription-only
preparation of the ENZYME cristantaspase. It
can be used as an ANTICANCER treatment of
acute lymphoblastic leukaemia, and is
available in a form for injection.
✚▲ Side-effects/warning: See
CRISTANTASPASE.

Erycen

(Berk) is a proprietary, prescription-only
preparation of the ANTIBACTERIAL and
(MACROLIDE) ANTIBIOTIC erythromycin. It can
be used to treat and prevent many forms of
infection, and is available as tablets.
✚▲ Side-effects/warning: See
ERYTHROMYCIN.

Erymax

(Elan) is a proprietary, prescription-only
preparation of the ANTIBACTERIAL and
(MACROLIDE) ANTIBIOTIC erythromycin. It can
be used to treat and prevent many forms of
infection, and is available as capsules.
✚▲ Side-effects/warning: See
ERYTHROMYCIN.

E

Erythrocin

(Abbott) is a proprietary, prescription-only preparation of the ANTIBACTERIAL and (MACROLIDE) ANTIBIOTIC erythromycin. It can be used to treat and prevent many forms of infection, and is available as tablets.

+▲ Side-effects/warning: See ERYTHROMYCIN.

Erythromid

(Abbott) is a proprietary, prescription-only preparation of the ANTIBACTERIAL and (MACROLIDE) ANTIBIOTIC erythromycin. It can be used to treat and prevent many forms of infection, and is available as tablets (there is also a stronger preparation, *Erythromid DS*).

+▲ Side-effects/warning: See ERYTHROMYCIN.

erythromycin

is an ANTIBACTERIAL and ANTIBIOTIC which is an original member of the MACROLIDE group. It has a similar spectrum of action to penicillin, but a different mechanism of action (macrolides work by inhibiting microbial protein synthesis). It is effective against many Gram-positive bacteria including streptococci (which causes infections of the soft tissue and respiratory tract), mycoplasma (which causes pneumonia), legionella (which causes legionnaires' disease) and chlamydia (which causes urethritis). It can also be used in the treatment of acne and chronic prostatitis and to prevent diphtheria and whooping cough. Its principal use is as an alternative to penicillin in individuals who are allergic to that drug. However, bacterial resistance to erythromycin is quite common. Administration is either oral or by injection (tablets are coated to prevent the drug being inactivated in the stomach).

+ Side-effects: Depending on the route of administration, there may be nausea and vomiting, abdominal discomfort and diarrhoea after large doses; allergic sensitivity reactions including rashes; reversible hearing loss after large doses;

jaundice on prolonged use.

▲ Warning: It should not be given to those with porphyria; certain forms that contain the estolate salt should not be given in liver disease. It must be used with caution in patients who have certain heart, liver or kidney disorders; or who are pregnant or breast-feeding.

✪ Related entries: Arpimycin; Benzamycin; Erycen; Erymax; Erythrocin; Erythromid; Erythroped; Erythroped A; Ilosone; Rommix; Stiemycin; Zineryt.

Erythroped

(Abbott) is a proprietary, prescription-only preparation of the ANTIBACTERIAL and (MACROLIDE) ANTIBIOTIC erythromycin. It can be used to treat and prevent many forms of infection, and is available as a suspension in several forms, *Erythroped SF, Forte* or *PI SF*, and as granules, *Erythroped PI* or *Forte*.

+▲ Side-effects/warning: See ERYTHROMYCIN.

Erythroped A

(Abbott) is a proprietary, prescription-only preparation of the ANTIBACTERIAL and (MACROLIDE) ANTIBIOTIC erythromycin. It can be used to treat and prevent many forms of infection, and is available as tablets and granules.

+▲ Side-effects/warning: See ERYTHROMYCIN.

eserine

see PHYSOSTIGMINE SULPHATE

Eskamel

(Goldshield) is a proprietary, non-prescription COMPOUND PREPARATION of the KERATOLYTIC agent resorcinol and sulphur. It can be used to treat acne, and is available as a cream.

+▲ Side-effects/warning: See RESORCINOL.

Eskazole

(SK&F) is a proprietary, prescription-only preparation of the ANTHELMINTIC drug albendazole. It can be used to provide cover during surgery for the removal of cysts caused by the tapeworm *Echinococcus*, as a treatment when surgery is not possible and also to treat strongyloidiasis. It is available as tablets.

✚▲ Side-effects/warning: See ALBENDAZOLE.

Eskornade Capsules

(Goldshield) is a proprietary, non-prescription COMPOUND PREPARATION of the SYMPATHOMIMETIC, VASOCONSTRICTOR and NASAL DECONGESTANT phenylpropanolamine hydrochloride and the ANTIHISTAMINE diphenylpyraline hydrochloride. It can be used for the symptomatic relief of the congestive symptoms of colds, allergy and flu. It is available as capsules and is not normally given to children under 12 years, except on medical advice.

✚▲ Side-effects/warning: See DIPHENYLPYRALINE HYDROCHLORIDE; PHENYLPROPANOLAMINE HYDROCHLORIDE.

Esmeron

(Organon-Teknika) is a proprietary, prescription-only preparation of the (*non-depolarizing*) SKELETAL MUSCLE RELAXANT rocuronium bromide. It can be used to induce muscle paralysis during surgery, and is available in a form for injection.

✚▲ Side-effects/warning: See ROCURONIUM BROMIDE.

esmolol hydrochloride

is a BETA-BLOCKER which can be used as an ANTIHYPERTENSIVE for raised blood pressure during operations and as an ANTIARRHYTHMIC, in the short term, to regularize heartbeat. Administration is by injection.

✚▲ Side-effects/warning: See PROPRANOLOL HYDROCHLORIDE.

✪ Related entry: Brevibloc.

Estracombi

(Ciba) is a proprietary, prescription-only COMPOUND PREPARATION of the female SEX HORMONES oestradiol (an OESTROGEN) and norethisterone (as acetate; a PROGESTOGEN). It can be used to treat menopausal problems, including in HRT, and is available as skin patches.

✚▲ Side-effects/warning: See NORETHISTERONE; OESTRADIOL.

Estracyt

(Pharmacia) is a proprietary, prescription-only preparation of the (CYTOTOXIC) ANTICANCER drug estramustine phosphate. It can be used to treat cancer of the prostate gland, and is available as capsules.

✚▲ Side-effects/warning: See ESTRAMUSTINE PHOSPHATE.

Estraderm MX

(Ciba) is a proprietary, prescription-only preparation of the OESTROGEN oestradiol. It can be used in HRT, and is available in the form of skin patches.

✚▲ Side-effects/warning: See OESTRADIOL.

Estraderm TTS

(Ciba) is a proprietary, prescription-only preparation of the OESTROGEN oestradiol. It can be used in HRT, and is available as skin patches.

✚▲ Side-effects/warning: See OESTRADIOL.

Estradurin

(Pharmacia) is a proprietary, prescription-only COMPOUND PREPARATION of the SEX HORMONE analogue polyestradiol phosphate (an OESTROGEN), the LOCAL ANAESTHETIC mepivacaine and the B vitamin nicotinamide. It can be used to treat cancer of the prostate gland, and is available in a form for injection.

✚▲ Side-effects/warning: See POLYESTRADIOL PHOSPHATE.

estramustine phosphate

is a CYTOTOXIC drug and an OESTROGEN. It can be used to treat cancer of the prostate gland, and is administered orally.

✚▲ Side-effects/warning: See CYTOTOXICS. It causes some feminization in men (eg growth of breasts), altered liver function

and cardiovascular disorders. It should not be used in patients with peptic ulcer or severe heart or liver disorders.
○ Related entry: Estracyt.

Estrapak 50

(Ciba) is a proprietary, prescription-only COMPOUND PREPARATION of the female SEX HORMONES oestradiol (an OESTROGEN) and norethisterone (a PROGESTOGEN). It can be used in HRT, and is available as tablets in a calendar pack and as skin patches.
✚▲ Side-effects/warning: See NORETHISTERONE; OESTRADIOL.

Estring

(Pharmacia) is a proprietary, prescription-only preparation of the female SEX HORMONE (an OESTROGEN) oestradiol. It can be used to treat urogenital complaints in postmenopausal women, and is available as a vaginal ring.
✚▲ Side-effects/warning: See OESTRADIOL.

etacrynic acid

see ETHACRYNIC ACID

etamsylate

see ETHAMSYLATE

ethacrynic acid

(etacrynic acid) is a powerful *loop* DIURETIC which can be used to treat oedema, particularly pulmonary (lung) oedema in patients with chronic heart failure or left ventricular heart failure and low urine production due to kidney failure (oliguria). Administration is by injection or infusion.
✚▲ Side-effects/warning: See FRUSEMIDE; but more gastrointestinal disturbances; also pain at injection site. Do not use when breast-feeding. Deafness may occur in renal failure.
○ Related entry: Edecrin.

ethambutol hydrochloride

is an ANTIBACTERIAL which is used as an ANTITUBERCULAR treatment for tuberculosis that is resistant to other types of drug. It is

used mainly in combination (to cover resistance and for maximum effect) with other antitubercular drugs, such as isoniazid or rifampicin. Administration is oral.
✚ Side-effects: These are rare and mostly in the form of visual disturbances (such as loss of acuity or colour-blindness).
▲ Warning: It should not be administered to children under six years or to patients who suffer from nervous disorders of the eyes. Administer with caution to patients with poor kidney function, the elderly or who are pregnant. Eye tests are advised during treatment.
○ Related entry: Myambutol.

ethamsylate

(etamsylate) is a HAEMOSTATIC agent that can be used in some situations where antifibrinolytic drugs might be used, though it appears not to work in the way such drugs normally do (ie preventing clot formation). It seems to improve platelet adhesion (stickiness) and reduce capillary bleeding, and can be used for bleeding in premature infants and menorrhagia (excessive periods bleeding). Administration is either oral or by injection.
✚ Side-effects: Headache, nausea and rashes.
▲ Warning: It should not be administered to patients with porphyria.
○ Related entry: Dicynene.

ethanol

see ETHYL ALCOHOL

ethanolamine oleate

(monoethanolamine oleate) is used in sclerotherapy, which is a technique to treat varicose veins by the injection of an irritant solution. Administration is by slow injection.
✚ Side-effects: Some patients experience allergic sensitivity reactions.
▲ Warning: Leakage of the drug into the tissues at the site of injection may cause tissue damage. It should not be injected into

patients whose varicose veins are already inflamed or so painful as to prevent walking, who are obese or are taking oral contraceptives.

○ Related entry: Ethanolamine Oleate Injection.

Ethanolamine Oleate Injection

(Evans) is a proprietary, prescription-only preparation of ethanolamine oleate. It can be used in sclerotherapy, which is a technique to treat varicose veins by the injection of an irritant solution.

✚▲ Side-effects/warning: See ETHANOLAMINE OLEATE.

ethinyloestradiol

is a female SEX HORMONE, a synthetic OESTROGEN, that has been used to make up hormonal deficiencies – sometimes in combination with a PROGESTOGEN – to treat menstrual, menopausal or other gynaecological problems, and is also a constituent of many ORAL CONTRACEPTIVES. It can also be used as an ANTICANCER drug in men with cancer of the prostate; and rarely (under specialist care) for hereditary haemorrhagic telangiectasia (hereditary condition of distended blood capillaries and bleeding). One form is available as a COMPOUND PREPARATION with CYPROTERONE ACETATE for the treatment of acne and abnormal bodily hair growth. Administration is oral.

✚▲ Side-effects/warning: These depend on use; also, see OESTROGENS. There may be nausea and vomiting. A common effect is weight gain, generally through fluid or sodium retention in the tissues. The breasts may become tender and enlarge slightly. There may also be headache and/or depression; sometimes a rash; thrombosis; in men, impotence and breast enlargement.

○ Related entries: BiNovum; Brevinor; Cilest; Dianette; Eugynon 30; Femodene; Femodene ED; Loestrin 20; Loestrin 30; Logynon; Logynon ED; Marvelon; Mercilon; Microgynon 30; Minulet; Normin; Ovran;

Ovran 30; Ovranette; Ovysmen; Schering PC4; Synphase; Triadene; Tri-Minulet; Trinordiol; TriNovum; TriNovum ED.

Ethmozine

(Monmouth) is a proprietary, prescription-only preparation of the ANTI-ARRHYTHMIC moracizine hydrochloride. It can be used to treat irregularities of the heartbeat, and is available as tablets.

✚▲ Side-effects/warning: See MORACIZINE HYDROCHLORIDE.

ethosuximide

is an ANTICONVULSANT and ANTI-EPILEPTIC which is used to treat absence (petit mal), myoclonic and some other types of seizure. Administration is oral.

✚ Side-effects: There may be gastrointestinal disturbances, drowsiness, dizziness, unsteady gait, movement disturbances, headache, hiccup, depression or mild euphoria, rashes, liver changes, effects on blood and psychotic states.

▲ Warning: It should be administered with caution to patients with porphyria, kidney or liver impairment, or who are pregnant or breast-feeding. The withdrawal of treatment should be gradual.

○ Related entries: Emeside; Zarontin.

ethyl alcohol

or ethanol, is the form of alcohol that is produced by the fermentation of sugar by yeast and which is found in alcoholic drinks. Therapeutically, it is used as a solvent in some medicines and as an ANTISEPTIC.

✚▲ Side-effects/warning: See ALCOHOL.

ethyl salicylate

like a number of other SALICYLATES, can exert a COUNTER-IRRITANT, or RUBEFACIENT, action on topical application to relieve inflammatory pain in joints and muscles.

✚▲ Side-effects/warning: On topical administration there may be local irritation. It should not be used on broken skin or mucous membranes.

E

○ Related entries: Aspellin; Dubam; Deep Heat Spray; Ralgex Stick; Transvasin Heat Rub.

ethynodiol diacetate
is a PROGESTOGEN which is used as a constituent of the combined ORAL CONTRACEPTIVES. Administration is oral.
✚▲ Side-effects/warning: See PROGESTOGEN.
○ Related entry: Femulen.

Ethyol
(Schering-Plough) is a proprietary, prescription-only preparation of amifostine, which is a specialist drug that is administered to reduce neutropenia-related risk of infection due to treatment of ovarian carcinoma with CYCLOPHOSPHAMIDE or CISPLATIN. It is available in a form for injection.
✚▲ Side-effects/warning: See AMIFOSTINE.

etodolac
is a (NSAID) NON-NARCOTIC ANALGESIC and ANTIRHEUMATIC drug. It is used primarily to treat the pain and inflammation of rheumatoid arthritis and osteoarthritis. Administration is oral.
✚▲ Side-effects/warning: See NSAID.
○ Related entry: Lodine.

etomidate
is a GENERAL ANAESTHETIC which is used for the initial induction of anaesthesia. The recovery from the effects of this drug after treatment is rapid and without any hangover symptoms, and it also causes less of a fall in blood pressure than many other anaesthetics. Administration is by intravenous infusion.
✚ Side-effects: Pain on injection, extraneous muscle movements; repeated doses may suppress the secretion of corticosteroid hormones by the adrenal glands.
▲ Warning: It is not to be used in patients with porphyria.
○ Related entry: Hypnomidate.

etoposide
is an ANTICANCER drug which is used primarily to treat small cell lung cancer, lymphomas and cancer of the testes. It works in much the same way as the VINCA ALKALOIDS by disrupting the replication of cancer cells and so preventing further growth. Administration is either oral or by injection.
✚▲ Side-effects/warning: See CYTOTOXICS.
○ Related entry: Vepesid.

Eucardic
(Boehringer Mannheim) is a proprietary, prescription-only preparation of the BETA-BLOCKER carvedilol. It can be used as an ANTIHYPERTENSIVE, and is available as tablets.
✚▲ Side-effects/warning: See CARVEDILOL.

Eudemine (injection)
(Link) is a proprietary, prescription-only preparation of diazoxide. It can be used, when administered by injection, as an ANTIHYPERTENSIVE to treat hypertensive crisis. It is available in a form for rapid intravenous injection.
✚▲ Side-effects/warning: See DIAZOXIDE.

Eudemine (tablets)
(Evans) is a proprietary, prescription-only preparation of diazoxide. It can be used, when taken orally, as a HYPOGLYCAEMIC to treat chronic hypoglycaemia. It is available as tablets.
✚▲ Side-effects/warning: See DIAZOXIDE.

Euglucon
(Roussel) is a proprietary, prescription-only preparation of the SULPHONYLUREA glibenclamide. It is used in DIABETIC TREATMENT of Type II diabetes (non-insulin-dependent diabetes mellitus; NIDDM; maturity-onset diabetes), and is available as tablets.
✚▲ Side-effects/warning: See GLIBENCLAMIDE.

Eugynon 30
(Schering) is a proprietary, prescription-

only COMPOUND PREPARATION which can be used as a (*monophasic*) ORAL CONTRACEPTIVE (and also for certain menstrual problems) of the type that combines an OESTROGEN and a PROGESTOGEN, in this case ethinyloestradiol and levonorgestrel. It is available as tablets in a calendar pack.

+▲ Side-effects/warning: See ETHINYLOESTRADIOL; LEVONORGESTREL.

Eumovate

(Glaxo) is a proprietary, prescription-only preparation of the CORTICOSTEROID and ANTI-INFLAMMATORY clobetasone butyrate. It can be used to treat non-infective and severe inflammation of the skin caused by conditions such as eczema and various forms of dermatitis. It is used particularly as a maintenance treatment between courses of more potent corticosteroids. It is available as a cream and an ointment.

+▲ Side-effects/warning: See CLOBETASONE BUTYRATE.

Eumovate-N

(Cusi) is a proprietary, prescription-only COMPOUND PREPARATION of the ANTI-INFLAMMATORY and CORTICOSTEROID clobetasone butyrate and the ANTIBACTERIAL and (AMINOGLYCOSIDE) ANTIBIOTIC neomycin sulphate. It can be used to treat inflammation of the eye when infection is also present, and is available as eye-drops.

+▲ Side-effects/warning: See CLOBETASONE BUTYRATE; NEOMYCIN SULPHATE.

Eurax

(Zyma) is a proprietary, non-prescription preparation of crotamiton. It can be used to treat itching, especially in scabies, and is available as a lotion and a cream; the cream is not normally given to children under ten years, except on medical advice.

+▲ Side-effects/warning: See CROTAMITON.

Eurax-Hydrocortisone

(Zyma) is a proprietary, prescription-only COMPOUND PREPARATION of the CORTICOSTEROID and ANTI-INFLAMMATORY hydrocortisone and crotamiton. It is used to treat itching (eg in scabies) and inflammation of the skin, and is available as a cream for topical application.

+▲ Side-effects/warning: See CROTAMITON; HYDROCORTISONE.

Evorel

(Cilag) is a proprietary, prescription-only preparation of the OESTROGEN oestradiol. It can be used in HRT, and is available in the form of skin patches.

+▲ Side-effects/warning: See OESTRADIOL.

Evorel Pak

(Cilag) is a proprietary, prescription-only COMPOUND PREPARATION of the OESTROGEN oestradiol and the PROGESTOGEN norethisterone. It can be used in HRT, and is available as skin patches.

+▲ Side-effects/warning: See NORETHISTERONE; OESTRADIOL.

Ex-Lax Chocolate

(Intercare) is a proprietary, non-prescription preparation of the (stimulant) LAXATIVE phenolphthalein. It can be used to relieve constipation, and is available as a chocolate bar. It is not normally given to children under six years, except on medical advice.

+▲ Side-effects/warning: See PHENOLPHTHALEIN.

Ex-Lax Pills

(Intercare) is a proprietary, non-prescription preparation of the (stimulant) LAXATIVE phenolphthalein. It can be used to relieve constipation, and is available as pills. It is not normally given to children under six years, except on medical advice.

+▲ Side-effects/warning: See PHENOLPHTHALEIN.

Exelderm

(Zeneca) is a proprietary, prescription-only preparation of the ANTIFUNGAL sulconazole nitrate. It can be used to treat fungal skin

E

infections, particularly tinea, and is available as a cream for topical application.
✚▲ Side-effects/warning: See SULCONAZOLE NITRATE.

Exirel

(3M) is a proprietary, prescription-only preparation of the BETA-RECEPTOR STIMULANT pirbuterol. It can be used as a BRONCHODILATOR in reversible obstructive airways disease, as an ANTI-ASTHMATIC treatment in severe acute asthma and for the alleviation of the symptoms of chronic bronchitis and emphysema. It is available as a metered aerosol inhalant and capsules.
✚▲ Side-effects/warning: See PIRBUTEROL.

Exocin

(Allergan) is a proprietary, prescription-only preparation of the ANTIBACTERIAL and (QUINOLONE) ANTIBIOTIC ofloxacin. It can be used to treat bacterial infections of the eye, and is available as eye-drops.
✚▲ Side-effects/warning: See OFLOXACIN.

expectorants ⚡

are medicated liquids intended to change the viscosity of sputum (phlegm), so making it more watery and easier to cough up (an action of MUCOLYTICS). In high dosage, most expectorants can be used as EMETICS (to provoke vomiting), which leads to the traditional suggestion that they act as expectorants by stimulating nerves in the stomach to cause reflex secretion of fluid by the bronchioles in the lungs. However, it is not known for sure how they act and, further, there is considerable doubt about their clinical efficacy. Examples include IPECACUANHA, GUAIPHENESIN and AMMONIUM CHLORIDE.

Expelix

(Cupal) is a proprietary, non-prescription preparation of the ANTHELMINTIC drug piperazine (as citrate). It can be used to treat infestation by threadworms or roundworms, and is available as an elixir.
✚▲ Side-effects/warning: See PIPERAZINE.

Expulin Children's Cough Linctus – Sugar Free

(Monmouth) is a proprietary, non-prescription COMPOUND PREPARATION of the ANTIHISTAMINE chlorpheniramine maleate and the (OPIOID) ANTITUSSIVE pholcodine. It can be used for the symptomatic relief of cough in children, and is available as an oral liquid. It is not normally given to children under one year, except on medical advice.
✚▲ Side-effects/warning: See CHLORPHENIRAMINE MALEATE; PHOLCODINE.

Expulin Cough Linctus – Sugar Free

(Monmouth) is a proprietary, non-prescription COMPOUND PREPARATION of the SYMPATHOMIMETIC and DECONGESTANT pseudoephedrine hydrochloride, the ANTIHISTAMINE chlorpheniramine maleate and the (OPIOID) ANTITUSSIVE pholcodine. It can be used for the symptomatic relief of congestion and cough associated with colds and flu. It is available as an oral liquid and is not normally given to children, except on medical advice.
✚▲ Side-effects/warning: See CHLORPHENIRAMINE MALEATE; PSEUDOEPHEDRINE HYDROCHLORIDE; PHOLCODINE.

Expulin Decongestant for Babies and Children (Linctus)

(Monmouth) is a proprietary, non-prescription COMPOUND PREPARATION of the SYMPATHOMIMETIC and DECONGESTANT ephedrine hydrochloride and the ANTIHISTAMINE chlorpheniramine maleate. It can be used for the symptomatic relief of congestion and runny nose associated with colds and flu. It is available as a liquid and is not normally given to children under three months, except on medical advice.
✚▲ Side-effects/warning: See CHLORPHENIRAMINE MALEATE; EPHEDRINE HYDROCHLORIDE.

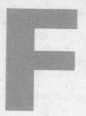

Expulin Dry Cough Linctus

(Monmouth) is a proprietary, non-prescription preparation of the (OPIOID) ANTITUSSIVE pholcodine. It can be used for the symptomatic relief of dry persistent cough, and is available as an oral liquid. It is not not normally given to children, except on medical advice.

✚▲ Side-effects/warning: See PHOLCODINE.

Exterol

(Dermal) is a proprietary, non-prescription preparation of the ANTISEPTIC agent HYDROGEN PEROXIDE in a complex with UREA in GLYCEROL. It can be used to dissolve and wash out earwax, and is available as ear-drops.

factor VIIA (recombinant)

is a preparation of recombinant human antihaemophilic factor VII. It acts as a HAEMOSTATIC drug to reduce or stop bleeding and is used to treat disorders in which bleeding is prolonged and potentially dangerous, usually patients with inhibitors to factors VIII and IX. Administration is by injection.

○ Related entry: NovoSeven.

factor VIII fraction (dried)

(human antihaemophilic fraction, dried) is a dried principle prepared from blood plasma obtained from healthy human donors. It acts as a HAEMOSTATIC drug to reduce or stop bleeding, and is administered by intravenous infusion or injection to treat disorders in which bleeding is prolonged and potentially dangerous (mainly haemophilia A).

✚ Side-effects: There may be allergic reactions with fever or chills; raised fibrin levels in the blood are rarely seen after extensive use.

▲ Warning: Clotting within blood vessels is possible after large or frequent doses (in blood groups A, B and AB).

○ Related entries: Alpha VIII; High Potency Factor VIII Concentrate; Kogenate; Monoclate-P; Recombinate; 8SM; 8Y.

factor VIII fraction (octocog alfa)

is a preparation of recombinant human antihaemophilic factor VIII. It acts as a HAEMOSTATIC drug to reduce or stop

235

F

bleeding, and is administered by
intravenous infusion or injection to treat
disorders in which bleeding is prolonged
and potentially dangerous (mainly
haemophilia A).

+▲ Side-effects/warning: See FACTOR VIII
FRACTION, DRIED.

○ Related entries: Kogenate; Recombinate.

factor VIII inhibitor bypassing fraction

is prepared from blood plasma obtained
from healthy human donors and used as a
HAEMOSTATIC in patients with factor VIII
inhibitors. It is available, only on
prescription, in a form for infusion.

○ Related entry: Hyate C.

factor IX fraction, dried

is prepared from human blood plasma. It
may also contain clotting factor II, VII and
X. It is used in treating patients with a
deficiency in factor IX (haemophilia B) and
hereditary deficiency of factor IX
(Christmas Factor). It is available only on
prescription and in a form for infusion.

+ Side-effects: There may be allergic
reactions with fever or chills.

▲ Warning: Risk of thrombosis (blood
clots); it should not be used in conditions of
uncontrolled generalized clotting
(disseminated intravascular coagulation).

○ Related entries: Alphanine; Mononine;
Replenine.

famciclovir

is an ANTIVIRAL drug similar to ACYCLOVIR, but
which can be given less often. It is used to
treat infection caused by herpes zoster.
Administration is oral.

+ Side-effects: Headache and nausea.

▲ Warning: It should be administered with
caution to patients who are pregnant or
breast-feeding, or who have impaired kidney
function.

○ Related entry: Famvir.

Famel Expectorant

(Seton) is a proprietary, non-prescription

preparation of the EXPECTORANT agent
GUAIPHENESIN. It can be used for the
symptomatic relief of chesty coughs,
bronchial congestion and catarrh. It is
available as a linctus and is not normally
given to children under one year, except on
medical advice.

Famel Linctus

(Seton) is a proprietary, non-prescription
preparation of the ANTITUSSIVE pholcodine.
It can be used for the relief of dry and
irritating coughs, and is available as a
linctus. It is not normally given to children
under five years, except on medical advice.

+▲ Side-effects/warning: See PHOLCODINE.

Famel Original Cough Syrup

(Seton) is a proprietary non-prescription
preparation of the OPIOID codeine
phosphate. It can be used as an ANTITUSSIVE
to relieve a dry, troublesome cough, and is
available as a linctus, together with
creosote. It is not normally given to
children under 12 years, except on medical
advice.

+▲ Side-effects/warning: See CODEINE
PHOSPHATE.

famotidine

is an H_2-ANTAGONIST and ULCER-HEALING DRUG.
It can be used to assist in the treatment of
benign peptic (gastric and duodenal)
ulcers, to relieve heartburn in cases of
reflux oesophagitis, Zollinger-Ellison
syndrome and a variety of conditions where
reduction of acidity is beneficial. It is now
also available without prescription – but in
a limited amount and for short-term uses
only – for the relief of heartburn, dyspepsia
and hyperacidity. It works by reducing the
secretion of gastric acid (by acting as a
histamine receptor H_2-receptor antagonist),
and therefore reducing erosion and
bleeding from peptic ulcers and allowing
them a chance to heal. However, treatment
with famotidine should not commence until
a full and thorough diagnosis of gastric
bleeding or serious pain has been

completed, because its action in restricting gastric secretions may possibly mask the presence of stomach cancer. Administration is oral.

✚▲ Side-effects/warning: See CIMETIDINE; but it does not significantly inhibit microsomal drug-metabolizing enzymes.
◐ Related entries: Pepcid; Pepcid AC.

Famvir
(SmithKline Beecham) is a proprietary, prescription-only preparation of the ANTIVIRAL drug famciclovir. It can be used to treat infections caused by herpes zoster, and is available as tablets.

✚▲ Side-effects/warning: See FAMCICLOVIR.

Fansidar
(Roche) is a proprietary, prescription-only COMPOUND PREPARATION of the ANTIMALARIAL drug pyrimethamine and the SULPHONAMIDE sulfadoxine. It can be used to treat patients who are seriously ill with malaria, and is available as tablets.

✚▲ Side-effects/warning: See
PYRIMETHAMINE; SULFADOXINE.

Fareston
(Orion) is a proprietary, prescription-only preparation of the sex HORMONE ANTAGONIST toremifene (as citrate). It inhibits the effect of OESTROGENS and because of this is used as an ANTICANCER treatment of hormone-dependent metastatic breast cancer in postmenopausal women. It is available as tablets.

✚▲ Side-effects/warning: See TOREMIFENE.

Farlutal
(Pharmacia) is a proprietary, prescription-only preparation of the SEX HORMONE medroxyprogesterone acetate (a synthetic PROGESTOGEN). It can be used as an ANTICANCER treatment in women for cancer of the breast or uterine endometrium. It is available as tablets and in a form for injection.

✚▲ Side-effects/warning: See
MEDROXYPROGESTERONE ACETATE.

Fasigyn
(Pfizer) is a proprietary, prescription-only preparation of the ANTIBACTERIAL and ANTIPROTOZOAL tinidazole. It can be used to treat anaerobic infections, such as bacterial vaginitis, and protozoal infections, such as giardiasis, trichomoniasis and amoebiasis. It can also be used to treat acute ulcerative gingivitis and to prevent infection following abdominal surgery. It is available as tablets.

✚▲ Side-effects/warning: See TINIDAZOLE.

Faverin
(Duphar) is a proprietary, prescription-only preparation of the (SSRI) ANTIDEPRESSANT fluvoxamine maleate, which has less sedative effects than some other antidepressants. It is available as tablets.

✚▲ Side-effects/warning: See FLUVOXAMINE MALEATE.

Fectrim
(DDSA) is a proprietary, prescription-only COMPOUND PREPARATION of the (SULPHONAMIDE) ANTIBACTERIAL sulphamethoxazole and the antibacterial trimethoprim, which is a combination called co-trimoxazole. It can be used to treat bacterial infections, particularly prostatitis, bronchitis and infections of the urinary tract. It is available as soluble tablets; a stronger preparation, *Fectrim Forte*, is also available.

✚▲ Side-effects/warning: See CO-TRIMOXAZOLE.

Fefol
(Evans) is a proprietary, non-prescription COMPOUND PREPARATION of ferrous sulphate and folic acid. It can be used as an IRON and folic acid supplement during pregnancy, and is available as capsules.

✚▲ Side-effects/warning: See FERROUS SULPHATE; FOLIC ACID.

Feldene
(Pfizer) is a proprietary, prescription-only preparation of the (NSAID) NON-NARCOTIC ANALGESIC and ANTIRHEUMATIC piroxicam. It

F

can be used to treat acute gout, arthritic and rheumatic pain and other musculoskeletal disorders. It is available as capsules, soluble tablets, as suppositories and in a form for injection. It is also available as a preparation called *Feldene Melt*, which can be taken by placing on the tongue.

+▲ Side-effects/warning: See PIROXICAM.

Feldene Gel

(Pfizer) is a proprietary, prescription-only preparation of the (NSAID) NON-NARCOTIC ANALGESIC and ANTIRHEUMATIC piroxicam, which also has COUNTER-IRRITANT, or RUBEFACIENT, actions. It can be applied topically to the skin for symptomatic relief of underlying muscle or joint pain, and is available as a gel.

+▲ Side-effects/warning: See PIROXICAM; but adverse effects on topical application are limited.

felodipine

is a CALCIUM-CHANNEL BLOCKER which is used as an ANTIHYPERTENSIVE. Administration is oral.

+ Side-effects: These include flushing, headache and fatigue; dizziness; palpitations; rashes; oedema. There may be an excessive growth of the gums.

▲ Warning: It should be administered with care to patients with certain liver disorders or who are breast-feeding; withdraw treatment if there is ischaemic pain (pain due to lack of blood supply). Do not use in pregnancy.

✪ Related entry: Plendil.

felypressin

is an analogue of vasopressin and is used as a VASOCONSTRICTOR and incorporated into LOCAL ANAESTHETIC preparations to prolong their duration of action.

+▲ Side-effects/warning: See VASOPRESSIN.
✪ Related entry: Citanest with Octapressin.

Femapak 80

(Solvay) is a proprietary, prescription-only

preparation that is a combination pack containing patches of *Fematrix*, which release the OESTROGEN oestradiol, and tablets of *Duphaston*, which release the PROGESTOGEN (dydrogesterone). It can be used to treat many conditions of hormonal deficiency in women, including menopausal symptoms as part of HRT.

+▲ Side-effects/warning: See DYDROGESTERONE, OESTRADIOL.

Femara

(Ciba) is a proprietary, prescription-only preparation of the sex HORMONE ANTAGONIST letrozole. It inhibits the effect of OESTROGENS and because of this is used as an ANTICANCER treatment of hormone-dependent breast cancer in postmenopausal women. It is available as tablets.

+▲ Side-effects/warning: See LETROZOLE.

Fematrix

(Solvay) is a proprietary, prescription-only preparation that releases the OESTROGEN oestradiol. It can be used to treat many conditions of hormonal deficiency in women, including menopausal symptoms as part of HRT. It is available as patches.

+▲ Side-effects/warning: See OESTRADIOL.

Femeron

(Janssen) is a proprietary, non-prescription preparation of the ANTIFUNGAL miconazole (as nitrate). It can be used to soothe and treat external vaginal itching due to *Candida* fungal infections (thrush), and is available as a cream.

+▲ Side-effects/warning: See MICONAZOLE.

Femeron Soft Pessary

(Janssen) is a proprietary, non-prescription preparation of the ANTIFUNGAL miconazole (as nitrate). It can be used to treat vaginal *Candida* fungal infections (thrush), and is available as soft, gelatin vaginal pessaries.

+▲ Side-effects/warning: See MICONAZOLE.

Femigraine

(Roche) is a proprietary, non-prescription

COMPOUND PREPARATION of the ANTIHISTAMINE cyclizine hydrochloride and the (NSAID) NON-NARCOTIC ANALGESIC and ANTIRHEUMATIC aspirin. It can be used as an ANTIMIGRAINE treatment for acute migraine attacks and associated nausea, but not prophylactically to prevent attacks. It is available as soluble (effervescent) tablets. The preparations are not normally given to children under 12 years, except on medical advice.

+▲ Side-effects/warning: See ASPIRIN; CYCLIZINE.

Feminax

(Roche) is a proprietary, non-prescription COMPOUND ANALGESIC preparation of the NON-NARCOTIC ANALGESIC paracetamol, the NARCOTIC ANALGESIC codeine phosphate, the STIMULANT caffeine and the ANTICHOLINERGIC and ANTISPASMODIC hyoscine hydrobromide. It can be used specifically for the relief of period pain, and is available as capsules.

+▲ Side-effects/warning: See CAFFEINE; CODEINE PHOSPHATE; HYOSCINE HYDROBROMIDE; PARACETAMOL.

Femodene

(Schering) is a proprietary, prescription-only COMPOUND PREPARATION which can be used as a (*monophasic*) ORAL CONTRACEPTIVE (and also for certain menstrual problems) of the type that combines an OESTROGEN and a PROGESTOGEN, in this case ethinyloestradiol and gestodene. It is available as tablets in a calendar pack.

+▲ Side-effects/warning: See ETHINYLOESTRADIOL; GESTODENE.

Femodene ED

(Schering) is a proprietary, prescription-only COMPOUND PREPARATION which can be used as a (*monophasic*) ORAL CONTRACEPTIVE (and also for certain menstrual problems) of the type that combines an OESTROGEN and a PROGESTOGEN, in this case ethinyloestradiol and gestodene. It is available as tablets in a calendar pack.

+▲ Side-effects/warning: See ETHINYLOESTRADIOL; GESTODENE.

Femoston

(Solvay) is a proprietary, prescription-only preparation that is a combination pack containing tablets of both the OESTROGEN oestradiol and the PROGESTOGEN dydrogesterone. They are available in various dosage combinations (called *1/10, 2/10* and *2/20*), and can be used to treat many conditions of hormonal deficiency in women, including menopausal symptoms as part of HRT.

+▲ Side-effects/warning: See DYDROGESTERONE; OESTRADIOL.

FemSeven

(Merck) is a proprietary, prescription-only preparation that releases the OESTROGEN oestradiol. It can be used to treat a wide range of hormonal deficiency conditions in women, such as menopausal symptoms as part of HRT (including the prevention of osteoporosis). It is available as patches.

+▲ Side-effects/warning: See OESTRADIOL.

Femulen

(Searle) is a proprietary, prescription-only preparation which can be used as an ORAL CONTRACEPTIVE of the PROGESTOGEN-only pill (POP) type and contains ethynodiol acetate. It is available as tablets in a calendar pack.

+▲ Side-effects/warning: See ETHYNODIOL ACETATE.

Fenbid

(Goldshield) is a proprietary, prescription-only preparation of the (NSAID) NON-NARCOTIC ANALGESIC and ANTIRHEUMATIC ibuprofen. It can be used to treat all kinds of pain and inflammation, especially pain from arthritis and rheumatism and other musculoskeletal disorders, and is available as modified-release capsules (*Spansules*).

+▲ Side-effects/warning: See IBUPROFEN.

fenbufen

is a (NSAID) NON-NARCOTIC ANALGESIC and ANTIRHEUMATIC drug. It has effects similar to those of aspirin and is used particularly in the treatment of pain associated with

F

rheumatoid arthritis and osteoarthritis.
✚▲ Side-effect/warning: See NSAID. It is thought to cause less gastrointestinal bleeding than other NSAIDs. However, it has a greater risk of causing rashes and may cause nasopharyngitis.
❍ Related entries: Fenbuzip; Lederfen; Traxam.

Fenbuzip

(Ashbourne) is a proprietary, prescription-only preparation of the (NSAID) NON-NARCOTIC ANALGESIC and ANTIRHEUMATIC fenbufen. It can be used to relieve pain and inflammation, particularly rheumatic and arthritic pain and to treat other musculoskeletal disorders, and is available as tablets and capsules.
✚▲ Side-effects/warning: See FENBUFEN.

fenfluramine hydrochloride

is an APPETITE SUPPRESSANT which is used in the short term to aid the slimming regimes of obese patients. It is not a stimulant (unlike most other appetite suppressants of this type) but has sedative properties that may affect a patient's intricacy of thought and movement.
✚ Side-effects: There may be depression; sedation with headache, disturbed sleep, drowsiness, irritability, impotence and loss of libido, effects on blood pressure, vertigo and gastric upsets. Sometimes there is insomnia, dry mouth, fluid retention, increased frequency of urination; and there may be blood disorders, rashes and schizophrenia-like behaviour. Treatment is only in the short term as tolerance and/or dependence may occur; dosage should be tapered off gradually to avoid withdrawal depression.
▲ Warning: It may affect mental concentration and enhances the effect of alcohol. It should not be used in patients with a history of drug abuse, psychiatric illness, epilepsy, glaucoma or alcoholism; or who are pregnant or breast-feeding.
❍ Related entry: Ponderax.

Fennings Children's Cooling Powders

(Fenning) is a proprietary, non-prescription preparation of the NON-NARCOTIC ANALGESIC paracetamol. It can be used for the relief of cold symptoms, teething pain, headache, feverishness and pain. It is available as a powder and is not normally given to babies under three months, except on medical advice.
✚▲ Side-effects/warning: See PARACETAMOL.

fenofibrate

can be used as a LIPID-LOWERING DRUG in hyperlipidaemia to reduce the levels, or change the proportions, of various lipids in the bloodstream. It is usually administered only to patients in whom a strict and regular dietary regime, alone, is not having the desired effect. Administration is oral.
✚▲ Side-effects/warning: See BEZAFIBRATE. It is not to be used in patients with gall bladder, severe kidney or liver disorders; or who are pregnant or breast-feeding.
❍ Related entry: Lipantil.

fenoprofen

is a (NSAID) NON-NARCOTIC ANALGESIC and ANTIRHEUMATIC drug. It can be used to treat and relieve pain and inflammation, particularly the pain of arthritis and rheumatism and other musculoskeletal disorders. Administration is oral.
✚▲ Side-effect/warning: See NSAID.
❍ Related entries: Fenopron 300; Fenopron 600; Progesic.

Fenopron 300

(Dista) is a proprietary, prescription-only preparation of the (NSAID) NON-NARCOTIC ANALGESIC and ANTIRHEUMATIC fenoprofen. It can be used to treat and relieve pain and inflammation, particularly the pain of arthritis and rheumatism and other musculoskeletal disorders. It is available as tablets.
✚▲ Side-effects/warning: See FENOPROFEN.

Fenopron 600

(Dista) is a proprietary, prescription-only preparation of the (NSAID) NON-NARCOTIC ANALGESIC and ANTIRHEUMATIC fenoprofen. It can be used to treat and relieve pain and inflammation, particularly the pain of arthritis and rheumatism and other musculoskeletal disorders. It is available as tablets.

+▲ Side-effects/warning: See FENOPROFEN.

fenoterol hydrobromide

is a SYMPATHOMIMETIC and BETA-RECEPTOR STIMULANT. It is mainly used as a BRONCHODILATOR in reversible obstructive airways disease and as an ANTI-ASTHMATIC treatment in severe acute asthma. It can also be used for the alleviation of symptoms of chronic bronchitis and emphysema. Administration is by aerosol. (Patients should be cautioned not to exceed the stated dose and if a previously effective dose fails to relieve symptoms, they must consult their doctor.)

+▲ Side-effects/warning: See SALBUTAMOL.
○ Related entries: Berotec; Duovent.

Fenox Nasal Drops

(Seton) is a proprietary, non-prescription preparation of the SYMPATHOMIMETIC and DECONGESTANT phenylephrine hydrochloride. It can be used for the symptomatic relief of nasal congestion associated with colds, catarrh, sinusitis and hay fever. It is available as viscous nose-drops and is not normally given to children under five years, except on medical advice.

+▲ Side-effects/warning: See PHENYLEPHRINE HYDROCHLORIDE.

Fenox Nasal Spray

(Seton) is a proprietary, non-prescription preparation of the SYMPATHOMIMETIC and DECONGESTANT phenylephrine hydrochloride. It can be used for the symptomatic relief of nasal congestion associated with colds, catarrh, sinusitis and hay fever. It is available as a nasal spray and is not normally given to children under five years, except on medical advice.

+▲ Side-effects/warning: See PHENYLEPHRINE HYDROCHLORIDE.

fentanyl

is an (OPIOID) NARCOTIC ANALGESIC which can be used to treat moderate to severe pain (mainly in operative procedures), to enhance general anaesthetics and to depress spontaneous respiration in patients having their breathing assisted. Administration is either by intravenous injection, with a relatively short duration of action, or transdermally as skin patches. Its proprietary preparations are on the Controlled Drugs List.

+▲ Side-effects/warning: See OPIOIDS.
○ Related entries: Durogesic; Sublimaze.

Fentazin

(Forley) is a proprietary, prescription-only preparation of the ANTIPSYCHOTIC perphenazine. It can be used to treat schizophrenia and other psychoses, and also as an ANTINAUSEANT and ANTI-EMETIC to relieve nausea and vomiting. It is available as tablets.

+▲ Side-effects/warning: See PERPHENAZINE.

fenticonazole nitrate

is an (IMIDAZOLE) ANTIFUNGAL drug. It can be used to treat fungal infections including vaginal candidiasis. Administration is by topical application.

+▲ Side-effects/warning: See CLOTRIMAZOLE. Occasionally, local irritation.
○ Related entry: Lomexin.

Feospan

(Evans) is a proprietary, non-prescription preparation of ferrous sulphate. It can be used as an IRON supplement in iron-deficiency ANAEMIA TREATMENT, and is available as modified-release capsules.

+▲ Side-effects/warning: SeeFERROUS SULPHATE.

Ferfolic SV

(Sinclair) is a proprietary, prescription-only COMPOUND PREPARATION of ferrous gluconate, folic acid and ascorbic acid. It can be used as an IRON and folic acid supplement during pregnancy, and is available as tablets.

✚▲ Side-effects/warning: See ASCORBIC ACID; FERROUS GLUCONATE; FOLIC ACID.

Fergon

(Sanofi Winthrop) is a proprietary, non-prescription preparation of ferrous gluconate. It can be used as an IRON supplement in iron-deficiency ANAEMIA TREATMENT, and is available as tablets.

✚▲ Side-effects/warning: See FERROUS GLUCONATE.

ferric ammonium citrate

is a drug rich in IRON which is used in iron-deficiency ANAEMIA TREATMENT to restore iron to the body, for example, to prevent deficiency in pregnancy.

✚▲ Side-effects/warning: See FERROUS SULPHATE.

✪ Related entries: Lexpec with Iron; Lexpec with Iron-M.

Ferrocontin Continus

(ASTA Medica) is a proprietary, non-prescription preparation of ferrous glycine sulphate. It can be used as an IRON supplement in iron-deficiency ANAEMIA TREATMENT and to prevent iron deficiency. It is available as modified-release tablets.

✚▲ Side-effects/warning: See FERROUS GLYCINE SULPHATE.

Ferrocontin Folic Continus

(ASTA Medica) is a proprietary, non-prescription COMPOUND PREPARATION of ferrous glycine sulphate and folic acid. It can be used as an IRON and folic acid supplement during pregnancy, and is available as capsules.

✚▲ Side-effects/warning: See FERROUS GLYCINE SULPHATE; FOLIC ACID.

Ferrograd

(Abbott) is a proprietary, non-prescription

proprietary preparation of the drug ferrous sulphate. It can be used as an IRON supplement in iron-deficiency ANAEMIA TREATMENT, and is available as modified-release tablets.

✚▲ Side-effects/warning: See FERROUS SULPHATE.

Ferrograd Folic

(Abbott) is a proprietary, non-prescription COMPOUND PREPARATION of ferrous sulphate and folic acid. It can be used as an IRON and folic acid supplement during pregnancy, and is available as modified-release capsules.

✚▲ Side-effects/warning: See FERROUS SULPHATE; FOLIC ACID.

ferrous fumarate

is a drug rich in IRON which is used in iron-deficiency ANAEMIA TREATMENT to restore iron to the body, for example, to prevent deficiency in pregnancy. Administration is oral.

✚▲ Side-effects/warning: See FERROUS SULPHATE.

✪ Related entries: Folex-350; Galfer; Galfer FA; Meterfolic; Pregaday; Slow-Fe Folic.

ferrous gluconate

is a drug rich in IRON which is used in iron-deficiency ANAEMIA TREATMENT to restore iron to the body, for example, to prevent deficiency in pregnancy. Administration is oral.

✚▲ Side-effects/warning: See FERROUS SULPHATE.

✪ Related entries: Ferfolic SV; Fergon.

ferrous glycine sulphate

is a drug rich in IRON which is used in iron-deficiency ANAEMIA TREATMENT to restore iron to the body, for example, to prevent deficiency in pregnancy.

✚▲ Side-effects/warning: See FERROUS SULPHATE.

✪ Related entries: Ferrocontin Continus; Ferrocontin Folic Continus; Plesmet.

ferrous sulphate

is a drug rich in IRON which is used in iron-deficiency ANAEMIA TREATMENT to restore iron, for example, to prevent deficiency in pregnancy. Administration is oral.

✚ Side-effects: Large doses may cause gastrointestinal upset and diarrhoea; there may be vomiting. Prolonged treatment may result in constipation.

▲ Warning: Iron preparations are best absorbed on an empty stomach, but may cause less gastrointestinal upsets if taken with food. Iron salts prevent the absorption of tetracycline antibiotics.

✪ Related entries: Fefol; Feospan; Ferrograd; Ferrograd Folic; Ferrous Sulphate Oral Solution, Paediatric, BP; Slow-Fe, Slow-Fe Folic.

Ferrous Sulphate Oral Solution, Paediatric, BP

(paediatric ferrous sulphate mixture) is a non-proprietary, non-prescription preparation of ferrous sulphate. It can be used as an IRON supplement in iron-deficiency ANAEMIA TREATMENT, and is available as modified-release tablets.

✚▲ Side-effects/warning: See FERROUS SULPHATE.

Fertiral

(Hoechst) is a proprietary preparation of gonadorelin (a synthetic analogue of the HORMONE gonadotrophin-releasing hormone; GnRH) and is available only on prescription at clinics and hospitals. It can be used to treat women for infertility and amenorrhoea due to hormonal insufficiency. In such cases, it is sometimes used in an attempt to determine the cause of infertility. Administration is by pulsatile infusion.

✚▲ Side-effects/warning: See GONADORELIN.

fexofenadine

is a recently developed ANTIHISTAMINE with less sedative side-effects than some older members of its class. In fact, it is an active metabolite of TERFENADINE. It can be used for the symptomatic relief of allergic symptoms, such as the rhinitis or hay fever. Administration is oral.

✚▲ Side-effects/warning: See ANTIHISTAMINES.

✪ Related entry: Telfast.

fibrinolytics ☒

(or thrombolytics) break up or disperse thrombi (blood clots). They are ENZYMES able to do this by breaking down the protein fibrin, which is the main constituent of many blood clots. They can be used rapidly in serious conditions, such as life-threatening venous thrombi, pulmonary embolism and clots in the eye. See ALTEPLASE; ANISTREPLASE; STREPTOKINASE; UROKINASE.

Filair Forte

(3M) is a proprietary, prescription-only preparation of the CORTICOSTEROID and ANTI-ASTHMATIC beclomethasone dipropionate. It can be used to prevent asthmatic attacks, and is available in an aerosol for inhalation.

✚▲ Side-effects/warning: See BECLOMETHASONE DIPROPIONATE.

finasteride

is an (indirect) ANTI-ANDROGEN, a SEX HORMONE ANTAGONIST, which can be used to treat benign prostatic hyperplasia in men. Administration is oral.

✚ Side-effects: Impotence, decreased libido and ejaculate volume.

▲ Warning: Use with caution in patients with urinary obstruction, or cancer of the prostate. It is recommended that a condom is used during sexual intercourse because the drug may enter the woman in semen and have adverse effects.

✪ Related entry: Proscar.

Fisherman's Friend

(Lofthouse of Fleetwood) is a proprietary, non-prescription lozenge for the relief of cold symptoms and contains liquorice, menthol and aniseed oil.

F

Flagyl

(Rhône-Poulenc Rorer) is a proprietary, prescription-only preparation of the ANTIMICROBIAL metronidazole, which has ANTIBACTERIAL and ANTIPROTOZOAL actions. It can be used to treat many types of anaerobic infection, including bacterial vaginitis, dental infections and following surgery. The antiprotozoal activity is effective against the micro-organisms that cause amoebic dysentery, giardiasis and trichomoniasis. It is available as tablets, suppositories and in a form for injection.

+▲ Side-effects/warning: See METRONIDAZOLE.

Flagyl Compak

(Rhône-Poulenc Rorer) is a proprietary, prescription-only COMPOUND PREPARATION of the ANTIMICROBIAL metronidazole, which has ANTIBACTERIAL properties and the ANTIFUNGAL and ANTIBIOTIC nystatin. It can be used to treat mixed infections of the vagina, including trichomoniasis and candidiasis, and is available as vaginal pessaries.

+▲ Side-effects/warning: See METRONIDAZOLE; NYSTATIN.

Flagyl S

(Rhône-Poulenc Rorer) is a proprietary, prescription-only preparation of the ANTIMICROBIAL metronidazole, which has ANTIBACTERIAL and ANTIPROTOZOAL properties. It can be used to treat anaerobic infections, including bacterial vaginitis, dental infections and following surgery. The antiprotozoal activity is effective against the organisms that cause amoebic dysentery, giardiasis and trichomoniasis. It is available as a suspension.

+▲ Side-effects/warning: See METRONIDAZOLE.

Flamatrol

(Berk) is a proprietary, prescription-only preparation of the (NSAID) NON-NARCOTIC ANALGESIC and ANTIRHEUMATIC piroxicam. It can be used to relieve pain and inflammation, particularly rheumatic and arthritic pain and to treat other musculoskeletal disorders (including juvenile arthritis) and acute gout. It is available as capsules.

+▲ Side-effects/warning: See PIROXICAM.

Flamazine

(Smith & Nephew) is a proprietary, prescription-only preparation of the ANTIBACTERIAL silver sulphadiazine. It can be used to treat wounds, burns and ulcers, bedsores and skin-graft donor sites. It is available as a cream.

+▲ Side-effects/warning: See SILVER SULPHADIAZINE.

Flamrase SR

(Berk) is a proprietary, prescription-only preparation of the (NSAID) NON-NARCOTIC ANALGESIC and ANTIRHEUMATIC diclofenac sodium. It can be used to treat pain and inflammation, particularly arthritic and rheumatic pain and other musculoskeletal disorders. It is available as modified-release capsules.

+▲ Side-effects/warning: See DICLOFENAC SODIUM.

flavoxate hydrochloride

is an ANTICHOLINERGIC drug which can be used as an ANTISPASMODIC to treat urinary frequency and incontinence. Administration is oral.

+▲ Side-effects/warning: See OXYBUTYNIN HYDROCHLORIDE; but it usually has fewer side-effects.

○ Related entry: Urispas.

Flaxedil

(Rhône-Poulenc Rorer) is a proprietary, prescription-only preparation of the (*non-depolarizing*) SKELETAL MUSCLE RELAXANT gallamine triethiodide. It can be used to induce muscle paralysis during surgery, and is available in a form for injection.

+▲ Side-effects/warning: See GALLAMINE TRIETHIODIDE.

flecainide acetate

is an ANTI-ARRHYTHMIC which is used to regularize the heartbeat in certain specific conditions. Administration is normally in hospital and is either oral or by slow intravenous injection.

✚ Side-effects: Dizziness; photosensitivity and cornea disturbances; nausea and vomiting; jaundice; changed liver enzymes.

▲ Warning: Administer with caution to patients with certain heart, kidney or liver disorders, jaundice, or who are pregnant or breast-feeding.

✪ Related entry: Tambocor.

Fleet Micro-enema

(De Witt) is a proprietary, non-prescription COMPOUND PREPARATION of the (*osmotic*) LAXATIVE sodium citrate with lauryl sulphoacetate, glycerol and other additives. It can be used to relieve constipation and to evacuate the rectum prior to abdominal procedures.

✚▲ Side-effects/warning: See SODIUM CITRATE.

Fleet Phospho-soda

(De Witt) is a proprietary, non-prescription COMPOUND PREPARATION of the (*osmotic*) LAXATIVE sodium phosphates (sodium dihydrogen phosphate dihydrate, disodium phosphate dodecahydrate). It can be used as a bowel-cleansing solution to ensure that the bowel is free of solid contents prior to, for example, colonic surgery, radiological examination or colonoscopy. It is available in the form of an oral solution.

✚▲ Side-effects/warning: See SODIUM ACID PHOSPHATE.

Fleet Ready-to-use Enema

(De Witt) is a proprietary, non-prescription COMPOUND PREPARATION of the (*osmotic*) LAXATIVES sodium phosphate and sodium acid phosphate. It can be used to relieve constipation and to evacuate the rectum prior to abdominal procedures.

✚▲ Side-effects/warning: See SODIUM ACID PHOSPHATE.

Fletchers' Arachis Oil Retention Enema

(Pharmax) is a proprietary, non-prescription preparation of arachis oil, which can be used as a (*faecal softener*) LAXATIVE.

✚▲ Side-effects/warning: See ARACHIS OIL.

Fletchers' Enemette

(Pharmax) is a proprietary, non-prescription preparation of the (*stimulant*) LAXATIVE docusate sodium and GLYCEROL (along with macrogol and sorbic acid). It can be used to relieve constipation and to evacuate the rectum prior to abdominal procedures.

✚▲ Side-effects/warning: See DOCUSATE SODIUM.

Fletchers' Phosphate Enema

(Pharmax) is a proprietary, non-prescription COMPOUND PREPARATION of the (*osmotic*) LAXATIVES sodium phosphate and sodium acid phosphate. It can be used to relieve constipation and to evacuate the rectum prior to abdominal procedures.

✚▲ Side-effects/warning: See SODIUM ACID PHOSPHATE.

Flexin Continus

(Napp) is a proprietary, prescription-only preparation of the (NSAID) NON-NARCOTIC ANALGESIC and ANTIRHEUMATIC indomethacin. It can be used to treat the pain and inflammation of rheumatic and other acute, severe musculoskeletal disorders. It is available as modified-release tablets.

✚▲ Side-effects/warning: See INDOMETHACIN.

Flexin-25 Continus

(Napp) is a proprietary, prescription-only preparation of the (NSAID) NON-NARCOTIC ANALGESIC and ANTIRHEUMATIC indomethacin. It can be used to treat the pain and inflammation of rheumatic and other acute, severe musculoskeletal disorders and also period pain. It is available as modified-release tablets.

+▲ Side-effects/warning: See INDOMETHACIN.

Flexin-LS Continus

(Napp) is a proprietary, prescription-only preparation of the (NSAID) NON-NARCOTIC ANALGESIC and ANTIRHEUMATIC indomethacin. It can be used to treat the pain and inflammation of rheumatic and other acute, severe musculoskeletal disorders. It is available as modified-release tablets.
+▲ Side-effects/warning: See INDOMETHACIN.

Flixonase

(Allen & Hanburys) is a proprietary, prescription-only preparation of the CORTICOSTEROID fluticasone propionate. It can be used to treat nasal allergy, such as hay fever, and is available as a nasal spray.
+▲ Side-effects/warning: See FLUTICASONE PROPIONATE.

Flixotide Accuhaler

(Allen & Hanburys) is a proprietary, prescription-only preparation of the CORTICOSTEROID fluticasone propionate. It can be used to treat nasal asthma, and is available as a dry powder for inhalation with an *Accuhaler* device.
+▲ Side-effects/warning: See FLUTICASONE PROPIONATE.

Flolan

(Wellcome) is a proprietary, prescription-only preparation of the ANTIPLATELET aggregation drug epoprostenol. It can be used to prevent formation of clots, for example, in conjunction with HEPARIN in kidney dialysis, and is available in a form for infusion.
+▲ Side-effects/warning: See EPOPROSTENOL.

Flomax MR

(Yamanouchi) is a proprietary, prescription-only preparation of the ALPHA-ADRENOCEPTOR BLOCKER tamsulosin hydrochloride. It can be used to treat urinary retention (eg in benign prostatic hyperplasia), and is available as capsules.
+▲ Side-effects/warning: See TAMSULOSIN HYDROCHLORIDE.

Florinef

(Squibb) is a proprietary, prescription-only preparation of the CORTICOSTEROID and ANTI-INFLAMMATORY fludrocortisone acetate, which can be used for its *mineralocorticoid* activity to treat adrenal gland insufficiency. It is available as tablets.
+▲ Side-effects/warning: See FLUDROCORTISONE ACETATE.

Floxapen

(Beecham) is a proprietary, prescription-only preparation of the ANTIBACTERIAL and (PENICILLIN) ANTIBIOTIC flucloxacillin. It can be used to treat bacterial infections, particularly staphylococcal infections that prove to be resistant to penicillin. It is available as capsules, a syrup and in a form for injection.
+▲ Side-effects/warning: See FLUCLOXACILLIN.

Flu-Amp

(Generics) is a proprietary prescription-only COMPOUND PREPARATION of the broad-spectrum ANTIBACTERIAL and (PENICILLIN) ANTIBIOTIC ampicillin and the *penicillinase-resistant*, antibacterial and (penicillin) antibiotic flucloxacillin (a combination called co-fluampicil). It can be used to treat severe infection where the causative organism has not been identified, but Gram-positive staphylococcal infection is suspected, or where penicillin-resistant bacterial infection is probable. It is available as capsules, a syrup and in a form for injection.
+▲ Side-effects/warning: See AMPICILLIN; FLUCLOXACILLIN.

Fluanxol

(Lundbeck) is a proprietary, prescription-only preparation of flupenthixol, which has ANTIPSYCHOTIC properties and also

ANTIDEPRESSANT actions. It can be used in the short-term treatment of depressive illness, and is available as tablets.
+▲ Side-effects/warning: See FLUPENTHIXOL.

Fluarix
(SmithKline Beecham) is a proprietary, prescription-only preparation of influenza VACCINE (split viron vaccine). It can be used for the prevention of influenza, and is available in a form for injection.
+▲ Side-effects/warning: See INFLUENZA VACCINE.

Fluclomix
(Ashbourne) is a proprietary, prescription-only preparation of the ANTIBACTERIAL and (PENICILLIN) ANTIBIOTIC flucloxacillin. It can be used to treat bacterial infections, particularly staphylococcal infections that prove to be resistant to penicillin, and is available as capsules.
+▲ Side-effects/warning: See FLUCLOXACILLIN.

flucloxacillin
is an ANTIBACTERIAL and ANTIBIOTIC drug of the PENICILLIN family. It can be used to treat bacterial infections, particularly those resistant to penicillin (eg penicillinase-producing staphylococcal infections) and in the treatment of ear infections, pneumonia, impetigo, cellulitis and staphylococcal endocarditis. Administration is either oral or by injection.
+▲ Side-effects/warning: See BENZYLPENICILLIN. Administer with caution to patients with porphyria. There have been reports of hepatic (liver) and cholestatic jaundice.
✪ Related entries: co-fluampicil; Floxapen; Flu-Amp; Fluclomix; Galfloxin; Ladropen; Magnapen; Stafoxil.

fluconazole
is an (AZOLE) ANTIFUNGAL drug which can be used in the treatment of many fungal infections of the mucous membranes, of the vagina (candidiasis) or mouth, oesophagitis, athlete's foot and cytococcal meningitis. It can also be used to prevent fungal infections in immunocompromised patients following chemotherapy or radiotherapy. Administration is either oral or by injection.
+ Side-effects: Nausea, abdominal discomfort and flatulence, diarrhoea, headaches, rash, angio-oedema, anaphylaxis and alteration in liver enzymes.
▲ Warning: It should be administered with care to patients with certain kidney disorders or who are pregnant or breast-feeding.
✪ Related entry: Diflucan.

flucytosine
is an (AZOLE) ANTIFUNGAL drug which can be used to treat systemic infections by yeasts, such as systemic candidiasis.
Administration is either oral or by injection.
+ Side-effects: There may be diarrhoea with nausea and vomiting; rashes may occur, and confusion, hallucinations and headaches may be experienced.
▲ Warning: It should be administered with caution to patients who suffer from certain kidney or liver disorders, blood disorders; or who are pregnant or breast-feeding. During treatment, there should be regular blood counts and liver-function tests.
✪ Related entry: Alcobon.

Fludara
(Schering) is a proprietary, prescription-only preparation of the (CYTOTOXIC) ANTICANCER drug fludarabine phosphate. It can be used in the treatment of acute leukaemia, and is available in a form for injection.
+▲ Side-effects/warning: See FLUDARABINE PHOSPHATE.

fludarabine phosphate
is a CYTOTOXIC drug which can be used as an ANTICANCER treatment primarily of certain leukaemias. Administration is by injection.
+▲ Side-effects/warning: See CYTOTOXICS.
✪ Related entry: Fludara.

F

fludrocortisone acetate

is a CORTICOSTEROID which is used for its *mineralocorticoid* activity to correct a deficiency of HORMONE from the adrenal gland, and is used to treat the resulting salt-and-water imbalance in the body. Administration is oral.

➕▲ Side-effects/warning: See CORTICOSTEROIDS.

⊙ Related entry: Florinef.

fludroxycortide

see FLURANDRENOLONE

flumazenil

is a BENZODIAZEPINE antagonist which can be used to reverse the sedative effects of benzodiazepine drugs on the central nervous system induced during anaesthesia, in intensive care or for diagnostic procedures. Administration is by intravenous infusion or injection.

➕ Side-effects: Nausea, vomiting, flushing; on waking rapidly, agitation, anxiety and fear; rarely, convulsions (particularly epileptics).

▲ Warning: It should be administered with caution to those with impaired liver function; or who are pregnant or breast-feeding.

⊙ Related entry: Anexate.

flumethasone pivalate

is a CORTICOSTEROID with ANTI-INFLAMMATORY properties. It is used in the treatment of inflammatory skin disorders, particularly eczema of the outer ear. Administration is by topical application.

➕▲ Side-effects/warning: See HYDROCORTISONE. There may be local sensitivity reactions; avoid prolonged use. Do not use in untreated infection.

⊙ Related entry: Locortan-Vioform.

flunisolide

is an ANTI-ALLERGIC and CORTICOSTEROID drug which is used to treat nasal allergy, such as hay fever. Administration is by nasal spray.

➕▲ Side-effects/warning: See

BECLOMETHASONE DIPROPIONATE.

⊙ Related entry: Syntaris.

flunitrazepam

is a BENZODIAZEPINE which is used as a HYPNOTIC in the short-term treatment of insomnia. Administration is oral.

➕▲ Side-effects/warning: See BENZODIAZEPINES.

⊙ Related entry: Rohypnol.

fluocinolone acetonide

is a CORTICOSTEROID with ANTI-INFLAMMATORY properties. It is used in the treatment of inflammatory skin disorders, such as eczema and psoriasis. Administration is by topical application. It is also a constituent in several COMPOUND PREPARATIONS that contain ANTIBACTERIALS or ANTIMICROBIALS.

➕▲ Side-effects/warning: See CORTICOSTEROIDS; though systemic effects are unlikely with topical application, but there may be local skin reactions.

⊙ Related entries: Synalar; Synalar C; Synalar N.

fluocinonide

is a CORTICOSTEROID with ANTI-INFLAMMATORY properties. It is used in the treatment of severe, acute inflammatory skin disorders, such as eczema and psoriasis, that are unresponsive to less powerful corticosteroids. Administration is by topical application.

➕▲ Side-effects/warning: See CORTICOSTEROIDS; though systemic effects are unlikely with topical application, but there may be local skin reactions.

⊙ Related entry: Metosyn.

fluocortolone

is a CORTICOSTEROID with ANTI-INFLAMMATORY properties. It is used in the treatment of severe, acute inflammatory skin disorders, such as eczema and psoriasis, that are unresponsive to less powerful corticosteroids. Administration is by topical application.

➕▲ Side-effects/warning: See

CORTICOSTEROIDS; though systemic effects are unlikely with topical application, but there may be local skin reactions.
⊕ Related entry: Ultralanum Plain.

fluorescein sodium

is a dye that is used on the surface of an eye in ophthalmic diagnostic procedures. Administration is topical as eye-drops.
⊕ Related entry: Minims Fluorescein Sodium.

fluorometholone

is a CORTICOSTEROID with ANTI-INFLAMMATORY properties which is used as a short-term treatment of inflammatory eye conditions. Administration is by eye-drops.
✚▲ Side-effects/warning: See CORTICOSTEROIDS; though systemic effects are unlikely with topical application, but there may be local skin reactions.
⊕ Related entries: FML; FML-Neo.

fluorouracil

is a CYTOTOXIC drug which is used as an ANTICANCER treatment primarily of solid tumours (eg of the colon and breast) and malignant skin lesions. It works by preventing the cancer cells from replicating and so prevents the growth of the cancer. Administration can be oral, topical or by injection.
✚▲ Side-effects/warning: See CYTOTOXICS.
⊕ Related entries: Efudix; Fluorouracil.

Fluorouracil

(Cambridge) is a non-proprietary, prescription-only preparation of the (CYTOTOXIC) ANTICANCER drug fluorouracil. It can be used to treat solid tumours (eg of the colon or breast), and is available as capsules and in a form for injection.
✚▲ Side-effects/warning: See FLUOROURACIL.

Fluothane

(Zeneca) is a proprietary preparation of the inhalant GENERAL ANAESTHETIC halothane. It can be used for the induction and maintenance of anaesthesia during surgery, and is available in a form for inhalation.
✚▲ Side-effects/warning: See HALOTHANE.

fluoxetine

is an ANTIDEPRESSANT of the SSRI group. It is used to treat depressive illness and has the advantage over some other antidepressants because it has relatively less SEDATIVE and ANTICHOLINERGIC side-effects. It has recently been used for bulimia nervosa and obsessive-compulsive disorders. The onset of action may take some weeks to reach full effect and offset on discontinuation is also slow. Administration is oral.
✚ Side-effects: Gastrointestinal symptoms, including nausea, vomiting and diarrhoea (which may be severe); abdominal pain, acid stomach, constipation, anorexia with weight loss, dry mouth, anxiety or drowsiness, tremor, palpitations, may cause a rash (if so, discontinue treatment), convulsions, fever, headache, tremor, insomnia, confusion, sweating, weakness, hypothermia, sexual dysfunction; occasionally, blood disorders including lowered sodium and liver dysfunction. A hypersensitivity syndrome has been described involving symptoms in the skin and inflammation of inner organs. A number of other disorders have been reported, including vaginal bleeding on withdrawal, several different blood disorders, violent behaviour and hair loss.
▲ Warning: Use with caution in patients with liver, kidney or heart disorders and those who have a history of mania (do not use during a manic phase), epilepsy, diabetes or who are pregnant or breast-feeding.
⊕ Related entry: Prozac.

flupenthixol

(flupentixol) is chemically one of the thioxanthenes, which have properties similar to the PHENOTHIAZINES. It is used as an ANTIPSYCHOTIC in the treatment of schizophrenia and other psychoses, particularly where there is apathy and

249

F

withdrawal, but not for mania or psychomotor hyperactivity. It is also used (at a lower dose) in the short-term treatment of depressive illness. Administration is oral. See also FLUPENTHIXOL DECANOATE.

✚▲ Side-effects/warning: See CHLORPROMAZINE HYDROCHLORIDE; but it is less sedating and extrapyramidal symptoms are more common; avoid its use in senile, overactive or excitable patients and in those with porphyria. There may be pain, redness and swelling at the injection site.

✪ Related entry: Fluanxol.

flupenthixol decanoate

(flupentixol deconate) is a salt of FLUPENTHIXOL and has a longer duration of action. It is used as an ANTIPSYCHOTIC drug for long-term maintenance in schizophrenia and other psychoses, particularly where there is apathy and withdrawal, but not for mania or psychomotor hyperactivity. Administration is by depot deep intramuscular injection.

✚▲ Side-effects/warning: See CHLORPROMAZINE HYDROCHLORIDE; but it may have mood-elevating effects and extrapyramidal symptoms are more common; avoid its use in senile, overactive or excitable patients and in those with porphyria.

✪ Related entries: Depixol; Depixol Conc; Depixol Low Volume.

flupentixol

see FLUPENTHIXOL

flupentixol deconate

see FLUPENTHIXOL DECONATE

fluphenazine decanoate

is a powerful ANTIPSYCHOTIC which is chemically one of the PHENOTHIAZINES group. It is used for the long-term treatment of psychoses, such as schizophrenia. The decanoate salt is administered by depot deep intramuscular injection.

✚▲ Side-effects/warning: See CHLORPROMAZINE HYDROCHLORIDE; but with less sedation, fewer anticholinergic and hypotensive side-effects; but there are extrapyramidal symptoms (muscle tremor and rigidity, and also dystonic and akinesic motor movements). Avoid its use in patients with depression.

✪ Related entries: Decazate; Modecate.

fluphenazine hydrochloride

is a powerful ANTIPSYCHOTIC which is chemically one of the PHENOTHIAZINES group. It is used in the treatment of psychoses, such as schizophrenia and for the short-term control of severe manic, violent or agitated states. It can also be used for the short-term treatment of severe anxiety. Administration of the hydrochloride salt is oral and the decanoate salt by depot deep intramuscular injection.

✚▲ Side-effects/warning: See CHLORPROMAZINE HYDROCHLORIDE; but with less sedation, fewer anticholinergic and hypotensive side-effects, but there are extrapyramidal symptoms (muscle tremor and rigidity, and also dystonic and akinesic motor movements). Avoid using it in patients with depression.

✪ Related entries: Moditen; Motipress; Motival.

flurandrenolone

(fludroxycortide) is a CORTICOSTEROID with ANTI-INFLAMMATORY properties. It is used in the treatment of inflammatory skin disorders, such as eczema, and is also a constituent in a COMPOUND PREPARATION with the ANTIBACTERIAL clioquinol. Administration is by topical application.

✚▲ Side-effects/warning: See CORTICOSTEROIDS; though systemic effects are unlikely with topical application, but there may be local skin reactions.

✪ Related entries: Haelan; Haelan-C.

flurazepam

is a BENZODIAZEPINE which is used as a HYPNOTIC to treat insomnia in cases where some degree of sedation during the daytime

is acceptable. Administration is oral.
+▲ Side-effects/warning: See
BENZODIAZEPINES.
○ Related entries: Dalmane; Dormonoct.

flurbiprofen

is a (NSAID) NON-NARCOTIC ANALGESIC and
ANTIRHEUMATIC with effects similar to those
of aspirin. It is used particularly in the
treatment of pain and inflammation in
musculoskeletal disorders, period pain and
postoperative pain. Administration can be
either oral or topical.
+▲ Side-effects/warning: See NSAID.
Suppositories may cause irritation.
○ Related entries: Froben; Ocufen.

Flurex Cold/Flu Capsules with Cough Suppressant

(Seton) is a proprietary, non-prescription
preparation of the SYMPATHOMIMETIC and
VASOCONSTRICTOR phenylephrine
hydrochloride, the NON-NARCOTIC ANALGESIC
and ANTIPYRETIC paracetamol and the
(OPIOID) NARCOTIC ANALGESIC and ANTITUSSIVE
dextromethorphan hydrobromide. It can be
used for the relief of nasal congestion
during colds and flu, aches, cough and
fever. It is available as a liquid and is not
normally given to children under six years,
except on medical advice.
+▲ Side-effects/warning: See
DEXTROMETHORPHAN HYDROBROMIDE;
PARACETAMOL; PHENYLEPHRINE HYDROCHLORIDE.

Flurex Tablets

(Seton) is a proprietary, non-prescription
COMPOUND PREPARATION of the NON-NARCOTIC
ANALGESIC and ANTIPYRETIC paracetamol, the
SYMPATHOMIMETIC and DECONGESTANT
phenylephrine hydrochloride and the
STIMULANT caffeine. It can be used for the
symptomatic relief of colds, flu, congested
and blocked nose and catarrh. It is
available in the form of a liquid and is not
normally given to children under six years,
except on medical advice.
+▲ Side-effects/warning: See CAFFEINE;
PARACETAMOL; PHENYLEPHRINE HYDROCHLORIDE.

flutamide

is a HORMONE ANTAGONIST (an anti-androgen)
which is used as an ANTICANCER drug for the
treatment of prostate cancer. Administration
is oral.
+ Side-effects: There may be gynaecomastia
(growth of breasts) and milk secretion,
diarrhoea, nausea and vomiting, increased
appetite, tiredness and sleep disturbances,
decreased libido, gastrointestinal and chest
pain, blurred vision, oedema, rashes, blood
disturbances, headache, dizziness, thirst,
rash, blood and liver disorders.
▲ Warning: It must be administered with
caution to patients suffering certain heart
disorders. Liver function should be
monitored.
○ Related entry: Drogenil.

fluticasone propionate

is a CORTICOSTEROID which is used as an
ANTI-INFLAMMATORY treatment for skin
disorders, such as dermatitis and eczema,
that are unresponsive to less potent
corticosteroids and also for psoriasis.
Administration is by topical application as a
cream. It can also be used as an ANTI-
ALLERGIC treatment for nasal allergy, such as
hay fever, and is administered by a nasal
spray.
+▲ Side-effects/warning: See
HYDROCORTISONE.
○ Related entries: Cultivate; Flixonase.

fluvastatin

can be used as a LIPID-LOWERING DRUG in
hyperlipidaemia to reduce the levels, or
change the proportions, of various lipids in
the bloodstream. It is usually administered
only to patients in whom a strict and
regular dietary regime, alone, is not having
the desired effect. Administration is oral.
+▲ Side-effects/warning: See SIMVASTATIN.
○ Related entry: Lescol.

Fluvirin

(Evans) is a proprietary, prescription-only
preparation of influenza VACCINE. It can be
used for the prevention of influenza, and is

available in a form for injection.

+▲ Side-effects/warning: See INFLUENZA VACCINE.

fluvoxamine maleate

is an ANTIDEPRESSANT of the SSRI group. It is used to treat depressive illness and has the advantage over some other antidepressants because it has less SEDATIVE and ANTICHOLINERGIC side-effects. Administration is oral.

+▲ Side-effects/warning: See FLUOXETINE; there may also be slowing of the heart.

✪ Related entry: Faverin.

Fluzone

(Servier) is a proprietary, prescription-only preparation of influenza VACCINE. It can be used for prevention of influenza, and is available in a form for injection.

+▲ Side-effects/warning: See INFLUENZA VACCINE.

FML

(Allergan) is a proprietary, prescription-only preparation of the CORTICOSTEROID and ANTI-INFLAMMATORY fluorometholone. It can be used for the short-term treatment of inflammatory eye conditions, and is available as eye-drops.

+▲ Side-effects/warning: See FLUOROMETHOLONE.

FML-Neo

(Allergan) is a proprietary, prescription-only COMPOUND PREPARATION of the ANTI-INFLAMMATORY and CORTICOSTEROID fluorometholone and the ANTIBACTERIAL and (AMINOGLYCOSIDE) ANTIBIOTIC neomycin sulphate. It can be used in cases where inflammation is not primarily caused by infection, and is available as eye-drops.

+▲ Side-effects/warning: See FLUOROMETHOLONE; NEOMYCIN SULPHATE.

Folex-350

(Rybar) is a proprietary, non-prescription COMPOUND PREPARATION of ferrous fumarate and folic acid. It can be used as an IRON and

folic acid supplement during pregnancy, and is available as tablets.

+▲ Side-effects/warning: See FERROUS FUMARATE; FOLIC ACID.

folic acid

is a vitamin of the B complex and is also known as pteroylglutamic acid. It has an important role in the synthesis of nucleic acids (DNA and RNA). Good food sources of folic acid include liver and vegetables and its consumption is particularly necessary during pregnancy. The Department of Health now agree that folic acid supplements help prevent neural tube defects when taken before and during pregnancy. There are also certain forms of anaemia (eg megaloblastic anaemia) that can be treated with folic acid (as well as supplements of cyanocobalamin). Administration is oral.

▲ Warning: Treatment with folic acid generally also indicates parallel treatment with cyanocobalamin (vitamin B_{12}).

✪ Related entries: Fefol; Ferfolic SV; Ferrocontin Folic Continus; Ferrograd Folic; Folex-350; Galfer FA; Lexpec; Lexpec with Iron; Lexpec with Iron-M; Meterfolic; Pregaday; Slow-Fe Folic.

folinic acid

is a derivative of FOLIC ACID (a vitamin of the vitamin B complex) and is used to counteract the folate-antagonist activity and resulting toxicity of certain ANTICANCER drugs, especially METHOTREXATE. Administration is either oral or by injection or intravenous infusion.

+ Side-effects: Rarely, fever after injections.

✪ Related entries: Calcium Leucovorin; Refolinon.

follicle-stimulating hormone

(FSH) is a HORMONE secreted by the anterior pituitary gland and is one of the gonadotrophin hormones, along with LUTEINISING HORMONE (LH). In women (in conjunction with LH), it causes the monthly ripening in one ovary of a follicle and stimulates ovulation. In men, it stimulates the production of sperm in the testes. It may be injected therapeutically in infertility treatment to stimulate ovulation. It is available in combination with LH, as HUMAN MENOPAUSAL GONADOTROPHIN. It is now available as a recently introduced recombinant (synthetic) form called FOLLITROPIN ALPHA. See also CHORIONIC GONADOTROPHIN.

follitropin alpha

is a recently introduced recombinant (synthetic) form of human FOLLICLE-STIMULATING HORMONE secreted by the anterior pituitary gland which is one of the gonadotrophin hormones (along with LUTEINISING HORMONE; LH). In women (in conjunction with LH), it causes the monthly ripening in one ovary of a follicle and stimulates ovulation. In men, it stimulates the production of sperm in the testes. It can be injected in infertility treatment to stimulate ovulation. It is available, in combination with LH, as HUMAN MENOPAUSAL GONADOTROPHIN. See also CHORIONIC GONADOTROPHIN.

+▲ Side-effects/warning: See HUMAN MENOPAUSAL GONADOTROPHINS.
○ Related entry: Gonal-F.

follitropin beta

is a recently introduced recombinant (synthetic) form of FOLLICLE-STIMULATING HORMONE (FSH), which is a HORMONE secreted by the anterior pituitary gland and is one of the gonadotrophin hormones (along with LUTEINISING HORMONE; LH). In women, in conjunction with LH, it causes the monthly ripening in one ovary of a follicle and stimulates ovulation. In men, it stimulates the production of sperm in the testes. It can be injected in infertility treatment to stimulate ovulation. It is available in combination with LH as HUMAN MENOPAUSAL GONADOTROPHIN. See also CHORIONIC GONADOTROPHIN.

+▲ Side-effects/warning: See HUMAN

MENOPAUSAL GONADOTROPHINS.
○ Related entry: Puregon.

Fomac

(Berk) is a proprietary, prescription-only preparation of the ANTISPASMODIC drug mebeverine hydrochloride. It can be used to treat gastrointestinal spasm, and is available as tablets.
+▲ Side-effects/warning: See MEBEVERINE HYDROCHLORIDE.

Foradil

(Geigy) is a proprietary, prescription-only preparation of the BETA-RECEPTOR STIMULANT eformoterol. It can be used as a BRONCHODILATOR in reversible obstructive airways disease and as an ANTI-ASTHMATIC treatment, and has a prolonged action. It is available as a powder for inhalation. Patients should be cautioned that this drug should not be used for the relief of acute attacks and that corticosteroid treatment must be continued. Patients should also be cautioned not to exceed the stated dose and if a previously effective dose fail to relieve symptoms, they should consult their doctor.
+▲ Side-effects/warning: See EFORMOTEROL.

formaldehyde

is a powerful KERATOLYTIC agent which is used in mild solution to dissolve away layers of toughened or warty skin, especially in the treatment of verrucas (plantar warts) on the soles of the feet.
+▲ Side-effects/warning: See SALICYLIC ACID.
○ Related entry: Veracur.

formestane

is an ANTICANCER drug which is used to treat advanced breast cancer in postmenopausal women. It works as an indirect HORMONE ANTAGONIST by inhibiting the conversion of the male SEX HORMONE androgen to the female sex hormone OESTROGEN. Administration is by deep intramuscular injection.

✚ Side-effects: There may be drowsiness and lethargy; rashes and allergic reactions; vomiting and constipation; hot flushes and headache, vaginal bleeding; joint pain, pelvic and muscle cramps; sore throat; growth of facial hair; emotional instability, clots in the blood vessels of the leg, or irritation at the site of injection.

▲ Warning: It should not be used in premenopausal women or in those who are pregnant of breast-feeding.

◑ Related entry: Lentaron.

Fortagesic

(Sanofi Winthrop) is a proprietary, prescription-only COMPOUND ANALGESIC preparation of the (OPIOID) NARCOTIC ANALGESIC pentazocine (as hydrochloride) and the NON-NARCOTIC ANALGESIC paracetamol. It can be used to relieve pain anywhere in the body, and is available as tablets. It is not normally given to children under seven years, except on medical advice.

✚▲ Side-effects/warning: See PARACETAMOL; PENTAZOCINE.

Fortral

(Sanofi Winthrop) is a proprietary, prescription-only preparation of the (OPIOID) NARCOTIC ANALGESIC pentazocine. It can be used to relieve pain, and is available as capsules, tablets, suppositories and in a form for injection.

✚▲ Side-effects/warning: See PENTAZOCINE.

Fortum

(Glaxo) is a proprietary, prescription-only preparation of the ANTIBACTERIAL and (CEPHALOSPORIN) ANTIBIOTIC ceftazidime. It can be used particularly to treat infections of the respiratory tract, in patients whose immune systems are defective and during surgery. It is available in a form for injection or infusion.

✚▲ Side-effects/warning: See CEFTAZIDIME.

Fosamax

(Merck Sharp & Dohme) is a recently introduced, proprietary, prescription-only preparation of alendronic acid. It can be used to treat postmenopausal osteoporosis, and is available as tablets.

✚▲ Side-effects/warning: See ALENDRONIC ACID.

foscarnet sodium

is an ANTIVIRAL drug which can be used to treat cytomegaloviral retinitis in patients with AIDS when the more commonly used antiviral GANCICLOVIR is inappropriate. Administration is by intravenous infusion.

✚ Side-effects: There may be various blood-cell deficiencies, effects on the functioning of the kidney and liver, gastrointestinal disturbances, nausea, vomiting, rash and fatigue.

▲ Warning: It should not be administered to patients who have impaired kidney function, or who are pregnant or breast-feeding.

◑ Related entry: Foscavir.

Foscavir

(Astra) is a proprietary, non-prescription preparation of the ANTIVIRAL drug foscarnet sodium. It can be used to treat viral infections, especially of the eye (cytomegaloviral retinitis) in patients with AIDS, and is available in a form for intravenous infusion.

✚▲ Side-effects/warning: See FOSCARNET SODIUM.

fosfestrol tetrasodium

is a drug that is converted in the body to STILBOESTROL, which has SEX HORMONE activity as an OESTROGEN. It is used in men as an ANTICANCER treatment for cancer of the prostate gland.

✚▲ Side-effects/warning: See STILBOESTROL.

◑ Related entry: Honvan.

fosfomycin

is an ANTIBACTERIAL and ANTIBIOTIC drug which is used mainly to treat urinary tract infections, including uncomplicated infections of the lower urinary tract, and to prevent infection during certain surgical procedures. Administration is oral as granules, which come in adult and paediatric strengths.

✚ Side-effects: Diarrhoea, heartburn, nausea or rash.

▲ Warning: It should be used with care in patients with severe kidney dysfunction, or who are pregnant or breast-feeding.

◎ Related entry: Monuril.

fosinopril

is an ACE INHIBITOR and acts as a VASODILATOR. It can be used as an ANTIHYPERTENSIVE, and often when other treatments cannot be used. It is frequently administered in conjunction with other classes of drug, particularly (THIAZIDE) DIURETICS. Administration is oral.

✚▲ Side-effects/warning: See CAPTOPRIL.

◎ Related entry: Staril.

Fragmin

(Pharmacia) is a proprietary, prescription-only preparation of the ANTICOAGULANT dalteparin, which is a low molecular weight version of heparin. It can be used for long-duration prevention of venous thrombo-embolism, particularly in orthopaedic use. It is available in a form for injection.

✚▲ Side-effects/warning: See DALTEPARIN.

framycetin sulphate

is a broad-spectrum ANTIBACTERIAL and ANTIBIOTIC drug of the AMINOGLYCOSIDE family. As with all aminoglycoside antibiotics, framycetin is active against some Gram-positive and many Gram-negative bacteria, and can be used in the treatment of infections of the eye, ear and open wounds (when it is used in a gauze dressing). Administration is largely restricted to topical application because of its toxicity.

✚▲ Side-effects/warning: See GENTAMICIN; but topical application limits its toxic side-effects.

◎ Related entries: Sofradex; Soframycin.

Franol

(Sanofi Winthrop) is a proprietary, prescription-only COMPOUND PREPARATION of the BRONCHODILATOR theophylline and the SYMPATHOMIMETIC ephedrine hydrochloride. It can be used as an ANTI-ASTHMATIC and to treat chronic bronchitis, and is available as tablets.

✚▲ Side-effects/warning: See EPHEDRINE HYDROCHLORIDE; THEOPHYLLINE.

Franol Plus

(Sanofi Winthrop) is a proprietary, prescription-only COMPOUND PREPARATION of the BRONCHODILATOR theophylline and the SYMPATHOMIMETIC ephedrine hydrochloride. It can be used as an ANTI-ASTHMATIC and to treat chronic bronchitis, and is available as tablets.

✚▲ Side-effects/warning: See EPHEDRINE HYDROCHLORIDE; THEOPHYLLINE.

Franolyn for Chesty Coughs

(Johnson & Johnson) is a proprietary, non-prescription COMPOUND PREPARATION of the BRONCHODILATOR and ANTI-ASTHMATIC theophylline, the SYMPATHOMIMETIC and DECONGESTANT ephedrine hydrochloride and the EXPECTORANT agent GUAIPHENSIN. It can be used for the symptomatic relief of coughs, especially when associated with asthma, bronchitis and hay fever. It is available as a liquid and is not normally used in children under seven years, except on medical advice.

✚▲ Side-effects/warning: See EPHEDRINE HYDROCHLORIDE; THEOPHYLLINE.

Franolyn for Dry Coughs

(Johnson & Johnson) is a proprietary, non-prescription preparation of the (OPIOID) ANTITUSSIVE and NARCOTIC ANALGESIC dextromethorphan hydrobromide. It can be used for the symptomatic relief of dry, irritating cough, and is available as a syrup. It is not normally given to children under seven years, except on medical advice.

✚▲ Side-effects/warning: See DEXTROMETHORPHAN HYDROBROMIDE.

F

Frisium

(Hoechst) is a proprietary, prescription-only preparation of the (BENZODIAZEPINE) ANXIOLYTIC clobazam. It can be used in the short-term treatment of anxiety and, in conjunction with other drugs, in ANTI-EPILEPTIC therapy. It is available as capsules.

+▲ Side-effects/warning: See CLOBAZAM.

Froben

(Boots) is a proprietary, prescription-only preparation of the (NSAID) NON-NARCOTIC ANALGESIC and ANTIRHEUMATIC flurbiprofen. It can be used to treat arthritic and rheumatic pain and inflammation, other musculoskeletal disorders, period pain and pain after surgical operations. It is available as tablets, as modified-release capsules (*Froben SR*) and as suppositories.

+▲ Side-effects/warning: See FLURBIPROFEN.

Froop

(Ashbourne) is a proprietary, prescription only preparation of the (*loop*) DIURETIC frusemide. It can be used to treat oedema, particularly pulmonary (lung) oedema in patients with chronic heart failure, and low urine production due to kidney failure (oliguria). It is available as tablets.

+▲ Side-effects/warning: See FRUSEMIDE.

Fru-Co

(Baker Norton) is a proprietary, prescription-only COMPOUND PREPARATION of the (*potassium-sparing*) DIURETIC amiloride hydrochloride and the (*loop*) diuretic frusemide (a combination called co-amilofruse 5/40). It can be used to treat oedema, and is available as tablets.

+▲ Side-effects/warning: See AMILORIDE HYDROCHLORIDE; FRUSEMIDE.

fructose

(laevulose; fruit sugar) is a simple sugar (a monosaccharide). Fructose and GLUCOSE make up the disaccharide sucrose when chemically combined, which is found naturally in cane sugar and sugar-beet and is a major source of carbohydrate and energy. In the body, sucrose is metabolized into the simple sugars. The glucose level in the blood is closely regulated by INSULIN and GLUCAGON. Fructose, as part of a normal diet, can therefore be used as a source of energy and is a constituent of honey and in certain fruits (such as figs). It offers no particular advantage in normal individuals, but medically may be recommended for use, without prescription, by patients who suffer from glucose or galactose intolerance.

Frumil

(Rhône-Poulenc Rorer) is a proprietary, prescription-only COMPOUND PREPARATION of the (*potassium-sparing*) DIURETIC amiloride hydrochloride and the (*loop*) diuretic frusemide (a combination called co-amilofruse 5/40). It can be used to treat oedema, and is available as tablets.

+▲ Side-effects/warning: See AMILORIDE HYDROCHLORIDE; FRUSEMIDE.

Frumil Forte

(Rhône-Poulenc Rorer) is a proprietary, prescription-only COMPOUND PREPARATION of the (*potassium-sparing*) DIURETIC amiloride hydrochloride and the (*loop*) diuretic frusemide (a combination called co-amilofruse 10/80). It can be used to treat oedema, and is available as tablets.

+▲ Side-effects/warning: See AMILORIDE HYDROCHLORIDE; FRUSEMIDE.

Frumil LS

(Rhône-Poulenc Rorer) is a proprietary, prescription-only COMPOUND PREPARATION of the (*potassium-sparing*) DIURETIC amiloride hydrochloride and the (*loop*) diuretic frusemide (a combination called co-amilofruse 2.5/20). It can be used to treat oedema, and is available as tablets.

+▲ Side-effects/warning: See AMILORIDE HYDROCHLORIDE; FRUSEMIDE.

frusemide

(furosemide) is a powerful DIURETIC of the

loop class. It can be used to treat oedema, particularly pulmonary (lung) oedema in patients with left ventricular or chronic heart failure, and low urine production due to kidney failure (oliguria). Administration can be oral or by injection or infusion.

✚ Side-effects: There may be lowered blood levels of potassium, sodium, magnesium and chloride. There may be an abnormally low blood pressure (hypotension), gastrointestinal disturbances, raised levels of urea in the blood, raised blood glucose, changes in fats in the blood, tinnitus and deafness. There may be skin rashes, photosensitivity, bone marrow depression, pancreatitis. Many of these effects are only seen with high or prolonged dosage.

▲ Warning: It should be administered with care to patients with certain kidney disorders, who are pregnant or breast-feeding, who have gout, diabetes, an enlarged prostate gland or liver failure or porphyria. It should not be used in patients with kidney failure and anuria (no urine produced).

✪ Related entries: Diumide-K Continus; Dryptal; Froop; Fru-Co; Frumil; Frumil Forte; Frumil LS; Frusene; Lasikal; Lasilactone; Lasix; Lasix+K; Lasix Paediatric Liquid; Lasoride; Min-I-Jet Frusemide; Rusyde.

Frusene

(Fisons) is a proprietary, prescription-only COMPOUND PREPARATION of the (*potassium-sparing*) DIURETIC triamterene and the (*loop*) diuretic frusemide. It can be used to treat oedema, and is available as tablets.
✚▲ Side-effects/warning: See FRUSEMIDE; TRIAMTERENE.

FSH

see FOLLICLE-STIMULATING HORMONE

Fucibet

(Leo) is a proprietary, prescription-only COMPOUND PREPARATION of the CORTICOSTEROID betamethasone and the ANTIBACTERIAL and ANTIBIOTIC fusidic acid. It can be used to treat skin disorders, such as psoriasis and eczema, in which bacterial infection is present, and is available as a cream.
✚▲ Side-effects/warning: See BETAMETHASONE; FUSIDIC ACID.

Fucidin

(Leo) is a proprietary, prescription-only preparation of the narrow-spectrum ANTIBACTERIAL and ANTIBIOTIC fusidic acid. It can be used against staphylococcal infections, especially infections of the skin and bone and also abscesses, that prove to be resistant to penicillin. It is available in many forms: for topical application as a gel, as a cream, as an ointment; for oral administration as tablets or suspension; and in a form for intravenous injection (all contain as their active constituent either fusidic acid or one of its salts).
✚▲ Side-effects/warning: See FUSIDIC ACID.

Fucidin H

(Leo) is a proprietary, prescription-only COMPOUND PREPARATION of the narrow-spectrum ANTIBACTERIAL and ANTIBIOTIC fusidic acid and the ANTI-INFLAMMATORY and CORTICOSTEROID hydrocortisone (as acetate). It can be used to treat skin inflammation where there is bacterial infection, such as eczema and nappy rash. It is available for topical application as a cream, ointment and a gel.
✚▲ Side-effects/warning: See FUSIDIC ACID; HYDROCORTISONE.

Fucidin Intertulle

(Leo) (Sodium Fusidate Gauze Dressing, BP) is a proprietary, prescription-only preparation of the narrow-spectrum ANTIBACTERIAL and ANTIBIOTIC fusidic acid (as sodium fusidate). It can be used to treat staphylococcal infections that prove to be resistant to penicillin, and is available as a gauze dressing.
✚▲ Side-effects/warning: See FUSIDIC ACID.

Fucithalmic

(Leo) is a proprietary, prescription-only preparation of the narrow-spectrum

ANTIBACTERIAL and ANTIBIOTIC fusidic acid. It can be used against staphylococcal infections of the eye that prove to be resistant to penicillin, and is available as eye-drops.

+▲ Side-effects/warning: See FUSIDIC ACID.

Fulcin

(Zeneca) is a proprietary, prescription-only preparation of the ANTIFUNGAL and ANTIBIOTIC griseofulvin. It can be used to treat fungal infections of the scalp, skin and nails, and is available as tablets and an oral suspension.

+▲ Side-effects/warning: See GRISEOFULVIN.

Full Marks Lotion

(Napp) is a proprietary, non-prescription preparation of the PEDICULICIDAL phenothrin. It can be used for the treatment of lice, and is available as a lotion. It is not normally given to infants under six months, except on medical advice.

+▲ Side-effects/warning: See PHENOTHRIN.

fungicidal

see ANTIFUNGAL

Fungilin

(Squibb) is a proprietary, prescription-only preparation of the ANTIFUNGAL and ANTIBIOTIC drug amphotericin. It can be used used to treat fungal infections, especially candidiasis (thrush) of the mouth and gastrointestinal tract. It is available as tablets, a liquid oral suspension and as lozenges.

+▲ Side-effects/warning: See AMPHOTERICIN.

Fungizone

(Squibb) is a proprietary, prescription-only preparation of the ANTIFUNGAL amphotericin. It can be used to treat systemic fungal infections, and is available in a form for intravenous infusion.

+▲ Side-effects/warning: See AMPHOTERICIN.

Furadantin

(Procter & Gamble) is a proprietary, prescription-only preparation of the ANTIBACTERIAL nitrofurantoin. It can be used to treat infections of the urinary tract, and is available as tablets and an oral suspension.

+▲ Side-effects/warning: See NITROFURANTOIN.

Furamide

(Boots) is a proprietary, prescription-only preparation of the ANTIPROTOZOAL and AMOEBICIDAL diloxanide furoate. It can be used to treat chronic intestinal infection by *Entamoeba histolytica*, and is available as tablets.

+▲ Side-effects/warning: See DILOXANIDE FUROATE.

furosemide

see FRUSEMIDE

fusafungine

is an ANTI-INFLAMMATORY and ANTIBIOTIC drug which is used in a proprietary preparation to treat infection and inflammation in the nose and throat. Administration is by topical application.

✪ Related entry: Locabiotal.

fusidic acid

(sodium fusidate) is a narrow-spectrum ANTIBACTERIAL and ANTIBIOTIC drug. It is commonly used in combination with other antibiotics to treat staphylococcal infections, especially infections of the skin, infections of the lining of the heart, infections of the bone (osteomyelitis) and the eye, that prove to be resistant to penicillin. The drug works by inhibiting protein synthesis at the ribosome level in sensitive organisms (Gram-positive bacteria). Administration can be oral, by infusion or by topical application. It is also used in the form of its salt sodium fusidate and as diethanolamine fusidate.

+ Side-effects: Nausea and vomiting; rash; jaundice.

▲ Warning: Regular monitoring of liver function during treatment is essential.
○ **Related entries:** Fucibet; Fucidin; Fucidin H; Fucidin Intertulle; Fucithalmic.

Fybogel

(Reckitt & Colman) is a proprietary, non-prescription preparation of the (*bulking-agent*) LAXATIVE ispaghula husk. It can be used to treat a number of gastrointestinal disorders, and is available as effervescent granules; another form, *Fybogel Orange*, is also available. It is not normally given to children under six years, except on medical advice.
✚▲ Side-effects/warning: See ISPAGHULA HUSK.

Fybogel Mebeverine

(Reckitt & Colman) is a proprietary, prescription-only COMPOUND PREPARATION of the ANTISPASMODIC mebeverine hydrochloride and the (*bulking-agent*) LAXATIVE ispaghula husk. It can be used to treat conditions characterized by gastrointestinal spasm, such as irritable bowel syndrome, and is available as effervescent granules.
✚▲ Side-effects/warning: See ISPAGHULA HUSK; MEBEVERINE HYDROCHLORIDE.

Fybozest Orange

(Reckitt & Colman) is a proprietary, non-prescription preparation of the (*bulking-agent*) LAXATIVE ispaghula husk. It can also be used in intestinal atony and to reduce cholesterol uptake in patients with hypercholesteraemia. It is available as effervescent granules.
✚▲ Side-effects/warning: See ISPAGHULA HUSK.

Fynnon Calcium Aspirin

(Seton) is a proprietary, non-prescription COMPOUND ANALGESIC preparation of the (NSAID) NON-NARCOTIC ANALGESIC and ANTIRHEUMATIC aspirin and the ANTACID calcium carbonate. It can be used to treat rheumatic pain, stiffness and swelling of the joints, and to provide relief from the symptoms of minor upper respiratory tract infections. It is available as tablets and is not normally given to children, except on medical advice.
✚▲ Side-effects/warning: See ASPIRIN; CALCIUM CARBONATE; PARACETAMOL.

Fynnon Salt

(Seton) is a proprietary, non-prescription preparation of the (OSMOTIC) *laxative* sodium sulphate. It can be used to relieve constipation, and is available as a powder. It is not normally given to children under 12 years, except on medical advice.

G

gabapentin

is an ANTICONVULSANT and ANTI-EPILEPTIC drug. It can be used to assist in the control of seizures that have not responded to other anti-epileptics. Administration is oral.

✚ Side-effects: Sleepiness, dizziness, unsteady gait, fatigue, eye-flicker and double vision, headache, tremor, nausea and vomiting, rhinitis, weight gain, convulsions, dyspepsia, cough, nervousness and amnesia.

▲ Warning: Administer with care in certain seizures, to patients with certain kidney disorders, or who are pregnant or breast-feeding. Withdrawal of treatment should be gradual.

✪ Related entry: Neurontin.

Galake

(Galen) is a proprietary, non-prescription COMPOUND ANALGESIC preparation of the (OPIOID) NARCOTIC ANALGESIC and ANTITUSSIVE dihydrocodeine tartrate and the NON-NARCOTIC ANALGESIC and ANTIPYRETIC paracetamol (in the ratio 500:10 (mg) – a combination known as co-dydramol). It can be used for pain and high body temperature, and is available as tablets.

✚▲ Side-effects/warning: See DIHYDROCODEINE TARTRATE; PARACETAMOL.

Galcodine

(Galen) is a proprietary, prescription-only preparation of the (OPIOID) ANTITUSSIVE codeine phosphate. It can be used to relieve a dry, painful cough, and is available as a sugar-free linctus.

✚▲ Side-effects/warning: See CODEINE PHOSPHATE.

Galcodine Paediatric

(Galen) is a proprietary, prescription-only preparation of the (OPIOID) ANTITUSSIVE codeine phosphate. It can be used to relieve a dry, painful cough, and is available as a sugar-free linctus. It is not normally given to children under one year, except on medical advice.

✚▲ Side-effects/warning: See CODEINE PHOSPHATE.

Galenamet

(Galen) is a proprietary preparation of the H_2-ANTAGONIST cimetidine, and is available on prescription or without a prescription in a limited amount and for short-term uses only. It can be used as an ULCER-HEALING DRUG for benign peptic ulcers (in the stomach or duodenum), gastro-oesophageal reflux and dyspepsia and associated conditions. It is available as tablets.

✚▲ Side-effects/warning: See CIMETIDINE.

Galenamox

(Galen) is a proprietary, prescription-only preparation of the broad-spectrum ANTIBACTERIAL and (PENICILLIN) ANTIBIOTIC amoxycillin. It can be used to treat systemic bacterial infections, infections of the upper respiratory tract, of the ear, nose and throat and of the urinogenital tracts. It is available as capsules and an oral suspension.

✚▲ Side-effects/warning: See AMOXYCILLIN.

Galenphol Linctus

(Galen) is a proprietary, non-prescription preparation of the (OPIOID) ANTITUSSIVE pholcodine. It can be used for a dry, painful cough, and is available as a sugar-free linctus.

✚▲ Side-effects/warning: See PHOLCODINE.

Galenphol Linctus, Strong

(Galen) is a proprietary, non-prescription preparation of the (OPIOID) ANTITUSSIVE

G

pholcodine. It can be used for a dry, painful cough, and is available as a sugar-free linctus.

+▲ Side-effects/warning: See PHOLCODINE.

Galenphol Paediatric Linctus

(Galen) is a proprietary, non-prescription preparation of the (OPIOID) ANTITUSSIVE pholcodine. It can be used for a dry, painful cough, and is available as a sugar-free linctus. It is not normally given to children under one year, except on medical advice.

+▲ Side-effects/warning: See PHOLCODINE.

Galfer

(Galen) is a proprietary, non-prescription preparation of ferrous fumarate. It can be used as an IRON supplement in iron-deficiency ANAEMIA TREATMENT, and is available as capsules and a syrup.

+▲ Side-effects/warning: See FERROUS FUMARATE.

Galfer FA

(Galen) is a proprietary, non-prescription COMPOUND PREPARATION of ferrous fumarate and folic acid. It can be used as an IRON and folic acid supplement during pregnancy, and is available as capsules.

+▲ Side-effects/warning: See FERROUS FUMARATE; FOLIC ACID.

Galfloxin

(Galen) is a proprietary, prescription-only preparation of the ANTIBACTERIAL and (PENICILLIN) ANTIBIOTIC flucloxacillin. It can be used to treat bacterial infections, especially staphylococcal infections that prove to be resistant to penicillin, and is available as capsules.

+▲ Side-effects/warning: See FLUCLOXACILLIN.

gallamine triethiodide

is a *non-depolarizing* SKELETAL MUSCLE RELAXANT which is used to induce muscle paralysis during surgery. Administration is by injection.

+▲ Side-effects/warning: See TUBOCURARINE CHLORIDE; but causes greater speeding of the heart. Avoid its use in patients with severe kidney disease.

○ Related entry: Flaxedil.

Galpseud

(Galen) is a proprietary, non-prescription preparation of the SYMPATHOMIMETIC pseudoephedrine hydrochloride. It can be used as a NASAL DECONGESTANT, and is available as tablets or an orange-flavoured, sugar-free linctus for dilution.

+▲ Side-effects/warning: See PSEUDOEPHEDRINE HYDROCHLORIDE.

Galpseud Plus

(Galen) is a proprietary, non-prescription COMPOUND PREPARATION of the SYMPATHOMIMETIC pseudoephedrine hydrochloride and the ANTIHISTAMINE chlorpheniramine maleate. It can be used as a NASAL DECONGESTANT and for the relief of cold symptoms, and is available as tablets or a linctus.

+▲ Side-effects/warning: See CHLORPHENIRAMINE MALEATE; PSEUDOEPHEDRINE HYDROCHLORIDE.

Gamanil

(Merck) is a proprietary, prescription-only preparation of the (TRICYCLIC) ANTIDEPRESSANT lofepramine (as hydrochloride). It can be used to treat depressive illness, and is available as tablets.

+▲ Side-effects/warning: See LOFEPRAMINE.

gamma globulin

see NORMAL IMMUNOGLOBULIN

Gammabulin

(Immuno) is a proprietary, prescription-only preparation of human NORMAL IMMUNOGLOBULIN. It can be used to confer immediate *passive immunity* against infection by viruses, including hepatitis A virus, rubeola (measles) and rubella (German measles). It is available in a form

G

for intramuscular injection.
+▲ Side-effects/warning: See
IMMUNIZATION.

gamolenic acid

is used in preparations that are taken by
mouth for the relief of atopic eczema and
breast pain.
+ Side-effects: There may be nausea,
headache or indigestion.
▲ Warning: Use with caution in patients
who are pregnant or epileptics.
○ Related entries: Efamast; Epogam.

ganciclovir

is an ANTIVIRAL drug related to acyclovir but
which is more toxic. Its use is therefore
restricted to the treatment of life-
threatening or sight-threatening
cytomegalovirus infections in
immunocompromised patients, and to
prevent cytomegalovirus disease during
immunosuppressive therapy following
organ transplant operations. Administration
is by intravenous infusion.
+ Side-effects: There are many side-effects;
various blood cell deficiencies; sore throat
and swelling of the face; fever and rash;
effects on liver function, gastrointestinal
disturbances; and a number of other
reactions.
▲ Warning: It should not be given to
patients who are pregnant or breast-feeding.
Blood monitoring is necessary. Administer
with caution to patients with blood-cell
deficiency or kidney impairment. An
adequate fluid intake must be maintained.
○ Related entry: Cymevene.

Ganda

(Smith & Nephew) is a proprietary,
prescription-only COMPOUND PREPARATION of
the ADRENERGIC-NEURONE BLOCKER
guanethidine monosulphate and the
SYMPATHOMIMETIC adrenaline. It can be used
as a GLAUCOMA TREATMENT, and is available as
eye-drops.
+▲ Side-effects/warning: See ADRENALINE;
GUANETHIDINE MONOSULPHATE.

ganglion-blockers 🔄

are drugs from a class of agents that block
transmission in the peripheral autonomic
nervous system at the nervous junction
called ganglia. These drugs work by
preventing the actions of ACETYLCHOLINE,
which is the NEUROTRANSMITTER at these
junctions and so, in effect, ganglion-
blockers are a type of ANTICHOLINERGIC drug.
The cholinergic receptors at which
ganglion-blockers act are called nicotinic
receptors (since NICOTINE is a strong
stimulant at such receptors) and these are
similar, but not identical, to the cholinergic
receptors of the same name that are found
at the skeletal neuromuscular junction. One
result of this is that some of the SKELETAL
MUSCLE RELAXANTS (eg TUBOCURARINE CHLORIDE
and GALLAMINE TRIETHIODIDE) have some
ganglion-blocking side-effects and vice
versa. The ganglion-blockers were
introduced as ANTIHYPERTENSIVES (and are
very effective as such), but their actions and
side-effects are so widespread that they are
now rarely used in medicine. However,
TRIMETAPHAN CAMSYLATE is still in use because
it reduces blood pressure by reducing
vascular tone normally induced by the
sympathetic nervous system, and as it is
short-acting it makes a useful HYPOTENSIVE
for controlling blood pressure during
surgery.
    A quite different group of
anticholinergic drugs, the ANTIMUSCARINICS,
have very extensive uses in medicine. For
this reason, the term 'anticholinergic' is
commonly used synonymously with
antimuscarinic, though this is not really
correct. (Examples of drugs that block the
actions of acetylcholine at muscarinic
receptors are ATROPINE SULPHATE, BENZHEXOL
HYDROCHLORIDE and HYOSCINE
HYDROBROMIDE.)

Garamycin

(Schering-Plough) is a proprietary,
prescription-only preparation of the
ANTIBACTERIAL and (AMINOGLYCOSIDE)
ANTIBIOTIC gentamicin (as sulphate). It can

be used to treat many forms of infection, particularly serious infections caused by Gram-negative bacteria, and is available as eye- and ear-drops.

+▲ Side-effects/warning: See GENTAMICIN.

Gardenal Sodium

(Rhône-Poulenc Rorer) is a proprietary, prescription-only preparation of the BARBITURATE phenobarbitone (as sodium) and is on the Controlled Drugs List. It can be used as an ANTICONVULSANT and ANTI-EPILEPTIC to treat most forms of epilepsy, and is available in a form for injection.

+▲ Side-effects/warning: See PHENOBARBITONE.

Gastrobid Continus

(Napp) is a proprietary, prescription-only preparation of the ANTI-EMETIC and ANTINAUSEANT metoclopramide hydrochloride. It can be used to treat nausea and vomiting, particularly in gastrointestinal disorders and after treatment with radiation or cytotoxic drugs. It also has gastric MOTILITY STIMULANT actions and can be used in the treatment of non-ulcer dyspepsia, gastric stasis and for the prevention of reflux oesophagitis. It is available as modified-release tablets.

+▲ Side-effects/warning: See METOCLOPRAMIDE HYDROCHLORIDE.

Gastrocote

(Boehringer Mannheim) is a proprietary, non-prescription COMPOUND PREPARATION of the ANTACIDS aluminium hydroxide, sodium bicarbonate and magnesium trisilicate and the DEMULCENT alginic acid. It can be used for the symptomatic relief of heartburn, reflux oesophagitis and hiatus hernia, and is available as chewable tablets.

+▲ Side-effects/warning: See ALUMINIUM HYDROXIDE; MAGNESIUM TRISILICATE; SODIUM BICARBONATE.

Gastroflux

(Ashbourne) is a proprietary, prescription-only preparation of the ANTI-EMETIC and ANTINAUSEANT metoclopramide hydrochloride. It can be used to treat nausea and vomiting, particularly of gastrointestinal disorders and after treatment with radiation or cytotoxic drugs. It also has gastric MOTILITY STIMULANT actions and can be used in the treatment of non-ulcer dyspepsia, gastric stasis and for the prevention of reflux oesophagitis. It is available as tablets.

+▲ Side-effects/warning: See METOCLOPRAMIDE HYDROCHLORIDE.

Gastromax

(Pharmacia) is a proprietary, prescription-only preparation of the ANTI-EMETIC and ANTINAUSEANT metoclopramide hydrochloride. It can be used to treat nausea and vomiting, particularly of gastrointestinal disorders and after treatment with radiation or cytotoxic drugs. It also has gastric MOTILITY STIMULANT actions and can be used in the treatment of non-ulcer dyspepsia, gastric stasis and for the prevention of reflux oesophagitis. It is available as modified-release capsules.

+▲ Side-effects/warning: See METOCLOPRAMIDE HYDROCHLORIDE.

Gaviscon 250

(Reckitt & Colman) is a proprietary, non-prescription COMPOUND PREPARATION of the ANTACIDS aluminium hydroxide, sodium bicarbonate and magnesium trisilicate and the DEMULCENT alginic acid. It can be used for the symptomatic relief of indigestion and heartburn, and is available as tablets.

+▲ Side-effects/warning: See ALUMINIUM HYDROXIDE; MAGNESIUM TRISILICATE; SODIUM BICARBONATE.

Gaviscon 500

(Reckitt & Colman) is a proprietary, non-prescription COMPOUND PREPARATION of the ANTACIDS aluminium hydroxide, sodium bicarbonate and magnesium trisilicate and the DEMULCENT alginic acid. It can be used for the symptomatic relief of indigestion and heartburn, and is available as tablets.

+▲ Side-effects/warning: See ALUMINIUM HYDROXIDE; MAGNESIUM TRISILICATE; SODIUM BICARBONATE.

Gaviscon Liquid

(Reckitt & Colman) is a proprietary, non-prescription COMPOUND PREPARATION of the ANTACIDS calcium carbonate and sodium bicarbonate and the DEMULCENT alginic acid (as sodium alginate). It can be used for the symptomatic relief of heartburn and indigestion due to gastric reflux, and is available as a liquid. It is not normally given to children, except on medical advice.
+▲ Side-effects/warning: See CALCIUM CARBONATE; SODIUM BICARBONATE.

Geangin

(Cusi) is a proprietary, prescription-only preparation of the CALCIUM-CHANNEL BLOCKER verapamil hydrochloride. It can be used as an ANTIHYPERTENSIVE, as an ANTI-ANGINA drug in the prevention of attacks and as an ANTI-ARRHYTHMIC to correct heart irregularities. It is available as tablets.
+▲ Side-effects/warning: See VERAPAMIL HYDROCHLORIDE.

Gelcosal

(Quinoderm) is a proprietary, non-prescription COMPOUND PREPARATION of salicylic acid and coal tar (and pine tar). It can be used to treat psoriasis or dermatitis, and is available as a gel and a liquid scalp preparation.
+▲ Side-effects/warning: See COAL TAR; SALICYLIC ACID.

Gelcotar

(Quinoderm) is a proprietary, non-prescription preparation of coal tar (and pine tar). It can be used to treat psoriasis and eczema, and is available as a gel (with pine tar) and a liquid (with cade oil).
+▲ Side-effects/warning: See COAL TAR.

GelTears

(Chauvin) is a proprietary, non-prescription preparation of carbomer. It can be used as artificial tears where there is dryness of the eye due to disease (eg ketanoconjunctivitis). It is available as a gel for application to the eye.
+▲ Side-effects/warning: See CARBOMER.

gemcitabine

is a CYTOTOXIC drug which is used as an ANTICANCER treatment of locally advanced or metastatic non-small cell lung cancer. Administration is by injection.
+▲ Side-effects/warning: See CYTOTOXICS.
✪ Related entry: Gemzar.

gemeprost

is a PROSTAGLANDIN (an analogue of prostaglandin E_1), which is a LOCAL HORMONE naturally involved in the control of uterine motility, that is used in early pregnancy in operative procedures. It is administered to the cervix by pessary to cause softening and dilation. It is also used as an ABORTIFACIENT to cause therapeutic abortion and to remove the foetus following intra-uterine death.
+ Side-effects: Vaginal bleeding and uterine pain; nausea, vomiting, flushing and shivering, headache and dizziness, a raised temperature and diarrhoea, muscle weakness, chills, backache, chest pain and breathing difficulties. Uterine rupture has been reported.
▲ Warning: It should not be administered to patients who have vaginal or cervical infections, or cardiovascular insufficiency. Administer with caution to those with asthma or glaucoma.
✪ Related entry: Gemeprost.

Gemeprost

(Farillon) is a proprietary, prescription-only preparation of the PROSTAGLANDIN analogue gemeprost. It is used during induction of labour and earlier in operative procedures, and is available as a pessary.
+▲ Side-effects/warning: See GEMEPROST.

gemfibrozil

can be used as a LIPID-LOWERING DRUG in

hyperlipidaemia to reduce the levels, or change the proportions, of various lipids in the bloodstream. It is usually administered only to patients in whom a strict and regular dietary regime, alone, is not having the desired effect. Administration is oral.

✚ Side-effects: Dizziness, blurred vision, gastrointestinal disturbances, skin disorders, pain in the extremities, muscle pain and impotence.

▲ Warning: It is not to be given to alcoholics, patients with liver damage, gallstones or who are pregnant. Blood and liver function should be monitored and eyes tested.

✪ Related entry: Lopid.

Gemzar

(Lilly) is a proprietary, prescription-only preparation of the (CYTOTOXIC) ANTICANCER drug gemcitabine (as hydrochloride). It is available in a form for injection.

✚▲ Side-effects/warning: See GEMCITABINE.

general anaesthetics ▨

are drugs that reduce sensation in the whole body with a loss of consciousness, and are used for surgical procedures. LOCAL ANAESTHETICS, in contrast, affect sensation in a specific, local area without the loss of consciousness. The general anaesthetic that is used to initially induce anaesthesia is often different from the drug, or drugs, administered to maintain the anaesthesia. For induction, short-acting general anaesthetics that can be injected are convenient (eg THIOPENTONE SODIUM, ETOMIDATE and METHOHEXITONE SODIUM), but for maintenance during long operations, inhalation anaesthetics are commonly used (eg HALOTHANE and ENFLURANE). In order to minimize the depth of anaesthesia necessary for a surgical procedure, premedication with, or concurrent use of, other drugs is usually necessary. A range of ancillary drugs are also valuable, including TRANQUILLIZERS or SEDATIVES (eg BENZODIAZEPINES), ANALGESICS (eg MORPHINE), SKELETAL MUSCLE RELAXANTS (eg TUBOCURARINE

CHLORIDE) and concurrent use of local anaesthetics (eg LIGNOCAINE HYDROCHLORIDE). See also CYCLOPROPANE; DESFLURANE; DIETHYL ETHER; ISOFLURANE; KETAMINE; PROPOFOL.

Genotropin

(Pharmacia) is a proprietary, prescription-only preparation of somatropin, which is the biosynthetic form of human growth hormone. It is used to treat growth hormone deficiency and associated symptoms (in particular, short stature). It is available in several forms for injection, including a powder for reconstitution, in cartridges (*KabiPen* and *KabiVial*) and in preloaded syringes (*KabiQuick*).

✚▲ Side-effects/warning: See SOMATROPIN.

gentamicin

is a broad-spectrum ANTIBACTERIAL and ANTIBIOTIC drug, which is the most widely used of the AMINOGLYCOSIDE family. Although it does have activity against Gram-positive bacteria, it is used primarily against serious infections caused by Gram-negative bacteria. It is not orally absorbed and is therefore given by injection or infusion for the treatment of, for example, septicaemia, meningitis, infections of the heart (usually in conjunction with penicillin), the kidney, prostate gland, eye and ear and skin infections. Because of its potential toxicity to the ear (ototoxicity), which could result in deafness, and its toxicity to the kidney (nephrotoxicity), treatment should be short term. It is also available in the form of drops, creams and ointments for topical application.

✚ Side-effects: Depending on the route of administration; prolonged or high dosage may be damaging to the ear (especially in the elderly, children and patients with renal damage) and cause deafness and balance disorders – treatment must be discontinued if this occurs; there may also be reversible kidney damage.

▲ Warning: Again, these depend on the route of administration. But it should not be

G

administered to patients who are pregnant or breast-feeding, or who suffer from myasthenia gravis or impaired kidney function. Kidney and neuronal function and gentamicin blood concentrations must be monitored.

✪ Related entries: Cidomycin; Cidomycin Topical; Garamycin; Genticin; Gentisone HC; Isotonic Gentamicin Injection; Minims Gentamicin.

gentian violet
see CRYSTAL VIOLET

Genticin
(Roche) is a proprietary, prescription-only preparation of the ANTIBACTERIAL and (AMINOGLYCOSIDE) ANTIBIOTIC gentamicin (as sulphate). It can be used to treat many forms of infection, particularly serious infections caused by Gram-negative bacteria, and is available in a form for injection and as eye- and ear-drops.
✚▲ Side-effects/warning: See GENTAMICIN.

Gentisone HC
(Roche) is a proprietary, prescription-only COMPOUND PREPARATION of the ANTIBACTERIAL and (AMINOGLYCOSIDE) ANTIBIOTIC gentamicin (as sulphate) and the ANTI-INFLAMMATORY and CORTICOSTEROID hydrocortisone (as acetate). It can be used to treat bacterial infections of the middle ear, and is available as ear-drops.
✚▲ Side-effects/warning: See GENTAMICIN; HYDROCORTISONE.

Geref 50
(Serono) is a proprietary, prescription-only preparation of sermorelin. It is used to test the release of GROWTH HORMONE, and is available in a for injection.
✚▲ Side-effects/warning: See SERMORELIN.

Germoline Cream
(SmithKline Beecham) is a proprietary, non-prescription COMPOUND PREPARATION of the ANTISEPTICS chlorhexidine (as gluconate) and phenol. It can be used for

cleaning all types of lesions, ranging from minor skin disorders or blisters to minor burns and small wounds, and preventing them from becoming infected. It is available as a cream.
✚▲ Side-effects/warning: See CHLORHEXIDINE; PHENOL.

Germoline Ointment
(SmithKline Beecham) is a proprietary, non-prescription COMPOUND PREPARATION of the ASTRINGENT agent ZINC OXIDE, the ANTISEPTICS phenol, octaphonium and methyl salicylate and the EMOLLIENTS white petroleum jelly, liquid paraffin and lanolin. It can be used for cleaning minor skin disorders, blisters, sunburn, minor burns and small wounds and preventing them from becoming infected. It is available as an ointment.
✚▲ Side-effects/warning: See LANOLIN; LIQUID PARAFFIN; METHYL SALICYLATE; PHENOL.

Germoloids
(SmithKline Beecham) is a proprietary, non-prescription COMPOUND PREPARATION of the LOCAL ANAESTHETIC lignocaine hydrochloride and the ASTRINGENT agent ZINC OXIDE. It can be used for the symptomatic relief of the pain and itching of haemorrhoids and pruritus ani. It is available as an ointment, a cream and as suppositories, and is not normally given to children, except on medical advice.
✚▲ Side-effects/warning: See LIGNOCAINE HYDROCHLORIDE.

gestodene
is a PROGESTOGEN which is used as a constituent of the combined ORAL CONTRACEPTIVES that contain OESTROGEN and a progestogen. Administration is oral.
✚▲ Side-effects/warning: See PROGESTOGEN.
✪ Related entries: Femodene; Femodene ED; Minulet; Tri-Minulet; Triadene.

Gestone
(Paines & Byrne) is a proprietary,

prescription-only preparation of the PROGESTOGEN progesterone. It can be used to treat many hormonal deficiency disorders in women, abnormal bleeding from the uterus and for maintenance of early pregnancy in recurrent miscarriage. It is available in a form for injection.
+▲ Side-effects/warning: See PROGESTERONE.

gestronol hexanoate
is a synthetic form of PROGESTOGEN, a SEX HORMONE, which is used primarily in women as an ANTICANCER treatment for cancer of the uterine lining (endometrium), but it can also be used to treat (malignant) enlargement of the kidneys (hypernephroma) and benign enlargement of the prostate gland in men. Administration is by intramuscular injection.
+▲ Side-effects/warning: See MEDROXYPROGESTERONE ACETATE.
✪ Related entry: Depostat.

Glandosane
(Fresenius) is a proprietary, non-prescription COMPOUND PREPARATION of CARMELLOSE SODIUM, SORBITOL, POTASSIUM CHLORIDE, sodium chloride and other salts. It can be used as a form of ARTIFICIAL SALIVA for application to the mouth and throat in conditions that make the mouth abnormally dry. It is available as an aerosol.
+▲ Side-effects/warning: See SODIUM CHLORIDE.

Glaucol
(Baker Norton) is a proprietary, prescription-only preparation of the BETA-BLOCKER timolol maleate. It can be used for GLAUCOMA TREATMENT, and is available as eye-drops.
+▲ Side-effects/warning: See TIMOLOL MALEATE.

glaucoma treatment ▨
involves the use of drugs to lower the raised intraocular pressure (pressure in

the eyeball) that is characteristic of the group of eye conditions in which the optic nerve, and so consequently vision, is damaged within the eye. A number of types of drug can help to reduce this pressure (which has nothing to do with blood pressure) and which one is administered depends on what sort of glaucoma is being treated (such as simple, open-angle, closed-angle, etc.). BETA-BLOCKERS are effective in most cases (eg BETAXOLOL HYDROCHLORIDE, CARTEOLOL HYDROCHLORIDE, LEVOBUNOLOL HYDROCHLORIDE and METIPRANOLOL), some SYMPATHOMIMETICS (eg APRACLONIDINE and DIPIVEFRINE HYDROCHLORIDE) and certain cholinergic drugs (eg CARBACHOL, PHYSOSTIGMINE SULPHATE and PILOCARPINE).

It is important to note that certain classes of drugs, such as the CORTICOSTEROIDS and ANTICHOLINERGICS (eg ATROPINE SULPHATE), cause a rise in intraocular pressure and if administered to patients predisposed to glaucoma may precipitate an acute attack.

glibenclamide
is one of the SULPHONYLUREAS and is used in DIABETIC TREATMENT of Type II diabetes (non-insulin-dependent diabetes mellitus; NIDDM; maturity-onset diabetes). It works by augmenting what remains of INSULIN production in the pancreas. Administration is oral.
+ Side-effects: These are generally minor and rare, but there may be some sensitivity reactions, such as a rash and also blood disorders. There may be headache and gastrointestinal upsets.
▲ Warning: It should not be administered to patients with certain liver, kidney or endocrine disorders, or who are under stress, pregnant or breast-feeding; and should be avoided in the elderly because of possible hypoglycaemia. There may be weight gain so diet should be controlled.
✪ Related entries: Calabren; Daonil; Diabetamide; Euglucon; Libanil; Malix; Semi-Daonil.

G

Glibenese

(Pfizer) is a proprietary, prescription-only preparation of the SULPHONYLUREA glipizide. It can be used in DIABETIC TREATMENT of Type II diabetes (non-insulin-dependent diabetes mellitus; NIDDM; maturity-onset diabetes), and is available as tablets.

✚▲ Side-effects/warning: See GLIPIZIDE.

gliclazide

is one of the SULPHONYLUREAS and is used in DIABETIC TREATMENT of Type II diabetes (non-insulin-dependent diabetes mellitus; NIDDM; maturity-onset diabetes). It works by augmenting what remains of INSULIN production in the pancreas. Administration is oral.

✚▲ Side-effects/warning: See GLIBENCLAMIDE; but, it may be used in renal impairment and the elderly.

⊘ Related entry: Diamicron.

glipizide

is one of the SULPHONYLUREAS and is used in DIABETIC TREATMENT of Type II diabetes (non-insulin-dependent diabetes mellitus; NIDDM; maturity-onset diabetes). It works by augmenting what remains of INSULIN production in the pancreas. Administration is oral.

✚▲ Side-effects/warning: See GLIBENCLAMIDE.

⊘ Related entries: Glibenese; Minodiab.

gliquidone

is one of the SULPHONYLUREAS and is used in DIABETIC TREATMENT of Type II diabetes (non-insulin-dependent diabetes mellitus; NIDDM; maturity-onset diabetes). It works by augmenting what remains of INSULIN production in the pancreas. Administration is oral.

✚▲ Side-effects/warning: See GLIBENCLAMIDE; but, it may be used in patients with kidney impairment.

⊘ Related entry: Glurenorm.

GlucaGen Kit

(Novo Nordisk) is a proprietary

prescription-only preparation of the HORMONE glucagon. It is used primarily as a diagnostic aid to test blood glucose control mechanisms and for emergency use in patients with low blood sugar levels. Administration is by injection.

✚▲ Side-effects/warning: See GLUCAGON.

glucagon

is a HORMONE produced and secreted by the pancreas in order to cause an increase in blood sugar levels, that is, it is a hyperglycaemic agent. It is normally part of a balancing mechanism with INSULIN, which has the opposite effect. Therapeutically, glucagon can be administered to patients with low blood sugar levels (hypoglycaemia) in an emergency, but it is mainly used for diagnostic purposes. Administration is by injection.

✚ Side-effects: Diarrhoea, nausea; vomiting; occasionally hypersensitivity reactions.

▲ Warning: It should not to be administered to patients with insulinoma, phaeochromocytoma or glucagonoma.

⊘ Related entry: GlucaGen Kit.

Glucobay

(Bayer) is a proprietary, prescription-only preparation of acarbose. It is used in DIABETIC TREATMENT, and is available as tablets.

✚▲ Side-effects/warning: See ACARBOSE.

Glucophage

(Lipha) is a proprietary, prescription-only preparation of the BIGUANIDE metformin hydrochloride. It is used in DIABETIC TREATMENT of Type II diabetes (non-insulin-dependent diabetes mellitus; NIDDM; maturity-onset diabetes), and is available as tablets.

✚▲ Side-effects/warning: See METFORMIN HYDROCHLORIDE.

glucose

or dextrose, is a simple sugar and is an important source of energy for the body –

and the sole source of energy for the brain. Once digested, it is stored in the liver and muscles in the form of glycogen and its break down in the muscles back into glucose produces energy. The level of glucose in the blood is critical and harmful symptoms can occur if the level is too high or too low. Therapeutically, it may be administered as a dietary supplement in conditions of low blood sugar level, to treat abnormally high acidity of body fluids (acidosis) or to increase glucose levels in the liver following liver damage. Administration is either oral or by intravenous infusion.

Glurenorm

(Sanofi Winthrop) is a proprietary, prescription-only preparation of the SULPHONYLUREA gliquidone. It is used in DIABETIC TREATMENT of Type II diabetes (non-insulin-dependent diabetes mellitus; NIDDM; maturity-onset diabetes), and is available as tablets.

+▲ Side-effects/warning: See GLIQUIDONE.

glutaraldehyde

is a DISINFECTANT, or ANTISEPTIC, which is similar to formaldehyde, but is stronger and faster-acting. It is mostly used to sterilize medical and surgical equipment. Therapeutically, it can be used in solution for warts (particularly verrucas) and as a KERATOLYTIC to remove hard, dead skin.

+▲ Side-effects/warning: See SALICYLIC ACID. Its effects as a treatment are not always predictable; skin treated may become irritated or sensitized.

✪ Related entries: Glutarol; Verucasep.

Glutarol

(Dermal) is a proprietary, non-prescription preparation of the KERATOLYTIC agent glutaraldehyde. It can be used to treat warts and to remove hard, dead skin, and is available as a solution for topical application.

+▲ Side-effects/warning: See GLUTARALDEHYDE.

glycerin(e)

see GLYCEROL

glycerol

or glycerin(e), is a colourless sweet viscous liquid that is chemically an alcohol. It is used therapeutically as a constituent in many EMOLLIENT skin preparations, as a sweetening agent for medications and as a LAXATIVE in the form of anal suppositories. Taken orally, glycerol can be used for short-term GLAUCOMA TREATMENT.

✪ Related entries: Compound Thymol Glycerin, BP; Exterol; Fletchers' Enemette; Massé Breast Cream; Micolette Micro-enema; Neutrogena Dematological Cream; Otex Ear Drops.

glyceryl trinitrate

is a short-acting VASODILATOR and ANTI-ANGINA drug. It is used to prevent attacks of angina pectoris (ischaemic heart pain) when taken before exercise, for symptomatic relief during an acute attack and to treat heart failure. It works by dilating the blood vessels returning blood to the heart and so reducing the workload of the heart. It is short-acting, but its effect is extended through use of modified-release tablets kept under the tongue (sublingual tablets). It is also administered by aerosol spray (which is sprayed under the tongue from where it is absorbed into the systemic circulation), by intravenous injection or in ointments and dressings placed on the surface of the chest so that it can be absorbed through the skin.

+ Side-effects: There may be a throbbing headache, flushing, dizziness; some patients experience an increase in heart rate and postural hypotension (fall in blood pressure on standing); when given by injection, there may be additional side-effects.

▲ Warning: It should be administered with caution to patients who suffer from hypotension and certain other cardiovascular disorders, and those with severe liver, kidney or thyroid impairment.

✪ Related entries: Coro-nitro Spray;

G

Deponit; Glytrin Spray; GTN 300 mcg;
Minitran; Nitro-Dur; Nitrocine; Nitrolingual
Pumpspray; Nitrolingual Spray; Nitromin;
Nitronal; Percutol; Suscard; Sustac;
Transiderm-Nitro.

glycol salicylate

like several SALICYLATES, has a COUNTER-
IRRITANT, or RUBEFACIENT, action on topical
application and can be used to relieve
inflammatory pain in joints and muscles.
+▲ Side-effects/warning: On topical
administration there may be some local
irritation. It should not be administered to
broken skin or mucous membranes.
✪ Related entries: Algipan Rub; Cremalgin
Balm; Dubam; Ralgex Cream; Ralgex Heat
Spray; Ralgex Stick.

glycopyrronium bromide

is an ANTICHOLINERGIC drug which is used in
preoperative medication for drying up
saliva and other secretions. Administration
is by injection.
+▲ Side-effects/warning: See ATROPINE
SULPHATE.
✪ Related entries: Robinul; Robinul-
Neostigmine.

Glypressin

(Ferring) is a proprietary preparation of
the pituitary HORMONE antidiuretic hormone
(ADH, or vasopressin). It is administered
as a VASOCONSTRICTOR to treat bleeding
from varices (varicose veins) in the
oesophagus, and is available in a form for
injection.
+▲ Side-effects/warning: See
TERLIPRESSIN.

Glytrin Spray

(Sherwin) is a proprietary, non-
prescription preparation of the VASODILATOR
and ANTI-ANGINA drug glyceryl trinitrate. It
can be used to treat and prevent angina
pectoris, and is available as a sublingual
aerosol spray in metered doses.
+▲ Side-effects/warning: See GLYCERYL
TRINITRATE.

GnRH

see GONADORELIN

Goddard's Embrocation

(LRC) is a proprietary, non-prescription
preparation of TURPENTINE OIL (with
ammonia and acetic acid), which has
COUNTER-IRRITANT, or RUBEFACIENT, action. It
can be applied to the skin for symptomatic
relief of underlying muscle or joint pain,
and is available as an embrocation for
topical application.
▲ Warning: Do not use on inflamed or
broken skin, or on mucous membranes.

gold

in the form of the chemical compounds
sodium aurothiomalate and auranofin, is
used therapeutically as an ANTIRHEUMATIC
treatment for rheumatoid arthritis and
juvenile arthritis. Gold compounds work
very slowly and it may take several months
of treatment before there are any beneficial
effects. Administration is by injection.
+▲ Side-effects/warning: See AURANOFIN;
SODIUM AUROTHIOMALATE.

Golden Eye Drops

(Typharm) is a proprietary, non-
prescription preparation of the
ANTIBACTERIAL propamidine isethionate. It
can be administered to treat infections of
the eyelids or conjunctiva (including
acanthamoeba keratitis), and is available as
eye-drops.
+▲ Side-effects/warning: See PROPAMIDINE
ISETHIONATE.

Golden Eye Ointment

(Typharm) is a proprietary, non-
prescription preparation of the
ANTIBACTERIAL drug dibromopropamidine
isethionate. It can be administered to treat
infections of the eyelids or conjunctiva
(specifically acanthamoeba keratitis), and
is available as an eye ointment and as eye-
drops.
+▲ Side-effects/warning: See
DIBROMOPROPAMIDINE ISETHIONATE.

gonadorelin

(gonadotrophin-releasing hormone; GnRH) is the hypothalamic HORMONE that acts on the pituitary gland to release the GONADOTROPHINS (luteinising hormone; LH, and follicle-stimulating hormone; FSH). It is therefore also known as luteinising-hormone releasing hormone, LH-RH, or more correctly LH-FSH-RH. Gonadorelin is in fact the synthetic analogue of the naturally occurring gonadotrophin-releasing hormone and is used for diagnostic purposes (to assess pituitary function) or as an infertility treatment, when it is given by pulsatile subcutaneous or intravenous infusion. Synthetic analogues of gonadorelin (BUSERELIN, GOSERELIN, LEUPRORELIN ACETATE and NAFARELIN) are used to treat endometriosis, infertility and breast and prostate cancer.

✚ Side-effects: Rarely, there may be headache, abdominal pain and nausea; the site of infusion may become painful.

▲ Warning: Administration of gonadorelin to treat infertility or absence of menstruation has to be by pulsed subcutaneous infusion, which is a form of treatment generally available only in specialist units.

⊙ Related entries: Fertiral; HRF; Relefact LH-RH; Relefact LH-RH/TRH.

Gonadotraphon LH

(Paines & Byrne) is a proprietary, prescription-only preparation of the HORMONE human chorionic gonadotrophin (HCG). It can be used to treat undescended testicles and delayed puberty in boys, and also women who are suffering from specific hormonal deficiency for infertility. It is available in a form for injection.

✚▲ Side-effects/warning: See CHORIONIC GONADOTROPHIN.

gonadotrophins ▣

is the name of a group of HORMONES that are produced and secreted by the anterior pituitary gland, and which act on the ovary in women and on the testes in men to promote the production in turn of other SEX HORMONES and of ova (eggs) or sperm, respectively. The major gonadotrophins are FOLLICLE-STIMULATING HORMONE (FSH) and LUTEINISING HORMONE (LH). In pregnancy, large amounts of a similar hormone are released by the placenta, so it is called CHORIONIC GONADOTROPHIN and this is the basis of most pregnancy tests. These hormones are used as an infertility treatment.

gonadotrophin-releasing hormone

see GONADORELIN

Gonal-F

(Serono) is a proprietary, prescription-only HORMONE preparation of follitropin alpha, which is a synthetic form of FOLLICLE-STIMULATING HORMONE (FSH). It can be used to treat infertile women with proven hypopituitarism and who do not respond to CLOMIPHENE CITRATE (another drug commonly used to treat infertility), and in superovulation treatment in assisted conception (as with *in vitro* fertilization; IVF). It is available in a form for injection.

✚▲ Side-effects/warning: See FOLLITROPIN ALPHA.

Gopten

(Knoll) is a proprietary, prescription-only preparation of the ACE INHIBITOR trandolapril. It can be used as an ANTIHYPERTENSIVE, often in conjunction with other classes of drug, and is available as capsules.

✚▲ Side-effects/warning: See TRANDOLAPRIL.

goserelin

is an analogue of GONADORELIN (gonadothrophin-releasing hormone; GnRH), which is a hypothalamic HORMONE. On prolonged administration it acts as an indirect HORMONE ANTAGONIST in that it reduces the pituitary gland's secretion of gonadotrophin (after an initial surge), which results in reduced secretion of SEX HORMONES by the ovaries or testes. It is used to treat endometriosis, and as an ANTICANCER drug for breast cancer and cancer of the prostate gland. Administration is by subcutaneous injection.

✚▲ Side-effects/warning: See BUSERELIN. Additionally, there may be rashes, bruises at the site of injection and rarely high blood calcium levels in patients with breast cancer.
✪ Related entry: Zoladex.

gramicidin

is an ANTIMICROBIAL and ANTIBIOTIC drug which is incorporated into a number of eye- and ear-drop preparations along with NEOMYCIN SULPHATE and NYSTATIN.
✪ Related entries: Adcortyl with Graneodin; Neosporin; Tri-Adcortyl; Tri-Adcortyl Otic.

Graneodin

(Squibb) is a proprietary, prescription-only preparation of the ANTIBACTERIAL and (AMINOGLYCOSIDE) ANTIBIOTIC neomycin sulphate. It can be used to treat bacterial infections of the skin and to prevent infection following minor surgery. It is available as an ointment for topical application.
✚▲ Side-effects/warning: See NEOMYCIN SULPHATE.

granisetron

is a recently introduced ANTI-EMETIC and ANTINAUSEANT which gives relief from nausea and vomiting, especially in patients receiving cytotoxic radiotherapy or chemotherapy. It acts by blocking the action of the natural mediator SEROTONIN. Administration is either oral or by intravenous injection or infusion.
✚ Side-effects: Headache, rash, constipation and change in liver function.
▲ Warning: Administer with care to patients who are pregnant or breast-feeding.
✪ Related entry: Kytril.

Gregoderm

(Unigreg) is a proprietary, prescription-

only COMPOUND PREPARATION of the ANTI-INFLAMMATORY and CORTICOSTEROID hydrocortisone, the ANTIBACTERIAL and (AMINOGLYCOSIDE) ANTIBIOTIC neomycin sulphate, the antibacterial and (POLYMYXIN) antibiotic polymyxin B sulphate and the ANTIFUNGAL and antibiotic nystatin. It can be used to treat inflammation of the skin in which infection is also present, and is available as an ointment for topical application.
✚▲ Side-effects/warning: See HYDROCORTISONE; NEOMYCIN SULPHATE; NYSTATIN; POLYMYXIN B SULPHATE.

griseofulvin

is a powerful ANTIFUNGAL and ANTIBIOTIC drug. It is most commonly used for large-scale skin infections, especially those that prove resistant to other treatments. During a course of treatment, which can often be quite prolonged, it is deposited selectively in the skin, hair and nails and so prevents further fungal invasion. Administration is oral.
✚ Side-effects: There may be headache with nausea and vomiting; some patients experience sensitivity to light, rash, dizziness, fatigue and blood disorders.
▲ Warning: It should not be administered to patients who suffer from liver failure, porphyria or who are pregnant. Administer with caution to patients who are breast-feeding. Avoid alcohol because its effects are enhanced.
✪ Related entries: Fulcin; Grisovin.

Grisovin

(Glaxo) is a proprietary, prescription-only preparation of the ANTIFUNGAL and ANTIBIOTIC drug griseofulvin. It can be administered to treat various fungal infections of the scalp, skin and nails, and is available as tablets.
✚▲ Side-effects/warning: See GRISEOFULVIN.

growth hormone

see SOMATOTROPIN; SOMATROPIN

GTN 300 mcg

(Martindale) is a proprietary, non-prescription preparation of the VASODILATOR and ANTI-ANGINA drug glyceryl trinitrate. It can be used to treat and prevent angina pectoris and in HEART FAILURE TREATMENT. It is available as short-acting sublingual tablets.

✚▲ Side-effects/warning: See GLYCERYL TRINITRATE.

guaiphenesin

is incorporated into a number of proprietary preparations as an EXPECTORANT, though evidence of its efficacy is lacking. Administration is oral.

✿ Related entries: Actifed Expectorant; Beechams All-In-One; Benylin Chesty Coughs Non-Drowsy; Boots Children's Chesty Cough Syrup; Covonia Bronchial Balsam; Dimotane Expectorant; Do-Do Expectorant Linctus; Famel Expectorant; Jackson's All Fours; Lemsip Chesty Cough; Meltus Adult Expectorant Linctus; Expectorant Linctus; Nirolex for Chesty Coughs; Robitussin Chesty Cough Medicine; Robitussin Chesty Cough with Congestion; Sudafed Expectorant; Tixylix Chesty Cough; Veno's Expectorant; Vicks Original Cough Syrup (Chesty); Vicks Vaposyrup for Chesty Coughs; Vicks Vaposyrup for Chesty Coughs and Nasal Congestion.

guanethidine monosulphate

is an ADRENERGIC-NEURONE BLOCKER, which is an ANTISYMPATHETIC class of drug that prevents release of noradrenaline from sympathetic nerves. It can be used as an ANTIHYPERTENSIVE for moderate to severe high blood pressure, especially when other treatments have failed and usually in conjunction with other antihypertensive drugs (eg a DIURETIC or BETA-BLOCKER). Administration can be either oral or by injection.

✚ Side-effects: Postural hypotension; fluid retention; nasal congestion; diarrhoea, failure to ejaculate; drowsiness.

▲ Warning: It should not be administered to patients with certain renal or heart disorders or phaeochromocytoma; it should be administered with caution to those who are elderly, pregnant or have peptic ulcers, asthma or coronary or cerebral arteriosclerosis.

✿ Related entries: Ganda; Ismelin.

guar gum

is a form of DIABETIC TREATMENT in as much that if it is taken in sufficient quantities it reduces the rise in blood glucose which occurs after meals, probably by delaying absorption of food. It may be used to relieve the symptoms of Dumping Syndrome. It is available as sachets of granules that are dissolved in fluid and drunk before a meal or sprinkled onto food.

✚ Side-effects: Flatulence, distension of the intestine with possible obstruction.

▲ Warning: Do not use when there is pre-existing intestinal obstruction. Fluid intake should be maintained. Gum preparations should usually be taken with plenty of water and not last thing at night.

✿ Related entry: Guarem.

Guarem

(Rybar) is a proprietary, non-prescription preparation of guar gum, which is a form of DIABETIC TREATMENT. It is available as sachets of granules that are dissolved in fluid and drunk before a meal or sprinkled onto food.

✚▲ Side-effects/warning: See GUAR GUM.

Gyno-Daktarin

(Janssen) is a proprietary, prescription-only range of preparations of the ANTIFUNGAL drug miconazole (as nitrate). The various preparations can be used to treat fungal infections of the vagina or vulva (eg candidiasis; thrush). They are available as an intravaginal cream (with its own applicator), vaginal inserts (pessaries), an *Ovule* (a vaginal capsule) called *Gyno-Daktarin 1* and a *Combipack* that

G

G

combines the cream and the pessaries. The preparations are also available, under certain conditions, without prescription.
+▲ Side-effects/warning: See MICONAZOLE.

Gyno-Pevaryl
(Cilag) is a proprietary, prescription-only range of preparations of the ANTIFUNGAL drug econazole nitrate. The various preparations can be used to treat fungal infections of the vagina or vulva (eg candidiasis; thrush) and the penis (applied under the foreskin). They are available as a cream for topical application to the anogenital area, as vaginal inserts (pessaries) in two formulations with one under the name *Gyno-Pevaryl 1* and *Combipacks* that combine the cream and one or other formulation of the pessaries. The cream is also available, under certain conditions, without prescription.
+▲ Side-effects/warning: See ECONAZOLE NITRATE.

Gynol II
(Ortho) is a proprietary, non-prescription SPERMICIDAL CONTRACEPTIVE for use in combination with barrier methods of contraception (such as a condom). It is available as a jelly containing nonoxinol.
+▲ Side-effects/warning: See NONOXINOL.

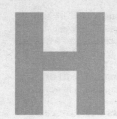

H₂-antagonists
are drugs that act to block the actions of histamine at a class of histamine receptor called H_2, which is found in the gastric mucosa (stomach lining) and promotes secretion of peptic (hydrochloric) acid. The over-production of peptic acid may be involved in ulceration of the gastric (stomach) and duodenal (first part of small intestine) linings, or be the cause of pain in reflux oesophagitis (regurgitation of acid and enzymes into the oesophagus). H_2-antagonists are commonly used as ULCER-HEALING DRUGS and for a wide variety of dyspepsia other peptic acid complaints. Technically, these drugs are ANTIHISTAMINES, but somewhat confusingly this term is not applied to them because it is reserved for the much earlier class of drugs that act at H_1 receptors and which have quite different actions (they are used, among other purposes, to treat allergic reactions). See CIMETIDINE; FAMOTIDINE; NIZATIDINE; RANITIDINE.

H-B-Vax II
(Merck Sharp & Dohme) is a proprietary, prescription-only VACCINE preparation of hepatitis B vaccine. It can be used to give protection from hepatitis B in people at risk, and is available in a form for injection.
+▲ Side-effects/warning: See HEPATITIS B VACCINE.

Haelan
(Dista) is a proprietary, prescription-only preparation of the CORTICOSTEROID and

ANTI-INFLAMMATORY drug flurandrenolone. It
can be used to treat inflammatory skin
disorders, such as eczema, and is available
as a cream and an ointment for topical
application.
✚▲ Side-effects/warning: See
FLURANDRENOLONE.

Haemophilus influenzae type B vaccine

(Hib) for IMMUNIZATION prevents
Haemophilus influenzae infection
(bacteria that cause respiratory infection).
It is given as a routine childhood preventive
vaccination, and is administered by
injection.
✚▲ Side-effects/warning: See VACCINES.
✪ Related entries: Act-HIB; Haemophilus
Influenzae Type B Vaccine; HibTITER.

Haemophilus Influenzae Type B Vaccine

(District Health Authorities) (Hib) is a non-
proprietary, prescription-only preparation
of the VACCINE used to prevent *Haemophilus
influenzae* infection, and is available in a
form for injection.
✚▲ Side-effects/warning: See HAEMOPHILUS
INFLUENZAE TYPE B VACCINE.

haemostatics ▣

are a wide range of drugs that act to slow or
prevent bleeding (haemorrhage). They are
used mostly to treat disorders in which
bleeding is prolonged and potentially
dangerous (eg haemophilia).

Halciderm Topical

(Squibb) is a proprietary, prescription-only
preparation of the CORTICOSTEROID and
ANTI-INFLAMMATORY halcinonide. It can be
used to treat inflammatory skin disorders,
such as eczema, and is available as a cream
for topical application.
✚▲ Side-effects/warning: See HALCINONIDE.

halcinonide

is a CORTICOSTEROID with ANTI-INFLAMMATORY
properties. It is used to treat inflammatory

skin disorders, such as recalcitrant eczema
and psoriasis, that are unresponsive to less
potent corticosteroids. Administration is by
topical application.
✚▲ Side-effects/warning: See
CORTICOSTEROIDS; though systemic effects
are unlikely with topical application, but
there may be local skin reactions.
✪ Related entry: Halciderm Topical.

Haldol

(Janssen) is a proprietary, prescription-
only preparation of the ANTIPSYCHOTIC
haloperidol. It can be used to treat
psychotic disorders, especially
schizophrenia or the hyperactive, euphoric
condition mania and to tranquillize patients
undergoing behavioural disturbance. It can
also be used for the short-term treatment of
severe anxiety and of some involuntary
motor (movement) disturbances.
Additionally, it can be used for intractable
hiccups. It is available as a liquid, tablets
and in a form for injection and depot deep
intramuscular injection.
✚▲ Side-effects/warning: See HALOPERIDOL.

Haldol Decanoate

(Janssen) is a proprietary, prescription-
only preparation of the ANTIPSYCHOTIC
haloperidol (as undecanoate). It can be
used in the maintenance of schizophrenia
and other psychoses, and is available in a
form for depot intramuscular injection.
✚▲ Side-effects/warning: See HALOPERIDOL.

Half Securon SR

(Knoll) is a proprietary, prescription-only
preparation of the CALCIUM-CHANNEL BLOCKER
verapamil hydrochloride. It can be used as
an ANTIHYPERTENSIVE and ANTI-ANGINA
treatment in the prevention of attacks. It is
available as modified-release tablets.
✚▲ Side-effects/warning: See VERAPAMIL
HYDROCHLORIDE.

Half Sinemet CR

(Du Pont) is a proprietary, prescription-
only COMPOUND PREPARATION of carbidopa

H

and levodopa, which is a combination known as co-careldopa (with a carbidopa/levodopa ratio of 25:100 mg). It can be administered to treat parkinsonism, but not the parkinsonian symptoms induced by drugs (see ANTIPARKINSONISM), and is available as modified-release tablets.

+▲ Side-effects/warning: See LEVODOPA.

Half-Beta-Prograne

(Tillomed) is a proprietary, prescription-only preparation of the BETA-BLOCKER propranolol hydrochloride. It can be used as an ANTIHYPERTENSIVE for raised blood pressure, as an ANTI-ANGINA treatment to relieve symptoms and improve exercise tolerance and as an ANTI-ARRHYTHMIC to regularize heartbeat and to treat myocardial infarction. It can also be used as an ANTITHYROID drug for short-term treatment of thyrotoxicosis, as an ANTIMIGRAINE treatment to prevent attacks, as an ANXIOLYTIC, particularly for symptomatic relief of tremor and palpitations, and, with an ALPHA-ADRENOCEPTOR BLOCKER, in the acute treatment of phaeochromocytoma. It is available as modified-release capsules.

+▲ Side-effects/warning: See PROPRANOLOL HYDROCHLORIDE.

Half-Betadur CR

(Monmouth) is a proprietary, prescription-only preparation of the BETA-BLOCKER propranolol hydrochloride. It can be used as an ANTIHYPERTENSIVE for raised blood pressure, as an ANTI-ANGINA treatment to relieve symptoms and improve exercise tolerance and as an ANTI-ARRHYTHMIC to regularize heartbeat and to treat myocardial infarction. It can also be used as an ANTITHYROID drug for short-term treatment of thyrotoxicosis, as an ANTIMIGRAINE treatment to prevent attacks, as an ANXIOLYTIC, particularly for symptomatic relief of tremor and palpitations, and, with an ALPHA-ADRENOCEPTOR BLOCKER, in the acute treatment of phaeochromocytoma. It is available as modified-release capsules.

+▲ Side-effects/warning: See PROPRANOLOL HYDROCHLORIDE.

Half-Inderal LA

(Zeneca) is a proprietary, prescription-only preparation of the BETA-BLOCKER propranolol hydrochloride. It can be used as an ANTIHYPERTENSIVE for raised blood pressure, as an ANTI-ANGINA treatment to relieve symptoms and improve exercise tolerance and as an ANTI-ARRHYTHMIC to regularize heartbeat and to treat myocardial infarction. It can also be used as an ANTITHYROID drug for short-term treatment of thyrotoxicosis, as an ANTIMIGRAINE treatment to prevent attacks, as an ANXIOLYTIC, particularly for symptomatic relief of tremor and palpitations, and, with an ALPHA-ADRENOCEPTOR BLOCKER, in the acute treatment of phaeochromocytoma. It is available as modified-release capsules.

+▲ Side-effects/warning: See PROPRANOLOL HYDROCHLORIDE.

Halfan

(SK&F) is a proprietary, prescription-only preparation of the ANTIMALARIAL halofantrine hydrochloride. It is available as tablets.

+▲ Side-effects/warning: See HALOFANTRINE HYDROCHLORIDE.

halibut-liver oil

is an excellent source of retinol (vitamin A) and also contains VITAMIN D. A non-proprietary preparation is available in the form of tablets, but it should not be taken without initial medical diagnosis. Retinol deficiency is rare and if any treatment should be required it must be under medical supervision in order to avoid the potentially unpleasant side-effects of excess vitamin A in the body. Administration is oral.

+▲ Side-effects/warning: See RETINOL.

halofantrine hydrochloride

is an ANTIMALARIAL drug. It is used to treat infection by uncomplicated, chloroquine-resistant *Plasmodium falciparum* species malaria, or chloroquine-resistant *Plasmodium vivax* species malaria in areas of the world where this is common. Administration is oral.

✚ Side-effects: Diarrhoea, nausea, vomiting, rash and pruritus and abdominal pain, elevation of certain blood enzymes, intravascular haemolysis and hypersensitivity reactions reported; ventricular arrhythmias.

▲ Warning: It may cause serious heart arrhythmias in susceptible patients; it should not be taken with food. It should not be administered to patients with certain heart disorders (such as arrhythmias), or with other drugs which may induce arrhythmias; it is not to be taken with drugs causing electrolyte disturbances, or by those who are pregnant or breast-feeding. Administer with care to those with certain heart disorders.

◎ Related entry: Halfan.

haloperidol

is a powerful ANTIPSYCHOTIC drug. It is used to treat and tranquillize patients with psychotic disorders (such as schizophrenia) and is particularly suitable for treating manic forms of behavioural disturbance, especially for emergency control. It can also be used in the short-term treatment of severe anxiety. Quite separately from the previous uses, it can be administered to treat other conditions that may cause tremor, tics, involuntary movements or involuntary utterances (eg Gilles de la Tourette syndrome). Administration can be either oral or by injection or depot deep intramuscular injection (in the form of the undecanoate salt).

✚▲ Side-effects/warning: See CHLORPROMAZINE HYDROCHLORIDE; but with less sedative effects, fewer anticholinergic and hypotensive symptoms and photosensitivity and skin pigmentation are rare. However, extrapyramidal symptoms are more frequent and there may be weight loss. Avoid in basal ganglia disease.

◎ Related entries: Dozic; Haldol; Haldol Decanoate; Serenace.

Halothane

(Rhône-Poulenc Rorer) is a proprietary preparation of the inhalant GENERAL ANAESTHETIC halothane. It can be used for the induction and maintenance of anaesthesia during surgery, and is available in a form for inhalation.

✚▲ Side-effects/warning: See HALOTHANE.

halothane

is an inhalant GENERAL ANAESTHETIC which is widely used both for induction and maintenance of anaesthesia during surgical operations. It is relatively non-irritant and does not induce coughing and seldom causes postoperative vomiting. Administration is by inhalation as a liquid through a calibrated vaporizer.

✚ Side-effects: There may be liver damage, cardiodepression and peripheral vasodilation.

▲ Warning: It should not be given to patients with porphyria.

◎ Related entries: Fluothane; Halothane.

Harmogen

(Upjohn) is a proprietary, prescription-only preparation of the OESTROGEN piperazine oestrone sulphate. It can be used in HRT, and is available as tablets.

✚▲ Side-effects/warning: See PIPERAZINE OESTRONE SULPHATE.

HAV

see HEPATITIS A VACCINE

Havrix

(SmithKline Beecham) is a proprietary, prescription-only VACCINE preparation of hepatitis A vaccine. It can be used to protect people at risk from infection with hepatitis A; there is also a paediatric preparation called *Havrix Junior*. It is available in a form for injection.

✚▲ Side-effects/warning: See HEPATITIS A VACCINE.

Havrix Monodose

(SmithKline Beecham) is a proprietary, prescription-only VACCINE preparation of the hepatitis A vaccine. It can be used to protect people at risk from infection with hepatitis A, and is available in a form for injection.

+▲ Side-effects/warning: See HEPATITIS A VACCINE.

Hay-Crom

(Baker Norton) is a proprietary, prescription-only preparation of the ANTI-ALLERGIC drug sodium cromoglycate. It can be used to treat allergic conjunctivitis, and is available as eye-drops and an eye ointment.

+▲ Side-effects/warning: See SODIUM CROMOGLYCATE.

Haymine

(Pharmax) is a proprietary, non-prescription COMPOUND PREPARATION of the ANTIHISTAMINE chlorpheniramine maleate and the SYMPATHOMIMETIC ephedrine hydrochloride. It can be used as a NASAL DECONGESTANT for the symptomatic relief of the allergic symptoms of hay fever and allergic rhinitis, and is available as tablets.

+▲ Side-effects/warning: See CHLORPHENIRAMINE MALEATE; EPHEDRINE HYDROCHLORIDE.

HBIG

see HEPATITIS B IMMUNOGLOBULIN (HBIG)

HCG

see CHORIONIC GONADOTROPHIN

Healonid

(Pharmacia) is a proprietary, prescription-only preparation of sodium hyaluronate, which is a visco-elastic polymer normally present in the aqueous and vitreous humour of the eye. It can be used during surgical procedures on the eye, and is available in a form for injection.

+▲ Side-effects/warning: See SODIUM HYALURONATE.

heart failure treatment ▨

is a therapy that used in order to rectify the functioning of a failing heart. It can involve the administration of a number of different drug types. There are various causes of heart failure which can include disease within the heart itself (mainly ischaemia – which is an inadequate supply of blood to the muscle that can cause angina pain) or an excessive load imposed on the heart by arterial and other forms of hypertension. CARDIAC GLYCOSIDE drugs increase the force of contraction of the heart and have been for some time extensively administered in congestive heart failure treatment, though nowadays they are usually used in conjunction with other drugs. The ANTIHYPERTENSIVES are frequently the first course of treatment to be used and here both the DIURETICS (eg AMILORIDE HYDROCHLORIDE, BUMETANIDE, CHLOROTHIAZIDE, ETHACRYNIC ACID, FRUSEMIDE, HYDROCHLOROTHIAZIDE and TRIAMTERENE) and the ACE INHIBITORS (eg CAPTOPRIL and ENALAPRIL MALEATE) may be valuable. Alternatively, VASODILATORS can be used, such as the NITRATES (eg GLYCERYL TRINITRATE, ISOSORBIDE DINITRATE, ISOSORBIDE MONONITRATE and PENTAERYTHRITOL TETRANITRATE) or HYDRALAZINE HYDROCHLORIDE. Lastly, CARDIAC STIMULANTS, such as the SYMPATHOMIMETIC drugs DOPEXAMINE HYDROCHLORIDE and DOBUTAMINE HYDROCHLORIDE, are usually reserved for emergencies.

Hedex Extra Tablets

(SmithKline Beecham) is a proprietary, non-prescription COMPOUND ANALGESIC preparation of the NON-NARCOTIC ANALGESIC and ANTIPYRETIC paracetamol and the STIMULANT caffeine. It can be used for the pain of headache (including migraine), neuralgia, period pain and to relieve cold symptoms. It is available as tablets and is not normally given to children under 12 years, except on medical advice.

+▲ Side-effects/warning: See CAFFEINE; PARACETAMOL.

Hedex Headcold Cherry Menthol Powders

(SmithKline Beecham) is a proprietary, non-prescription COMPOUND ANALGESIC preparation of the NON-NARCOTIC ANALGESIC and ANTIPYRETIC paracetamol and the DECONGESTANT phenylephrine hydrochloride with VITAMIN C. It can be used for the relief of sinus pain and cold and flu symptom. It is available as tablets and is not normally given to children under 12 years, except on medical advice.

+▲ Side-effects/warning: See PARACETAMOL; PHENYLEPHRINE HYDROCHLORIDE.

Hedex Ibuprofen Tablets

(SmithKline Beecham) is a proprietary, non-prescription preparation of the NON-NARCOTIC ANALGESIC and ANTIPYRETIC ibuprofen. It can be used for the pain of headache (including migraine), tension headaches, backache, period pain and to relieve cold and flu symptoms. It is available as tablets and is not normally given to children, except on medical advice.

+▲ Side-effects/warning: See IBUPROFEN.

Hedex Tablets

(SmithKline Beecham) is a proprietary, non-prescription preparation of the NON-NARCOTIC ANALGESIC and ANTIPYRETIC paracetamol. It can be used for the pain of headache (including migraine), tension headaches, backache, period pain and to relieve cold and flu symptoms. It is available as tablets and is not normally given to children under six years, except on medical advice.

+▲ Side-effects/warning: See PARACETAMOL.

Hemabate

(Upjohn) is a proprietary, prescription-only preparation of the PROSTAGLANDIN analogue carboprost. It can be used to treat haemorrhage following childbirth, especially where other drugs have proved to be ineffective, and is available in a form for injection.

+▲ Side-effects/warning: See CARBOPROST.

Heminevrin

(Astra) is a proprietary, prescription-only preparation of chlormethiazole (as base or edisylate). It can be used as a HYPNOTIC for treating severe insomnia (especially in the elderly), as an ANTICONVULSANT and ANTI-EPILEPTIC for treating status epilepticus, eclampsia, the symptoms caused by withdrawal from alcohol and for maintaining unconsciousness under regional anaesthesia. It is available as capsules, a syrup and in a form for intravenous infusion.

+▲ Side-effects/warning: See CHLORMETHIAZOLE.

Hemocane

(Intercare) is a proprietary, non-prescription COMPOUND PREPARATION of the LOCAL ANAESTHETIC lignocaine hydrochloride and the ASTRINGENT agents BENZOIC AICD, BISMUTH OXIDE and ZINC OXIDE. It can be used for the symptomatic relief of the pain and itching of haemorrhoids and other ano-rectal conditions. It is available as a cream and is not normally given to children, except on medical advice.

+▲ Side-effects/warning: See LIGNOCAINE HYDROCHLORIDE.

heparin

is a natural ANTICOAGULANT which is produced mainly by the liver, leucocytes (white blood cells) and at some other sites. It inhibits the action of the enzyme thrombin, which is needed for the final stages of blood coagulation. For therapeutic use, it is purified after extraction from bovine lungs and bovine and porcine intestinal mucosa. It is available in several forms, including low molecular-weight forms CERTOPARIN SODIUM, DALTEPARIN, ENOXAPARIN and TINZAPARIN. Also there are heparinoid forms (DANAPAROID SODIUM. Administration is generally by injection (eg during surgery) to prevent or treat thrombosis and similar conditions. It is short-acting and so it may be administered frequently or by constant infusion.

✚ Side-effects: Should haemorrhage occur, it may be difficult to stop the bleeding for a time – although, because heparin is so short-acting, merely discontinuing treatment is usually effective fairly quickly. There may be sensitivity reactions. Prolonged use may cause a loss of calcium from the bones and of hair from the head. There may be skin damage.

▲ Warning: It should not be administered to patients with haemophilia, thrombocytopenia, peptic ulcer, hypertension, severe kidney or liver disorders, or who have recently undergone eye surgery. It should be administered with caution to those who are pregnant.

⊙ Related entries: Calciparine; Minihep; Minihep Calcium; Monoparin; Monoparin Calcium; Multiparin; Pump-Hep; Unihep; Uniparin; Uniparin Calcium.

heparinoid

compounds are chemically similar to the HEPARIN type ANTICOAGULANTS. The version called DANAPAROID SODIUM is thought to have some advantages over heparin as an anticoagulant and is used to prevent deep vein thrombosis, particularly in orthopaedic surgery, and may be used in some patients who are hypersensitive to heparin. Other heparinoids are used to improve circulation in the skin in the treatment of conditions such as bruising, chilblains, thrombophlebitis, varicose veins and also in haemorrhoids, though it is not entirely clear how they work.

✚▲ Side-effects/warning: See HEPARIN for intravenous use; by topical application it is relatively free of side-effects.

⊙ Related entries: Anacal Suppositories; Anacal Rectal Ointment; Hirudoid; Lasonil; Movelat Relief Cream.

hepatitis A vaccine

consists of a VACCINE, used for IMMUNIZATION, that is prepared from biosynthetic inactivated hepatitis A virus (HAV). It is an alternative to human NORMAL IMMUNOGLOBULIN for frequent travellers to

moderate to high risk areas. Administration is by intramuscular injection.

✚▲ Side-effects/warning: See VACCINES.

Hepatitis B Immunoglobulin

(Public Health Laboratory Service) (Antihepatatis B Immunoglobulin) is a non-proprietary, prescription-only preparation of HEPATITIS B IMMUNOGLOBULIN, which is a SPECIFIC IMMUNOGLOBULIN used to give immediate immunity against infection by the hepatitis B virus. It is available in a form for intramuscular injection.

✚▲ Side-effects/warning: See IMMUNIZATION.

hepatitis B immunoglobulin (HBIG)

(HBIG) is a SPECIFIC IMMUNOGLOBULIN that is used for IMMUNIZATION to give immediate *passive immunity* against infection by the hepatitis B virus. It is used specifically to immunize personnel in medical laboratories and hospitals who may be infected and to treat babies of mothers infected by the virus during pregnancy. Administration is by intramuscular injection. See HEPATITIS B VACCINE.

✚▲ Side-effects/warning: See IMMUNIZATION.

⊙ Related entry: Hepatitis B Immunoglobulin.

hepatitis B vaccine

consists of a VACCINE, used for IMMUNIZATION, that is prepared from biosynthetic inactivated hepatitis B virus surface antigen (HBsAg). It is given to patients with a high risk of infection from the hepatitis B virus mostly through contact with a carrier. Administration is by intramuscular injection.

✚▲ Side-effects/warning: See VACCINES.

⊙ Related entries: Engerix B; H-B-Vax II.

heroin

is the common term for DIAMORPHINE HYDROCHLORIDE.

Herpid

(Yamanouchi) is a proprietary, prescription-only preparation of the ANTIVIRAL idoxuridine. It can be used to treat infections of the skin by herpes simplex or herpes zoster, and is available in a form for topical application with its own applicator.

✚▲ Side-effects/warning: See IDOXURIDINE.

Hewletts Cream

(Bioglan) is a proprietary, non-prescription preparation of ZINC OXIDE in hydrous wool fat. It can be used for minor abrasions and burns, and is available as a cream for topical application to the skin.

✚▲ Side-effects/warning: See WOOL FAT.

hexachlorophane

(hexachlorophene) is an ANTISEPTIC agent. It can be used on the skin for many purposes, including to prevent staphylococcal infections of the skin in newborn babies and to treat recurrent boils. Administration is topical.

✚ Side-effects: Rarely, there may be sensitivity reactions and increased sensitivity to light.

▲ Warning: It should not be used on areas of raw or badly burned skin. It is not for use by pregnant women.

✪ Related entry: Dermalex.

hexachlorophene

see HEXACHLOROPHANE

hexamine hippurate

(methenamine hippurate) is an ANTIBACTERIAL drug which is used to treat recurrent infections of the urinary tract and to prevent infections during urinogenital surgery. Administration is oral.

✚ Side-effects: Gastrointestinal upsets, rash and bladder irritation.

▲ Warning: It should not be used in patients with severe kidney impairment; administer with care to those who are pregnant.

✪ Related entry: Hiprex.

hexetidine

is an ANTISEPTIC mouthwash or gargle which is used for routine oral hygiene and to cleanse and freshen the mouth.

✪ Related entry: Oraldene.

Hexopal

(Sanofi Winthrop) is a proprietary, non-prescription preparation of the VASODILATOR inositol nicotinate. It can be used to help improve blood circulation to the hands and feet when this is impaired, for instance, in peripheral vascular disease (Raynaud's phenomenon). It is available as tablets and a suspension.

✚▲ Side-effects/warning: See INOSITOL NICOTINATE.

Hib

is an abbreviation for HAEMOPHILUS INFLUENZAE TYPE B VACCINE.

Hibicet Hospital Concentrate

(Zeneca) is a proprietary, non-prescription COMPOUND PREPARATION of the ANTISEPTICS chlorhexidine (as gluconate) and cetrimide. It can be used, after dilution, for cleaning, disinfecting and swabbing wounds, and is available as a cream.

✚▲ Side-effects/warning: See CETRIMIDE; CHLORHEXIDINE.

Hibisol

(Zeneca) is a proprietary, non-prescription preparation of the ANTISEPTIC chlorhexidine (as gluconate). It can be used to treat minor wounds and burns on the skin and hands, and is available as a solution.

✚▲ Side-effects/warning: See CHLORHEXIDINE.

Hibitane

(Zeneca) is the name of a range of proprietary, non-prescription ANTISEPTIC preparations that are based on solutions of chlorhexidine. The standard preparation is a powder which is used to prepare solutions of chlorhexidine and powdered

H

antiseptic compounds. There are two solutions: *Hibitane 5% Concentrate*, which is diluted in water or alcohol and then used to disinfect the skin, and *Hibitane Gluconate 20%*, which can be used to disinfect cavities and the bladder and to treat urethral infections. Also available is *Hibitane Antiseptic* which is a cream and can be used to treat minor wounds and burns.

➕▲ Side-effects/warning: See CHLORHEXIDINE.

HibTiter

(Lederle) is a proprietary, prescription-only VACCINE preparation which is used to provide protection against *Haemophilus influenzae* infection. It is available in a form for injection.

➕▲ Side-effects/warning: See HAEMOPHILUS INFLUENZAE TYPE B VACCINE.

High Potency Factor VIII Concentrate

(SNBTS) is a proprietary, prescription-only preparation of dried human factor VIII fraction. It acts as a HAEMOSTATIC to reduce or stop bleeding in the treatment of disorders in which bleeding is prolonged and potentially dangerous (mainly haemophilia A). It is available in a form for infusion or injection.

➕▲ Side-effects/warning: See FACTOR VIII FRACTION, DRIED.

Hioxyl

(Quinoderm) is a proprietary, non-prescription preparation of the ANTISEPTIC agent HYDROGEN PEROXIDE. It can be used to treat bedsores, leg ulcers, minor wounds and burns, and is available as a cream for topical application.

Hiprex

(3M) is a proprietary, non-prescription preparation of the ANTIBACTERIAL drug hexamine hippurate. It can be administered to treat various infections of the urinary and gastrointestinal tracts and also to prevent infections during urinogenital surgery. It is available as capsules.

➕▲ Side-effects/warning: See HEXAMINE HIPPURATE.

Hirudoid

(Panpharma) is a proprietary, non-prescription preparation of HEPARINOID. It can be administered to improve a patient's circulation in conditions such as bruising, haematoma, chilblains, thrombophlebitis and varicose veins. It is available as a cream.

➕▲ Side-effects/warning: See HEPARINOID.

Hismanal

(Johnson & Johnson) is a proprietary, non-prescription preparation of the ANTIHISTAMINE astemizole. It can be used to treat the symptoms of allergic disorders, such as hay fever and urticaria, and is available as tablets and a sugar-free suspension.

➕▲ Side-effects/warning: See ASTEMIZOLE.

Hivid

(Roche) is a proprietary, prescription-only preparation of zalcitabine (DDC). It can be administered as an ANTIVIRAL drug in the treatment of AIDS, and is available as tablets.

➕▲ Side-effects/warning: See ZALCITABINE.

HNIG

see NORMAL IMMUNOGLOBULIN

homatropine hydrobromide

is an ANTICHOLINERGIC drug which can be used to dilate the pupil and paralyse the focusing of the eye for ophthalmic examination. Administration is by topical application.

➕▲ Side-effects/warning: See ATROPINE SULPHATE. When applied locally it has few side-effects, but it should not be used in patients with raised intraocular pressure (it may precipitate glaucoma).

✪ Related entry: Minims Homatropine Hydrobromide.

Honvan

(ASTA Medica) is a proprietary, prescription-only preparation of fosfestrol tetrasodium, which is converted in the body to STILBOESTROL (which has OESTROGEN activity as a SEX HORMONE). It can be used in men as an ANTICANCER treatment for cancer of the prostate gland, and is available as tablets and in a form for injection.

+▲ Side-effects/warning: See FOSFESTROL TETRASODIUM.

hormone antagonists ▣

are a class of drugs that prevent the action of HORMONES at their receptors (special recognition sites on cells). They act either directly by competing for these sites (eg TAMOXIFEN at oestrogen receptors and CYPROTERONE ACETATE at androgen receptors), or indirectly where the antagonist acts on other receptors to inhibit the production, or the release, of the hormone (eg OCTREOTIDE inhibits the release of hormones from cancerous cells).

hormone replacement therapy

see HRT

hormones ▣

are substances produced and secreted by glands. In the case of endocrine hormones they are carried by the bloodstream to the organs on which they have their effect. Hormones can be divided into several families. The *adrenal hormones* are secreted by the adrenal glands (a small paired-gland just above the kidneys), of which there are two distinct types: adrenal cortical hormones and adrenal medullary hormones. The adrenocortical hormones come from the cortical (outer) region of the adrenal gland (eg CORTICOSTEROID hormones, which are STEROIDS with glucocorticoid or mineralocorticoid activity). The adrenalomedullary hormones come from the medullary (outer) region of the adrenal gland (eg ADRENALINE and NORADRENALINE).

The THYROID HORMONES and the *parathyroid hormones* come from the thyroid and parathyroid glands at the base of the neck (eg CALCITONIN, parathormone, THYROXINE and TRIIODOTHYRONINE). The *glucose-regulatory hormones* are produced by the pancreas (eg GLUCAGON and INSULIN). The SEX HORMONES come mainly from the ovaries or the testes (eg the ANDROGENS, such as TERSTOSTERONE; the OESTROGENS, such as OESTRADIOL and OESTRIOL; and the PROGESTOGENS, such as PROGESTERONE).

The *pituitary gland*, situated at the base of the skull, is an important producer of several vital hormones. There are two distinct classes of pituitary hormones: the posterior pituitary hormones OXYTOCIN and VASOPRESSIN (antidiuretic hormone; ADH); and the anterior pituitary hormones, which include CORTICOTROPHIN (adrenocorticotrophic hormone; ACTH), SOMATOTROPIN (growth hormone; GH); PROLACTIN and THYROTROPHIN (thyroid-stimulating hormone; TSH); or the GONADOTROPHINS – follicle-stimulating hormone (FSH) AND luteinising hormone (LH).

The release of anterior pituitary hormones is controlled, in turn, by factors that travel, in a specialized system of portal blood vessels, the short distance from the hypothalamus (an adjacent brain area). These *hypothalamic hormones* include corticotrophin-releasing hormone (CRH; or corticotrophin-releasing factor, CRF); GONADORELIN (gonadotrophin-releasing hormone, GnRH; or gonadotropin-releasing factor, GRF; LH-RH); growth hormone-releasing hormone (GHRH, or growth hormone-releasing factor, GRF); growth hormone release-inhibiting hormone (GHRIH; somatostatin, or growth hormone-release-inhibiting factor, GHRIF); and PROTIRELIN (thyrotrophin-releasing hormone; TRH). Many of these hormones can be administered therapeutically to people with a hormonal deficiency, sometimes in synthetic form. Synthetic

H

HORMONE ANTAGONISTS have been developed either to reduce the release of hormones (eg in cancers of endocrine glands) or, with sex hormones, to reduce normal release or the effects of normal levels of hormone, for example, where this inhibition benefits cancers of certain organs such as the prostate gland, the endometrium of the uterus or of the breast (eg TAMOXIFEN).

Hormonin

(Shire) is a proprietary, prescription-only COMPOUND PREPARATION of the natural, OESTROGEN SEX HORMONES oestradiol and oestriol. It can be used in HRT, and is available as tablets.

+▲ Side-effects/warning: See OESTRADIOL; OESTRIOL.

HRF

(Monmouth) is a proprietary, prescription-only preparation of the HORMONE gonadorelin (gonadotrophin-releasing hormone, GnRH). It can be used as a diagnostic aid in assessing the functioning of the pituitary gland, and is available in a form for injection or infusion.

+▲ Side-effects/warning: See GONADORELIN.

HRT ▣

(hormone replacement therapy) is a term commonly applied to drug treatment for women to supplement the diminished production of OESTROGEN, a major SEX HORMONE, by the body during the menopause. In a more general sense the term refers to the use of any synthetic or natural hormone to supplement a deficiency in the body (eg THYROID HORMONES, GROWTH HORMONE, ANTIDIURETIC HORMONE and INSULIN).

HRT in women is essentially *oestrogen replacement therapy*, and consists of the administration of small amounts of natural or synthetic oestrogens (eg CONJUGATED OESTROGENS, DIENOESTROL, MESTRANOL, OESTRADIOL, PIPERAZINE OESTRONE SULPHATE,

STILBOESTROL), which are used to alleviate menopausal vasometer symptoms (eg flushing), night sweats and vaginitis (thinning and drying of the vagina) in women whose lives are inconvenienced by these conditions. Additionally, there is good evidence that HRT will reduce post-menopausal osteoporosis (brittle bones) and often is beneficial in reducing the risk of atherosclerosis, myocardial infarction and stroke. However, a number of risk factors need to be taken into account (particularly a possible increase in blood clotting) according to the individual's medical background (including previous drug treatments, familial and genetic traits, history of stroke or hypertension, smoking habits, exercise and body weight), so expert counselling is necessary. In those at risk of osteoporosis, treatment may be advised to start prior to the menopause. In women who have had a hysterectomy, long-term treatment with oestrogen alone may be used, but otherwise a PROGESTOGEN (eg DYDROGESTERONE, LEVONORGESTREL, NORETHISTERONE, NORGESTREL) may also be prescribed (to reduce the risk of endometrial cystic hyperplasia and possible cancer of the uterus). Administration of HRT drug, often cyclically, can be oral as tablets, by topical application (eg vaginal cream, skin gels or skin patches) or implants. Possible side-effects are given under oestrogen or progestogen.

HTIG

see TETANUS IMMUNOGLOBULIN, HUMAN

Humalog

(Lilly) is a proprietary, non-prescription preparation of INSULIN LISPRO, which is a recombinant human insulin analogue. It is used to treat and maintain diabetic patients, and is available in vials for injection.

+▲ Side-effects/warning: See INSULIN.

Human Actraphane 30/70

(Novo Nordisk) is a proprietary, non-prescription preparation of human BIPHASIC

ISOPHANE INSULIN. It is used in DIABETIC TREATMENT to treat and maintain diabetic patients. It contains both isophane and neutral insulins in a proportion of 70% to 30% respectively. It is available in vials for injection and has an intermediate duration of action.

✚▲ Side-effects/warning: See INSULIN.

Human Actrapid

(Novo Nordisk) is a proprietary, non-prescription preparation of synthesized neutral SOLUBLE INSULIN. It is used in DIABETIC TREATMENT to treat and maintain diabetic patients. It is available in vials for injection, in cartridges (*Penfil*) for use with *NovoPen* injectors and as prefilled disposable injectors (*Actrapid*). It has a short duration of action.

✚▲ Side-effects/warning: See INSULIN.

human antihaemophilic fraction, dried

see FACTOR VIII FRACTION, DRIED

human chorionic gonadotrophin

see CHORIONIC GONADOTROPHIN

human growth hormone

see SOMATOTROPIN; SOMATROPIN

Human Initard 50/50

(Novo Nordisk, Wellcome) is a proprietary, non-prescription preparation of BIPHASIC ISOPHANE INSULIN. It is used to treat and maintain diabetic patients and contains isophane and neutral insulins in equal proportions. It is available in vials for injection and has an intermediate duration of action.

✚▲ Side-effects/warning: See INSULIN.

Human Insulatard

(Novo Nordisk, Wellcome) is a proprietary, non-prescription preparation of human ISOPHANE INSULIN. It is used to treat and maintain diabetic patients, and is available in vials for injection and has an

intermediate duration of action.

✚▲ Side-effects/warning: See INSULIN.

human menopausal gonadotrophins

is a pituitary HORMONE preparation and is a collective name for combinations of the gonadotrophins FOLLICLE-STIMULATING HORMONE (FSH) and LUTEINISING HORMONE (LH) (one form of which is called MENOTROPHIN). It is extracted from the urine of postmenopausal women and has various uses, including as an infertility treatment for women with proven hypopituitarism, or who do not respond to the drug CLOMIPHENE CITRATE (another drug commonly used to treat infertility) and in superovulation treatment in assisted conception (as with IN VITRO fertilization; IVF). Administration is by injection.

✚ Side-effects: Hyperstimulation of the ovaries, multiple pregnancy and local reactions.

▲ Warning: It should be given with caution to women with ovarian cysts, thyroid, adrenal or pituitary gland tumours or certain other disorders.

✪ Related entries: Humegon; Normegon; Pergonal.

Human Mixtard 30/70

(Novo Nordisk, Wellcome) is a proprietary, non-prescription preparation of BIPHASIC ISOPHANE INSULIN. It is used to treat and maintain diabetic patients and contains both isophane and neutral insulins in a proportion of 70% to 30% respectively. It is available in vials for injection and has an intermediate duration of action.

✚▲ Side-effects/warning: See INSULIN.

Human Monotard

(Novo Nordisk) is a proprietary, non-prescription preparation of human INSULIN ZINC SUSPENSION. It is used in DIABETIC TREATMENT to treat and maintain diabetic patients, and is available in vials for injection and has a long duration of action.

✚▲ Side-effects/warning: See INSULIN.

H

human normal immunoglobulin
see NORMAL IMMUNOGLOBULIN

Human Protaphane
(Novo Nordisk) is a proprietary, non-prescription preparation of human ISOPHANE INSULIN. It is used in DIABETIC TREATMENT to maintain diabetic patients, and is available in vials for injection and as cartridges (*Penfill*) for *Human Protaphane Novopen* injection devices. It has an intermediate duration of action.

+▲ Side-effects/warning: See INSULIN.

Human Ultratard
(Novo Nordisk) is a proprietary, non-prescription preparation of human INSULIN ZINC SUSPENSION (CRYSTALLINE). It is used in DIABETIC TREATMENT to treat and maintain diabetic patients, and is available in vials for injection and has a long duration of action.

+▲ Side-effects/warning: See INSULIN.

Human Velosulin
(Novo Nordisk, Wellcome) is a proprietary, non-prescription preparation of human SOLUBLE INSULIN. It is used in DIABETIC TREATMENT to treat and maintain diabetic patients, and is available in vials for injection and has a short duration of action.

+▲ Side-effects/warning: See INSULIN.

Humatrope
(Lilly) is a proprietary, prescription-only preparation of somatropin, which is the biosynthetic form of the pituitary HORMONE human growth hormone. It can be used to treat hormonal deficiency and associated symptoms (in particular, short stature), and is available in a form for injection.

+▲ Side-effects/warning: See SOMATROPIN.

Humegon
(Organon) is a proprietary, prescription-only HORMONE preparation of human menopausal gonadotrophins, which contains FOLLICLE-STIMULATING HORMONE (FSH) and LUTEINISING HORMONE (LH). It can be used to treat infertile women with proven hypopituitarism and who do not respond to CLOMIPHENE CITRATE (which is another drug commonly administered to treat infertility) and in superovulation treatment in assisted conception (as with *in vitro* fertilization; IVF). It is available in a form for injection.

+▲ Side-effects/warning: See HUMAN MENOPAUSAL GONADOTROPHINS.

Humiderm
(BritCair) is a proprietary, non-prescription preparation of pyrrolidone carboxylic acid. It can be used as an EMOLLIENT to treat dry skin, and is available as a cream.

Humulin I
(Lilly) is a proprietary, non-prescription preparation of human ISOPHANE INSULIN. It is used in DIABETIC TREATMENTto treat and maintain diabetic patients, and is available in vials for injection and as cartridges for the *B-D Pen* device. It has an intermediate duration of action.

+▲ Side-effects/warning: See INSULIN.

Humulin Lente
(Lilly) is a proprietary, non-prescription preparation of human INSULIN ZINC SUSPENSION. It is used in DIABETIC TREATMENT to treat and maintain diabetic patients. It is available in vials for injection and has a relatively long duration of action.

+▲ Side-effects/warning: See INSULIN.

Humulin M1
(Lilly) is a proprietary, non-prescription preparation of BIPHASIC ISOPHANE INSULIN, human insulins. It is used in DIABETIC TREATMENT to treat and maintain diabetic patients and contains both isophane and neutral insulins in a proportion of 90% to 10% respectively. It is available in vials for injection or as cartridges for the *B-D Pen* device and has an intermediate duration of action.

+▲ Side-effects/warning: See INSULIN.

Humulin M2

(Lilly) is a proprietary, non-prescription preparation of BIPHASIC ISOPHANE INSULIN, human insulins. It is used in DIABETIC TREATMENT to treat and maintain diabetic patients and contains both isophane and neutral insulins in a proportion of 80% to 20% respectively. It is available in vials for injection or as cartridges for the *B-D Pen* device and has an intermediate duration of action.

✚▲ Side-effects/warning: See INSULIN.

Humulin M3

(Lilly) is a proprietary, non-prescription preparation of BIPHASIC ISOPHANE INSULIN, human insulins. It is used in DIABETIC TREATMENT to treat and maintain diabetic patients and contains human isophane insulin (30% soluble/70% isophane). It is available in vials for injection or as cartridges for the *B-D pen* device and has an intermediate duration of action.

✚▲ Side-effects/warning: See INSULIN.

Humulin M4

(Lilly) is a proprietary, non-prescription preparation of BIPHASIC ISOPHANE INSULIN, mixed human insulins. It is used in DIABETIC TREATMENT to treat and maintain diabetic patients and contains human isophane insulin (40% soluble/60% isophane). It has a short duration of action.

✚▲ Side-effects/warning: See INSULIN.

Humulin M5

(Lilly) is a proprietary, non-prescription preparation of BIPHASIC ISOPHANE INSULIN, mixed human insulins. It is used in DIABETIC TREATMENT to treat and maintain diabetic patients and contains human isophane insulin (50% soluble/50% isophane). It is in a form for injection.

✚▲ Side-effects/warning: See INSULIN.

Humulin S

(Lilly) is a proprietary, non-prescription preparation of human synthesized neutral SOLUBLE INSULIN. It is used in DIABETIC TREATMENT to treat and maintain diabetic patients, and is available in vials for injection or as cartridges for the *B-D Pen* device. It has a short duration of action.

✚▲ Side-effects/warning: See INSULIN.

Humulin Zn

(Lilly) is a proprietary, non-prescription preparation of human INSULIN ZINC SUSPENSION (CRYSTALLINE). It is used in DIABETIC TREATMENT to treat and maintain diabetic patients, and is available in vials for injection. It has an intermediate duration of action.

✚▲ Side-effects/warning: See INSULIN.

Hyalase

(CP) is a proprietary, prescription-only preparation of the ENZYME hyaluronidase. It can be used to increase the permeability of soft tissues to injected drugs, and is available in a form for injection.

✚▲ Side-effects/warning: See HYALURONIDASE.

hyaluronidase

is an ENZYME which can be used to increase the permeability of soft tissues to injected drugs. Administration is by injection.

✚ Side-effects: Sometimes there are allergic sensitivity reactions.

▲ Warning: It should not be administered directly to the cornea of the eye, or where there is malignant infection; it is not to be used to reduce swelling in stings and bites.

✪ Related entries: Hyalase; Lasonil.

Hyate C

(Porton) is a porcine, prescription-only preparation of factor VIII inhibitor bypassing fraction, and is used in patients with factor VIII inhibitors.

✚▲ Side-effects/warning: See FACTOR VIII INHIBITOR BYPASSING FRACTION.

Hydergine

(Sandoz) is a proprietary, prescription-only preparation of the mixture of drugs known as co-dergocrine mesylate, which has

H

ALPHA-ADRENOCEPTOR BLOCKER properties, and is a VASODILATOR of blood vessels in the brain. It is used primarily to assist in the management of elderly patients with mild to moderate dementia. It is available as tablets.

✚▲ Side-effects/warning: See CO-DERGOCRINE MESYLATE.

hydralazine hydrochloride

is a VASODILATOR drug which is used to treat acute and chronic cardiovascular disorders, such as a hypertensive crisis and as an ANTIHYPERTENSIVE for long-term high blood pressure (where it is often administered with a BETA-BLOCKER and a DIURETIC). Administration is either oral or by injection or infusion.

✚ Side-effects: There may be nausea and vomiting. Prolonged high-dosage may cause lupus erythematosus, blood disorders, headache, fast heartbeat and fluid retention.

▲ Warning: There may be a swift and severe fall in blood pressure. Special care must be taken when used with certain cardiovascular disorders, in pregnancy and when breast-feeding.

✪ Related entry: Apresoline.

hydrating agents ▨

are drugs that soothe and soften the skin. They are incorporated into ointments and skin creams that are used to treat conditions where the skin is dry or flaky (eg eczema). They are usually fats or oils, such as LANOLIN and LIQUID PARAFFIN and can be combined with other hydrating agents such as UREA. In conditions where there is a skin infection, hydrating agents can be combined with ANTIMICROBIALS or ANTIFUNGALS, and ANTI-INFLAMMATORY and CORTICOSTEROID drugs can be added where there is inflammation.

Hydrea

(Squibb) is a proprietary, prescription-only preparation of the (CYTOTOXIC) ANTICANCER drug hydroxyurea. It can be administered in the treatment of myeloid leukaemia, and is available as capsules.

✚▲ Side-effects/warning: See HYDROXYUREA.

Hydrenox

(Boots) is a proprietary, prescription-only preparation of the (THIAZIDE) DIURETIC hydroflumethiazide. It can be used in the treatment of oedema, either alone or in conjunction with other drugs, and as an ANTIHYPERTENSIVE. It is available as tablets.

✚▲ Side-effects/warning: See HYDROFLUMETHIAZIDE.

Hydrocal

(Bioglan) is a proprietary, prescription-only COMPOUND PREPARATION of the CORTICOSTEROID and ANTI-INFLAMMATORY hydrocortisone (as acetate) and the ASTRINGENT agent CALAMINE. It can be used to treat mild inflammatory skin conditions (such as eczema), and is available as a cream for topical application.

✚▲ Side-effects/warning: See HYDROCORTISONE.

hydrochloric acid

is a strong acid that, within the body, is part of the gastric juice secreted from special cells within the mucosal lining of the stomach. It provides the acid environment that is essential for the working of the enzyme pepsin, which begins the process of digestion that then continues within the small intestine. Over-production of acid (known as hyperacidity) can cause the symptoms of dyspepsia (commonly called indigestion) and this can be exacerbated by alcohol and NSAID drugs. ANTACIDS provide symptomatic relief of acute dyspepsia and gastritis. But for long-term problems associated with peptic ulcers (gastric or duodenal ulcers) and oesophagitis ULCER-HEALING DRUGS are required (see H_2-ANTAGONISTS and PROTON-PUMP INHIBITORS). The under-production of acid (hypochlorhydria and achlorhydria) can also be a problem.

hydrochlorothiazide

is a DIURETIC of the THIAZIDE class. It can be used as an ANTIHYPERTENSIVE, either alone or in conjunction with other drugs, and in the treatment of oedema associated with congestive heart failure. Administration is usually oral.

+▲ Side-effects/warning: See BENDROFLUAZIDE.

✿ Related entries: Accuretic; Acezide; Adizem-XL Plus; Amil-Co; Capozide; Carace Plus; Delvas; Dyazide; HydroSaluric; Innozide; Kalten; Moducren; Moduret-25; Moduretic; Monozide 10; Secadrex; Triam-Co; TrimaxCo; Zestoretic.

hydrocortisone

is a CORTICOSTEROID with ANTI-INFLAMMATORY properties, which can be administered therapeutically (sometimes in COMPOUND PREPARATIONS with ANTIBACTERIAL, ANTIBIOTIC or ANTIFUNGAL drugs) to treat any kind of inflammation, including arthritis, to treat allergic conditions, adrenocortical insufficiency, shock, inflammatory bowel disease, haemorrhoids, eye and skin inflammation and hypersensitivity reactions. It can be administered in a number of forms: hydrocortisone, hydrocortisone acetate, hydrocortisone butyrate, hydrocortisone sodium phosphate or hydrocortisone sodium succinate; and by several different routes, including by topical application as a lotion, ointment, eye ointment, cream, lozenge, gel, suppositories, spray, foam, ear-drops or scalp lotion, or as tablets or by injection.

+▲ Side-effects/warning: See CORTICOSTEROIDS. Side-effects depend on the route of administration, but are unlikely with topical application.

✿ Related entries: Actinac; Alphaderm; Alphosyl HC; Anugesic-HC; Anusol-HC; Calmurid HC; Canesten-HC; Carbo-Cort; Chloromycetin Hydrocortisone; Cobadex; Corlan; Daktacort; Dioderm; Econacort; Efcortelan; Efcortesol; Eurax-Hydrocortisone; Fucidin H; Gentisone HC; Gregoderm; Hydrocal; Hydrocortistab; Hydrocortisyl; Hydrocortone; Locoid; Locoid C; Mildison; Neo-Cortef; Nystaform-HC; Otosporin; Perinal; Proctofoam HC; Proctosedyl; Quinocort; Solu-Cortef; Tarcortin; Terra-Cortril; Terra-Cortril Nystatin; Timodine; Uniroid-HC; Vioform-Hydrocortisone; Xyloproct.

hydrocortisone acetate

see HYDROCORTISONE

hydrocortisone butyrate

see HYDROCORTISONE

hydrocortisone sodium phosphate

see HYDROCORTISONE

hydrocortisone sodium succinate

see HYDROCORTISONE

Hydrocortistab

(Boots) is a proprietary, prescription-only preparation of the CORTICOSTEROID and ANTI-INFLAMMATORY hydrocortisone (as acetate). It can be used to treat local inflammation in joints, and is available in a form for injection.

+▲ Side-effects/warning: See HYDROCORTISONE.

Hydrocortisyl

(Roussel) is a proprietary, prescription-only preparation of the CORTICOSTEROID and ANTI-INFLAMMATORY hydrocortisone. It can be used to treat mild inflammatory skin conditions, such as eczema, and is available as a cream and an ointment.

+▲ Side-effects/warning: See HYDROCORTISONE.

Hydrocortone

(Merck Sharp & Dohme) is a proprietary, prescription-only preparation of the CORTICOSTEROID and ANTI-INFLAMMATORY hydrocortisone. It can be used to make up hormonal deficiency and to treat inflammation, shock and certain allergic

H

conditions. It is available as tablets.

+▲ Side-effects/warning: See HYDROCORTISONE.

hydroflumethiazide

is a DIURETIC of the THIAZIDE class. It can be used, either alone or with other drugs, as an ANTIHYPERTENSIVE and in the treatment of oedema associated with congestive heart failure. Administration is oral.

+▲ Side-effects/warning: See BENDROFLUAZIDE.

✪ Related entries: Aldactide 25; Aldactide 50; Hydrenox; Spiro-Co; Spiro-Co 50.

hydrogen peroxide

is a general ANTISEPTIC which can be used for a wide range of purposes and is available in several forms: in solution and as a cream to cleanse and deodorize wounds and ulcers; as drops to clean ears; and as a mouthwash and gargle for oral hygiene.

✪ Related entries: Exterol; Hioxyl; Otex Ear Drops.

Hydromol

(Quinoderm) is a proprietary, non-prescription COMPOUND PREPARATION of LIQUID PARAFFIN and arachis oil (and several other constituents). It has EMOLLIENT properties and can be used for treating dry skin. It is available as a cream and a bath additive (*Emollient*).

+▲ Side-effects/warning: See ARACHIS OIL.

HydroSaluric

(Merck Sharp & Dohme) is a proprietary, prescription-only preparation of the (THIAZIDE) DIURETIC hydrochlorothiazide. It can be used, either alone or in conjunction with other drugs, in the treatment of oedema and as an ANTIHYPERTENSIVE. It is available as tablets.

+▲ Side-effects/warning: See HYDROCHLOROTHIAZIDE.

hydrotalcite

is an ANTACID complex of aluminium

magnesium carbonate hydroxide hydrate. It is used for the relief of dyspepsia and also reduces flatulence. Administration is oral in the form of chewable tablets or a suspension.

✪ Related entries: Altacite Plus; Altacite Suspension; Altacite Tablets.

hydroxocobalamin

is the form of vitamin B_{12} that is now used therapeutically, having replaced CYANOCOBALAMIN. Supplements of hydroxocobalamin are administered only by injection, because vitamin B_{12} deficiency is usually caused by malabsorption, which renders oral administration futile.

✪ Related entries: Cobalin-H; Neo-Cytamen.

hydroxychloroquine sulphate

is a drug that has ANTI-INFLAMMATORY and ANTIRHEUMATIC properties. It can be used primarily to treat rheumatoid arthritis (including juvenile arthritis) and is usually used when other, more common treatments (eg with NSAIDs) are unsuccessful. Its effects may not be seen for four to six months. Administration is oral.

+▲ Side-effects/warning: See CHLOROQUINE. (Although it is not used for malaria, it is a similar chemical and has similar side-effects and warnings.)

✪ Related entry: Plaquenil.

hydroxyethylcellulose

is a constituent of a preparation that is used as artificial tears and which is given to patients with dry eyes due to disease. Administration is topical.

✪ Related entry: Minims Artificial Tears.

hydroxyprogesterone caproate

see HYDROXYPROGESTERONE HEXANOATE

hydroxyprogesterone hexanoate

(hydroxyprogesterone caproate) is a PROGESTOGEN which can be used to treat recurrent abortion (habitual abortion). Administration is by long-lasting, intramuscular depot injection.

+▲ Side-effects/warning: See PROGESTOGEN.

✪ Related entry: Proluton Depot.

hydroxyurea

is a CYTOTOXIC drug which is used as an ANTICANCER treatment for chronic myeloid leukaemia and sometimes for polycythaemia. Administration is oral.

+▲ Side-effects/warning: See CYTOTOXICS.

✪ Related entry: Hydrea.

hydroxyzine hydrochloride

is an ANTIHISTAMINE that also has some additional ANXIOLYTIC properties. It can be administered for the relief of allergic symptoms, such as itching and mild rashes, and also for short-term treatment of anxiety. Administration is oral.

+▲ Side-effects/warning: See ANTIHISTAMINES. Because of its sedative side-effects, the performance of skilled tasks, such as driving, may be impaired.

✪ Related entries: Atarax; Ucerax.

Hygroton

(Geigy) is a proprietary, prescription-only preparation of the (THIAZIDE-like) DIURETIC chlorthalidone. It can be used, either alone or in conjunction with other drugs, in the treatment of oedema and as an ANTIHYPERTENSIVE. It is available as tablets.

+▲ Side-effects/warning: See CHLORTHALIDONE.

hyoscine butylbromide

is an ANTICHOLINERGIC drug which can be used as an ANTISPASMODIC for the symptomatic relief of smooth muscle spasm in the gastrointestinal tract. Administration is either oral or by injection.

+▲ Side-effects/warning: See ATROPINE SULPHATE; but with less actions on the central nervous system. Avoid it use in patients with porphyria.

✪ Related entry: Buscopan.

hyoscine hydrobromide

(known as scopolamine hydrobromide in the USA) is a BELLADONNA ALKALOID derived from plants of the belladonna family and is a powerful ANTICHOLINERGIC . By itself it is an effective SEDATIVE and is commonly used for premedication prior to surgery and in obstetric practice. It also has ANTINAUSEANT properties and can be administered to prevent motion sickness. In a solution, it can be used in ophthalmic treatments in order to paralyse the muscles of the pupil either prior to surgery or to rest the eye following surgery. Administration is either topical or by injection. See HYOSCINE BUTYLBROMIDE for use as an ANTISPASMODIC.

+ Side-effects: Depending on the route of administration, there may be drowsiness, dry mouth, dizziness, blurred vision and difficulty in urination; in doses for premedication and obstetrics it may cause confusion, hallucinations, behavioural disturbances, amnesia, ataxia, occasionally excitement and slowing of the heartbeat (especially in the elderly).

▲ Warning: It is not to be given to patients with porphyria or closed-angle glaucoma. Administer with caution to those who are pregnant or breast-feeding, elderly or have urinary retention, cardiovascular disease, or liver or kidney impairment. Because it has sedative properties, the performance of skilled tasks, such as driving, may be impaired.

✪ Related entries: Boots Travel Calm Tablets; Feminax; Joy-Rides; Kwells Junior; Kwells Tablets; Scopoderm TTS.

hyoscyamine

see ATROPINE SULPHATE

Hypnomidate

(Janssen) is a proprietary, prescription-only preparation of the GENERAL ANAESTHETIC etomidate. It can be used for the induction of anaesthesia, and is available in a form for injection.

+▲ Side-effects/warning: See ETOMIDATE.

H

hypnotics ▨

are drugs that induce sleep by an action on the brain. They are used mainly to treat insomnia and to calm patients who are mentally ill, but can also be used for the short-term treatment of insomnia due to jet lag, shiftwork, emotional problems or serious illness. The best-known and most-used hypnotics are the BENZODIAZEPINES (which can also be used as ANXIOLYTICS) such as DIAZEPAM, NITRAZEPAN, FLUNITRAZEPAM and FLURAZEPAM, which have a relatively long duration of action and may cause drowsiness the next day. There are some more recently introduced benzodiazepines that have a comparatively short duration of action and cause less drowsiness, eg LOPRAZOLAM, LORMETAZEPAM and TEMAZEPAM. Other types of drug that are used as hypnotics include CHLORAL HYDRATE, TRICLOFOS SODIUM and CHLORMETHIAZOLE. The BARBITURATES (eg AMYLOBARBITONE) are now rarely used, because they can readily cause dependence and are extremely dangerous in overdose.

Hypnovel

(Roche) is a proprietary, prescription-only preparation of the BENZODIAZEPINE midazolam. It can be used as an ANXIOLYTIC and SEDATIVE, where its ability to cause amnesia is useful in preoperative medication, dental surgery and local anaesthesia, because the patient forgets the unpleasant procedure. It is available in a form for injection.

✚▲ Side-effects/warning: See MIDAZOLAM.

hypoglycaemics ▨

are drugs reduce the levels of glucose (sugar) in the bloodstream. They are used mainly in the treatment of diabetes mellitus. The ORAL HYPOGLYCAEMICS are primarily used to treat Type II diabetes (non-insulin-dependent diabetes mellitus; NIDDM; maturity-onset diabetes), for example, the SULPHONYLUREAS (eg CHLORPROPAMIDE and GLIBENCLAMIDE), the BIGUANIDE drug METFORMIN HYDROCHLORIDE and ACARBOSE and

GUAR GUM. Administration of INSULIN, which is mainly used in Type I diabetes (insulin-dependent diabetes mellitus; IDDM; juvenile-onset diabetes), is by injection.

Hypotears

(CIBA Vision) is a proprietary, non-prescription preparation of POLYVINYL ALCOHOL. It can be used as artificial tears in conditions where there is dryness of the eye due to disease. It is available as eye-drops.

hypotensives ▨

lower blood pressure and there are many drugs that have such an action. Some drugs do so on acute (short-term) administration as a deliberate part of their medical use. For instance, NITRATES, which are used to treat angina attacks, have an immediate and powerful VASODILATOR action which redistributes blood flow in the body and beneficially reduces the workload of the heart. In a hypertensive crisis the aim is an immediate fall in blood pressure and this can be achieved by the injection of a vasodilator, such as HYDRALAZINE HYDROCHLORIDE. However, other types of drug may cause an unwanted fall in blood pressure to below normal levels as one of their side-effects, which may limit their usefulness in susceptible patients. This undesirable side-effect usually occurs as postural hypotension (a fall in blood pressure on standing quickly, where the brain is starved of blood causing the patient to feel dizzy or faint) and can be minimized, or avoided, by taking the drug in question on retiring to bed. Also, this side-effect often becomes less of a problem if the drug is taken as part of a chronic (long-term) treatment.

The term ANTIHYPERTENSIVE is, by convention, commonly used in medicine to describe drugs that are used to lower abnormally high blood pressure (hypertension) and which are usually administered on a long-term basis. Such drugs are not necessarily hypotensive in normal individuals.

Hypovase

(Invicta) is a proprietary, prescription-only preparation of the ALPHA-ADRENOCEPTOR BLOCKER prazosin hydrochloride. It can be used as an ANTIHYPERTENSIVE treatment, in peripheral vascular disease and in congestive HEART FAILURE TREATMENT. It is available as tablets.

+▲ Side-effects/warning: See PRAZOSIN HYDROCHLORIDE.

Hypovase Benign Prostatic Hypertrophy

(Invicta) is a proprietary, prescription-only preparation of the ALPHA-ADRENOCEPTOR BLOCKER prazosin hydrochloride. It can be used to treat urinary retention (eg in benign prostatic hypertrophy), and is available as tablets.

+▲ Side-effects/warning: See PRAZOSIN HYDROCHLORIDE.

hypromellose

is a constituent of artificial tears, which are used to treat extremely dry eyes due to certain disorders. It is available as eye-drops and often in combination with a variety of drugs.

✪ Related entries: Ilube; Isopto Alkaline; Isopto Carpine; Isopto Frin; Isopto Plain; Maxidex; Maxitrol; Moisture-eyes; Tears Naturale.

Hypurin Isophane

(CP) is a proprietary, non-prescription preparation of highly purified bovine ISOPHANE INSULIN It is used in DIABETIC TREATMENT to treat and maintain diabetic patients, and is available in vials for injection. It has an intermediate duration of action.

+▲ Side-effects/warning: See INSULIN.

Hypurin Lente

(CP) is a proprietary, non-prescription preparation of highly purified bovine INSULIN ZINC SUSPENSION. It is used in DIABETIC TREATMENT to treat and maintain diabetic patients, and is available in vials for

injection. It has a relatively long duration of action.

+▲ Side-effects/warning: See INSULIN.

Hypurin Neutral

(CP) is a proprietary, non-prescription preparation of highly purified bovine SOLUBLE INSULIN. It is used in DIABETIC TREATMENT to treat and maintain diabetic patients, and is available in vials for injection. It has a relatively short duration of action.

+▲ Side-effects/warning: See INSULIN.

Hypurin Protamine Zinc

(CP) is a proprietary, non-prescription preparation of highly purified bovine PROTAMINE ZINC INSULIN. It is used in DIABETIC TREATMENT to treat and maintain diabetic patients, and is available in vials for injection. It has a long duration of action.

+▲ Side-effects/warning: See INSULIN.

Hytrin

(Abbott) is a proprietary, prescription-only preparation of the ALPHA-ADRENOCEPTOR BLOCKER terazosin (as terazosin hydrochloride). It can be used as an ANTIHYPERTENSIVE, and is available as tablets.

+▲ Side-effects/warning: See TERAZOSIN.

Hytrin BPH

(Abbott) is a proprietary, prescription-only preparation of the ALPHA-ADRENOCEPTOR BLOCKER terazosin (as terazosin hydrochloride). It can be used to treat urinary retention (eg in benign prostatic hyperplasia), and is available as tablets.

+▲ Side-effects/warning: See TERAZOSIN.

Ibugel

(Dermal) is a proprietary, prescription-only preparation of the (NSAID) NON-NARCOTIC ANALGESIC and ANTIRHEUMATIC ibuprofen, which has COUNTER-IRRITANT, or RUBEFACIENT, actions. It can be applied to the skin for symptomatic relief of underlying rheumatic and muscular pain, sprains and neuralgia. It is available as a gel for topical application to the skin and is not normally used for children, except on medical advice.

➕▲ Side-effects/warning: See IBUPROFEN; but adverse effects on topical application are limited.

Ibular

(Lagap) is a proprietary, prescription-only preparation of the (NSAID) NON-NARCOTIC ANALGESIC and ANTIRHEUMATIC ibuprofen. It can be used to relieve pain, particularly the pain and inflammation of rheumatic disease and other musculoskeletal disorders, and is available as tablets.

➕▲ Side-effects/warning: See IBUPROFEN.

Ibuleve Gel

(DDD) is a proprietary, non-prescription preparation of the (NSAID) NON-NARCOTIC ANALGESIC and ANTIRHEUMATIC ibuprofen, which has COUNTER-IRRITANT, or RUBEFACIENT, actions. It can be used for the symptomatic relief of rheumatic and muscular pain, backache, sprains, strains and neuralgia. It is available as a massage gel and is not normally used for children under 14 years, except on medical advice.

➕▲ Side-effects/warning: See IBUPROFEN.

Ibuleve Sports Gel

(DDD) is a proprietary, non-prescription preparation of the (NSAID) NON-NARCOTIC ANALGESIC and ANTIRHEUMATIC ibuprofen, which has COUNTER-IRRITANT, or RUBEFACIENT, actions. It can be used for the symptomatic relief of muscular aches, sprains and strains, and is available as a non-greasy massage gel, in a pump-action tube. It is not normally used for children under 14 years, except on medical advice.

➕▲ Side-effects/warning: See IBUPROFEN.

Ibuleve Spray

(DDD) is a proprietary, non-prescription preparation of the (NSAID) NON-NARCOTIC ANALGESIC and ANTIRHEUMATIC ibuprofen, which has COUNTER-IRRITANT, or RUBEFACIENT, actions. It can be used for the symptomatic relief of rheumatic and muscular pain, backache, sprains, strains and neuralgia. It is available as a spray for the effected area and is not normally used for children under 14 years, except on medical advice.

➕▲ Side-effects/warning: See IBUPROFEN.

Ibumed

(Medipharma) is a proprietary, prescription-only preparation of the (NSAID) NON-NARCOTIC ANALGESIC and ANTIRHEUMATIC drug ibuprofen, which also has valuable ANTIPYRETIC properties. It can be used to relieve pain, particularly the pain of rheumatic disease and other musculoskeletal disorders, and is available as tablets.

➕▲ Side-effects/warning: See IBUPROFEN.

ibuprofen

is a (NSAID) NON-NARCOTIC ANALGESIC and ANTIRHEUMATIC drug. It is used primarily to treat the pain of rheumatism and other musculoskeletal disorders, moderate pain of inflammatory origin and postoperative pain. Although its anti-inflammatory property is not as powerful as a number of other NSAIDs, its side-effects tend to be relatively well tolerated, so higher dosage may be used to compensate. Accordingly, it was the first and only modern NSAID administered orally licensed for non-prescription, over-the-counter sale in the UK. It has extensive use both in its own right and as the major active constituent in COMPOUND ANALGESIC preparations for the treatment of minor to moderate pain, including headache, period pain, toothache and muscle ache. Its ANTIPYRETIC action helps symptomatic relief of the fever associated with colds and flu. It is also available for use in babies and children (including juvenile arthritis), and also during breast-feeding. Administration can be oral or by topical application.

+▲ Side-effects/warning: See NSAID; but ibuprofen is better tolerated and causes less gastrointestinal disturbances than the majority of its class.

○ Related entries: Apsifen; Arthrofen; Brufen; Brufen Retard; Codafen Continus; Cuprofen Ibuprofen Tablets; Cuprofen Tablets Maximum Strength; Ebufac; Fenbid; Hedex Ibuprofen Tablets; Ibugel; Ibular; Ibuleve Gel; Ibuleve Sports Gel; Ibuleve Spray; Ibumed; Inoven; Isisfen; Junifen Suspension; Lemsip Power+; Librofem (200 mg); Lidifen; Motrin; Nurofen; Nurofen 400; Nurofen Cold & Flu; Nurofen Micro-granules; Nurofen Plus; Nurofen Soluble; Pacifene; Pacifene Maximum Strength; PhorPain; PhorPain Double Strength; Proflex Pain Relief; Proflex Sustained Relief Capsules; Proflex Tablets; Rimafen.

Ibuspray

(Dermal) is a proprietary, prescription-only preparation of the (NSAID) NON-NARCOTIC ANALGESIC and ANTIRHEUMATIC ibuprofen, which has COUNTER-IRRITANT, or RUBEFACIENT, actions. It can be used for the symptomatic relief of underlying rheumatic and muscular pain, sprains and neuralgia. It is available as a spray for topical application to the skin and is not normally used for children, except on medical advice.

+▲ Side-effects/warning: See IBUPROFEN; but any adverse effects on topical application are limited.

ichthammol

is a thick, dark brown liquid derived from bituminous oils. It is used in ointments or in glycerol solution for the topical treatment of ulcers and inflammation of the skin. It is milder than coal tar and is useful in treating the less-severe forms of eczema. A common mode of administration is as an impregnated bandage with ZINC PASTE.

+▲ Side-effects/warning: See COAL TAR. Some patients may experience skin irritation; the skin may become sensitized. It must not be placed in contact with broken skin surfaces.

idarubicin hydrochloride

is a recently introduced CYTOTOXIC drug (of ANTIBIOTIC origin) with properties similar to doxorubicin hydrochloride, and which is used as an ANTICANCER drug, particularly for acute leukaemia and breast cancer. Administration can be oral or by infusion.

+▲ Side-effects/warning: See CYTOTOXICS. Administer with care to patients with liver or kidney impairment.

○ Related entry: Zavedos.

Idoxene

(Spodefell) is a proprietary, prescription-only preparation of the ANTIVIRAL idoxuridine. It can be used to treat local viral infections, particularly herpes simplex eye infections, and is available as an eye ointment.

+▲ Side-effects/warning: See IDOXURIDINE.

idoxuridine

is an ANTIVIRAL drug which can be used in solution to treat infections caused by herpes viruses in and around the mouth or eye, on external genitalia and the skin. It has rather weak and variable results when used topically and is too toxic to be used systemically. It works by stopping the virus multiplying by interfering with DNA synthesis. Administration is by topical application.

+ Side-effects: It may cause initial irritation and/or stinging on application;

changes in taste; over-use may cause softening of the skin.

▲ Warning: Avoid contact with the eyes and mucous membranes. It should not be administered to patients who are pregnant or when breast-feeding. It will damage fabrics.

○ Related entries: Herpid; Idoxene; Iduridin.

Iduridin

(Ferring) is a proprietary, prescription-only preparation of the ANTIVIRAL idoxuridine (in the organic solvent dimethyl sulphoxide; DMSO). It can be used to treat infections of the skin by herpes simplex (cold sores) or by herpes zoster, and is available as a solution for topical application either with a dropper or its own applicator.

+▲ Side-effects/warning: See IDOXURIDINE.

ifosfamide

is a CYTOTOXIC drug which is used in ANTICANCER treatment. It works by interfering with cellular DNA and so inhibits cell replication. Administration is by injection or infusion, and often simultaneously with the synthetic drug MESNA which reduces the toxic side-effects.

+▲ Side-effects/warning: See CYTOTOXICS.

○ Related entry: Mitoxana.

Ikorel

(Rhône-Poulenc Rorer) is a proprietary, prescription-only preparation of the POTASSIUM-CHANNEL ACTIVATOR and VASODILATOR nicorandil. It can be used as an ANTI-ANGINA drug to prevent and treat angina pectoris, and is available as tablets.

+▲ Side-effects/warning: See NICORANDIL.

Ilosone

(Dista) is a proprietary, prescription-only preparation of the ANTIBACTERIAL and (MACROLIDE) ANTIBIOTIC erythromycin. It can be used to treat and prevent many forms of infection, and is available as capsules and tablets.

+▲ Side-effects/warning: See ERYTHROMYCIN.

Ilube

(Cusi) is a proprietary, prescription-only preparation of the MUCOLYTIC acetylcysteine and a small proportion of the synthetic tear fluid HYPROMELLOSE. It can be used to treat a deficiency of tears in the eyes (eg in rheumatoid arthritis), which may lead to eye dryness and inflammation, and is available as eye-drops.

+▲ Side-effects/warning: See ACETYLCYSTEINE.

Imbrilon

(Berk) is a proprietary, prescription-only preparation of the (NSAID) NON-NARCOTIC ANALGESIC and ANTIRHEUMATIC indomethacin. It can be used to treat the pain and inflammation of rheumatic disease and other musculoskeletal disorders (including gout). It is available as capsules and suppositories.

+▲ Side-effects/warning: See INDOMETHACIN.

Imdur

(Astra) is a proprietary, prescription-only preparation of the VASODILATOR and ANTI-ANGINA drug isosorbide mononitrate. It can be used to treat and prevent angina pectoris, and is available as modified-release tablets (*Durules*).

+▲ Side-effects/warning: See ISOSORBIDE MONONITRATE.

imidazoles ▨

(or AZOLES) are a chemical group that includes drugs with a variety of ANTIMICROBIAL and ANTIPROTOZOAL actions, but the term is mainly used as a convenient, collective description of a group of broad-spectrum ANTIFUNGALS that are active against most fungi and yeasts. The most common conditions that they are used to treat are vaginal infections (such as candidiasis; thrush), infections of the skin surface, of the mucous membranes, the hair and the nails. The best-known and most-used imidazoles include CLOTRIMAZOLE, MICONAZOLE, KETOCONAZOLE, ISOCONAZOLE and

ECONAZOLE NITRATE. Miconazole and ketoconazole can be used systemically, though the latter can cause hepatoxicity (liver damage). They work by interfering with fungal enzymes, causing a lethal accumulation of hydrogen peroxide, and by interfering with the fungal cell wall.

Imigran

(Glaxo) is a proprietary, prescription-only preparation of the ANTIMIGRAINE drug sumatriptan. It can be used to treat acute migraine attacks and cluster headaches, and is available as tablets and in a form for self-injection.

✚▲ Side-effects/warning: See SUMATRIPTAN.

imipenem with cilastin

is an ANTIBACTERIAL and ANTIBIOTIC drug which is a new sort of BETA-LACTAM with a broad-spectrum of activity against many Gram-positive and Gram-negative bacteria. However, it is partly degraded by an enzyme in the kidney and is therefore combined with CILASTIN, which is an ENZYME INHIBITOR. It can be used to treat infections in the periphery, such as the urethra and cervix, and to prevent infection during surgery. Administration is by injection or infusion.

✚ Side-effects: Vomiting and nausea, diarrhoea and abdominal pain; altered taste and mouth ulcers; skin rashes; hepatitis, jaundice and blood disorders; pain at site of injection; brain and nerve disturbances. The urine may be coloured red.

▲ Warning: Administer with caution to those who have impaired kidney function, who are pregnant or have brain disorders, such as epilepsy

○ Related entry: Primaxin.

imipramine hydrochloride

is an ANTIDEPRESSANT of the TRICYCLIC class, but which has fewer SEDATIVE properties than many other tricyclics. It is therefore more suited for the treatment of withdrawn and apathetic patients, rather than those who are agitated and restless. As is the case with many such drugs, it can also be used

to treat bed-wetting at night by children. Administration is oral.

✚▲ Side-effects/warning: See AMITRIPTYLINE HYDROCHLORIDE.

○ Related entry: Tofranil.

Immukin

(Boehringer Ingelheim) is a proprietary, prescription-only preparation of the IMMUNOMODULATOR interferon (in the form of gamma-1b). It can be used in conjunction with ANTIMICROBIAL and ANTIBIOTIC drugs to reduce the frequency of serious infections in patients with chronic glanulomatous disease. It is available in a form for injection.

✚▲ Side-effects/warning: See INTERFERON.

immunization 🔲

agents are used in the immunization procedure, which can be used to prevent an individual from contracting specific infections, or help treat existing infection. This is achieved by using one of two methods, providing *active* or *passive* immunity.

Active immunity is conferred by vaccination (that is, administering a VACCINE), which involves the injection or administration of bacterial or viral agents that are live (but weakened, 'attenuated'), dead or of *toxoids* (chemically-modified microbial toxins). These agents act as *antigens* to trigger the body's own defence mechanisms to manufacture antibodies. This method gives long-lasting, but not necessarily permanent, protection.

Passive immunity is conferred by the injection of a quantity of prepared blood serum already containing mixed antibodies (NORMAL IMMUNOGLOBULIN) or selected antibodies (SPECIFIC IMMUNOGLOBULIN), and so helps to prevent the person contracting the infection or helps an treat an already existing infection. This method gives immediate but short-lived protection. See ANTISERUM and IMMUNOGLOBULIN

✚▲ Side-effects/warning: These vary greatly depending on the particular vaccine or immunoglobulin and the individual. However, all involve administering foreign protein and so some sort of sensitivity reaction is usual. Commonly, there is malaise, fever and chills. Expert advice is required.

immunoglobulin

is a term used to describe any of five-or-so classes of proteins in the immune system that naturally act as antibodies in the bloodstream. They are created in response to the presence of a specific *antigen* (any substance the body regards as foreign or dangerous) and circulate within the blood. Immunoglobulin deficiencies are often associated with increased risk of infection. These antibodies can be administered therapeutically, by injection or infusion, to confer immediate immunity, commonly known as *passive immunity*, against certain diseases. To minimize the risk of allergic reactions, immunoglobulins are normally of human origin rather than from an animal (when they are usually referred to as *antiserum* or *antisera*). Two classes of human immunoglobulins are used to protect either patients suffering from infection or individuals exposed to infection: NORMAL IMMUNOGLOBULIN and SPECIFIC IMMUNOGLOBULIN. Normal immunoglobulin is prepared from the pooled serum of at least 1000 donors who have antibodies to viruses prevalent in a normal population (including for hepatitis A, measles and rubella). *Specific immunoglobulin* is prepared in a similar way, except that the pooled blood plasma used to obtain the immunoglobulins is taken from donors with high levels of the particular antibody that is required (eg for hepatitis B, rabies, rubella, tetanus or varicella-zoster). See ANTISERUM; IMMUNIZATION.

✪ Related entries: anti-D (Rh₀) immunoglobulin; hepatitis B immunoglobulin (HBIG); rabies immunoglobulin, human; rubella immunoglobulin, human; tetanus immunoglobulin, human; varicella-zoster immunoglobulin (VZIG).

immunomodulators ⁊

are agents that are used to modify the activity of the body's immune system, normally improving defences against infections and possibly malignant growths. INTERFERONS are inducible proteins synthesized by mammalian cells, though they can now be produced by recombinant technology. There are three or more types, alpha-, beta- and gamma-interferons. They can modify the host response by inducing production of enzymes, for instance, that inhibit translocation of viral mRNA into viral protein, and thus prevent virus reproduction. They are administered by intravenous or intramuscular injection in the treatment of AIDS, cancer, multiple sclerosis and for other chemotherapy. Interleukins (ALDESLEUKIN, or interleukin-2, is the first used), can help in ANTICANCER therapy, for instance, in treating metastatic renal cell carcinoma. Administration is by injection.

Immunoprin

(Ashbourne) is a proprietary, prescription-only preparation of the IMMUNOSUPPRESSANT azathioprine. It can be used to treat a variety of autoimmune diseases and also tissue rejection in transplant patients, and is available as tablets.
✚▲ Side-effects/warning: See AZATHIOPRINE.

immunostimulants ⁊

are agents that are used to boost the efficiency of the body's immune sytem, and thus inprove defence against infections and possibly malignant growths. In the recent past, preparations of inactivated bacteria, *Corynebacterium parvum* (Coparvax), for example, were injected into the pleural cavity of the chest or the abdominal peritoneal cavity to treat the collection of fluids (effusion) there, with the intension of increasing the local activity of the natural immune system. This particular therapy did not prove to be very successful and has largely been discontinued, though a number of similar agents are currently being evaluated or are licenced in other countries (some for use against certain forms of cancer). VACCINES are used for systemic long-term immunostimulation against specific bacterial or viral organisms, through administration of live but weakened (attenuated) organisms, dead but immunogenic organisms or live non-pathogenic organisms closely related to the invading microbe. Many vaccines are administered with *immunoadjuvant* drugs (eg aluminium phosphate) to enhance their immunostimulant actions. INTERFERONS and interleukins are discussed under IMMUNOMODULATORS.

immunosuppressants ⁊

are drugs that are used to inhibit the body's resistance to the presence of infection or foreign bodies. Because of this property, such drugs can be used to prevent tissue rejection following donor grafting or transplant surgery (although there is then the risk of unopposed infection). They are also commonly used to treat autoimmune disease (when the immune system is triggered into acting against part of the body itself). Immunosuppressant drugs can be used to treat conditions such as rheumatoid arthritis, lupus erythematosus and collagen disorders. The best-known and most-used immunosuppressants are theCORTICOSTEROIDS (eg PREDNISOLONE), the non-steroid drugs AZATHIOPRINE, CHLORAMBUCIL, CYCLOPHOSPHAMIDE and CYCLOSPORIN, and the recently introduced specialist drug MYCOPHENOLATE MOFETIL.

Imodium Capsules

(Johnson & Johnson) is a proprietary, non-prescription preparation of the (OPIOID) ANTIDIARRHOEAL loperamide hydrochloride. It can be used for the symptomatic relief of acute diarrhoea and its associated pain and discomfort, and is available as capsules.

✚▲ Side-effects/warning: See LOPERAMIDE HYDROCHLORIDE.

Improvera

(Upjohn) is a proprietary, prescription-only preparation of the OESTROGEN piperazine oestrone sulphate and the PROGESTOGEN medroxyprogesterone acetate. It can be used to treat menopausal symptoms (including osteoporosis prophylaxis) in HRT, and is available as tablets.

✚▲ Side-effects/warning: See PIPERAZINE OESTRONE SULPHATE; MEDROXYPROGESTERONE ACETATE.

Imtack Spray

(Astra) is a proprietary, non-prescription preparation of the VASODILATOR and ANTI-ANGINA drug isosorbide dinitrate. It can be used to treat and prevent angina pectoris and also in HEART FAILURE TREATMENT, and is available as an aerosol spray.

✚▲ Side-effects/warning: See ISOSORBIDE DINITRATE.

Imunovir

(Leo) is a proprietary, prescription-only preparation of the ANTIVIRAL drug inosine pranobex. It can be used to treat herpes simplex infections and warts in mucous membranes and adjacent skin (eg genital warts). It is available as tablets.

✚▲ Side-effects/warning: See INOSINE PRANOBEX.

Imuran

(Wellcome) is a proprietary, prescription-only preparation of the IMMUNOSUPPRESSANT azathioprine. It can be used to treat a variety of autoimmune diseases and tissue rejection in transplant patients. It is available as tablets and in a form for injection.

✚▲ Side-effects/warning: See AZATHIOPRINE.

Inactivated Influenza Vaccine (Split Virion)

(Mérieux) is a proprietary, prescription-only VACCINE preparation of influenza vaccine (split virion vaccine). It can be used to prevent an individual from contracting influenza, and is available in a form for injection.

✚▲ Side-effects/warning: See INFLUENZA VACCINE.

indapamide

is a DIURETIC of the THIAZIDE-like class which can be used as an ANTIHYPERTENSIVE, either alone or in conjunction with other drugs. Administration is oral.

✚ Side-effects: Headache, dizziness, fatigue; nausea and anorexia; muscle cramps; gastrointestinal upsets; skin rashes and other disorders; hypotension; low blood potassium; raised blood urea and glucose; loss of feeling in the extremities; photosensitivity; impotence; kidney impairment, myopia (reversible shortsightedness).

▲ Warning: It is not to be used after recent stroke, or where there is severe liver impairment; care must be taken when administering to patients with certain kidney disorders, parathyroid disease (blood electrolytes must be measured), or who are pregnant or breast-feeding.

○ Related entries: Indaxa 25; Natrilix.

Indaxa 25

(Ashbourne) is a proprietary, prescription-only preparation of the (THIAZIDE-like) DIURETIC indapamide. It can be used, either alone or in conjunction with other drugs, as an ANTIHYPERTENSIVE, and is available as tablets .

✚▲ Side-effects/warning: SeeINDAPAMIDE.

Inderal

(Zeneca) is a proprietary, prescription-only preparation of the BETA-BLOCKER propranolol hydrochloride. It can be used as an ANTIHYPERTENSIVE for raised blood pressure, as an ANTI-ANGINA treatment to relieve symptoms and improve exercise tolerance and as an ANTI-ARRHYTHMIC to regularize heartbeat and to treat myocardial

infarction. It can also be used as an ANTITHYROID drug for short-term treatment of thyrotoxicosis, as an ANTIMIGRAINE treatment to prevent attacks, as an ANXIOLYTIC, particularly for symptomatic relief of tremor and palpitations, and, with an ALPHA-ADRENOCEPTOR BLOCKER, in the acute treatment of phaeochromocytoma. It is available as tablets and in a form for injection.

✚▲ Side-effects/warning: See PROPRANOLOL HYDROCHLORIDE.

Inderal-LA

(Zeneca) is a proprietary, prescription-only preparation of the BETA-BLOCKER propranolol hydrochloride. It can be used as an ANTIHYPERTENSIVE for raised blood pressure, as an ANTI-ANGINA treatment to relieve symptoms and improve exercise tolerance and as an ANTI-ARRHYTHMIC to regularize heartbeat and to treat myocardial infarction. It can also be used as an ANTITHYROID drug for short-term treatment of thyrotoxicosis, as an ANTIMIGRAINE treatment to prevent attacks, as an ANXIOLYTIC, particularly for symptomatic relief of tremor and palpitations, and, with an ALPHA-ADRENOCEPTOR BLOCKER, in the acute treatment of phaeochromocytoma. It is available as modified-release capsules.

✚▲ Side-effects/warning: See PROPRANOLOL HYDROCHLORIDE.

Inderetic

(Zeneca) is a proprietary, prescription-only COMPOUND PREPARATION of the BETA-BLOCKER propranolol hydrochloride and the (THIAZIDE) DIURETIC bendrofluazide. It can be used as an ANTIHYPERTENSIVE for raised blood pressure, and is available as capsules.

✚▲ Side-effects/warning: See BENDROFLUAZIDE; PROPRANOLOL HYDROCHLORIDE.

Inderex

(Zeneca) is a proprietary, prescription-only COMPOUND PREPARATION of the BETA-BLOCKER propranolol hydrochloride and the (THIAZIDE) DIURETIC bendrofluazide. It can be used as an ANTIHYPERTENSIVE for raised blood pressure, and is available as capsules.

✚▲ Side-effects/warning: See BENDROFLUAZIDE; PROPRANOLOL HYDROCHLORIDE.

indinavir

is a (*protease inhibitor*) ANTIVIRAL drug which is often used together with (*reverse transcriptase*) antivirals. It can be used in the treatment of progressive or advanced AIDS. Administration is oral.

✚ Side-effects: Nausea, vomiting, diarrhoea, abdominal pain; taste disturbance and dry mouth; headache, insomnia, dizziness, muscle weakness and loss of sensation in the extremities; dry skin, pruritis, rash; changes in kidney function, blood changes, blood in the urine, vision disturbances.

▲ Warning: It should not be given to patients who are breast-feeding. Administer with caution where there is impaired liver function, certain kidney disturbances, haemophilia or pregnancy.

✪ Related entry: Crixivan.

Indocid

(Morson) is a proprietary, prescription-only preparation of the (NSAID) NON-NARCOTIC ANALGESIC and ANTIRHEUMATIC indomethacin. It can be used to treat the pain of rheumatic disease and other musculoskeletal disorders. It is available as capsules, as modified-release capsules (under the name *Indocid-R*), as suppositories and as a sugar-free suspension.

✚▲ Side-effects/warning: See INDOMETHACIN.

Indocid PDA

(Morson) is a proprietary, prescription-only preparation of the (NSAID) NON-NARCOTIC ANALGESIC and ANTIRHEUMATIC indomethacin. It can be used (in this preparation only) for specialist, emergency, short-term treatment of premature infants with a heart defect (patent ductus arteriosus), while preparations are being made for surgery. It is available in a form for intravenous infusion.

✚▲ Side-effects/warning: See INDOMETHACIN.

Indolar SR

(Lagap) is a proprietary, prescription-only preparation of the (NSAID) NON-NARCOTIC ANALGESIC and ANTIRHEUMATIC indomethacin. It can be used to relieve the pain of rheumatic disease, gout and other inflammatory musculoskeletal disorders, and is available as modified-release capsules.

✚▲ Side-effects/warning: See INDOMETHACIN.

Indomax

(Ashbourne) is a proprietary, prescription-only preparation of the (NSAID) NON-NARCOTIC ANALGESIC and ANTIRHEUMATIC indomethacin. It can be used to relieve the pain of rheumatic disease and other musculoskeletal disorders, and is available as capsules.

✚▲ Side-effects/warning: See INDOMETHACIN.

indometacin

see INDOMETHACIN

indomethacin

(indometacin) is a (NSAID) NON-NARCOTIC ANALGESIC and ANTIRHEUMATIC drug which can be used to treat rheumatic and muscular pain caused by inflammation and/or bone degeneration, particularly at the joints. It can also be used to treat period pain and acute gout. Administration is mainly oral as tablets, capsules, modified-release capsules or a liquid; but its use in suppositories is especially effective for the relief of overnight pain and stiffness in the morning. Most of its proprietary preparations are not normally given to children, but one form is used (under specialist supervision with extensive monitoring) in premature babies who have patent ductus arteriosus (failure of this connecting vessel between the pulmonary artery and aorta to close after birth).

✚▲ Side-effects/warning: See NSAID; there may also be pronounced intestinal disturbances; headaches, dizziness and, though rarely, drowsiness, confusion, insomnia, depression, convulsions, blood disorders, blurred vision, blood pressure changes. It is not to be used in patients who are breast-feeding, who have blood coagulation defects, or kidney and certain other disorders.

✪ Related entries: Artracin; Flexin Continus; Flexin-25 Continus; Flexin-LS Continus; Imbrilon; Indocid; Indocid PDA; Indolar SR; Indomax; Indomod; Mobilan; Rheumacin LA; Rimacid; Slo-Indo.

Indomod

(Pharmacia) is a proprietary, prescription-only preparation of the (NSAID) NON-NARCOTIC ANALGESIC and ANTIRHEUMATIC indomethacin. It can be used to treat the pain of rheumatic disease and other musculoskeletal disorders, and is available as modified-release capsules.

✚▲ Side-effects/warning: See INDOMETHACIN.

indoramin

is a selective ALPHA-ADRENOCEPTOR BLOCKER drug. It is used as an ANTIHYPERTENSIVE treatment, often in conjunction with other classes of drug (eg BETA-BLOCKERS or DIURETICS), and can be used to treat urinary retention in benign prostatic hypertrophy. Administration is oral.

✚▲ Side-effects/warning: See PRAZOSIN HYDROCHLORIDE.

✪ Related entries: Baratol; Doralese.

Infacol

(Pharmax) is a proprietary, non-prescription preparation of the ANTIFOAMING AGENT dimethicone (as simethicone). It can

be used for the relief of infant colic and griping pain, and is available as an oral liquid.

✚▲ Side-effects/warning: See DIMETHICONE.

Infadrops

(Goldshield) is a proprietary, non-prescription preparation of the NON-NARCOTIC ANALGESIC paracetamol. It can be used to treat mild to moderate pain (including teething pain) and as an ANTIPYRETIC (for instance, to reduce fever after vaccination, when it can be used in two-month-old babies). It is available as a liquid suspension and is not normally given to infants under three months, except on medical advice.

✚▲ Side-effects/warning: See PARACETAMOL.

influenza vaccine

for IMMUNIZATION helps protect people from catching influenza. It is recommended only for persons at high risk of catching known strains of influenza, such as the elderly. This is because, unlike some viruses, the influenza viruses A and B are constantly changing in physical form and antibodies manufactured in the body to deal with one strain at one time will have no effect at all on the same strain at another time. Administration is by injection.

✚▲ Side-effects/warning: See VACCINES. Because these vaccines are prepared from virus strains grown in chicken embryos, they should be used with caution in individuals known to be sensitive to eggs.

✪ Related entries: Fluarix; Fluvirin; Fluzone; Inactivated Influenza Vaccine (Split Viron); Influvac Sub-unit.

Influvac Sub-unit

(Duphar) is a proprietary, prescription-only VACCINE preparation of influenza vaccine (surface antigen). It can be used to prevent an individual from contracting influenza, and is available in a form for injection.

✚▲ Side-effects/warning: See INFLUENZA VACCINE.

Initard 50/50

(Novo Nordisk; Wellcome) is a proprietary, non-prescription preparation of (mixed) BIPHASIC ISOPHANE UNSULIN. It is used in DIABETIC TREATMENT to treat and maintain diabetic patients, and contains both neutral and isophane porcine insulins in equal proportions. It is available in vials for injection and has an intermediate duration of action.

✚▲ Side-effects/warning: See INSULIN.

Innohep

(Leo) is a proprietary, prescription-only preparation of the ANTICOAGULANT drug tinzaparin, which is a low molecular weight version of heparin. It can be administered for long-duration prevention of venous thrombo-embolism, particularly in orthopaedic use, and is available in a form for injection.

✚▲ Side-effects/warning: See TINZAPARIN.

Innovace

(Merck Sharp & Dohme) a proprietary, prescription-only preparation of the ACE INHIBITOR enalapril maleate. It can be used as an ANTIHYPERTENSIVE and in HEART FAILURE TREATMENT, and is available as tablets.

✚▲ Side-effects/warning: See ENALAPRIL MALEATE.

Innozide

(Merck Sharp & Dohme) is a proprietary, prescription-only COMPOUND PREPARATION of the ACE INHIBITOR enalapril maleate and the (THIAZIDE) DIURETIC hydrochlorothiazide. It can be used as an ANTIHYPERTENSIVE, and is available as tablets.

✚▲ Side-effects/warning: See ENALAPRIL MALEATE; HYDROCHLOROTHIAZIDE.

inosine pranobex

is an ANTIVIRAL drug which is used to treat herpes simplex infections in mucous membranes and adjacent skin (eg genital warts). Administration is oral.

✚ Side-effects: Increased uric acid levels in the blood and urine.

▲ Warning: It should not be administered to patients with impaired kidney function or high blood levels of uric acid (for instance in gout).

○ Related entry: Imunovir.

inositol nicotinate

is a VASODILATOR drug which can be administered to help improve blood circulation to the hands and feet when this is impaired, for example, in peripheral vascular disease (Raynaud's phenomenon). Administration is oral.

✚▲ Side-effects/warning: See NICOTINIC ACID.

○ Related entry: Hexopal.

Inoven

(Johnson & Johnson) is a proprietary, non-prescription preparation of the (NSAID) NON-NARCOTIC ANALGESIC and ANTIRHEUMATIC ibuprofen. It can be used for the relief of headache, period pain, muscular pain, dental pain and feverishness. It is available as tablets and is not normally given to children under 12 years, except on medical advice.

✚▲ Side-effects/warning: See IBUPROFEN.

Instillagel

(CliniFlex) is a proprietary, non-prescription COMPOUND PREPARATION of the ANTISEPTIC chlorhexidine (as gluconate) and the LOCAL ANAESTHETIC lignocaine hydrochloride. It can be used to treat painful inflammations of the urethra, and is available as a gel in disposable syringes.

✚▲ Side-effects/warning: See CHLORHEXIDINE; LIGNOCAINE HYDROCHLORIDE.

Insulatard

(Novo Nordisk, Wellcome) is a proprietary, non-prescription preparation of porcine isophane insulin. It is used in DIABETIC TREATMENT to treat and maintain diabetic patients, and is available in vials for injection and has an intermediate duration of action.

✚▲ Side-effects/warning: See INSULIN.

insulin

is a protein HORMONE produced and secreted by the Islets of Langerhans within the pancreas. It has the effect of reducing the level of glucose (blood sugar) in the bloodstream and is part of a balancing mechanism with the opposing hormone glycogen (which increases blood sugars). Its deficiency (in the disorder called diabetes mellitus) results in high levels of blood sugar, which can rapidly lead to severe symptoms and potentially coma and death. Patients suffering from diabetes can be divided into two groups, which largely determines the nature of their treatment. Those who have Type I diabetes (insulin-dependent diabetes mellitus; IDDM; juvenile-onset diabetes) are generally maintained for life on one or other of the insulin preparations. Those who develop Type II diabetes (non-insulin-dependent diabetes mellitus; NIDDM; maturity-onset diabetes) can usually be managed by treatment with ORAL HYPOGLYCAEMIC drugs or by diet alone and less commonly require insulin injections. Most diabetics take some form of insulin on a regular (daily) basis, generally by subcutaneous injection. Modern genetic engineering has enabled the production of quantities of the human form of insulin, which is now replacing the former insulins extracted from cows (bovine insulin) or pigs (porcine insulin). There are marked differences in absorption time – which dictates both the rate of onset and duration of action – between insulin preparations. This depends on their pH and whether preparations are solutions, suspensions or complexes with zinc or protamine. Consequently, forms are available that are short-acting (eg SOLUBLE INSULIN) or intermediate-acting (eg INSULIN ZINC SUSPENSION (AMORPHOUS)), or long-acting (eg INSULIN ZINC SUSPENSION (CRYSTALLINE)). Many diabetic patients use more than one type of insulin in proportions that are appropriate to their own specific requirements. Insulin is usually administered by patients themselves, by subcutaneous injection into the thigh, buttock, upper arm or abdomen.

✚ Side-effects: Hypoglycaemia in overdose. Local reactions at the injection site.

▲ Warning: Expert counselling, initial training and blood-glucose monitoring is required because it is essential that patients maintain a stable blood-glucose level over long periods. Choice of suitable preparations, or combination of preparations, for injection may take some time to establish. Patients should be warned of possible hazards in driving over long periods and should only drive if *hypoglycaemic aware*.

✪ Related entries: biphasic insulin; biphasic isophane insulin; Human Actraphane 30/70; Human Actrapid; Human Initard 50/50; Human Insulatard; Human Mixtard 30/70; Human Monotard; Human Protaphane; Human Ultratard; Human Velosulin; Humulin I; Humulin Lente; Humulin M1; Humulin M2; Humulin M3; Humulin M4; Humulin S; Humulin Zn; Hypurin Isophane; Hypurin Lente; Hypurin Neutral; Hypurin Protamine Zinc; Initard 50/50; Insulatard; insulin zinc suspension; Lentard MC; Mixtard 30/70; PenMix 10/90; PenMix 20/80; PenMix 30/70; PenMix 40/60; PenMix 50/50; protamine zinc insulin; Pur-In Isophane; Pur-In Mix 15/85; Pur-In Mix 25/75; Pur-In Mix 50/50; Pur-In Neutral; Rapitard MC; Semitard MC; Velosulin.

insulin injection

see SOLUBLE INSULIN

insulin lispro

is a recombinant (biosynthetic) human insulin analogue, which is used in DIABETIC TREATMENT to maintain diabetic patients. It has a more rapid onset of action than soluble insulin (so can be given subcutaneously soon after a meal), and has a shorter duration of action than soluble insulin. Administration is by injection.

✚▲ Side-effects/warning: See INSULIN.

✪ Related entry: Humalog.

insulin zinc suspension

(Insulin Zinc Suspension (Mixed); I.Z.S.) is a form of highly purified purified bovine and/or porcine insulin, prepared as a sterile neutral complex with zinc salts, which is used in DIABETIC TREATMENT to maintain diabetic patients. Administration is by injection and it has a long duration of action.

+▲ Side-effects/warning: See INSULIN.

✪ Related entries: Human Monotard; Humulin Lente; Humulin M1; Hypurin Lente; Lentard MC.

insulin zinc suspension (amorphous)

(Amorph.I.Z.S.) is a form of highly purified purified animal (porcine or bovine) insulin, prepared as a sterile neutral complex with zinc salts, which is used in DIABETIC TREATMENT to maintain diabetic patients. It is available in vials for injection and has an intermediate duration of action.

+▲ Side-effects/warning: See INSULIN.

✪ Related entry: Semitard MC.

insulin zinc suspension (crystalline)

(Cryst.I.Z.S.) is a form of highly purified bovine or human insulin, prepared as a sterile complex with zinc salts, which is used in DIABETIC TREATMENT to maintain diabetic patients. It is available in vials for injection and has a medium to long duration of action.

+▲ Side-effects/warning: See INSULIN.

✪ Related entries: Human Ultratard; Humulin Zn.

Intal

(Fisons) is a proprietary, prescription-only preparation of sodium cromoglycate (sodium cromoglicate). It can be used as a prophylactic (preventive) ANTI-ASTHMATIC treatment. It is available as a liquid in aerosol units (available with a spacer device, *Syncroner* and large volume inhaler, *Fisonair*), as a nebulizer solution or as a powder for inhalation in *Spincaps*

(which can be used with the *Spinhaler Insufflator*).

+▲ Side-effects/warning: See SODIUM CROMOGLYCATE.

interferon

is a protein produced in tiny quantities by cells infected by a virus and which has the ability to inhibit further growth of the virus. Genetic engineering, including the use of bacteria as host cells has enabled interferons to be mass-produced, but they have been less effective against viruses than was hoped. They also have complex effects on cells, cell function and immunity, which has limited their use. *Interferon alpha* is used as an ANTICANCER treatment for particular cancers, particularly lymphomas (eg AIDS-related Kaposi's sarcoma), certain cancers of the kidney, some solid tumours and other conditions including chronic active hepatitis B. *Interferon beta-1b* can be used to treat Relapsing-Remitting Multiple Sclerosis. *Interferon gamma* is used in conjunction with ANTIMICROBIALS and ANTIBIOTICS to reduce the frequency of serious infection in patients with chronic granulatomatous disease.

+ Side-effects: Severe flu-like symptoms; there may also be lethargy and depression. The blood-producing capacity of the bone marrow may be reduced. Some patients experience high or low blood pressure and heartbeat irregularities. Liver toxicity has been reported. There may be thyroid abnormalities, rashes and confusion.

▲ Warning: Regular blood counts are essential during treatment, particularly to check the levels of white blood cells.

✪ Related entries: Betaferon; Immukin; Intron A; Roferon-A; Viraferon; Wellferon.

Intralgin

(3M) is a proprietary, non-prescription COMPOUND PREPARATION of the LOCAL ANAESTHETIC benzocaine with salicylamide, which has a COUNTER-IRRITANT, or RUBEFACIENT, action. It can be applied topically to the skin for symptomatic relief of underlying muscle or joint pain, and is available as a gel.

+▲ Side-effects/warning: See BENZOCAINE.

Intraval Sodium

(Rhône-Poulenc Rorer) is a proprietary, prescription-only preparation of the BARBITURATE thiopentone sodium. It can be used as a GENERAL ANAESTHETIC for the induction of anaesthesia, and is available in a form for injection.

+▲ Side-effects/warning: See THIOPENTONE SODIUM.

Intron A

(Schering-Plough) is a proprietary, prescription-only preparation of the IMMUNOMODULATOR interferon (in the form alpha-2b, rbe). It can be used as an ANTICANCER treatment mainly for leukaemia, AIDS-related Kaposi's sarcoma and chronic active hepatitis B, and is available in a form for injection.

+▲ Side-effects/warning: See INTERFERON.

Intropin

(Du Pont) is a proprietary, prescription-only preparation of the SYMPATHOMIMETIC and CARDIAC STIMULANT dopamine hydrochloride. It can be used to treat cardiogenic shock following a heart attack or during heart surgery, and is available as a liquid in vials for dilution and infusion.

+▲ Side-effects/warning: See DOPAMINE.

Invirase

(Roche) is a proprietary, prescription-only preparation of the ANTIVIRAL saquinavir (as mesylate). It can be used in the treatment of AIDS, and is available as capsules.

+▲ Side-effects/warning: See SAQUINAVIR.

iodine

is a non-metallic element which is accumulated by the body in the thyroid gland (situated at the base of the neck) and is used by the cells of this gland to synthesize the thyroid HORMONES THYROXINE and TRIIODOTHYRONINE, which control a

number of normal metabolic processes and growth. Nutritional sources of iodine include seafood, vegetables grown in soil containing iodine and iodinated table salt. A deficiency is one of the possible causes of goitre, where the thyroid gland becomes enlarged. Therapeutically, iodine (as AQUEOUS IODINE ORAL SOLUTION) can be used in thyrotoxicosis prior to surgery and in solution as an ANTISEPTIC.

Ionamin

(Lipha) is a proprietary preparation of the APPETITE SUPPRESSANT phentermine. It can be used, in the short term only, to assist in the medical treatment of obesity. It is on the Controlled Drugs List, and is available as modified-release capsules.

+▲ Side-effects/warning: See PHENTERMINE.

Ionax Scrub

(Novex) is a proprietary, non-prescription preparation of the ANTISEPTIC benzalkonium chloride with abrasive polyethylene granules within a foaming aqueous-alcohol base. It can be used in the treatment of acne.

+▲ Side-effects/warning: See BENZALKONIUM CHLORIDE.

Ionil T

(Novex) is a proprietary, non-prescription COMPOUND PREPARATION of the ANTISEPTIC benzalkonium chloride, the KERATOLYTIC salicylic acid and coal tar. It can be used as a treatment for dandruff and other scalp conditions, and is available as a shampoo.

+▲ Side-effects/warning: See BENZALKONIUM CHLORIDE; COAL TAR; SALICYLIC ACID.

ipecac

see IPECACUANHA

ipecacuanha

is an extract from the ipecac plant. It contains two ALKALOIDS (emetine and cephaeline) that have an irritant action on the gastrointestinal tract and is therefore a powerful EMETIC. It can be used to clear the stomach in certain cases of non-corrosive poisoning when the patient is conscious (particularly in children). In smaller doses it can also be used as an EXPECTORANT in non-proprietary mixtures and proprietary tinctures and syrups. Emetine (and certain derivatives) has been used as an AMOEBICIDAL.

✚ Side-effects: Excessive vomiting, effects on the heart (if absorbed), damage to epithelium (surface tissues) of the gastrointestinal tract.

▲ Warning: In high dosage it can cause severe gastric upset.

⊙ Related entries: Ammonia and Ipecacuanha Mixture, BP; Ipecacuanha and Morphine Mixture, BP; Mu-Cron Syrup, Junior.

Ipecacuanha and Morphine Mixture, BP

is a non-proprietary, non-prescription COMPOUND PREPARATION that combines the (OPIOID) NARCOTIC ANALGESIC morphine (anhydrous) as a tincture with chloroform. It is used as an ANTITUSSIVE in combination with a tincture of the EMETIC ipecacuanha, and liquorice liquid extract. Administration is oral as a liquid.

✚▲ Side-effects/warning: See IPECACUANHA; MORPHINE SULPHATE.

Ipral

(Squibb) is a proprietary, prescription-only preparation of the ANTIBACTERIAL trimethoprim. It can be used to treat infections of the upper respiratory tract, particularly bronchitis, and the urinary tract, and is available as tablets.

✚▲ Side-effects/warning: See TRIMETHOPRIM.

ipratropium bromide

is an ANTICHOLINERGIC drug with BRONCHODILATOR properties. It can be used to treat obstructive airways disease, where it is more often used for chronic bronchitis than as an ANTI-ASTHMATIC treatment. For this treatment it is administered by inhalation from an aerosol or a nebulizer. It is also used, in the form of a nasal spray, as a NASAL DECONGESTANT to treat watery rhinitis.

✚ Side-effects: There may be dryness of mouth; rarely, there is urinary retention and/or constipation.

▲ Warning: Administer with caution to patients with glaucoma or enlargement of the prostate gland, or who are pregnant.

⊙ Related entries: Atrovent; Duovent; Rinatec; Steri-Neb Ipratropium.

iron

is a metallic element essential to the body in several ways, particularly its role, as the red blood cell constituent haemoglobin, as the transporter of oxygen around the body and in a similar form in muscle to accept the oxygen. Iron deficiency due to disease states that prevent its proper absorption or because of its deficiency in the diet, lead to forms of anaemia (*iron-deficiency anaemia*). It is used therapeutically usually to treat anaemia caused by dietary deficiency. Supplements can be administered orally (in the form of FERROUS FUMARATE, FERROUS GLUCONATE, FERROUS GLYCINE SULPHATE, FERROUS SULPHATE and other salts) or by injection or intravenous infusion (in the form of iron dextran and other preparations). There are numerous iron-and-vitamin supplements available, which can be particularly useful during pregnancy. Excellent foods sources of iron include meat and liver.

Isclofen

(Isis) is a prescription-only, non-proprietary version of the (NSAID) NON-NARCOTIC ANALGESIC and ANTIRHEUMATIC drug diclofenac sodium. It can be administered to treat the pain and inflammation of arthritis and rheumatism and other musculoskeletal disorders. It is available as tablets.

✚▲ Side-effects/warning: See DICLOFENAC SODIUM.

Isisfen

(Isis) is a proprietary, prescription-only preparation of the (NSAID) NON-NARCOTIC ANALGESIC and ANTIRHEUMATIC drug ibuprofen. It can be administered to relieve the pain of rheumatism and other musculoskeletal disorders, and is available as tablets.

✚▲ Side-effects/warning: See IBUPROFEN.

Ismelin

(Ciba) is a proprietary, prescription-only preparation of the ADRENERGIC-NEURONE BLOCKER guanethidine monosulphate. It can be used as an ANTIHYPERTENSIVE for moderate to severe high blood pressure, and is available as tablets and in a form for injection.

✚▲ Side-effects/warning: See GUANETHIDINE MONOSULPHATE.

Ismo

(Boehringer Mannheim) is a proprietary, non-prescription preparation of the VASODILATOR and ANTI-ANGINA isosorbide mononitrate. It can be used to treat and prevent angina pectoris and in HEART FAILURE TREATMENT. It is available as tablets.

✚▲ Side-effects/warning: See ISOSORBIDE MONONITRATE.

Ismo Retard

(Boehringer Mannheim) is a proprietary, non-prescription preparation of the VASODILATOR and ANTI-ANGINA drug isosorbide mononitrate. It can be used to treat and prevent angina pectoris, and is available as modified-release tablets.

✚▲ Side-effects/warning: See ISOSORBIDE MONONITRATE.

isocarboxazid

is an ANTIDEPRESSANT of the MONOAMINE-OXIDASE INHIBITOR (MAOI) class. It can be used to treat depressive illness. Administration is oral.

✚▲ Side-effects/warning: See PHENELZINE; but it has a more stimulant action.

○ Related entry: Marplan.

isoconazole

is an (IMIDAZOLE) ANTIFUNGAL drug which is used particularly to treat fungal infections (candidiasis) of the vagina. Administration is in the form of vaginal tablets (pessaries).

✚ Side-effects: There may be local irritation.

○ Related entry: Travogyn.

isoflurane

is an inhalant GENERAL ANAESTHETIC which is similar to ENFLURANE. It can be used with nitrous oxide-oxygen for the induction and maintenance of anaesthesia during surgical operations. Administration is by inhalation.

✚ Side-effects: There may be an increase in heart rate accompanied by a fall in blood pressure; it may depress respiration.

○ Related entry: Isoflurane.

Isoflurane

(Abbott) is a proprietary, prescription-only preparation of the inhalant GENERAL ANAESTHETIC isoflurane. It can be used for the induction and maintenance of anaesthesia, and is available in a form for inhalation.

✚▲ Side-effects/warning: See ISOFLURANE.

Isogel

(Pfizer) is a proprietary, non-prescription preparation of the (*bulking-agent*) LAXATIVE ispaghula husk. It can be used to treat a number of gastrointestinal disorders, including irritable bowel syndrome, and is available as granules.

✚▲ Side-effects/warning: See ISPAGHULA HUSK.

Isoket

(Schwarz) is a proprietary, prescription-only preparation of the VASODILATOR and ANTI-ANGINA drug isosorbide dinitrate. It can be used in HEART FAILURE TREATMENT and to treat and, in particular, prevent angina pectoris. It is available in a form for injection.

✚▲ Side-effects/warning: See ISOSORBIDE DINITRATE.

Isoket Retard

(Schwarz) is a proprietary, non-prescription preparation of the VASODILATOR and ANTI-ANGINA drug isosorbide dinitrate. It can be used to prevent angina pectoris, and is available as modified-release tablets in two strengths, *Isoket Retard-20* and *Isoket Retard-20*.

✚▲ Side-effects/warning: See ISOSORBIDE DINITRATE.

isometheptene mucate

is a SYMPATHOMIMETIC drug which is used as an ANTIMIGRAINE treatment for acute attacks. Administration is oral.

✚ Side-effects: Dizziness, peripheral circulation disturbances and rashes; blood disturbances have been reported.

▲ Warning: Administer with caution to patients with cardiovascular disease, diabetes or hyperthyroidism; do not administer to those with glaucoma, severe heart, liver or kidney disorders, porphyria, or who are pregnant or breast-feeding.

✪ Related entry: Midrid.

Isomide CR

(Monmouth) is a proprietary, prescription-only preparation of the ANTI-ARRHYTHMIC drug disopyramide (as disopyramide phosphate). It is available as modified-release tablets.

✚▲ Side-effects/warning: See DISOPYRAMIDE.

isoniazid

is an ANTIBACTERIAL drug which is used, in combination with other drugs, as an ANTITUBERCULAR treatment. It can also be administered to prevent the contraction of tuberculosis by close associates of an infected patient. Administration is either oral or by injection.

✚ Side-effects: These include nausea and vomiting; sensitivity reactions, including rash and fever and peripheral neuritis (which may be prevented by taking vitamin B_6), convulsions and/or psychotic episodes, blood disorders and other complications.

▲ Warning: It is not to be administered to patients with liver disease induced by drug treatment; administer with caution to patients with impaired kidney or liver function, epilepsy, alcoholism, who are pregnant or breast-feeding or who have porphyria. (Patients with abnormal metabolism (slow acetylators) are known to need the dose to be adjusted to avoid unacceptable side-effects.)

✪ Related entries: Rifater; Rifinah; Rimactazid; Rimifon.

isophane insulin

is a form of purified bovine, porcine or human insulin, prepared as a sterile complex with protamine, that is used in DIABETIC TREATMENT to maintain diabetic patients. It is available in vials for injection and has an intermediate duration of action.

✚▲ Side-effects/warning: See INSULIN.

✪ Related entries: Human Insulatard; Human Protaphane; Humulin I; Hypurin Isophane; Insulatard; Pur-In Isophane.

isoprenaline

is a synthetic SYMPATHOMIMETIC substance similar to ADRENALINE. As isoprenaline sulphate, it is used as a BETA-RECEPTOR STIMULANT and SMOOTH MUSCLE RELAXANT. These properties have allowed its administration, in a form suitable for use in an aerosol inhalant, as a BRONCHODILATOR in ANTI-ASTHMATIC treatment. However, isoprenaline's use for this purpose has largely been superseded by drugs that are more selective of the beta$_2$-receptors of the airways and therefore are far less likely to produce cardiac arrhythmias by stimulating the beta$_1$-receptors of the heart. Since isoprenaline does stimulate the heart, it may be used as a CARDIAC STIMULANT to produce an increased rate and force of contraction (eg in heart block or severe bradycardia), when it is administered (as isoprenaline hydrochloride) orally or by injection.

✚▲ Side-effects/warning: See SALBUTAMOL. There may be headache, tremor, sweating,

increased heart rate and heartbeat irregularities and a decrease in blood pressure. Administer with caution to patients with certain heart diseases or excessive secretion of thyroid hormones (hyperthyroidism), or who are diabetic.
۞ Related entries; Medihaler-iso; Min-I-Jet Isoprenaline; Saventrine.

Isopto Alkaline
(Alcon) is a proprietary, non-prescription preparation of HYPROMELLOSE. It can be used as artificial tears to treat dryness of the eyes due to disease, and is available as eye-drops.

Isopto Atropine
(Alcon) is a proprietary, prescription-only preparation of the ANTICHOLINERGIC drug atropine sulphate. It can be used to dilate the pupil and so facilitate inspection of the eye and for refraction procedures in young children. It is available as eye-drops.
✚▲ Side-effects/warning: See ATROPINE SULPHATE.

Isopto Carbachol
(Alcon) is a proprietary, prescription-only preparation of the PARASYMPATHOMIMETIC drug carbachol. It can be used in GLAUCOMA TREATMENT because it lowers intraocular pressure (pressure in the eyeball) and constics the pupil. It is available as eye-drops.
✚▲ Side-effects/warning: See CARBACHOL.

Isopto Carpine
(Alcon) is a proprietary, prescription-only COMPOUND PREPARATION of the PARASYMPATHOMIMETIC pilocarpine and HYPROMELLOSE. It can be used in GLAUCOMA TREATMENT because it lowers intraocular pressure (pressure in the eyeball) and constics the pupil. It is available as eye-drops.
✚▲ Side-effects/warning: See PILOCARPINE.

Isopto Frin
(Alcon) is a proprietary, non-prescription

preparation of the SYMPATHOMIMETIC phenylephrine hydrochloride and HYPROMELLOSE. It can be used to treat tear deficiency, and is available as eye-drops.
✚▲ Side-effects/warning: See PHENYLEPHRINE HYDROCHLORIDE.

Isopto Plain
(Alcon) is a proprietary, non-prescription preparation of HYPROMELLOSE. It can be used as artificial tears to treat dryness of the eyes due to disease, and is available as eye-drops.

Isordil
(Monmouth) is a proprietary, non-prescription preparation of the VASODILATOR and ANTI-ANGINA drug isosorbide dinitrate. It can be used in HEART FAILURE TREATMENT and to treat and prevent angina pectoris. It is available as short-acting oral and sublingual tablets.
✚▲ Side-effects/warning: See ISOSORBIDE DINITRATE.

Isordil Tembids
(Monmouth) is a proprietary, non-prescription preparation of the VASODILATOR and ANTI-ANGINA drug isosorbide dinitrate. It can be used to prevent angina pectoris, and is available as modified-release capsules.
✚▲ Side-effects/warning: See ISOSORBIDE DINITRATE.

isosorbide dinitrate
is a short-acting VASODILATOR and ANTI-ANGINA drug. It is used to prevent attacks of angina pectoris (ischaemic heart pain) when taken before exercise, for symptomatic relief during an acute attack and to treat left ventricular heart failure. It works by dilating the veins returning blood to the heart and so reducing the heart's workload. It is short-acting, but its effect can be extended through the use of modified-release tablets kept under the tongue (sublingual tablets). Administration can be oral as tablets (for swallowing, chewing or holding under the tongue), as modified-

release capsules, as a spray or aerosol (applied under the tongue) or in a form for injection or infusion.

+▲ Side-effects/warning: See GLYCERYL TRINITRATE.

✪ Related entries: Cedocard; Cedocard-Retard; Imtack Spray; Isoket; Isoket Retard; Isordil; Isordil Tembids; Sorbichew; Sorbid SA; Sorbitrate.

isosorbide mononitrate

is a short-acting VASODILATOR and ANTI-ANGINA drug. It is used to prevent attacks of angina pectoris (ischaemic heart pain) when taken before exercise, for symptomatic relief during an acute attack and in HEART FAILURE TREATMENT. It works by dilating the blood vessels returning blood to the heart and so reducing the heart's workload. It is short-acting, but its effect is extended through the use of modified-release tablets kept under the tongue (sublingual tablets).
Administration is oral.

+▲ Side-effects/warning: See GLYCERYL TRINITRATE.

✪ Related entries: Elantan; Elantan LA; Imdur; Ismo; Ismo Retard; Isotrate; MCR-50; Monit; Monit SR; Mono-Cedocard.

Isotonic Gentamicin Injection

(Baxter) is a proprietary, prescription-only preparation of the ANTIBACTERIAL and (AMINOGLYCOSIDE) ANTIBIOTIC gentamicin (as sulphate). It can be used to treat many forms of infection, particularly serious infections by Gram-negative bacteria, and is available in a form for intravenous infusion.

+▲ Side-effects/warning: See GENTAMICIN.

Isotrate

(Bioglan) is a proprietary, non-prescription preparation of the VASODILATOR and ANTI-ANGINA drug isosorbide mononitrate. It can be used to treat and prevent angina pectoris and in HEART FAILURE TREATMENT, and is available as tablets.

+▲ Side-effects/warning: See ISOSORBIDE MONONITRATE.

isotretinoin

is chemically a retinoid (a derivative of RETINOL, or vitamin A) and has a marked effect on the cells that make up the skin epithelium (surface tissues). It can be used for the long-term, systemic treatment of severe acne. Administration is either oral or by topical application.

+▲ Side-effects/warning: See TRETINOIN for the side-effects of topical application. There are many side-effects with oral administration, including effects on the skin, mucous membranes (eg nasal mucosa), visual disturbances and other effects on the eyes, hair thinning, headache, nausea, drowsiness, sweating, muscle and joint pain, effects on the liver and blood function.

▲ Warning: See TRETINOIN for topical application. For oral administraion, do not use when pregnant (or one month before or after treatment), breast-feeding or in certain liver or kidney disorders.

✪ Related entries: Isotrex; Roaccutane.

Isotrex

(Stiefel) is a proprietary, prescription-only preparation of isotretinoin (a retinoid). It can be used for the long-term treatment of severe acne, and is available as tablets and a gel.

+▲ Side-effects/warning: See ISOTRETINOIN.

ispaghula husk

is a *bulking-agent* LAXATIVE which works by increasing the overall mass of faeces (and retaining a lot of water) and so stimulating bowel movement (the full effect may not be achieved for many hours). It can be used in patients who cannot tolerate bran for treating a range of bowel conditions, including diverticular disease and irritable bowel syndrome. Administration is oral as granules or a powder for dissolving in water.

+ Side-effects: There may be flatulence, abdominal distention, faecal impaction and lack of tone in the colon. Hypersensitivity reactions have been reported.

▲ Warning: Preparations of ispaghula husk should not be administered to patients with obstruction of the intestines, lack of tone in the colon or faecal impaction. Fluid intake during treatment should be higher than usual. Preparations containing ispaghula husk swell on contact with liquids and should be carefully swallowed with water, and should not be taken last thing at night.
✪ Related entries: Fybogel; Fybogel Mebeverine; Fybozest Orange; Isogel; Manevac; Metamucil; Regulan.

isradipine

is a CALCIUM-CHANNEL BLOCKER which is used as an ANTIHYPERTENSIVE. Administration is oral.
✚ Side-effects: These include flushing, headache; dizziness, hypotension and palpitations; rashes and itching; rarely, increased body weight, oedema and gastrointestinal upsets.
▲ Warning: The dose should be reduced when treating patients with certain liver or kidney disorders and avoided if possible in pregnancy. It should be given with caution to patients with some types of heart defect.
✪ Related entry: Prescal.

Istin

(Pfizer) is a proprietary, prescription-only preparation of the CALCIUM-CHANNEL BLOCKER amlodipine besylate. It can be used as an ANTIHYPERTENSIVE and as an ANTI-ANGINA drug in the prevention of attacks. It is available as tablets.
✚▲ Side-effects/warning: See AMLODIPINE BESYLATE.

itraconazole

is a broad-spectrum (AZOLE) ANTIFUNGAL drug which can be used to treat resistant forms of candidiasis (thrush) of the vagina, vulva or oropharyngeal region, infections of the skin and mucous membranes and infections of the fingernails by tinea organisms, including ringworm and athlete's foot. Administration is oral.

✚ Side-effects: Nausea and gastrointestinal disturbances, abdominal pains, dyspepsia, skin disorders, headaches and liver disorders.
▲ Warning: It should not be administered to patients with certain liver or kidney disorders, or who are pregnant or breast-feeding.
✪ Related entry: Sporanox.

ivermectin

is an ANTHELMINTIC drug which, although it is not available in the UK, is very effective in the treatment of the tropical disease onchocerciasis (infestation by the filarial worm-parasite Onchocerca volvulus). The destruction of the worms, however, may cause an allergic response. It is now the drug of choice because a single treatment produces a large reduction in the level of parasites, though more than one course of treatment with ivermectin may be necessary to eradicate the infestation. Administration is oral.
✚ Side-effects: Headache with nausea and vomiting; the dermatitis associated with onchocerciasis may temporarily be aggravated, causing itching and rash, as may any associated conjunctivitis or other eye inflammation.
▲ Warning: Medical supervision is essential during treatment.
✪ Related entry: Mectizan.

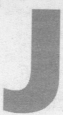

J Collis Browne's Mixture

(Seton) is a proprietary, non-prescription preparation of the (OPIOID) ANTIDIARRHOEAL morphine anhydrous and peppermint oil. It can be used for the symptomatic relief of occasional diarrhoea and its associated pain and discomfort, and is also an effective ANTITUSSIVE. It is available as a liquid.
+▲ Side-effects/warning: See MORPHINE HYDROCHLORIDE; PEPPERMINT OIL.

J Collis Browne's Tablets

(Napp) is a proprietary, non-prescription preparation of the (OPIOID) ANTIDIARRHOEAL morphine (as hydrochloride), kaolin and calcium carbonate. It can be used for the symptomatic relief of occasional diarrhoea and its associated pain and discomfort, and is available as tablets. It is not normally given to children under six years, except on medical advice.
+▲ Side-effects/warning: See CALCIUM CARBONATE; KAOLIN; MORPHINE SULPHATE.

Jackson's All Fours

(Waterhouse) is a proprietary, non-prescription preparation of the EXPECTORANT agent GUAIPHENESIN. It can be used for the symptomatic relief of coughs, and is available as a syrup. It is not normally given to children under 12 years, except on medical advice.

Jackson's Febrifuge

(Waterhouse) is a proprietary, non-prescription preparation of the (NSAID) NON-NARCOTIC ANALGESIC and ANTIRHEUMATIC sodium salicylate. It can be used for the symptomatic relief of flu, sore throat, feverish colds and muscle pains. It is available as a liquid preparation and is not normally given to children under 12 years, except on medical advice.
+▲ Side-effects/warning: See SODIUM SALICYLATE.

Japps Health Salts

(Roche) is a proprietary, non-prescription COMPOUND PREPARATION of the ANTACID and (*osmotic*) LAXATIVE sodium bicarbonate with sodium potassium tartrate and tartaric acid. It can be used for the symptomatic relief of indigestion and heartburn, and for the mild relief of constipation. It is available as an effervescent powder.
+▲ Side-effects/warning: See SODIUM BICARBONATE.

Joy-Rides

(Stafford Miller) is a proprietary, non-prescription preparation of the ANTICHOLINERGIC drug hyoscine hydrobromide. It can be used as an ANTINAUSEANT in the treatment of motion sickness, and is available as chewable tablets. It is not normally given to children under three years, except on medical advice.
+▲ Side-effects/warning: See HYOSCINE HYDROBROMIDE.

Junifen Suspension

(Crookes) is a proprietary, non-prescription preparation of the (NSAID) NON-NARCOTIC ANALGESIC, ANTIRHEUMATIC and ANTIPYRETIC ibuprofen. It can be used to relieve pain such as earache, sore throats, minor aches and sprains and flu and cold symptoms in children. It is available as a sugar-free, oral suspension and is not normally given to children under one year, except on medical advice.
+▲ Side-effects/warning: See IBUPROFEN.

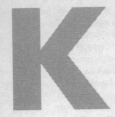

ANTIHYPERTENSIVE for raised blood pressure, and is available as capsules.

+▲ Side-effects/warning: See AMILORIDE HYDROCHLORIDE; ATENOLOL: HYDROCHLOROTHIAZIDE.

Kamillosan

(Norgine) is a proprietary, non-prescription COMPOUND PREPARATION of arachis oil and liquid paraffin (and some other constituents). It can be used as an EMOLLIENT to treat and soothe nappy rash, sore nipples, chapped hands and dry skin. It is available as an ointment.

+▲ Side-effects/warning: See ARACHIS OIL; LIQUID PARAFFIN.

kanamycin

is a broad-spectrum ANTIBACTERIAL and (AMINOGLYCOSIDE) ANTIBIOTIC. Although it does have activity against Gram-positive bacteria, it is primarily used against serious infections caused by Gram-negative bacteria. It has, however, largely been replaced by other aminoglycosides. Administration is by injection.

+▲ Side-effects/warning: See GENTAMICIN.

۞ Related entry: Kannasyn.

Kannasyn

(Sanofi Winthrop) is a proprietary, prescription-only preparation of the ANTIBACTERIAL and (AMINOGLYCOSIDE) ANTIBIOTIC kanamycin. It can be used to treat many forms of bacterial infection, particularly serious Gram-negative ones, and is available in a form for injection.

+▲ Side-effects/warning: See KANAMYCIN.

kaolin

is a purified and sometimes powdered white clay (china clay) which is used as an adsorbent, particularly in ANTIDIARRHOEAL preparations (with or without OPIOIDS, such as CODEINE PHOSPHATE or MORPHINE SULPHATE), and also to treat food poisoning and some digestive disorders. Additionally, it can be used in some poultices and dusting powders.

Kabiglobulin

(Pharmacia) is a proprietary, prescription-only preparation of human NORMAL IMMUNOGLOBULIN. It can be used in IMMUNIZATION to confer immediate *passive immunity* to infection by viruses such as hepatitis A virus, rubeola (measles) and rubella (German measles). It is available in a form for intramuscular injection.

+▲ Side-effects/warning: See IMMUNIZATION.

Kabikinase

(Pharmacia) is a proprietary, prescription-only preparation of the FIBRINOLYTIC drug streptokinase. It can be used to treat thrombosis and embolism, and is available in a form for injection.

+▲ Side-effects/warning: See STREPTOKINASE.

Kalspare

(Cusi) is a proprietary, prescription-only COMPOUND PREPARATION of the (THIAZIDE-related) DIURETIC chlorthalidone and the (*potassium-sparing*) diuretic triamterene. It can be used as an ANTIHYPERTENSIVE, and is available as tablets.

+▲ Side-effects/warning: See CHLORTHALIDONE; TRIAMTERENE.

Kalten

(Stuart) is a proprietary, prescription-only COMPOUND PREPARATION of the BETA-BLOCKER drug atenolol and the DIURETICS hydrochlorothiazide and amiloride hydrochloride. It can be used as an

+▲ Side-effects/warning: Because it is applied topically or taken by mouth, it is normally free of adverse reactions.

✪ Related entries: J Collis Browne's Tablets; Enterosan; Kaodene; Enterosan; Kaopectate; KLN Suspension.

Kaolin and Morphine Mixture, BP

ia COMPOUND PREPARATION that combines KAOLIN, the white clay (china clay), and the ANTIDIARRHOEAL and antimotility drug tincture of morphine (anhydrous). It is available as a suspension.

+▲ Side-effects/warning: See MORPHINE SULPHATE.

Kaopectate

(Upjohn) is a proprietary, non-prescription preparation of kaolin, the white clay (china clay). It can be used as an absorbent in ANTIDIARRHOEAL treatment, and is available as a suspension.

+▲ Side-effects/warning: See KAOLIN.

Kapake

(Galen) is a proprietary, prescription-only COMPOUND PREPARATION of the (OPIOID) NARCOTIC ANALGESIC codeine phosphate and the NON-NARCOTIC ANALGESIC paracetamol (which is a combination known as co-codamol 30/500). It can be administered to relieve pain, and is available in as tablets.

+▲ Side-effects/warning: See CODEINE PHOSPHATE; PARACETAMOL.

Karvol Decongestant Capsules

(Crookes) is a proprietary, non-prescription preparation of MENTHOL, CHLORBUTOL and THYMOL (with aromatic oils). It can be used as a NASAL DECONGESTANT for the symptomatic relief of colds. It is available as capsules which are sprinkled over bedding or added to hot water for the essences to be inhaled. It is not normally given to children under three months, except on medical advice.

Kefadim

(Lilly) is a proprietary, prescription-only preparation of the ANTIBACTERIAL and (CEPHALOSPORIN) ANTIBIOTIC ceftazidime. It can be used to treat many infections, particularly of the respiratory tract, and to prevent infection during surgery and in patients whose immune systems are defective. It is available in a form for injection or infusion.

+▲ Side-effects/warning: See CEFTAZIDIME.

Kefadol

(Dista) is a proprietary, prescription-only preparation of the ANTIBACTERIAL and (CEPHALOSPORIN) ANTIBIOTIC cephamandole. It can be used to treat infections caused by both Gram-positive and Gram-negative bacteria and also to prevent infections following abdominal surgery. It is available in a form for injection or infusion.

+▲ Side-effects/warning: See CEPHAMANDOLE.

Keflex

(Lilly) is a proprietary, prescription-only preparation of the ANTIBACTERIAL and (CEPHALOSPORIN) ANTIBIOTIC cephalexin. It can be used to treat many forms of infection, including of the urinogenital tract, and is available as capsules, tablets and an oral suspension.

+▲ Side-effects/warning: See CEPHALEXIN.

Kefzol

(Lilly) is a proprietary, prescription-only preparation of the ANTIBACTERIAL and (CEPHALOSPORIN) ANTIBIOTIC cephazolin. It can be used used to treat bacterial infections and to prevent infection during surgery, and is available in a form for injection or infusion.

+▲ Side-effects/warning: See CEPHAZOLIN.

Kelfizine W

(Pharmacia) is a proprietary, prescription-only preparation of the (SULPHONAMIDE) ANTIBACTERIAL sulfametopyrazine. It can be used primarily to treat chronic bronchitis

K

and infections of the urinary tract, and is available as tablets.

+▲ Side-effects/warning: See SULFAMETOPYRAZINE.

Kelocyanor

(Lipha) is a proprietary, prescription-only preparation of the CHELATING AGENT dicobalt edetate. It can be used as an ANTIDOTE to acute cyanide poisoning, and is available in a form for injection.

+▲ Side-effects/warning: See DICOBALT EDETATE.

Kemadrin

(Wellcome) is a proprietary, prescription-only preparation of the ANTICHOLINERGIC procyclidine hydrochloride. It can be used in the treatment of parkinsonism, and is available as tablets and in a form for injection.

+▲ Side-effects/warning: See PROCYCLIDINE HYDROCHLORIDE.

Kemicetine

(Pharmacia) is a proprietary, prescription-only preparation of the broad-spectrum ANTIBACTERIAL and ANTIBIOTIC chloramphenicol. It can be used to treat life-threatening infections, and is available in a form for injection.

+▲ Side-effects/warning: See CHLORAMPHENICOL.

Kenalog

(Squibb) is a proprietary, prescription-only preparation of the CORTICOSTEROID and ANTI-INFLAMMATORY triamcinolone acetonide. It can be used to treat inflammation and allergic conditions, and is available in a form for injection.

+▲ Side-effects/warning: See TRIAMCINOLONE ACETONIDE.

Kenalog Intra-articular/Intramuscular

(Squibb) is a proprietary, prescription-only preparation of the CORTICOSTEROID and ANTI-INFLAMMATORY triamcinolone acetonide. It

can be used to treat inflammation of the joints and the soft tissues, and is available in a form for injection.

+▲ Side-effects/warning: See TRIAMCINOLONE ACETONIDE.

keratolytics

(desquamating agents) are agents used to clear the skin of hyperkeratoses (thickened and horny patches) and scaly areas that occur in some forms of eczema, ichthyosis and psoriasis, and also in the treatment of acne. The standard keratolytic is SALICYLIC ACID, but there are others such as BENZOIC ACID, COAL TAR, DITHRENOL, ICHTHAMMOL and ZINC PASTE (several of which can usefully be applied in the form of a paste inside an impregnated bandage).

Keri

(Bristol-Myers) is a proprietary, non-prescription COMPOUND PREPARATION of liquid paraffin and lanolin oil. It can be used as an EMOLLIENT to soften dry skin, relieve itching and to treat nappy rash. It is available as a lotion.

+▲ Side-effects/warning: See LANOLIN; LIQUID PARAFFIN.

Kerlone

(Lorex) is a proprietary, prescription-only preparation of the BETA-BLOCKER betaxolol hydrochloride. It can be used as an ANTIHYPERTENSIVE for raised blood pressure, as an ANTI-ANGINA treatment to relieve symptoms and improve exercise tolerance and as an ANTI-ARRHYTHMIC to regularize heartbeat and to treat myocardial infarction. It is available as tablets.

+▲ Side-effects/warning: See BETAXOLOL HYDROCHLORIDE.

Keromask

(Network Management) is a proprietary, non-prescription preparation which is used to mask scars and other skin disfigurements. It is available as a cream and a powder and may be obtained on prescription under certain circumstances.

Ketalar

(Parke-Davis) is a proprietary, prescription-only preparation of the GENERAL ANAESTHETIC ketamine (as hydrochloride). It is available in a form for injection.

✚▲ Side-effects/warning: See KETAMINE.

ketamine

is a GENERAL ANAESTHETIC which can be used for the induction or maintenance of anaesthesia. Administration is by intramuscular or intravenous injection or infusion.

✚ Side-effects: Transient psychotic episodes, such as hallucinations, may occur. There is cardiovascular stimulation and blood pressure may rise.

▲ Warning: It should not be administered to patients with hypertension or prone to hallucinations. Recovery is slow.

❍ Related entry: Ketalar.

ketoconazole

is an (IMIDAZOLE) ANTIFUNGAL drug which can be used to treat deep-seated, serious fungal infections (mycoses) and to prevent infection in immunosuppressed patients. In particular, it is used to treat resistant candidiasis (thrush), gastrointestinal infections and serious infections of the skin (including the scalp) and fingernails. Administration is either oral or by topical application.

✚ Side-effects: Depending on the route of administration, serious liver damage may occur, there may be an itching skin rash, nausea, abdominal pain, blood disorders and breast enlargement in men.

▲ Warning: It should not be administered to patients who have impaired liver function or who are pregnant. Because it may cause serious liver toxicity, it should not be used for minor fungal infections. Liver function should be monitored.

❍ Related entry: Nizoral.

ketoprofen

is a (NSAID) NON-NARCOTIC ANALGESIC and ANTIRHEUMATIC drug which can be used to treat rheumatic and muscular pain caused by inflammation, pain after orthopaedic surgery, acute gout and period pain. Administration is either oral or by injection.

✚▲ Side-effects/warning: See NSAID. There is also an intermediate risk of gastrointestinal disturbances; there may be pain at the site of injection, or irritation with suppositories.

❍ Related entries: Ketoprofen CR; Ketovail; Larafen CR; Orudis; Oruvail Gel 2.5%; Powergel.

Ketoprofen CR

(Du Pont) is a proprietary, prescription-only preparation of the (NSAID) NON-NARCOTIC ANALGESIC and ANTIRHEUMATIC ketoprofen. It can be used to relieve the pain of arthritis and rheumatism and other musculoskeletal disorders, and is available as modified-release capsules.

✚▲ Side-effects/warning: See KETOPROFEN.

ketorolac trometamol

is a (NSAID) NON-NARCOTIC ANALGESIC which is used in the short-term management of moderate to severe, acute postoperative pain and to prevent and reduce inflammation following eye surgery. Administration can be oral, by topical application or injection.

✚▲ Side-effects/warning: See NSAID; but use with care, because it is a recently introduced drug and its side-effects have not been thoroughly established. (There are reports of anaphylaxis, gastrointestinal bleeding, pancreatitis, mental and sensory changes, convulsions, acute renal failure, pulmonary oedema, skin reactions and liver function changes.)

❍ Related entries: Acular; Toradol.

ketotifen

is an ANTIHISTAMINE which has additional ANTI-ALLERGIC properties somewhat like those of SODIUM CROMOGLYCATE, and can be used as an ANTI-ASTHMATIC drug to prevent asthmatic attacks. Administration is oral.

K

✚ Side-effects: It may cause drowsiness with dryness in the mouth; dizziness and weight gain.

▲ Warning: It may impair the performance of skilled tasks, such as driving; effects of alcohol are enhanced.

✪ Related entry: Zaditen.

Ketovail

(APS) is a proprietary, prescription-only preparation of the (NSAID) NON-NARCOTIC ANALGESIC and ANTIRHEUMATIC ketoprofen. It can be used to relieve the pain of arthritis and rheumatism and other musculoskeletal disorders, and is available as modified-release capsules.

✚▲ Side-effects/warning: See KETOPROFEN.

Kinidin Durules

(Astra) is a proprietary, prescription-only preparation of the ANTI-ARRHYTHMIC drug quinidine (as quinidine bisulphate). It can be used to treat heartbeat irregularities, and is available as modified-release tablets.

✚▲ Side-effects/warning: See QUINIDINE.

Klaricid

(Abbott) is a proprietary, prescription-only preparation of the ANTIBACTERIAL and (MACROLIDE) ANTIBIOTIC clarithromycin. It can be used to treat and prevent many forms of infection, including of the respiratory tract, skin and soft tissues. It is available as tablets, a paediatric suspension and in a form for intravenous infusion.

✚▲ Side-effects/warning: See CLARITHROMYCIN.

Klean-Prep

(Norgine) is proprietary, non-prescription preparation of macrogol (polyethylene glycol) with sodium and potassium salts. It can be used as a bowel-cleansing solution prior to colonic surgery, colonoscopy or a barium enema to ensure that the bowel is free of solid contents. It is available in a form to make up in water.

✚▲ Side-effects/warning: See BOWEL-CLEANSING SOLUTIONS.

Kliofem

(Novo Nordisk) is a proprietary, prescription-only preparation of the PROGESTOGEN norethisterone. It can be used to treat menopausal symptoms (including osteoporosis prophylaxis) as HRT, and is available as tablets.

✚▲ Side-effects/warning: See NORETHISTERONE.

KLN Suspension

(Roche) is a proprietary, non-prescription COMPOUND PREPARATION of kaolin, peppermint oil and sodium citrate (with pectin). It can be administered as an absorbent in ANTIDIARRHOEAL treatment for children and for minor stomach upsets caused by diet. It is available as an oral suspension.

✚▲ Side-effects/warning: See KAOLIN; PEPPERMINT OIL; SODIUM CITRATE.

Kogenate

(Bayer) is a proprietary, prescription-only preparation of factor VIII fraction (octocog alfa), which acts as a HAEMOSTATIC to reduce or stop bleeding in the treatment of disorders in which bleeding is prolonged and potentially dangerous (mainly haemophilia A). It is available in a form for infusion or injection.

✚▲ Side-effects/warning: See FACTOR VIII FRACTION (DRIED).

Kolanticon Gel

(Hoechst Marrion Roussel) is a proprietary, non-prescription COMPOUND PREPARATION of the ANTACID agents aluminium hydroxide and magnesium oxide, the ANTICHOLINERGIC drug dicyclomine hydrochloride and the ANTIFOAMING AGENT dimethicone. It can be administered to treat gastrointestinal spasm, hyperacidity, flatulence and the symptoms of peptic ulceration. It is available as a gel and is not normally given to children, except on medical advice.

✚▲ Side-effects/warning: See ALUMINIUM HYDROXIDE; DICYCLOMINE HYDROCHLORIDE; DIMETHICONE.

Konakion

(Roche) is a proprietary, preparation of vitamin K₁ (phytomenadione). It can be used to treat deficiency of VITAMIN K and is available without a prescription as *Konakion Tablets* and in prescription-only forms for injection, as *Konakion Injection*, *Konakion MM* and *Konakion MM Paediatric*.

✚▲ Side-effects/warning: See PHYTOMENADIONE.

Kwells Junior

(Roche) is a proprietary, non-prescription preparation of the ANTICHOLINERGIC hyoscine hydrobromide. It can be used as an ANTINAUSEANT in the treatment of motion sickness, and is available as chewable tablets. It is not normally given to children under four years, except on medical advice.

✚▲ Side-effects/warning: See HYOSCINE HYDROBROMIDE.

Kwells Tablets

(Roche) is a proprietary, non-prescription preparation of the ANTICHOLINERGIC hyoscine hydrobromide. It can be used as an ANTINAUSEANT in the treatment of motion sickness, and is available as chewable tablets. It is not normally given to children under ten years, except on medical advice.

✚▲ Side-effects/warning: See HYOSCINE HYDROBROMIDE.

Kytril

(SmithKline Beecham) is a proprietary, prescription-only preparation of the ANTI-EMETIC and ANTINAUSEANT granisetron. It can be used to give relief from nausea and vomiting, especially in patients receiving radiotherapy or chemotherapy. It is available as tablets and in a form for intravenous injection or infusion.

✚▲ Side-effects/warning: See GRANISETRON.

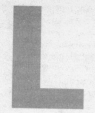

labetalol hydrochloride

is an unusual drug that combines both BETA-BLOCKER and ALPHA-ADRENOCEPTOR BLOCKER properties. It can be used as an ANTIHYPERTENSIVE to reduce high blood pressure, including in pregnancy, after myocardial infarction, in angina and during surgery. Administration is either oral or by injection.

✚ Side-effects: There may be lethargy, weakness, headache, and/or tingling of the scalp, nausea and vomiting; rashes may occur; there may be liver damage; pain in the upper body; difficulty in urinating. Higher dosages may lead to postural hypotension.

▲ Warning: See PROPRANOLOL HYDROCHLORIDE. Also, it should be administered with caution to patients who are in late pregnancy or who are breast-feeding. It should not be given to patients with certain liver disorders. Withdrawal of treatment must be gradual.

❂ Related entry: Trandate.

Labosept Pastilles

(LAB) is a proprietary, non-prescription preparation of the ANTISEPTIC dequalinium chloride which can be used to treat sore throats.

✚▲ Side-effects/warning: See: DEQUALINIUM CHLORIDE.

lacidipine

is a CALCIUM-CHANNEL BLOCKER which is used as an ANTIHYPERTENSIVE treatment. Administration is oral.

+ Side-effects: Include flushing, headache; dizziness, palpitations; rashes and itching; gastrointestinal upsets and increased production of urine; chest pains. There may be an excessive growth of the gums.

▲ Warning: Administer with caution to patients with certain heart and liver disorders, or who are breast-feeding. Do not use in pregnancy.

○ Related entry: Motens.

Lacri-Lube

(Allergan) is a proprietary, non-prescription COMPOUND PREPARATION of liquid paraffin and white soft paraffin. It can be used as an eye lubricant in patients with tear deficiency, and is available as an eye ointment.

+▲ Side-effects/warning: See LIQUID PARAFFIN.

Lacticare

(Stiefel) is a proprietary, non-prescription COMPOUND PREPARATION of sodium pyrrolidone carboxylate and lactic acid. It can be used as an EMOLLIENT for dry skin conditions, and is available as a lotion for topical application.

lactilol

is an *osmotic* LAXATIVE and is a sugar-like compound. It can be used to relieve constipation and works by retaining fluid in the intestine and may take up to 48 hours to have full effect. Administration is oral.

+▲ Side-effects/warning: See LACTULOSE.

Lactugal

(Galen) is a proprietary, non-prescription preparation of the (*osmotic*) LAXATIVE lactulose. It can be used to relieve constipation, and is available as a solution.

+▲ Side-effects/warning: See LACTULOSE.

lactulose

is an *osmotic* LAXATIVE and is a sugar-like compound. It can be used to relieve constipation by retaining fluid in the intestine and may take 48 hours to have full

effect. It can also be used to treat hepatic encephalopathy. Administration is oral.

+ Side-effects: There may be flatulence, intestinal cramps and abdominal discomfort.

▲ Warning: It should not be administered to patients with any form of intestinal obstruction. Because lactulose is itself a form of sugar, patients who have blood sugar abnormalities should be checked before using it.

○ Related entries: Duphalac; Lactugal; Laxose; Osmolax; Regulose.

Ladropen

(Berk) is a proprietary, prescription-only preparation of the ANTIBACTERIAL and (PENICILLIN) ANTIBIOTIC flucloxacillin. It can be used to treat bacterial infections, especially staphylococcal infections that prove to be resistant to penicillin, and is available as capsules, an oral solution and in a form for injection.

+▲ Side-effects/warning: See FLUCLOXACILLIN.

Lamictal

(Wellcome) is a proprietary, prescription-only preparation of the ANTICONVULSANT and ANTI-EPILEPTIC lamotrigine. It can be used to treat partial and tonic-clonic seizures that have not responded to other drugs. It is available as tablets and dispersible tablets.

+▲ Side-effects/warning: See LAMOTRIGINE.

Lamisil

(Sandoz) is a proprietary, prescription-only preparation of the ANTIFUNGAL terbinafine. It can be used to treat fungal infections of the nails and ringworm, and is available as tablets and a cream.

+▲ Side-effects/warning: See TERBINAFINE.

lamivudine

(3TC) is a recently introduced (*reverse transcriptase*) ANTIVIRAL drug which can be used in the treatment of AIDS, normally in combination with other antiviral drugs. Administration is oral.

✚ Side-effects: Nausea and vomiting,
diarrhoea, abdominal pain; headache,
cough, malaise, insomnia; muscular pain,
nasal symptoms; also reports of peripheral
neuropathy, rarely pancreatitis, blood
disturbances or changes liver enzymes.
▲ Warning: It should not be used in breast-
feeding. Administer with caution in kidney
impairment, where there is a history of
pancreatitis or in pregnancy.
◑ Related entry: Epivir.

lamotrigine

is a recently introduced ANTICONVULSANT and
ANTI-EPILEPTIC drug. It is used, in
conjunction with other drugs, to treat
partial and tonic-clonic seizures that have
not responded to other drugs.
Administration is oral.
✚ Side-effects: Rashes, fever, malaise, flu-
like symptoms, drowsiness; rarely, liver
dysfunction, blood changes, blurred vision,
headache, drowsiness, gastrointestinal
upsets and nausea.
▲ Warning: It should not be administered
to patients with kidney or liver impairment.
Administer with caution to those who are
pregnant or breast-feeding. All the body
functions known to be influenced by the
drug should be monitored.
◑ Related entry: Lamictal.

Lamprene

(Geigy) is a proprietary, prescription-only
preparation of the ANTIBACTERIAL drug
clofazimine. It can be used, in combination
with other drugs, to treat the major form of
leprosy, and is available as capsules.
✚▲ Side-effects/warning: See CLOFAZIMINE.

lanolin

is a non-proprietary constituent of WOOL FAT
and is incorporated into several EMOLLIENT
preparations. It can be is used on cracked,
dry or scaling skin, where it encourages
hydration and is commonly combined with
LIQUID PARAFFIN.
✚▲ Side-effects/warning: Some people are
sensitive to wool fat preparations; there may

be an eczematous rash.
◑ Related entries: Alpha Keri Bath; Bengués
Balsam; Germoline Ointment; Keri; Panda
Baby Cream & Castor Oil Cream with
Lanolin; Sudocrem Antiseptic Cream.

Lanoxin

(Wellcome) is a proprietary, prescription-
only preparation of the CARDIAC GLYCOSIDE
digoxin. It can be used in congestive HEART
FAILURE TREATMENT and as an ANTI-
ARRHYTHMIC to treat heartbeat irregularities.
It is available as tablets and in a form for
injection.
✚▲ Side-effects/warning: See DIGOXIN.

Lanoxin-PG

(Wellcome) is a proprietary, prescription-
only preparation of the CARDIAC GLYCOSIDE
digoxin. It can be used in congestive HEART
FAILURE TREATMENT and as an ANTI-
ARRHYTHMIC to treat heartbeat irregularities.
It is available as tablets and an elixir.
✚▲ Side-effects/warning: See DIGOXIN.

lansoprazole

is an ULCER-HEALING DRUG. It works as an
inhibitor of gastric acid secretion in the
parietal (acid-producing) cells of the
stomach lining by acting as a PROTON-PUMP
INHIBITOR. It is used for the treatment of
benign gastric and duodenal ulcers
(including those complicating NSAID
therapy), Zollinger-Ellison syndrome and
reflux oesophagitis. Administration is oral.
✚▲ Side-effects/warning: See OMEPRAZOLE.
◑ Related entry: Zoton.

Lanvis

(Wellcome) is a proprietary, prescription-
only preparation of the (CYTOTOXIC)
ANTICANCER drug thioguanine. It can be used
in the treatment of leukaemia, and is
available as tablets.
✚▲ Side-effects/warning: See THIOGUANINE.

Laractone

(Lagap) is a proprietary, prescription-only
preparation of the (*aldosterone-*

L

antagonist and *potassium-sparing*) DIURETIC spironolactone. It can be used, in conjunction with other types of diuretic (such as the THIAZIDES, which cause loss of potassium) to treat oedema associated with aldosteronism, heart disease or kidney disease; and fluid retention and ascites caused by cirrhosis of the liver. It is available as tablets.

+▲ Side-effects/warning: See SPIRONOLACTONE.

Larafen CR

(Lagap) is a proprietary, prescription-only preparation of the (NSAID) NON-NARCOTIC ANALGESIC and ANTIRHEUMATIC ketoprofen. It can be used to relieve arthritic and rheumatic pain and to treat other musculoskeletal disorders. It is available as modified-release capsules.

+▲ Side-effects/warning: See KETOPROFEN.

Laraflex

(Lagap) is a proprietary, prescription-only preparation of the (NSAID) NON-NARCOTIC ANALGESIC and ANTIRHEUMATIC naproxen. It can be used to relieve pain, particularly rheumatic and arthritic pain and to treat other musculoskeletal disorders, and is available as tablets.

+▲ Side-effects/warning: See NAPROXEN.

Larapam

(Lagap) is a proprietary, prescription-only preparation of the (NSAID) NON-NARCOTIC ANALGESIC and ANTIRHEUMATIC piroxicam. It can be used to relieve pain, particularly rheumatic and arthritic pain and inflammation and to treat other musculoskeletal disorders (including juvenile arthritis) and acute gout. It is available as tablets.

+▲ Side-effects/warning: See PIROXICAM.

Laratrim

(Lagap) is a proprietary, prescription-only COMPOUND PREPARATION of the (SULPHONAMIDE) ANTIBACTERIAL sulphamethoxazole and the antibacterial

trimethoprim, which is a combination called co-trimoxazole. It can be used to treat bacterial infections, especially infections of the urinary tract, prostatitis and bronchitis. It is available as soluble tablets, a suspension and a paediatric suspension.

+▲ Side-effects/warning: See CO-TRIMOXAZOLE.

Largactil

(Rhône-Poulenc Rorer) is a proprietary, prescription-only preparation of the (PHENOTHIAZINE) ANTIPSYCHOTIC chlorpromazine hydrochloride. It can be used to treat patients undergoing behavioural disturbances, who are psychotic (especially schizophrenics), or with severe anxiety where a degree of sedation is useful. It can also be used as an ANTINAUSEANT and ANTI-EMETIC to relieve nausea and vomiting, particularly in terminal illness, as a preoperative medication and for intractable hiccup. It is available as tablets, a syrup, a suspension, as suppositories and in a form for injection.

+▲ Side-effects/warning: See CHLORPROMAZINE HYDROCHLORIDE.

Lariam

(Roche) is a proprietary, prescription-only preparation the ANTIMALARIAL drug mefloquine. It can be used to prevent or treat malaria, and is available as tablets.

+▲ Side-effects/warning: See MEFLOQUINE.

Larodopa

(Cambridge) is a proprietary, prescription-only preparation of the ANTIPARKINSONISM drug levodopa. It can be used to treat parkinsonism, and is available as tablets.

+▲ Side-effects/warning: See LEVODOPA.

Laryng-O-Jet

(IMS) is a proprietary, prescription-only preparation of the LOCAL ANAESTHETIC lignocaine hydrochloride. It can be used instilled into lumen of larynx and trachea, and is available in a form of a jet spray.

L

+▲ Side-effects/warning: See LIGNOCAINE HYDROCHLORIDE.

Lasikal

(Hoechst) is a proprietary, prescription-only COMPOUND PREPARATION of the (*loop*) DIURETIC frusemide and the potassium supplement POTASSIUM CHLORIDE. It can be used to treat oedema, and is available as tablets which should be swallowed whole with plenty of fluid at mealtimes, or when in an upright posture.

+▲ Side-effects/warning: See FRUSEMIDE.

Lasilactone

(Hoechst) is a proprietary, prescription-only COMPOUND PREPARATION of the (*aldosterone-antagonist* and *potassium-sparing*) DIURETIC spironolactone and the (*loop*) diuretic frusemide. It can be used to treat resistant oedema, and is available as capsules.

+▲ Side-effects/warning: See FRUSEMIDE; SPIRONOLACTONE.

Lasix

(Hoechst) is a proprietary, prescription-only preparation of the (*loop*) DIURETIC frusemide. It can be used to treat oedema, particularly pulmonary (lung) oedema in patients with chronic heart failure, and low urine production due to kidney failure (oliguria). It is available as tablets and in a form for injection or infusion.

+▲ Side-effects/warning: See FRUSEMIDE.

Lasix+K

(Hoechst) is a proprietary, prescription-only COMPOUND PREPARATION of the (*loop*) DIURETIC frusemide and the potassium supplement POTASSIUM CHLORIDE. It can be used to treat oedema, and is available as tablets which should be swallowed whole with plenty of fluid at mealtimes, or when in an upright posture.

+▲ Side-effects/warning: See FRUSEMIDE.

Lasix Paediatric Liquid

(Hoechst) is a proprietary, prescription-only preparation of the (*loop*) DIURETIC frusemide. It can be used to treat oedema, and is available as an oral solution.

+▲ Side-effects/warning: See FRUSEMIDE.

Lasma

(Pharmax) is a proprietary, non-prescription preparation of the BRONCHODILATOR theophylline. It can be used as an ANTI-ASTHMATIC and to treat chronic bronchitis, and is available as modified-release tablets.

+▲ Side-effects/warning: See THEOPHYLLINE.

Lasonil

(Bayer) is a proprietary, non-prescription COMPOUND PREPARATION of a heparinoid (HDB-U 500) and the ENZYME hyaluronidase (which helps the heparinoid to reach the affected area). It can be used in treating superficial soft-tissue injuries, such as bruising, chilblains, thrombophlebitis and varicose veins. It is available as an ointment.

+▲ Side-effects/warning: See HEPARINOID; HYALURONIDASE.

Lasoride

(Hoechst) is a proprietary, prescription-only COMPOUND PREPARATION of the (*potassium-sparing*) DIURETIC amiloride hydrochloride and the (*loop*) diuretic frusemide (a combination called co-amilofruse 5/40). It can be used to treat oedema, and is available in as tablets.

+▲ Side-effects/warning: See AMILORIDE HYDROCHLORIDE; FRUSEMIDE.

Lassar's paste

see ZINC AND SALICYLIC ACID PASTE, BP

latanoprost

is a PROSTAGLANDIN analogue which has been recently introduced as a novel GLAUCOMA TREATMENT in open-angle glaucoma and ocular hypertension in patients for whom other drugs are not suitable. Administration is topical in the form of eye-drops.

L

✚ Side-effects: Brown pigmentation of the
iris, irritation of the eye, hyperaemia or
epithelial erosions.
▲ Warning: Patients should be advised of
possible iris colouration; administer with
care in patients with asthma, or who are
pregnant or breast-feeding.
✪ Related entry: Xalatan.

laxatives

(or purgatives) are preparations that
promote defecation and so relieve
constipation. They can be divided into
several different types. The *faecal softener*
laxatives (eg LIQUID PARAFFIN) soften the
faeces for easier evacuation. The *bulking-
agent* laxatives increase the overall volume
of the faeces, which then stimulates bowel
movement. Bulking agents are more often
than not some form of fibre, eg BRAN,
ISPAGHULA HUSK, METHYLCELLULOSE and
STERCULIA. The *stimulant* type of laxatives
act on the intestinal muscles to increase
motility. Many of the traditional remedies
for constipation have a stimulant action, for
instance, cascara, CASTOR OIL, SENNA and
elixir of figs. However, there are modern
variants of stimulant laxatives with less of a
stimulant action and which also have other
properties, eg BISACODYL, DANTHRON,
DOCUSATE SODIUM (dioctyl sodium
sulphosuccinate) and SODIUM PICOSULPHATE.
Finally, the *osmotic* laxatives, which are
chemical salts that work by retaining water
in the intestine so increasing overall
liquidity, eg LACTULOSE, MAGNESIUM HYDROXIDE
and MAGNESIUM SULPHATE (note that
magnesium salts are also used as ANTACIDS).
Suppositories and enemas also aid in
promoting defecation.

Laxoberal

(Windsor) is a proprietary, non-
prescription preparation of the
(*stimulant*) LAXATIVE sodium picosulphate.
It can be used for the relief of constipation,
and is available as an elixir.
✚▲ Side-effects/warning: See SODIUM
PICOSULPHATE.

Laxose

(Berk) is a proprietary, non-prescription
preparation of the (*osmotic*) LAXATIVE
lactulose. It can be used to relieve
constipation, and is available as an oral
solution.
✚▲ Side-effects/warning: See LACTULOSE.

Ledclair

(Sinclair) is a proprietary, prescription-
only preparation of the CHELATING AGENT
sodium calciumedetate. It can be used as
an ANTIDOTE to poisoning by heavy metals,
especially by lead, and is available in a form
for injection.
✚▲ Side-effects/warning: See SODIUM
CALCIUMEDETATE.

Ledercort

(Lederle) is a proprietary, prescription-only
preparation of the CORTICOSTEROID and
ANTI-INFLAMMATORY drug triamcinolone. It
can be administered to treat severe
inflammatory and allergic disorders of the
skin, such as severe eczema, and is
available as tablets.
✚▲ Side-effects/warning: See
TRIAMCINOLONE.

Lederfen

(Lederle) is a proprietary, prescription-only
preparation of the (NSAID) NON-NARCOTIC
ANALGESIC and ANTIRHEUMATIC fenbufen. It
can be used to relieve pain, particularly
rheumatic and arthritic pain and
inflammation and to treat other
musculoskeletal disorders. It is available as
tablets and capsules.
✚▲ Side-effects/warning: See FENBUFEN.

Ledermycin

(Lederle) is a proprietary, prescription-only
preparation of the ANTIBACTERIAL and
(TETRACYCLINE) ANTIBIOTIC demeclocycline
hydrochloride. It can be used to treat a
wide range of infections and is available, as
capsules.
✚▲ Side-effects/warning: See
DEMECLOCYCLINE HYDROCHLORIDE.

Lederspan

(Lederle) is a proprietary, prescription-only preparation of the CORTICOSTEROID and ANTI-INFLAMMATORY triamcinolone hexacetonide. It can be used to treat inflammation of the joints and the soft tissues, and is available in a form for injection.

+▲ Side-effects/warning: See TRIAMCINOLONE HEXACETONIDE.

Lemsip Chesty Cough

(Reckitt & Colman) is a proprietary, non-prescription preparation of the EXPECTORANT agent GUAIPHENESIN. It can be used for the relief of sore throats and deep chesty coughs. It is available as a linctus and is not normally given to children under two years, except on medical advice.

Lemsip Cold Relief Capsules

(Reckitt & Colman) is a proprietary, non-prescription preparation of the NON-NARCOTIC ANALGESIC and ANTIPYRETIC paracetamol, the SYMPATHOMIMETIC and DECONGESTANT phenylephrine hydrochloride and the STIMULANT caffeine. It can be used for the relief of cold and flu symptoms, and is available as capsules. It is not normally given to children under 12 years, except on medical advice.

+▲ Side-effects/warning: See CAFFEINE; PARACETAMOL; PHENYLEPHRINE HYDROCHLORIDE.

Lemsip Flu Strength Pseudoephedrine Formula

(Reckitt & Colman) is a proprietary, non-prescription preparation of the NON-NARCOTIC ANALGESIC and ANTIPYRETIC paracetamol, the SYMPATHOMIMETIC and DECONGESTANT pseudoephedrine hydrochloride (and vitamin C). It can be used for the relief of flu and cold symptoms, including aches and pains, nasal congestion and fever. It is available as sachets for making up in hot water and is not normally given to children under, except on medical advice.

+▲ Side-effects/warning: See PARACETAMOL; PSEUDOEPHEDRINE HYDROCHLORIDE; VITAMIN C.

Lemsip Maximum Strength

L

(Reckitt & Colman) is a proprietary, non-prescription preparation of the NON-NARCOTIC ANALGESIC and ANTIPYRETIC paracetamol, the SYMPATHOMIMETIC and DECONGESTANT phenylephrine hydrochloride (and vitamin C). It can be used for the relief of cold and flu symptoms, and nasal congestion. It is available as sachets of powder for making up in hot water and is not normally given to children, except on medical advice.

+▲ Side-effects/warning: See PARACETAMOL; PHENYLEPHRINE HYDROCHLORIDE; VITAMIN C.

Lemsip Menthol Extra

(Reckitt & Colman) is a proprietary, non-prescription preparation of the NON-NARCOTIC ANALGESIC and ANTIPYRETIC paracetamol, the DECONGESTANT phenylephrine hydrochloride (and vitamin C). It can be used for the relief of flu and cold symptoms, including aches and pains, nasal congestion and fever, and is available as sachets for making up in hot water. It is not to be given to children under 12 years, except on medical advice.

+▲ Side-effects/warning: See PARACETAMOL; PHENYLEPHRINE HYDROCHLORIDE; VITAMIN C.

Lemsip Night-time

(Reckitt & Colman) is a proprietary, non-prescription preparation of the ANTIHISTAMINE chlorpheniramine maleate, the SYMPATHOMIMETIC and VASOCONSTRICTOR phenylpropanolamine hydrochloride, the NON-NARCOTIC ANALGESIC and ANTIPYRETIC paracetamol and the NARCOTIC ANALGESIC and ANTITUSSIVE dextromethorphan hydrobromide (with alcohol). It can be used as a NASAL DECONGESTANT during colds and flu, and provides symptomatic relief of aches, cough and fever. It is available as a liquid and is not normally given to children under 13 years, except on medical advice.

+▲ Side-effects/warning: See CHLORPHENIRAMINE MALEATE; DEXTROMETHORPHAN HYDROBROMIDE;

L

PARACETAMOL; PHENYLPROPANOLAMINE HYDROCHLORIDE.

Lemsip Original

(Reckitt & Colman) is a proprietary, non-prescription preparation of the NON-NARCOTIC ANALGESIC and ANTIPYRETIC paracetamol, the SYMPATHOMIMETIC and DECONGESTANT phenylephrine hydrochloride (and vitamin C). It can be used for the relief of cold and flu symptoms, and is available as sachets of powder for making up in hot water. It is not normally given to children, except on medical advice.
+▲ Side-effects/warning: See PARACETAMOL; PHENYLEPHRINE HYDROCHLORIDE; VITAMIN C.

Lemsip Power+

(Reckitt & Colman) is a proprietary, non-prescription preparation of the NON-NARCOTIC ANALGESIC and ANTIPYRETIC drug ibuprofen and the SYMPATHOMIMETIC and DECONGESTANT pseudoephedrine hydrochloride. It can be used for the relief of cold and flu symptoms and nasal congestion. It is available as sachets of powder for making up in hot water and is not normally given to children, except on medical advice.
+▲ Side-effects/warning: See IBUPROFEN; PSEUDOEPHEDRINE HYDROCHLORIDE.

Lenium

(Cilag) is a proprietary, non-prescription preparation of selenium sulphide. It can be used as an antidandruff agent, and is available as a cream.
+▲ Side-effects/warning: See SELENIUM SULPHIDE.

Lentard MC

(Novo Nordisk) is a proprietary, non-prescription preparation of INSULIN ZINC SUSPENSION. It is used in DIABETIC TREATMENT to treat and maintain diabetic patients and contains highly purified bovine and porcine insulin. It is available in vials for injection and has a relatively long duration of action.
+▲ Side-effects/warning: See INSULIN.

Lentaron

(Ciba) is a proprietary, prescription-only preparation of the sex HORMONE ANTAGONIST formestane. It can be used as an ANTICANCER drug in the advanced stages of breast cancer, and is available in a form for injection.
+▲ Side-effects/warning: See FORMESTANE.

Lentizol

(Parke-Davis) is a proprietary, prescription-only preparation of the (TRICYCLIC) ANTIDEPRESSANT amitriptyline hydrochloride. It can be used to treat depressive illness, particularly in cases where some degree of sedation is required, and is available as capsules.
+▲ Side-effects/warning: See AMITRIPTYLINE HYDROCHLORIDE.

Lescol

(Sandoz) is a proprietary, prescription-only preparation of fluvastatin. It can be used as a LIPID-LOWERING DRUG in hyperlipidaemia to reduce the levels, or change the proportions, of various lipids in the bloodstream. It is available as capsules.
+▲ Side-effects/warning: See FLUVASTATIN.

letrozole

is an ANTICANCER drug which is used to treat advanced breast cancer in postmenopausal women. It is a non-steroidal compound, an *aromatase inhibitor* that works as an indirect HORMONE ANTAGONIST by inhibiting the conversion of the male SEX HORMONE androgen to the female sex hormone OESTROGEN. Administration is oral.
+ Side-effects: Hot flushes; nausea and vomiting; dyspepsia, diarrhoea, constipation, abdominal pain, anorexia; chest pain, shortness of breath, coughing; dizziness, fatigue, headache; infection; muscle pain, oedema, rash and pruritus.
▲ Warning: It should not be administered to pre-menopausal women or to women who are pregnant or breast-feeding, or with severely impaired liver function; and it should be administered with care to those

with impaired kidney function.
○ Related entry: Femara.

Leukeran

(Wellcome) is a proprietary, prescription-only preparation of the IMMUNOSUPPRESSANT and CYTOTOXIC (ANTICANCER) drug chlorambucil. It can be used to treat various forms of cancer and rheumatoid arthritis, and is available as tablets.
✛▲ Side-effects/warning: See CHLORAMBUCIL.

leuprorelin acetate

is an analogue of GONADORELIN (gonadothrophin-releasing hormone; GnRH), which is a hypothalamic HORMONE. On prolonged administration it acts as an indirect HORMONE ANTAGONIST in that it reduces the pituitary gland's secretion of gonadotrophin (after an initial surge), which results in reduced secretion of SEX HORMONES by the ovaries or testes. It can be used to treat endometriosis (a growth of the lining of the uterus at inappropriate sites) and is also used as an ANTICANCER drug for cancer of the prostate gland. Administration is by injection.
✛▲ Side-effects/warning: See BUSERELIN. There may also be fatigue, peripheral oedema, nausea and irritation at the injection site.
○ Related entry: Prostap SR.

Leustat

(Janssen-Cilag) is a proprietary, prescription-only preparation of the (CYTOTOXIC) ANTICANCER drug cladribine. It can be used to treat of hairy cell leukaemia, and is available in a form for intravenous infusion.
✛▲ Side-effects/warning: See CLADRIBINE.

levamisole

is an ANTHELMINTIC drug which, although not available in the UK, is very effective in treating infestation by roundworms (*Ascaris lumbricoides*) and is well tolerated with rarely any side-effects.

Administration is oral.
✛▲ Side-effects/warning: Rarely, mild nausea and vomiting.

levobunolol hydrochloride

is a BETA-BLOCKER which can be used as a GLAUCOMA TREATMENT for chronic simple glaucoma. It is thought to work by slowing the rate of production of the aqueous humour in the eye. Administration is as eye-drops.
✛ Side-effects: There may be some systemic absorption after using eye-drops, so some of the side-effects listed under PROPRANOLOL HYDROCHLORIDE may be seen. Also, dry eyes and some local allergic reactions, including conjunctivitis, may occur.
▲ Warning: In view of possible absorption, dangerous side-effects should be borne in mind, particularly bronchospasm in asthmatics and interactions with calcium-channel blockers.
○ Related entry: Betagen.

levocabastine

is an ANTIHISTAMINE which can be used for the symptomatic relief of allergic rhinitis and allergic conjunctivitis. Administration is topical.
✛▲ Side-effects/warning: See ANTIHISTAMINES; but any adverse effects are less severe when given locally. Local application to the nasal mucosa may cause irritation and taste disturbances; to the eye it may cause blurred vision and irritation. There may be headache and tiredness.
○ Related entry: Livostin.

levodopa

is a powerful ANTIPARKINSONISM drug which is used to treat parkinsonism, but not the symptoms of parkinsonism induced by drugs. Levodopa is converted into the NEUROTRANSMITTER DOPAMINE within the brain and works by replenishing dopamine levels in the part of the brain (striatum) where there is depletion in Parkinson's disease. It is effective in reducing the slowness of movement and rigidity associated with parkinsonism, but is not as successful in controlling the tremor. Administration is oral. It is often combined with other types of drug (eg CARBIDOPA) that inhibit the conversion of levodopa to dopamine outside the brain, therefore enabling as much levodopa as possible to reach the brain before it is converted and so maximizing its effect. It is the presence of such an inhibitor that may produce involuntary movements.

✚ Side-effects: Anorexia, nausea, vomiting, insomnia, agitation, postural hypotension (or sometimes short-lived hypertension), dizziness, heart rate changes, red discolouration of the urine and other fluids, rarely sensitivity reactions, abnormal involuntary muscle movements, psychiatric changes, depression, drowsiness, headache, flushing, sweating, gastrointestinal bleeding, changes in liver enzymes and peripheral nerve disturbances.

▲ Warning: It is not to be administered to patients with closed-angle glaucoma; administer with caution to those with lung disease, peptic ulcers, cardiovascular disease, diabetes, certain bone disorders, open-angle glaucoma, skin melanoma or psychiatric disorders; or who are pregnant or breast-feeding. Monitoring of heart, blood, liver and kidney functions is advisable during prolonged treatment.

⊕ Related entries: co-beneldopa; co-careldopa; Half Sinemet CR; Larodopa; Madopar; Sinemet; Sinemet CR; Sinemet LS; Sinemet-Plus.

levomepromazine

see METHOTRIMEPRAZINE

levonorgestrel

is a PROGESTOGEN which is used as a constituent of the *combined* ORAL CONTRACEPTIVES that contain OESTROGEN with a progesterone and also in progesterone-only pills. It is also used (in combination with oestrogens) in HRT and as an emergency 'morning-after' pill. Administration is either oral as tablets or as

capsules for implanting.

✚▲ Side-effects/warning: See PROGESTOGEN.

⊕ Related entries: Eugynon 30; Logynon; Logynon ED; Microgynon 30; Microval; Mirena; Norgeston; Norplant; Nuvelle; Ovran; Ovran 30; Ovranette; Schering PC4; Trinordiol.

Levophed

(Sanofi Winthrop) is a proprietary, prescription-only preparation of the VASOCONSTRICTOR and SYMPATHOMIMETIC noradrenaline (as noradrenaline acid tartrate). It can be used in emergencies to raise the blood pressure in cases of dangerous hypotension and cardiac arrest, and is available in a form for injection.

✚▲ Side-effects/warning: See NORADRENALINE.

Lexotan

(Roche) is a proprietary, prescription-only preparation of the (BENZODIAZEPINE) ANXIOLYTIC bromazepam. It can be used in the short-term treatment of anxiety, and is available as tablets.

✚▲ Side-effects/warning: See BROMAZEPAM.

Lexpec

(RP) is a proprietary, prescription-only preparation of folic acid. It can be used as a VITAMIN supplement, for example, during pregnancy or to treat a deficiency, and is available as a syrup.

✚▲ Side-effects/warning: See FOLIC ACID.

Lexpec with Iron

(RP) is a proprietary, prescription-only COMPOUND PREPARATION of ferric ammonium citrate and folic acid. It can be used as an IRON and folic acid supplement during pregnancy, and is available as a syrup.

✚▲ Side-effects/warning: See FERRIC AMMONIUM CITRATE; FOLIC ACID.

Lexpec with Iron-M

(RP) is a proprietary, prescription-only COMPOUND PREPARATION of ferric ammonium citrate and folic acid. It can be used as an IRON and folic acid supplement during pregnancy, and is available as a syrup.

+▲ Side-effects/warning: See FERRIC AMMONIUM CITRATE; FOLIC ACID.

LH
see LUTEINISING HORMONE

Li-Liquid
(RP) is a proprietary, prescription-only preparation of the ANTIMANIA drug lithium (as lithium citrate). It can be used to prevent and treat mania, manic-depressive bouts and recurrent depression, and is available as an oral solution.

+▲ Side-effects/warning: See LITHIUM.

Libanil
(APS) is a proprietary, prescription-only preparation of the SULPHONYLUREA glibenclamide. It is used in DIABETIC TREATMENT of Type II diabetes (non-insulin-dependent diabetes mellitus; NIDDM; maturity-onset diabetes), and is available as tablets.

+▲ Side-effects/warning: See GLIBENCLAMIDE.

Librium
(Roche) is a proprietary, prescription-only preparation of the (BENZODIAZEPINE) ANXIOLYTIC chlordiazepoxide. It can be used in the short-term treatment of anxiety and acute alcohol withdrawal symptoms, and is available as capsules and tablets.

+▲ Side-effects/warning: See CHLORDIAZEPOXIDE.

Librofem (200 mg)
(Zyma) is a proprietary, non-prescription preparation of the (NSAID) NON-NARCOTIC ANALGESIC, ANTIRHEUMATIC and ANTIPYRETIC ibuprofen. It can be used to relieve period pain and also for headache, muscular pain and feverishness. It is available as tablets and is not to be given to children under 12 years, except on medical advice.

+▲ Side-effects/warning: See IBUPROFEN.

Lidifen
(Berk) is a proprietary, prescription-only preparation of the (NSAID) NON-NARCOTIC ANALGESIC and ANTIRHEUMATIC ibuprofen. It can be used to relieve pain and inflammation, particularly the pain of rheumatic disease and other musculo-skeletal disorders, and is available as tablets.

+▲ Side-effects/warning: See IBUPROFEN.

lignocaine hydrochloride
is the most commonly used of all the various LOCAL ANAESTHETIC drugs. It can be administered by a number of routes and always close to its site of action. When administered by injection or infiltration, it can be used for dental and minor surgery (such as sutures). When given by an epidural injection (into a space surrounding the nerves of the spinal cord), it is used in childbirth or major surgery (sometimes in combination with a GENERAL ANAESTHETIC). When injected into a vascular region, it is co-injected with ADRENALINE which acts as a VASOCONSTRICTOR and so limits the rate at which the lignocaine is washed away. When applied topically, it is well absorbed from mucous membranes and abraded skin and so can be administered to treat discomfort at many sites. It is also used in eye-drops as an anaesthetic for minor surgery on the eye. Additionally, lignocaine is used as an ANTI-ARRHYTHMIC (particularly in the emergency treatment of arrhythmias and fibrillation following heart attack), when it is administered by intravenous injection. It is available in a variety of forms suitable for infiltration, injection or infusion, or topically as a gel, ointment, spray, lotion, lozenges or eye-drops.

+ Side-effects: These depend on what it is being used for and the route of administration. There may be a slowing of the heartbeat, a fall in blood pressure and depression of respiration. There may be allergic hypersensitivity reactions, tingling in the extremities, dizziness and confusion.

L

▲ Warning: Depending on the route of administration; it should not be administered to patients with certain heart disorders or porphyria. It should be administered with caution to patients with liver or respiratory impairment, or epilepsy.
✪ Related entries: Anbesol Adult Strength Gel; Anbesol Liquid; Anbesol Teething Gel; Anodesyn; Betnovate; Bonjela Antiseptic Pain-Relieving Pastilles; Bradosol Plus; Calgel Teething Gel; Dentinox Teething Gel; Depo-Medrone with Lidocaine; Emla; Germoloids; Hemocane; Instillagel; Laryng-O-Jet; Lignocaine in Glucose Injection; Medijel Gel; Min-I-Jet Lignocaine; Min-I-Jet Lignocaine Hydrochloride with Adrenaline; Minims Lignocaine and Fluorescein; Perinal; Rinstead Teething Gel; Ulc-Aid Gel; Xylocaine; Xylocard; Xyloproct.

Lignocaine in Glucose Injection

(Baxter) is a prescription-only preparation of the LOCAL ANAESTHETIC lignocaine hydrochloride, which can be used as an ANTI-ARRHYTHMIC to treat irregularities in the heartbeat, especially after a heart attack, and is available in a form for infusion.
✚▲ Side-effects/warning: See LIGNOCAINE HYDROCHLORIDE.

Limclair

(Sinclair) is a proprietary, prescription-only preparation of trisodium edetate. It can be used to treat the symptoms of hypercalcaemia (excess calcium in the blood) and calcification of the cornea, or lime burns, of the eyeball. It is available in a form for injection.
✚▲ Side-effects/warning: See TRISODIUM EDETATE.

lindane

is a SCABICIDAL and PEDICULICIDAL drug which is used to treat parasitic infestation by itch-mites (scabies) on the skin surface, particularly under the hair, and crab lice (pubic lice). Administration is topical.
✚ Side-effects: Skin irritation.

▲ Warning: Avoid contact with the eyes and do not use on broken or infected skin. It should not be used on patients who are pregnant or breast-feeding, or who are epileptics.
✪ Related entry: Quellada.

Lingraine

(Sanofi Winthrop) is a proprietary, prescription-only preparation of the VASOCONSTRICTOR ergotamine tartrate. It can be used as an ANTIMIGRAINE treatment for acute attacks, and is available as tablets.
✚▲ Side-effects/warning: See ERGOTAMINE TARTRATE.

Lioresal

(Geigy) is a proprietary, prescription-only preparation of the SKELETAL MUSCLE RELAXANT baclofen. It can be used to treat muscle spasm caused by an injury to or a disease of the central nervous system. It is available as tablets, an oral liquid and in a form for intrathecal injection.
✚▲ Side-effects/warning: See BACLOFEN.

liothyronine sodium

is a form of the natural THYROID HORMONE l-tri-iodothyronine sodium which can be administered to make up a hormonal deficiency (hypothyroidism). It is rapidly absorbed by the body and is administered by intravenous injection in emergency treatment of hypothyroid coma. Administration can be either oral or by intravenous injection.
✚▲ Side-effects/warning: See THYROXINE SODIUM.
✪ Related entries: Tertroxin; Triiodothyronine.

Lipantil

(Fournier) is a proprietary, prescription-only preparation of fenofibrate. It can be used as a LIPID-LOWERING DRUG in hyperlipidaemia to reduce the levels, or change the proportions, of various lipids in the bloodstream. It is available as capsules.
✚▲ Side-effects/warning: See FENOFIBRATE.

lipid-lowering drugs ▣

are used in clinical conditions of hyperlipidaemia; where the blood plasma contains very high levels of the lipids cholesterol and/or triglycerides (natural fats of the body). Current medical opinion suggests that if diet, or drugs, can be used to lower levels of LDL-cholesterol (low-density lipoprotein) while raising HDL-cholesterol (high-density lipoprotein), then there may be a regression of the progress of coronary atherosclerosis (a diseased state of the arteries of the heart where plaques of lipid material narrow blood vessels, which contributes to angina pectoris attacks and the formation of abnormal clots that go on to cause heart attacks and strokes). Currently, lipid-lowering drugs are generally only used where there is a family history of hyperlipidaemia, or clinical signs indicating the need for intervention. In most individuals, an appropriate low-fat diet can adequately do what is required.

Lipid-lowering drugs work in a number of ways: CHOLESTYRAMINE and COLESTIPOL HYDROCHLORIDE lower LDL-cholesterol production. The *clofibrate group* of drugs (BEZAFIBRATE, CIPROFIBRATE, CLOFIBRATE, FENOFIBRATE and GEMFIBROZIL) reduce triglycerides, increase LDL-cholesterol and raise HDL-cholesterol. The *nicotinic acid group* (ACIPIMOX and NICOTINIC ACID) can lower cholesterol and triglyceride levels by an action on enzymes in the liver. The *fish oils* (eg OMEGA-3 MARINE TRIGLYCERIDES) are dietary supplements that may be useful in treating hypertriglyceridaemia. FLUVASTATIN, PRAVASTATIN and SIMVASTATIN are recently introduced drugs that inhibit an enzyme in the liver so lowering LDL-cholesterol.

Lipostat

(Squibb) is a proprietary, prescription-only preparation of the LIPID-LOWERING DRUG pravastatin. It can be used in hyperlipidaemia to reduce the levels, or change the proportions, of various lipids in the bloodstream. It is available as tablets.
+▲ Side-effects/warning: See PRAVASTATIN.

liquid paraffin

is a traditional (*faecal-softener*) LAXATIVE which can be used to relieve constipation. It is a constituent of a number of proprietary laxatives and some non-proprietary preparations. It is also incorporated into many skin treatment preparations as an EMOLLIENT.
+ Side-effects: Because only a little of the paraffin is absorbed in the intestines, seepage may occur from the anus causing local irritation. Prolonged use may interfere with the internal absorption of fat-soluble vitamins.
▲ Warning: Prolonged or continuous use of liquid paraffin as a laxative is to be avoided.
○ Related entries: Agarol; Alcoderm; Alpha Keri Bath; Calamine Cream, Aqueous, BP; Calamine Lotion, Aqueous, BP; Diprobase; Diprobath; E45 Cream; Emmolate; Emulsiderm; Emulsifying Ointment, BP; Germoline Ointment; Hydromol; Kamillosan; Keri; Lacri-Lube; Mil-Par; simple eye ointment; Unguentum Merck.

Liquifilm Tears

(Allergan) is a proprietary, non-prescription preparation of POLYVINYL ALCOHOL. It can be used as artificial tears where there is dryness of the eyes due to disease, and is available as an ophthalmic eye solution.

liquorice

is an extract from a leguminous plant. It has a strong flavour and can be used in medicines with unpleasant tastes. Liquorice extract also has a weak EXPECTORANT activity and is therefore incorporated into a number of cough remedies. There are certain preparations of liquorice that are used to treat peptic ulcers, some are prepared from LIQUORICE, DEGLYCYRRHIZINISED and others are a synthetic chemical derivative of glycyrrhizinic acid (CARBENOXOLONE SODIUM).
○ Related entries: Caved-S; Fisherman's Friend.

L

liquorice, deglycyrrhizinised

is a constituent of some preparations that are used to treat peptic ulcers, particularly in the stomach but also in the duodenum.
○ Related entry: Caved-S.

lisinopril

is an ACE INHIBITOR and acts as a VASODILATOR. It can be used as an ANTIHYPERTENSIVE and is often administered in conjunction with other classes of drug, particularly (THIAZIDE) DIURETICS. Administration is oral.
✚▲ Side-effects/warning: See CAPTOPRIL.
○ Related entries: Carace; Carace Plus; Zestoretic; Zestril.

Liskonum

(SK&F) is a proprietary, prescription-only preparation of the ANTIMANIA drug lithium (as lithium carbonate). It can be used to prevent and treat mania, manic-depressive bouts and recurrent depression, and is available as tablets.
✚▲ Side-effects/warning: See LITHIUM.

lisuride maleate

see LYSURIDE MALEATE

Litarex

(CP) is a proprietary, prescription-only preparation of the ANTIMANIA drug lithium (as lithium citrate). It can be used to treat acute mania, manic-depressive bouts and recurrent depression, and is available as tablets.
✚▲ Side-effects/warning: See LITHIUM.

lithium

in the form of lithium carbonate or lithium citrate, is singularly effective as an ANTIMANIA drug to control or prevent the hyperactive manic episodes in manic-depressive illness. It may also reduce the frequency and severity of depressive episodes. How it works remains imperfectly understood, but its use is so successful that the side-effects caused by its toxicity are

deemed to be justified. Administration is oral.
✚ Side-effects: Many long-term patients experience nausea, thirst and excessive urination, gastrointestinal disturbance, weakness and tremor. There may be fluid retention and consequent weight gain. Visual disturbances, worsening gastric problems, muscle weakness and lack of coordination indicate lithium intoxication.
▲ Warning: It should not be administered to patients with certain heart or kidney disorders, or imperfect sodium balance in the bloodstream. It should be administered with caution to those who are pregnant or breast-feeding, who are elderly, taking diuretics or have myasthenia gravis. Prolonged treatment may cause kidney and thyroid gland dysfunction; prolonged overdosage eventually causes serious effects on the brain. Consequently, blood levels of lithium must be regularly checked for toxicity, thyroid function must be monitored and there must be adequate intake of fluids and sodium.
○ Related entries: Camcolit 250 Camcolit 400; Li-Liquid; Liskonum; Litarex; Phasal; Priadel.

lithium succinate

is a constituent of an ointment for seborrhoeic dermatitis.
○ Related entry: Efalith.

Lithofalk

(Thames) is a proprietary, prescription-only COMPOUND PREPARATION of chenodeoxycholic acid and ursodeoxycholic acid. It can be used to dissolve gallstones, and is available as tablets.
✚▲ Side-effects/warning: See CHENODEOXYCHOLIC ACID; URSODEOXYCHOLIC ACID.

Livial

(Organon) is a proprietary, prescription-only preparation of the drug tibolone, which has both OESTROGEN and PROGESTOGEN activity. It can be used in HRT, and is available as tablets.

Livostin

(Ciba) is proprietary, prescription-only preparation of the ANTIHISTAMINE levocabastine. It can be used for the symptomatic relief of allergic rhinitis and allergic conjunctivitis, and is available as a nasal spray and as eye-drops.

+▲ Side-effects/warning: See LEVOCABASTINE.

Lloyd's Cream

(Seton) is a proprietary, non-prescription preparation of the COUNTER-IRRITANT, or RUBEFACIENT, diethylamine salicylate. It can be applied to the skin for symptomatic relief of underlying muscle or joint pain, and is available as a cream.

+▲ Side-effects/warning: See DIETHYLAMINE SALICYLATE.

Lobak

(Sanofi Winthrop) is a proprietary, prescription-only COMPOUND PREPARATION of the SKELETAL MUSCLE RELAXANT and ANXIOLYTIC chlormezanone and the NON-NARCOTIC ANALGESIC paracetamol. It is used to relieve muscle pain, and is available as tablets.

+▲ Side-effects/warning: See CHLORMEZANONE; PARACETAMOL.

Locabiotal

(Servier) is a proprietary, prescription-only preparation of the ANTI-INFLAMMATORY and ANTIBIOTIC drug fusafungine. It can be used to treat infection and inflammation in the nose and throat, and is available as an aerosol with a nose and mouth adapter. It is not normally given to children under three years, except on medical advice.

+▲ Side-effects/warning: See FUSAFUNGINE.

local anaesthetics ⚕

are drugs used to reduce sensation (especially pain) in a specific, local area of the body and without loss of consciousness. GENERAL ANAESTHETICS, in contrast, decrease

sensation only because of a loss of consciousness. Local anaesthetics work by reversibly blocking the transmission of impulses in nerves. They can be administered by a number of routes and always close to their site of action. By local injection or infiltration, they can be used for dental and minor surgery (such as sutures). A more extensive loss of sensation with nerve block (eg injected near to the nerve supplying a limb) or with spinal anaesthesia (eg epidural injection in childbirth) or intrathecal block (for extensive procedures) produces a loss of sensation in whole areas of the body sufficient to allow major surgery (though with some, quickly reversible paralysis). Local anaesthetics are particularly valuable where the use of a general anaesthetic carries a high risk, or when the cooperation of the patient is required. When administered into a vascular region, ADRENALINE is co-injected and acts as a VASOCONSTRICTOR to limit the rate at which the anaesthetic is washed away. When applied topically, certain local anaesthetics are well absorbed from mucous membranes and abraded skin and can be used to treat discomfort at many sites. See AMETHOCAINE HYDROCHLORIDE; BENZOCAINE; BUPIVACAINE HYDROCHLORIDE; CINCHOCAINE; COCAINE; LIGNOCAINE HYDROCHLORIDE; OXETHAZAINE; OXYBUPROCAINE HYDROCHLORIDE; PRILOCAINE HYDROCHLORIDE; PROCAINAMIDE HYDROCHLORIDE; PROCAINE; PROXYMETACAINE; TOCAINIDE HYDROCHLORIDE.

local hormones ⚕

are mediators that are released within the body to act at a site local to their point of release. In this respect, as mediators of body signals, they differ from blood-borne (*endocrine*) HORMONES, which are released from specific glands and generally act remote to the point of release, and NEUROTRANSMITTERS, which are released only from nerves and act very close to the point of release. Local hormones have many functions in the body.

L

One of their best-understood functions is their role in inflammation. It is known that local hormones are often released as a result of an injury to tissues or because of an allergic reaction and mediate responses in the body that are pro-inflammatory (cause inflammation). Reactions such as these are generally intended to protect the body, but if too extreme or inappropriate they can cause adverse effects on health and need to be controlled with drugs. Many of the ANTI-INFLAMMATORY and ANTI-ALLERGIC drugs in common medical use work by preventing the formation, release or actions of local hormones. Examples of pro-inflammatory local hormones are histamine and the members of the PROSTAGLANDIN family. ANTIHISTAMINES inhibit the effects in the body of the local hormone histamine by blocking its RECEPTORS, whereas the NSAID drugs (eg ASPIRIN and IBUPREFEN) work by preventing the formation, and hence release, of the prostaglandin local hormones. CORTICOSTEROIDS and SODIUM CROMOGLYCATE-related drugs are also of value in treating allergic conditions where local hormones are released; for example, for asthma and skin conditions such as eczema and psoriasis.

By no means all actions of local hormones are undesirable and many are part of normal body function. For instance, the prostaglandins play a part in controlling the blood flow in the mucosal lining of the stomach and intestine and act as CYTOPROTECTANTS and ULCER-HEALING DRUGS. Prostaglandins may also have a role in controlling motility and other functions of the intestine and uterus. The latter actions are used in obstetrics by the administration of synthetic preparations of the naturally occurring members of the prostaglandin family, such as prostaglandin E_2 (DINOPROSTONE), prostaglandin $F_{2\alpha}$ (DINOPROST) or prostacyclin (EPOPROSTENOL), or synthetic analogues (eg MISOPROSTOL), which mimic the actions where prostaglandins are potent in contraction of the uterus, softening and dilation of the cervix and dilation of blood vessels. These actions can be used for abortion and in aiding labour.

There are many other local hormones and drugs that modify their actions are continually being developed. For example, the recently introduced ANTINAUSEANT drug ONDANSETRON, blocks and mimics some actions of SEROTONIN where it acts as a local hormone in the gastrointestinal tract.

Loceryl

(Roche) is a proprietary, prescription-only preparation of the ANTIFUNGAL drug AMOROLFINE. It can be used topically to treat fungal skin infections, and is available as a cream and a nail lacquer.

Locoid

(Yamanouchi) is a proprietary, prescription-only preparation of the CORTICOSTEROID hydrocortisone (as butyrate). It can be used for serious inflammatory skin conditions, such as eczema and psoriasis, and is available as a cream (*Lipocream*), an ointment and a scalp lotion, and a lotion for topical application (*Locoid Crelo*).
➕▲ Side-effects/warning: See HYDROCORTISONE.

Locoid C

(Yamanouchi) is a proprietary, prescription-only COMPOUND PREPARATION of the CORTICOSTEROID hydrocortisone (as butyrate) and the ANTIMICROBIAL chlorquinaldol. It can be used to treat inflammatory skin conditions, such as eczema, and is available as a cream and an ointment.
➕▲ Side-effects/warning: See CHLORQUINALDOL; HYDROCORTISONE.

Locorten-Vioform

(Zyma) is a proprietary, prescription-only COMPOUND PREPARATION of the CORTICOSTEROID flumethasone pivalate and the ANTIMICROBIAL drug clioquinol. It can be be used to treat mild infections of the outer ear, and is available as ear-drops.

✚▲ Side-effects/warning: See CLIOQUINOL; FLUMETHASONE PIVALATE.

Lodine

(Wyeth) is a proprietary, prescription-only preparation of the (NSAID) NON-NARCOTIC ANALGESIC and ANTIRHEUMATIC etodolac. It can be used to treat the pain of osteoarthritis and rheumatoid arthritis, and is available as capsules and tablets.

✚▲ Side-effects/warning: See ETODOLAC.

Loestrin 20

(Parke-Davis) is a proprietary, prescription-only COMPOUND PREPARATION that can be used as a (MONOPHASIC) ORAL CONTRACEPTIVE (and also for certain menstrual problems) of the type that combines an OESTROGEN and a PROGESTOGEN, in this case ethinyloestradiol and norethisterone. It is available as tablets in a calendar pack.

✚▲ Side-effects/warning: See ETHINYLOESTRADIOL; NORETHISTERONE.

Loestrin 30

(Parke-Davis) is a proprietary, prescription-only COMPOUND PREPARATION that can be used as a (*monophasic*) ORAL CONTRACEPTIVE (and also for certain menstrual problems) of the type that combines an OESTROGEN and a PROGESTOGEN, in this case ethinyloestradiol and norethisterone. It is available as tablets in a calendar pack.

✚▲ Side-effects/warning: See ETHINYLOESTRADIOL; NORETHISTERONE.

lofepramine

is an ANTIDEPRESSANT of the TRICYCLIC group. It has less SEDATIVE properties than other antidepressants and is therefore more suitable for the treatment of withdrawn and apathetic patients, rather than those who are agitated and restless. Administration is oral.

✚▲ Side-effects/warning: See AMITRIPTYLINE HYDROCHLORIDE; but is less

sedating. It should not be prescribed to patients with severe liver or kidney damage.

○ Related entry: Gamanil.

lofexidine hydrochloride

is a recently introduced drug that is used to alleviate OPIOID withdrawal symptoms. It appears to have actions that are similar to those of CLONIDINE, but is less effective. Administration is oral.

✚ Side-effects: Drowsiness, dry mouth, throat and nose, hypotension, slowing of the heart and hypertension on withdrawal.

▲ Warning: Use with caution in patients with certain heart disorders, kidney impairment, a history of depression or who are pregnant or breast-feeding.

○ Related entry: BritLofex.

Logynon

(Schering) is a proprietary, prescription-only COMPOUND PREPARATION that can be used as a (*triphasic*) ORAL CONTRACEPTIVE (and also for certain menstrual problems) of the type that combines an OESTROGEN and a PROGESTOGEN, in this case ethinyloestradiol and levonorgestrel. It is available as tablets in a calendar pack.

✚▲ Side-effects/warning: See ETHINYLOESTRADIOL; LEVONORGESTREL.

Logynon ED

(Schering) is a proprietary, prescription-only COMPOUND PREPARATION that can be used as a (*triphasic*) ORAL CONTRACEPTIVE (and also for certain menstrual problems) of the type that combines an OESTROGEN and a PROGESTOGEN, in this case ethinyloestradiol and levonorgestrel. It is available as tablets in a calendar pack.

✚▲ Side-effects/warning: See ETHINYLOESTRADIOL; LEVONORGESTREL.

Lomexin

(Upjohn) is a proprietary, non-prescription preparation of the ANTIFUNGAL drug fenticonazole nitrate. It can be used to treat vaginal candidiasis (thrush), and is available as vaginal pessaries.

L

➕▲ Side-effects/warning: See
FENTICONAZOLE NITRATE.

Lomotil

(Searle) is a proprietary, prescription-only
COMPOUND PREPARATION of the
ANTICHOLINERGIC drug atropine sulphate and
the (OPIOID) ANTIDIARRHOEAL diphenoxylate
hydrochloride, which is a combination
called co-phenotrope. It can be used to
treat chronic diarrhoea (eg in mild chronic
ulcerative colitis), and is available as a
liquid and as tablets.

➕▲ Side-effects/warning: See ATROPINE
SULPHATE; DIPHENOXYLATE HYDROCHLORIDE.

lomustine

is a CYTOTOXIC drug which is used as an
ANTICANCER treatment, particularly for
Hodgkin's disease (cancer of the lymphatic
tissues) and some solid tumours. It works
by disrupting cellular DNA and so inhibiting
cell replication. Administration is oral.

➕▲ Side-effects/warning: See CYTOTOXICS.
Nausea and vomiting can be quite severe.

○ Related entry: CCNU.

Loniten

(Upjohn) is a proprietary, prescription-only
preparation of the VASODILATOR minoxidil. It
can be used as an ANTIHYPERTENSIVE to treat
severe acute hypertension (usually in
combination with a DIURETIC or BETA-
BLOCKER), and is available as tablets.

➕▲ Side-effects/warning: See MINOXIDIL.

loperamide hydrochloride

is an (OPIOID) ANTIDIARRHOEAL drug which
acts on the nerves of the intestine to inhibit
peristalsis (the waves of muscular activity
that move along the contents of the
intestines), so reducing motility, and also
decreases fluid secretion in the intestines.
Administration is oral. (Preparations
containing loperamide hydrochloride are
available without prescription for the
treatment of acute diarrhoea only.)

➕▲ Side-effects/warning: See OPIOIDS; but
when used to treat acute diarrhoea there is

little or no risk of dependence and it is less
sedative.

○ Related entries: Arret; Diareze; Diocalm
Ultra; Diocaps; Imodium Capsules.

Lopid

(Parke-Davis) is a proprietary,
prescription-only preparation of the LIPID-
LOWERING DRUG gemfibrozil. It can be used
in hyperlipidaemia to reduce the levels, or
change the proportions, of various lipids in
the bloodstream. It is available as capsules
(*Lopid 300*) and tablets (*Lopid 600*).

➕▲ Side-effects/warning: See GEMFIBROZIL.

Lopidine

(Alcon) is a proprietary, prescription-only
preparation of the SYMPATHOMIMETIC
apraclonidine. It can be used to control or
prevent postoperative elevation of
intraocular pressure (pressure of the
eyeball) after laser surgery, and is available
as eye-drops.

➕▲ Side-effects/warning: See
APRACLONIDINE.

loprazolam

is a BENZODIAZEPINE which is used as a
relatively short-acting HYPNOTIC for the
short-term treatment of insomnia.
Administration is oral.

➕▲ Side-effects/warning: See
BENZODIAZEPINES.

○ Related entry: Loprazolam.

Loprazolam

(Hoechst Marion Roussel) is a non-
proprietary, prescription-only preparation
of the BENZODIAZEPINE loprazolam. It can be
used as a relatively short-acting HYPNOTIC
for the short-term treatment of insomnia,
and is available as tablets.

➕▲ Side-effects/warning: See LOPRAZOLAM.

Lopresor

(Geigy) is a proprietary, prescription-only
preparation of the BETA-BLOCKER metoprolol
tartrate. It can be used as an
ANTIHYPERTENSIVE for raised blood pressure,

as an ANTI-ANGINA treatment to relieve symptoms and improve exercise tolerance and as an ANTI-ARRHYTHMIC to regularize heartbeat and to treat myocardial infarction. It can also be used as an ANTITHYROID drug for short-term treatment of thyrotoxicosis and as an ANTIMIGRAINE treatment to prevent attacks. It is available as tablets.

✚▲ Side-effects/warning: See METOPROLOL TARTRATE.

Lopresor SR

(Geigy) is a proprietary, prescription-only preparation of the BETA-BLOCKER metoprolol tartrate. It can be used as an ANTIHYPERTENSIVE for raised blood pressure, as an ANTI-ANGINA treatment to relieve symptoms and improve exercise tolerance and as an ANTI-ARRHYTHMIC to regularize heartbeat and to treat myocardial infarction. It can also be used as an ANTITHYROID drug for short-term treatment of thyrotoxicosis and as an ANTIMIGRAINE treatment to prevent attacks. It is available as modified-release tablets.

✚▲ Side-effects/warning: See METOPROLOL TARTRATE.

loratadine

is a recently developed ANTIHISTAMINE which has less sedative side-effects than some older members of its class and can be used for the symptomatic relief of allergic symptoms, such as hay fever and urticaria. Administration is oral.

✚▲ Side-effects/warning: See ANTIHISTAMINES. But the incidence of sedative and anticholinergic effects is low; nevertheless, it may impair the performance of skilled tasks, such as driving. It should not be given to patients who are pregnant.

✪ Related entry: Clarityn.

lorazepam

is a BENZODIAZEPINE with a number of applications. It is used as an ANXIOLYTIC in the short-term treatment of anxiety, as a HYPNOTIC for insomnia, as an ANTI-EPILEPTIC

in status epilepticus and as a SEDATIVE in pre-operative medication, because its ability to cause amnesia means that the patient forgets the unpleasant procedure. Administration is either oral or by injection.

✚▲ Side-effects/warning: See BENZODIAZEPINES.

✪ Related entry: Ativan.

lormetazepam

is a BENZODIAZEPINE which is used as a relatively short-acting HYPNOTIC for the short-term treatment of insomnia. Administration is oral.

✚▲ Side-effects/warning: See BENZODIAZEPINES.

Loron

(Boehringer Mannheim) is a recently introduced proprietary, prescription-only preparation of the CALCIUM METABOLISM MODIFIER sodium chlodronate. It can be used to treat high calcium levels associated with malignant tumours and bone lesions. It is available in a form for intravenous infusion (*Loron for infusion*), as capsules (*Loron capsules*) and as tablets (*Loron 520*).

✚▲ Side-effects/warning: See SODIUM CHLODRONATE.

losartan potassium

is a recently introduced drug, the first of the ANGIOTENSIN-RECEPTOR BLOCKERS which work by blocking angiotensin receptors. Angiotensin II is a circulating HORMONE that is a powerful VASOCONSTRICTOR and blocking its effects leads to a fall in blood pressure. Losartan potassium can therefore be used as an ANTIHYPERTENSIVE. Administration is oral.

✚ Side-effects: Orthostatic hypotension, dizziness; raised blood potassium, rash, taste disturbance and changes in liver function have been reported.

▲ Warning: It should not be administered to patients who are pregnant or breast-feeding. Administer with care to those who have liver impairment, and to the elderly

337

with kidney impairment.
○ **Related entry: Cozaar.**

Losec

(Astra) is a proprietary, prescription-only
preparation of the PROTON-PUMP INHIBITOR
omeprazole. It can be used as an ULCER-
HEALING DRUG and for associated conditions,
and is available as capsules.
✚▲ Side-effects/warning: See OMEPRAZOLE.

Lotriderm

(Schering-Plough) is a proprietary,
prescription-only COMPOUND PREPARATION of
the CORTICOSTEROID betamethasone (as
dipropionate) and the ANTIFUNGAL
clotrimazole. It can be used to treat fungal
infections, particularly those associated
with inflammation, and is available as a
cream for topical application.
✚▲ Side-effects/warning: See
BETAMETHASONE; CLOTRIMAZOLE.

low molecular weight heparins ▨

are forms of ANTICOAGULANTS of the HEPARIN
type which have a smaller chemical size but
have certain advantages over heparin. They
are as effective in the prevention of venous
thrombo-embolism, particularly in
orthopaedic practice. They have a longer
duration of action than unfractionated
heparin. Some low molecular weight
heparins can be used in the treatment of
deep-vein thrombosis and for the
prevention of clotting in extracorporeal
circuits. See CERTOPARIN SODIUM; DALTEPARIN;
ENOXAPARIN; TINZAPARIN.

Loxapac

(Novex) is a proprietary, prescription-only
preparation of the ANTIPSYCHOTIC drug
loxapine. It can be used to treat acute and
chronic psychoses, and is available as
capsules.
✚▲ Side-effects/warning: See LOXAPINE.

loxapine

is an ANTIPSYCHOTIC drug which is used to

treat acute and chronic psychoses.
Administration is oral.
✚▲ Side-effects/warning: See
CHLORPROMAZINE HYDROCHLORIDE; but there is
also nausea and vomiting, weight gain or
weight loss, shortness of breath, drooping of
the eyelids, raised body temperature, loss of
sensation in the extremities, flushing and
headache.
○ **Related entry: Loxapac.**

Luborant

(Antigen) is a proprietary, non-prescription
COMPOUND PREPARATION of CARMELLOSE
SODIUM, POTASSIUM CHLORIDE, SORBITOL and
other salts. It can be used as a form of
ARTIFICIAL SALIVA for application to the mouth
and throat in conditions that make the
mouth abnormally dry. It is available as an
aerosol.

Ludiomil

(Ciba) is a proprietary, prescription-only
preparation of the TRICYCLIC-related
ANTIDEPRESSANT maprotiline hydrochloride.
It can be used to treat depressive illness,
especially in cases where sedation is
required, and is available as tablets.
✚▲ Side-effects/warning: See MAPROTILINE
HYDROCHLORIDE.

Lugol's solution

see AQUEOUS IODINE ORAL SOLUTION

Lustral

(Invicta) is a proprietary, prescription-only
preparation of the (SSRI) ANTIDEPRESSANT
sertraline. It has less sedative effects than
some other antidepressants, and is available
as tablets.
✚▲ Side-effects/warning: See SERTRALINE.

luteinising hormone

(LH) is a HORMONE secreted by the anterior
pituitary gland and (along with FOLLICLE-
STIMULATING HORMONE; FSH) is a
gonadotrophin hormone. In women, in
conjunction with FSH, it causes the monthly
ripening in one ovary of a follicle and

stimulates ovulation. In men, it facilitates the production of sperm in the testes (hence its alternative name interstitial cell-stimulating hormone; ICSH). It may be injected therapeutically, along with FSH, in infertility treatment to stimulate ovulation. It is available, in combination with FSH, as HUMAN MENOPAUSAL GONADOTROPHIN. See also CHORIONIC GONADOTROPHIN.

○ Related entries: Gonadotraphon LH; Humegon; Normegon; Pergonal.

Lyclear

(Wellcome) is a proprietary, non-prescription preparation of the SCABICIDAL and PEDICULICIDAL drug permethrin. It can be used for the treatment of head-louse infestation, and is available as a cream rinse and a skin cream; the cream rinse is not normally used on infants under six months, except on medical advice.

✚▲ Side-effects/warning: See PERMETHRIN.

lymecycline

is a broad-spectrum ANTIBACTERIAL and (TETRACYCLINE) ANTIBIOTIC which can be used to treat infections of many kinds, for example, of the respiratory and genital tracts. Administration is oral.

✚▲ Side-effects/warning: See TETRACYCLINE.

○ Related entry: Tetralysal 300.

lypressin

is an analogue of the antidiuretic HORMONE vasopressin. It can be used as a DIABETES INSIPIDUS TREATMENT in pituitary-originated diabetes insipidus. Administration is as a nasal spray (it is absorbed into the systemic circulation from the nasal mucosa).

✚▲ Side-effects/warning: See VASOPRESSIN; but with less hypersensitivity. Also, with the nasal spray there may be ulceration of the nasal mucosa and nasal congestion.

○ Related entry: Syntopressin.

lysuride maleate

(lisuride maleate) is a recently introduced ANTIPARKINSONISM drug that is an ERGOT ALKALOID derivative. It has actions that are similar to those of BROMOCRIPTINE and is particularly useful in patients who cannot tolerate levodopa. Administration is oral as tablets.

✚ Side-effects: Headache, nausea and vomiting, dizziness, lethargy, malaise, drowsiness, psychotic reactions (including hallucinations), occasional hypotension, rashes, constipation and abdominal pain.

▲ Warning: It should be administered with caution to patients with a history of psychosis, who have had a pituitary tumour; or are pregnant or breast-feeding. It should not be given to patients with certain, severe cardiovascular disorders or porphyria. It may impair the performance of skilled tasks, such as driving.

○ Related entry: Revanil.

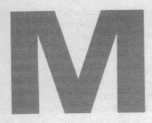

Maalox Plus Suspension

(Rhône-Poulenc Rorer) is a proprietary, non-prescription COMPOUND PREPARATION of the ANTACIDS magnesium hydroxide and aluminium hydroxide and the ANTIFOAMING AGENT dimethicone. It can be used for the symptomatic relief of dyspepsia, heartburn and flatulence, and is available as a suspension.

+▲ Side-effects/warning: See ALUMINIUM HYDROXIDE; DIMETHICONE; MAGNESIUM HYDROXIDE.

Maalox Plus Tablets

(Rhône-Poulenc Rorer) is a proprietary, non-prescription COMPOUND PREPARATION of the ANTACIDS magnesium hydroxide and aluminium hydroxide and the ANTIFOAMING AGENT dimethicone. It can be used for the symptomatic relief of dyspepsia, heartburn and flatulence, and is available as tablets. It is not normally given to children, except on medical advice.

+▲ Side-effects/warning: See ALUMINIUM HYDROXIDE; DIMETHICONE; MAGNESIUM HYDROXIDE.

Maalox Suspension

(Rhône-Poulenc Rorer) is a proprietary, non-prescription COMPOUND PREPARATION of the ANTACIDS magnesium hydroxide and aluminium hydroxide. It can be used for the symptomatic relief of dyspepsia, gastric hyperacidity and gastritis. It is available as a suspension and is not normally given to children under 14 years, except on medical advice.

+▲ Side-effects/warning: See ALUMINIUM HYDROXIDE; MAGNESIUM HYDROXIDE.

Maalox TC Suspension

(Rhône-Poulenc Rorer) is a proprietary, non-prescription COMPOUND PREPARATION of the ANTACIDS magnesium hydroxide and aluminium hydroxide. It can be used for the symptomatic relief of heartburn, gastric hyperacidity and gastritis. It is available as a suspension and is not normally given to children, except on medical advice.

+▲ Side-effects/warning: See ALUMINIUM HYDROXIDE; MAGNESIUM HYDROXIDE.

Maalox TC Tablets

(Rhône-Poulenc Rorer) is a proprietary, non-prescription COMPOUND PREPARATION of the ANTACIDS magnesium hydroxide and aluminium hydroxide. It can be used for the symptomatic relief of dyspepsia, gastric hyperacidity and gastritis. It is available as tablets, and is not normally given to children under 14 years, except on medical advice.

+▲ Side-effects/warning: See ALUMINIUM HYDROXIDE; MAGNESIUM HYDROXIDE.

Maclean Indigestion Tablets

(SmithKline Beecham) is a proprietary, non-prescription COMPOUND PREPARATION of the ANTACIDS calcium carbonate, magnesium carbonate and aluminium hydroxide. It can be used for the symptomatic relief of indigestion, flatulence and nausea, and is available as tablets. It is not normally given to children, except on medical advice.

+▲ Side-effects/warning: See ALUMINIUM HYDROXIDE; CALCIUM CARBONATE; MAGNESIUM CARBONATE.

Macrobid

(Procter & Gamble) is a proprietary, prescription-only preparation of the ANTIBACTERIAL drug nitrofurantoin. It can be used to treat infections of the urinary tract, and is available as capsules.

+▲ Side-effects/warning: See NITROFURANTOIN.

Macrodantin

(Procter & Gamble) is a proprietary, prescription-only preparation of the ANTIBACTERIAL drug nitrofurantoin. It can be used to treat infections of the urinary tract, and is available as capsules.
+▲ Side-effects/warning: See NITROFURANTOIN.

macrolides 🛈

are a chemical class of ANTIBIOTICS that are used for their ANTIBACTERIAL action. They have a similar spectrum of action to penicillin, but a different mechanism of action; they work by inhibiting microbial protein synthesis – they are *bacteriostatic*. Their principal use is as an alternative antibiotic in patients who are allergic to penicillin. The original and best-known, member of the group is ERYTHROMYCIN, which is effective against many Gram-positive bacteria, including streptococci (which can cause soft tissue and respiratory tract infections), legionella (legionnaires' disease) and chlamydia (urethritis), and is also used in the treatment of acne, chronic prostatitis, diphtheria and whooping cough. The macrolides are relatively non-toxic and serious side-effects are rare. See AZITHROMYCIN; CLARITHROMYCIN.

Madopar

(Roche) is a proprietary, prescription-only COMPOUND PREPARATION of levodopa and BENSERAZIDE HYDROCHLORIDE, which is a combination called co-beneldopa. It can be used to treat parkinsonism, but not the parkinsonian symptoms induced by drugs (see ANTIPARKINSONISM). It is available as tablets, capsules (both in several preparations of different strengths) and modified-release capsules, as *Madopar CR*.
+▲ Side-effects/warning: See LEVODOPA.

magaldrate

is an ANTACID complex that is used to treat severe dyspepsia. It is a combination of aluminium and magnesium hydroxides (with sulphuric acid).

+▲ Side-effects/warning: See ALUMINIUM HYDROXIDE; MAGNESIUM HYDROXIDE.
✪ Related entries: Bisodol Heartburn; Dynese.

Magnapen

(Beecham) is a proprietary, prescription-only COMPOUND PREPARATION of the broad-spectrum ANTIBACTERIAL (PENICILLIN) ANTIBIOTIC ampicillin and the *penicillinase-resistant*, antibacterial and (penicillin) antibiotic flucloxacillin, which is a combination called co-fluampicil. It can be used to treat severe infection where the causative organism has not been identified, but Gram-positive staphylococcal or a penicillin-resistant bacterial infection is probable. It is available as capsules, a syrup and in a form for injection.
+▲ Side-effects/warning: See AMPICILLIN; FLUCLOXACILLIN.

Magnatol

(Sterling) is a proprietary, non-prescription COMPOUND PREPARATION of the ANTACIDS potassium bicarbonate, magnesium carbonate and ALEXITOL SODIUM (with xanthan gum). It can be used for the symptomatic relief of heartburn and is available as a suspension. It is not normally given to children, except on medical advice.
+▲ Side-effects/warning: See MAGNESIUM CARBONATE.

magnesium

is a metallic element necessary to the body and is ingested as a trace element in a well-balanced diet (a good source is green vegetables). It is essential to the bones and important for the proper functioning of nerves and muscles. Therapeutically, magnesium is used in the form of its salts: MAGNESIUM CARBONATE, MAGNESIUM HYDROXIDE, magnesium oxide (magnesia) and MAGNESIUM TRISILICATE are ANTACIDS; MAGNESIUM SULPHATE (Epsom salt/salts) is a LAXATIVE. Magnesium deficiency is usually treated with supplements of MAGNESIUM CHLORIDE.

M

magnesium carbonate

is an ANTACID that also has LAXATIVE properties. It is a mild antacid but fairly long-acting and is a constituent of many proprietary preparations that are used for the relief of hyperacidity and dyspepsia and for the symptomatic relief of heartburn or a peptic ulcer. Administration is oral.

✚ Side-effects: There may be belching due to the internal liberation of carbon dioxide and diarrhoea.

▲ Warning: It should be administered with caution to patients with impaired function of the kidneys, or who are taking certain other drugs. It is not to be taken by those with low phosphate levels.

❍ Related entries: Algicon; Aludrox Tablets; Andrews Antacid; Bismag Tablets; Bisodol Antacid Powder; Bisodol Antacid Tablets; Bisodol Extra Tablets; Caved-S; Digestif Suspension; Dijex Tablets; Maclean Indigestion Tablets; Magnatol; Nulacin Tablets; Rennie Tablets; Topal.

magnesium chloride

is the form of MAGNESIUM that is most commonly used to make up a magnesium deficiency in the body, which may result from either prolonged diarrhoea or vomiting or due to alcoholism.

❍ Related entry: Balanced Salt Solution.

magnesium hydroxide

or hydrated magnesium oxide (*magnesia*), is an ANTACID that also has LAXATIVE properties. As an antacid it is comparatively weak but fairly long-acting and is a constituent of many proprietary preparations that are used for the relief of hyperacidity and dyspepsia and for the symptomatic relief of heartburn or a peptic ulcer. It can also be used to treat constipation. Administration is oral.

✚ Side-effects: There may be diarrhoea.

▲ Warning: It should be administered with caution to patients with impaired function of the kidneys, certain gastrointestinal conditions or who are also taking a course of certain other drugs.

❍ Related entries: Algicon; Aludrox Tablets; Asilone Liquid; Asilone Suspension; Caved-S; Dijex Suspension; Dijex Tablets; Diovol; Maalox Plus Suspension; Maalox Plus Tablets; Maalox Suspension; Maalox TC Suspension; Maalox TC Tablets; Milk of Magnesia Liquid; Milk of Magnesia Tablets; Mil-Par; Mucaine; Mucogel Suspension; Pyrogastrone; Topal.

magnesium sulphate

or Epsom salt(s), is an *osmotic* LAXATIVE. It works by preventing the reabsorption of water within the intestines and can be used to facilitate rapid bowel evacuation. Occasionally, it can also be used as a MAGNESIUM supplement and to treat boils and carbuncles when it is applied topically as a paste with glycerol.

✚ Side-effects: Colitis when taken orally.

▲ Warning: When administered orally, care must be taken in patients with renal or liver impairment and do not use in severe gastrointestinal impairment.

❍ Related entries: Original Andrews Salts; Picolax.

magnesium trisilicate

is used as an ANTACID and has a long duration of action. It is a constituent of many proprietary preparations that are used to relieve hyperacidity and dyspepsia and for the symptomatic relief of heartburn or a peptic ulcer. Administration is oral.

✚ Side-effects: It may cause diarrhoea.

▲ Warning: It should be administered with caution to patients with impaired function of the kidneys, or who are taking certain other drugs.

❍ Related entries: Gastrocote; Gaviscon 250; Gaviscon 500; Nulacin Tablets; Pyrogastrone.

major tranquillizers

see ANTIPSYCHOTICS

malathion

is an insecticidal drug which is used as a PEDICULICIDAL to treat infestations by head and pubic lice, or as a SCABICIDAL to treat skin infestation by mites (scabies). Administration is topical.

✚ Side-effects: Skin irritation.

▲ Warning: Avoid contact with the eyes and do not use on broken or infected skin. It should not be used by asthmatics.

✪ Related entries: Derbac-M; Prioderm; Quellada M; Suleo-M.

malic acid

is a weak organic acid found in apples and some fruits. It is incorporated into some medicinal preparations, such as ARTIFICIAL SALIVA and skin treatments, to adjust their acidity.

✪ Related entry: Aserbine.

Malix

(Lagap) is a proprietary, prescription-only preparation of the SULPHONYLUREA glibenclamide. It is used in DIABETIC TREATMENT for Type II diabetes (non-insulin-dependent diabetesmellitus; NIDDM; maturity-onsetdiabetes), and is available as tablets.

✚▲ Side-effects/warning: See GLIBENCLAMIDE.

Maloprim

(Wellcome) is a proprietary, prescription-only COMPOUND PREPARATION of the ANTIBACTERIAL and ANTIMALARIAL dapsone and the antimalarial pyrimethamine. It can be used to prevent travellers to tropical regions from contracting malaria, and is available as tablets.

✚▲ Side-effects/warning: See DAPSONE; PYRIMETHAMINE.

Manerix

(Roche) is a proprietary, prescription-only preparation of the MONOAMINE-OXIDASE INHIBITOR (MAOI) ANTIDEPRESSANT moclobemide. It can be used to treat major depressive illness, and is available as tablets.

✚▲ Side-effects/warning: See MOCLOBEMIDE.

Manevac

(Galen) is a proprietary, non-prescription COMPOUND PREPARATION of the (*bulking-agent*) LAXATIVE ispaghula husk and the (*stimulant*) laxative senna. It can be used to treat a number of gastrointestinal disorders and is available as granules. It is not normally given to children under five years, except on medical advice.

✚▲ Side-effects/warning: See ISPAGHULA HUSK; SENNA.

mannitol

is one of the *osmotic* class of DIURETICS. It consists of substances secreted into the kidney proximal tubules, which are not resorbed and so carry water and mineral salts into the urine, therefore increasing the volume produced. Therapeutically, it is used primarily to treat oedema, particularly cerebral (brain) oedema. It may also be used in GLAUCOMA TREATMENT to decrease pressure within the eyeball in acute attacks. Administration is by intravenous infusion.

✚ Side-effects: There may be chills and fever.

▲ Warning: Treatment may, in the short term, expand the overall blood volume and therefore it should not be administered to patients with congestive heart failure or fluid on the lungs (pulmonary oedema). An escape of mannitol into the tissues from the site of infusion (vein) causes inflammation and thrombosis.

✪ Related entry: Min-I-Jet Mannitol (25%).

MAOI

see MONOAMINE-OXIDASE INHIBITORS

maprotiline hydrochloride

is a TRICYCLIC-related ANTIDEPRESSANT drug which is administered to treat depressive illness, particularly in cases where some degree of sedation is called for. Administration is oral

✚▲ Side-effects/warning: See AMITRIPTYLINE HYDROCHLORIDE; but some anticholinergic actions are less marked. Rashes are common and there is a danger of

M

convulsions and precipitated epileptic episodes; it is therefore not recommended for epileptics.
○ Related entry: Ludiomil.

Marcain
(Astra) is a proprietary, prescription-only preparation of the LOCAL ANAESTHETIC bupivacaine hydrochloride. It can be used particularly when a prolonged course of treatment is required. It is available in several forms for injection, for example, *Marcain Heavy*.
✚▲ Side-effects/warning: See BUPIVACAINE HYDROCHLORIDE.

Marcain with Adrenaline
(Astra) is a proprietary, prescription-only COMPOUND PREPARATION of the LOCAL ANAESTHETIC bupivacaine hydrochloride and the VASOCONSTRICTOR adrenaline, which prolongs the anaesthetic's duration of action. It is available in a range of forms for injection.
✚▲ Side-effects/warning: See ADRENALINE; BUPIVACAINE HYDROCHLORIDE.

Marevan
(Goldshield) is a proprietary, prescription-only preparation of the synthetic ANTICOAGULANT warfarin sodium. It can be used to prevent clot formation in heart disease, following heart surgery (especially following implantation of prosthetic heart valves), to prevent venous thrombosis and pulmonary embolism. It is available as tablets.
✚▲ Side-effects/warning: See WARFARIN SODIUM.

Marplan
(Cambridge) is a proprietary, prescription-only preparation of the MONOAMINE-OXIDASE INHIBITOR (MAOI) ANTIDEPRESSANT isocarboxazid. It can be used to treat depressive illness, and is available as tablets.
✚▲ Side-effects/warning: See ISOCARBOXAZID.

Marvelon
(Organon) is a proprietary, prescription-only COMPOUND PREPARATION that can be used as a (*monophasic*) ORAL CONTRACEPTIVE (and also for certain menstrual problems) of the type that combines an OESTROGEN and a PROGESTOGEN, in this case ethinyloestradiol and desogestrel. It is available as tablets.
✚▲ Side-effects/warning: See DESOGESTREL; ETHINYLOESTRADIOL.

Masnoderm
(Cusi) is a proprietary, non-prescription preparation of the ANTIFUNGAL drug clotrimazole. It can be used to treat fungal (particularly *Candida*) skin infections, and is available as a cream for topical application.
✚▲ Side-effects/warning: See CLOTRIMAZOLE.

Massé Breast Cream
(Cilag) is a proprietary, non-prescription COMPOUND PREPARATION of arachis oil, wool fat, GLYCEROL, glyceryl monostearate and other constituents. It can be used as an EMOLLIENT for sore nipples, and is available as a cream.
✚▲ Side-effects/warning: See ARACHIS OIL; WOOL FAT.

Matrex
(Pharmacia) is a proprietary, prescription-only preparation of the IMMUNOSUPPRESSANT and (CYTOTOXIC) ANTICANCER drug methotrexate. It can be used to treat rheumatoid arthritis and lymphoblastic leukaemia, other lymphomas and solid tumours. It is available in a form for injection.
✚▲ Side-effects/warning: See METHOTREXATE.

Maxepa
(Innovex) is a proprietary, prescription-only preparation of the LIPID-LOWERING DRUG omega-3 marine triglycerides. It can be used in hyperlipidaemia to reduce the levels, or change the proportions, of

various lipids. It is available as capsules, an emulsion and a liquid.

➕▲ Side-effects/warning: See OMEGA-3 MARINE TRIGLYCERIDES.

Maxidex

(Alcon) is a proprietary, prescription-only COMPOUND PREPARATION of the CORTICOSTEROID and ANTI-INFLAMMATORY dexamethasone and the artificial tear medium HYPROMELLOSE. It can be used to treat inflammation of the eye, and is available as eye-drops.

➕▲ Side-effects/warning: See DEXAMETHASONE.

Maximum Strength Aspro Clear

(Roche) is a proprietary, non-prescription preparation of the (NSAID) NON-NARCOTIC ANALGESIC, ANTIRHEUMATIC and ANTIPYRETIC aspirin. It can be used to relieve pain, including headache, neuralgia, period and dental pain, for the relief of cold and flu symptoms, sore throats and to treat musculoskeletal pain. It is available as effervescent tablets and is not normally given to children, except on medical advice.

➕▲ Side-effects/warning: See ASPIRIN.

Maxitrol

(Alcon) is a proprietary, prescription-only COMPOUND PREPARATION of the ANTI-INFLAMMATORY and CORTICOSTEROID dexamethasone, the ANTIBACTERIAL and (AMINOGLYCOSIDE) ANTIBIOTIC neomycin sulphate and the antibacterial and (POLYMYXIN) antibiotic polymyxin B sulphate and HYPROMELLOSE ('artificial tears'). It can be used to treat inflammation of the eye when infection is also present, and is available as eye-drops.

➕▲ Side-effects/warning: See DEXAMETHASONE; NEOMYCIN SULPHATE; POLYMYXIN B SULPHATE.

Maxivent

(Ashbourne) is a proprietary, prescription-only preparation of the BETA-RECEPTOR STIMULANT salbutamol. It can be used as a BRONCHODILATOR in reversible obstructive airways disease, as an ANTI-ASTHMATIC treatment in severe acute asthma and for the alleviation of symptoms of chronic bronchitis and emphysema. It is available in an aerosol inhalant.

➕▲ Side-effects/warning: See SALBUTAMOL.

Maxolon

(Beecham) is a proprietary, prescription-only preparation of the ANTI-EMETIC and ANTINAUSEANT metoclopramide hydrochloride. It can be used for the treatment of nausea and vomiting, particularly when associated with gastrointestinal disorders and after treatment with radiation or cytotoxic drugs. It also has gastric MOTILITY STIMULANT actions and can be used in the treatment of non-ulcer dyspepsia, gastric stasis and to prevent reflux oesophagitis. It is available as tablets, a syrup, a liquid form (*Maxolon Paediatric Liquid*), as modified-release capsules (*Maxolon SR*) and in several forms for injection (eg *Maxolon High Dose*).

➕▲ Side-effects/warning: See METOCLOPRAMIDE HYDROCHLORIDE.

MCR-50

(Pharmacia) (Mono-Cedocard Retard-50) is a proprietary, non-prescription preparation of the VASODILATOR and ANTI-ANGINA drug isosorbide mononitrate. It can be used to treat and prevent angina pectoris and in HEART FAILURE TREATMENT. It is available as modified-release capsules.

➕▲ Side-effects/warning: See ISOSORBIDE MONONITRATE.

measles vaccine

is a VACCINE used for IMMUNIZATION which has almost entirely been replaced by a combined measles/mumps/rubella vaccine (MMR) and a measles/rubella (MR) vaccine for use in children. It is available as a single vaccine under special circumstances only.

➕▲ Side-effects/warning: See MMR VACCINE.

M

mebendazole

is an (AZOLE) ANTHELMINTIC drug which can be used in the treatment of infections by roundworm, threadworm, whipworm and hookworm. Administration is oral.

✚ Side-effects: These are rare, but there may be diarrhoea and abdominal pain; hypersensitivity reactions (rash, urticaria and angio-oedema).

▲ Warning: Administer with caution to those who are pregnant or breast-feeding.

○ Related entries: Ovex Tablets; Pripsen Mebendazole; Vermox.

mebeverine hydrochloride

is an ANTISPASMODIC drug which is used to treat muscle spasm in the gastrointestinal tract, which causes abdominal pain and constipation, eg irritable bowel syndrome. Administration is oral.

✚▲ Side-effects/warning: It should not be taken by patients with paralytic ileus. Avoid in porphyria.

○ Related entries: Colofac; Fomac; Fybogel Mebeverine.

meclozine hydrochloride

is an ANTIHISTAMINE which is used primarily as an ANTINAUSEANT in the treatment or prevention of motion sickness and vomiting. Administration is oral.

✚▲ Side-effects/warning: See CYCLIZINE.

○ Related entry: Sea-Legs.

Mectizan

(Merck Sharp & Dohme) is a proprietary preparation of the ANTHELMINTIC drug ivermectin, which (though not available in the UK) is effective in treating the tropical disease onchocerciasis (infestation by the filarial worm-parasite *Onchocerca volvulus*. Administration is oral.

✚▲ Side-effects/warning: See IVERMECTIN.

mecyteine hydrochloride

see METHYL CYSTEINE HYDROCHLORIDE

Mediclear 10 Acne Cream

(Boots) is a proprietary, non-prescription preparation of the KERATOLYTIC and ANTIMICROBIAL drug benzoyl peroxide (5%). It can be applied topically for the treatment of acne and spots, and is available as a cream. It is not normally used on children under 12 years, except on medical advice.

✚▲ Side-effects/warning: See BENZOYL PEROXIDE.

Mediclear 5 Acne Cream

(Boots) is a proprietary, non-prescription preparation of the KERATOLYTIC and ANTIMICROBIAL drug benzoyl peroxide (5%). It can be applied topically for the treatment of acne and spots, and is available as a cream. It is not normally used on children under 12 years, except on medical advice.

✚▲ Side-effects/warning: See BENZOYL PEROXIDE.

Mediclear Acne Lotion

(Boots) is a proprietary, non-prescription preparation of the KERATOLYTIC and ANTIMICROBIAL drug benzoyl peroxide (5%). It can be applied topically for the treatment of acne and spots, and is available as a cream. It is not normally used on children under 12 years, except on medical advice.

✚▲ Side-effects/warning: See BENZOYL PEROXIDE.

Medicoal

(Torbet) is a proprietary, non-prescription preparation of the adsorbent material ACTIVATED CHARCOAL. It can be administered to treat patients suffering from poisoning or a drug overdose. It is available as a granules.

Medihaler-epi

(3M) is a proprietary, prescription-only preparation of the SYMPATHOMIMETIC adrenaline acid tartrate. It can be used as a BRONCHODILATOR, administered in the form of an aerosol inhalant, for emergency treatment of acute and severe allergic reactions, cardiopulmonary resuscitation and angio-oedema.

✚▲ Side-effects/warning: See ADRENALINE.

Medihaler-Ergotamine

(3M) is a proprietary, prescription-only preparation of the VASOCONSTRICTOR ergotamine tartrate. It can be used as an ANTIMIGRAINE treatment for acute attacks, and is available as an inhalant aerosol.
✚▲ Side-effects/warning: See ERGOTAMINE TARTRATE.

Medihaler-iso

(3M) is a proprietary, prescription-only preparation of the BETA-RECEPTOR STIMULANT isoprenaline (as isoprenaline sulphate). It can be used as a BRONCHODILATOR in reversible obstructive airways disease and as an ANTI-ASTHMATIC in severe acute asthma. It is available in a metered-dosage aerosol in two strengths (the stronger under the trade name *Medihaler-iso Forte*).
✚▲ Side-effects/warning: See ISOPRENALINE.

Medijel Gel

(DDD) is a proprietary, non-prescription COMPOUND PREPARATION of the LOCAL ANAESTHETIC lignocaine hydrochloride and the ANTISEPTIC aminacrine hydrochloride. It can be used for the temporary relief of pain caused by mouth ulcers, denture rubbing and sore gums, and is available as a gel for topical application.
✚▲ Side-effects/warning: See AMINACRINE HYDROCHLORIDE; LIGNOCAINE.

Medilave

(Martindale) is a proprietary, non-prescription COMPOUND PREPARATION of the ANTISEPTIC agent CETYLPYRIDINIUM CHLORIDE and the LOCAL ANAESTHETIC benzocaine. It can be used to relieve the pain of sores and ulcers in the mouth, and is available as a gel for topical application. It is not normally used on children under 12 years, except on medical advice.
✚▲ Side-effects/warning: See BENZOCAINE.

Medinol over 6

(Seton) is a proprietary, non-prescription preparation of the NON-NARCOTIC ANALGESIC paracetamol. It can be used for relieving the symptoms of pain and feverish conditions, and is available as an oral suspension. It is not normally given to adults and children under six years.
✚▲ Side-effects/warning: See PARACETAMOL.

Medinol Under 6

(Seton) is a proprietary, non-prescription preparation of the NON-NARCOTIC ANALGESIC paracetamol. It can be used for relieving the symptoms of pain and feverish conditions, and is available as an oral suspension. It is not normally given to children under one year, except on medical advice.
✚▲ Side-effects/warning: See PARACETAMOL.

Medised

(Seton) is a proprietary, non-prescription COMPOUND PREPARATION of the NON-NARCOTIC ANALGESIC paracetamol and the SEDATIVE and ANTIHISTAMINE drug promethazine hydrochloride. It can be used for reducing temperature and relieving the symptoms of painful or feverish conditions, such as toothache, headache, sore throats, colds and flu and nasal irritation. It is available as a suspension and is not normally given to children under one year, except on medical advice.
✚▲ Side-effects/warning: See PARACETAMOL; PROMETHAZINE HYDROCHLORIDE.

Medrone

(Upjohn) is a proprietary, prescription-only preparation of the CORTICOSTEROID and ANTI-INFLAMMATORY drug methylprednisolone. It can be used to treat allergic disorders, shock and cerebral oedema, and is available as tablets.
✚▲ Side-effects/warning: See METHYLPREDNISOLONE.

medroxyprogesterone acetate

is a SEX HORMONE, a synthetic PROGESTOGEN. One of its uses is as an ORAL CONTRACEPTIVE, for a short period of time or by deep

M

intramuscular injection every three months for a longer duration of action. It can also be used as a hormonal supplement in women whose progestogen level requires boosting (such as in endometriosis or dysfunctional uterine bleeding).
Additionally, it can be used in the treatment of cancer of the breast, uterine endometrium and, less commonly, of the prostate gland in men. Administration is either oral or by injection.

✚ Side-effects: Fluid retention and weight gain, acne and urticaria, gastrointestinal disturbances, PMS and irregular periods, changes in libido, breast tenderness; also insomnia, depression and sleepiness; loss or growth of hair; rarely, jaundice.

▲ Warning: It should not be administered to patients with certain liver disorders, undiagnosed vaginal haemorrhage or sex hormone-linked cancer; who are pregnant; or have porphyria. Administer with caution to those with diabetes, certain heart or kidney disorders or hypertension.

○ Related entries: Depo-Provera; Farlutal; Improvera; Provera; Tridestra.

mefenamic acid

is a (NSAID) NON-NARCOTIC ANALGESIC and ANTIRHEUMATIC drug which is used primarily to treat mild to moderate pain and inflammation in rheumatoid arthritis, osteoarthritis and other musculoskeletal disorders, including juvenile arthritis. It is also used to treat dysmenorrhoea. Administration is oral.

✚▲ Side-effects/warning: See NSAID. It has weaker anti-inflammatory properties than most drugs of this class and a higher incidence of diarrhoea. There may be blood disturbances.

○ Related entries: Contraflam; Dysman 250; Dysman 500; Ponstan.

mefloquine

is an ANTIMALARIAL drug which is used to prevent and treat malaria infection, including uncomplicated falciparum malaria and chloroquine-resistant vivax

malaria. Administration is oral.

✚ Side-effects: There may be nausea and vomiting, visual disturbances, rash and itching; diarrhoea, abdominal pain and disturbances of the gastrointestinal tract and liver, dizziness, loss of balance, headache, somnolence, sleep disorders (insomnia, abnormal dreams). Susceptible patients may undergo psychotic episodes and neuropsychiatric reactions (including motor and sensory neuropathies, anxiety, depression, hallucinations, overt psychosis and convulsions), tinnitus and vestibular disorders and visual disturbances. Also circulatory disorders (hypotension and hypertension), bradycardia, tachycardia, heart disorders, muscle weakness, myalgia, arthralgia, urticaria, pruritus, alopecia, disturbances in liver function, asthenia, malaise, fatigue, fever, loss of appetite, disturbed blood counts and AV block and encephalopathy. The performance of skilled tasks, such as driving, may be impaired. Patients must consult their doctor if adverse symptoms are experienced after discontinuation of treatment.

▲ Warning: These depend on whether it is used to prevent or to treat malaria. It should not be used in patients with certain kidney, liver or heart disorders. It should not be given to those who are breast-feeding or pregnant (and avoid getting pregnant for three months after treatment with mefloquine), or to those with a history of convulsions. There may be serious psychiatric disorders, or hypersensitivity to quinine.

○ Related entry: Lariam.

Mefoxin

(Merck Sharp & Dohme) is a proprietary, prescription-only preparation of the ANTIBACTERIAL and (CEPHALOSPORIN) ANTIBIOTIC cefoxitin. It can be used to treat many types of bacterial infection, including peritonitis, and also to prevent infection following surgery. It is available in a form for injection or infusion.

✚▲ Side-effects/warning: See CEFOXITIN.

mefruside

is one of the THIAZIDE class of DIURETICS. It can be used as an ANTIHYPERTENSIVE, either alone or in conjunction with other types of drugs, and also in the treatment of oedema associated with congestive heart failure. Administration is oral.
+▲ Side-effects/warning: See BENDROFLUAZIDE.
O Related entry: Baycaron.

Megace

(Bristol-Myers) is a proprietary, prescription-only preparation of the PROGESTOGEN megestrol acetate, which is a female SEX HORMONE. It can be used to treat oestrogen-linked cancers (such as cancer of the breast or of the endometrium of the uterus), and is available as tablets.
+▲ Side-effects/warning: See MEGESTROL ACETATE.

megestrol acetate

is a PROGESTOGEN, a female SEX HORMONE, which is used primarily as an ANTICANCER treatment when the presence of OESTROGENS is significant (eg breast cancer or cancer of the endometrium of the uterus). Administration is oral.
+▲ Side-effects/warning: See MEDROXYPROGESTERONE ACETATE.
O Related entry: Megace.

Meggezones

(Schering-Plough) is a proprietary, non-prescription preparation of the aromatic oil MENTHOL. It can be used for the symptomatic relief of sore throat, coughs, colds, catarrh and nasal congestion, and is available as pastilles.

Melleril

(Sandoz) is a proprietary, prescription-only preparation of the ANTIPSYCHOTIC thioridazine. It can be used to treat and tranquillize patients with psychotic disorders (such as schizophrenia), particularly manic forms of behavioural disturbance, and also in the short-term

treatment of anxiety. It is available as tablets, a suspension and a syrup.
+▲ Side-effects/warning: See THIORIDAZINE.

meloxicam

is a (NSAID) NON-NARCOTIC ANALGESIC and ANTIRHEUMATIC drug which is used to treat pain and inflammation in rheumatoid arthritis, and for short-term exacerbation of osteoarthritis. Administration is either oral or by suppositories.
+▲ Side-effects/warning: See NSAID. Avoid suppositories if there are haemorrhoids, and use with caution in those with impaired kidneys.
O Related entry: Mobic.

melphalan

is a CYTOTOXIC drug which is used as an ANTICANCER treatment of various forms of cancers, especially cancer of the bone marrow (myelomatosis). It works by a direct action on the DNA of the cancer cells and so prevents cell replication. Administration is either oral or by injection.
+▲ Side-effects/warning: See CYTOTOXICS.
O Related entry: Alkeran.

Meltus Adult Expectorant Linctus

(Seton) is a proprietary, non-prescription preparation of the EXPECTORANT agent GUAIPHENESIN, the ANTISEPTIC agent CETYLPYRIDINIUM CHLORIDE, sucrose and honey. It can be used for the symptomatic relief of coughs and catarrh associated with flu, colds and mild cold infections. It is available as a liquid and is not normally given to children, except on medical advice.

Meltus Dry Cough Elixir, Adult

(Seton) is a proprietary, non-prescription preparation of the SYMPATHOMIMETIC and DECONGESTANT pseudoephedrine hydrochloride and the NARCOTIC ANALGESIC and ANTITUSSIVE dextromethorphan hydrobromide. It can be used for the

M

symptomatic relief of dry, painful, tickly cough and catarrh. It is available in the form of a liquid and is not to be given to children.

+▲ Side-effects/warning: See DEXTROMETHORPHAN HYDROBROMIDE; PSEUDOEPHEDRINE HYDROCHLORIDE.

Meltus Junior Dry Cough Elixir

(Seton) is a proprietary, non-prescription preparation of the SYMPATHOMIMETIC and DECONGESTANT pseudoephedrine hydrochloride and the NARCOTIC ANALGESIC and ANTITUSSIVE dextromethorphan hydrobromide. It can be used for the symptomatic relief of unproductive coughs and congestion of the upper airways. It is available as a liquid and is not normally given to children under two years, except on medical advice.

+▲ Side-effects/warning: See DEXTROMETHORPHAN HYDROBROMIDE; PSEUDOEPHEDRINE HYDROCHLORIDE.

Meltus Junior Expectorant Linctus

(Seton) is a proprietary, non-prescription preparation of the EXPECTORANT agent GUAIPHENESIN, the ANTISEPTIC agent CETYLPYRIDINIUM CHLORIDE, sucrose and honey. It can be used for the symptomatic relief of coughs and catarrh associated with flu, colds and mild cold infections. It is available as a liquid and is not normally given to children under two years, except on medical advice.

menadiol sodium phosphate

(vitamin K_3) is a synthetic form of VITAMIN K. It is sometimes used in medicine in preference to vitamins K_1 and K_2, because these natural forms are only fat-soluble, whereas vitamin K_3 is water-soluble and is therefore effective when taken by mouth to treat vitamin deficiency caused by fat malabsorption syndromes (eg due to obstruction of the bile ducts or in liver

disease). In malabsorption syndromes it is important to make up a deficiency on a regular basis, because vitamin K is essential for maintaining the clotting factors in the blood and for calcification of bone. Administration is oral.

+▲ Side-effects/warning: see VITAMIN K.
✪ Related entry: Synkavit.

Mengivac (A+C)

(Mérieux) is a proprietary, prescription-only preparation of a VACCINE that is used to give protection against the organism meningococcus (*Neisseria meningitidis* groups A and C), which can cause serious infections such as meningitis. It is available in a form for injection.

+▲ Side-effects/warning: See MENINGOCOCCAL POLYSACCHARIDE VACCINE.

meningococcal polysaccharide vaccine

is a VACCINE that is used for IMMUNIZATION against infection from the organism meningococcus (*Neisseria meningitidis*), which can cause a serious infection, such as meningitis. It may be given to those intending to travel 'rough' through parts of the world where the risk of meningococcal infection is much higher than in the UK (eg parts of India and much of Africa). Administration is by subcutaneous or intramuscular injection.

+▲ Side-effects/warning: See VACCINES.
✪ Related entries: AC Vax ; Mengivac (A+C).

Menorest

(Rhône-Poulenc Rorer) is a proprietary, prescription-only preparation of the OESTROGEN oestradiol. It can be used in HRT, and is available as a gel.

+▲ Side-effects/warning: See OESTRADIOL.

menotropin

is a HORMONE preparation and is a collective name for combinations of the gonadotrophin hormones – FOLLICLE-STIMULATING HORMONE (FSH) and LUTEINISING HORMONE (LH) – in a particular activity ratio (1:1).

✚▲ Side-effects/warning: See HUMAN MENOPAUSAL GONADOTROPHINS.

menthol

is a white, crystalline substance derived from peppermint oil (an essential oil extracted from a plant of the mint family) and is chemically a TERPENE. It is commonly used, with or without the volatile substance eucalyptus oil, in inhalations intended to clear the nasal or catarrhal congestion associated with colds, rhinitis (inflammation of the nasal mucous membrane) or sinusitis. It is also included in some COUNTER-IRRITANT, or RUBEFACIENT, preparations that are rubbed into the skin to relieve muscle or joint pain, and in preparations used to treat gallstones or kidney stones.

❂ Related entries: Aspellin; Balmosa Cream; Bengué's Balsam; Benylin Chesty Coughs Non-Drowsy; Benylin Dry Coughs Original; Benylin with Codeine; Copholco; Copholcoids Cough Pastilles; Covonia Bronchial Balsam; Deep Heat Massage Liniment; Deep Heat Maximum Strength; Fisherman's Friend; Karvol Decongestant Capsules; Meggezones; Merothol Lozenges; Nirolex for Chesty Coughs; Penetrol Catarrh Lozenges; Penetrol Inhalant; Radian B Heat Spray; Radian B Muscle Lotion; Radian B Muscle Rub; Ralgex Stick; Rowachol; Tixylix Inhalant; Vicks Sinex Decongestant Nasal Spray.

Menzol

(Swarz) is a proprietary, prescription-only preparation of the PROGESTOGEN norethisterone. It can be used to treat uterine bleeding, abnormally heavy menstruation, premenstrual tension, endometriosis and other menstrual problems, and also for contraception. It is available as tablets.

✚▲ Side-effects/warning: See NORETHISTERONE.

mepacrine hydrochloride

has ANTIPROTOZOAL properties and is used primarily to treat infection of the small intestine by the intestinal protozoan *Giardia lamblia*. Giardiasis (lambliasis) occurs throughout the world, particularly in children, and is contracted by eating contaminated food. However, mepacrine has largely been superseded by METRONIDAZOLE, which is now the drug of choice. It is still sometimes used to treat discoid lupus erythematosus. Administration is oral.

✚ Side-effects: Gastrointestinal disturbances, nausea and vomiting; headache and dizziness; stimulation of the central nervous system and psychoses; discolouration of the skin and dermatitis (with prolonged use); blood disturbances; discolouration of nails, palate and cornea (with vision disturbances).

▲ Warning: It should not be administered to patients with psoriasis; and with care to those with liver impairment or psychosis.

mepenzolate bromide

is an ANTICHOLINERGIC drug which can be used as an ANTISPASMODIC for the symptomatic relief of smooth muscle spasm in the gastrointestinal tract. Administration is oral.

✚▲ Side-effects/warning: See ATROPINE SULPHATE.

❂ Related entry: Cantil.

Mepranix

(Ashbourne) is a proprietary, prescription-only preparation of the BETA-BLOCKER metoprolol tartrate. It can be used as an ANTIHYPERTENSIVE for raised blood pressure, as an ANTI-ANGINA treatment to relieve symptoms and improve exercise tolerance and as an ANTI-ARRHYTHMIC to regularize heartbeat and to treat myocardial infarction. It can also be used as an ANTITHYROID drug for short-term treatment of thyrotoxicosis and as an ANTIMIGRAINE treatment to prevent attacks. It is available as tablets.

✚▲ Side-effects/warning: See METOPROLOL TARTRATE.

M

meprobamate

is an ANXIOLYTIC which is used in the short-term treatment of anxiety. It is also used in some SKELETAL MUSCLE RELAXANT and COMPOUND ANALGESIC preparations. It is potentially more hazardous than the BENZODIAZEPINES in overdose and can cause dependence (addiction). Administration is oral. Preparations containing meprobamate are on the Controlled Drugs List.

✚ Side-effects: See BENZODIAZEPINES; but there are also gastrointestinal disturbances, hypotension, disturbed peripheral nerve function, weakness, headache, disturbances of vision and blood changes. Drowsiness is a very common side-effect.

▲ Warning: It should not be administered to patients with porphyria, who have certain lung and breathing disorders or who are breast-feeding. It should be administered with caution to those with respiratory difficulties, epilepsy, impaired liver or kidney function, drug or alcohol abuse, personality disorders or who are pregnant. Withdrawal of treatment must be gradual otherwise convulsions may occur.

✪ Related entries: Equagesic; Equanil.

meptazinol

is a powerful, synthetic (OPIOID) NARCOTIC ANALGESIC which is used to treat moderate to severe pain, including pain in childbirth, renal colic or following surgery. Administration can be either oral or by injection.

✚▲ Side-effects/warning: See OPIOIDS; but less respiratory depression.

✪ Related entry: Meptid.

Meptid

(Monmouth) is a proprietary, prescription-only preparation of the (OPIOID) NARCOTIC ANALGESIC meptazinol (as hydrochloride). It can be used to treat moderate to severe pain, particularly during or following surgical procedures and also in childbirth. It is available as tablets and in a form for injection.

✚▲ Side-effects/warning: See MEPTAZINOL.

mequitazine

is an ANTIHISTAMINE which is used to treat the symptoms of allergic conditions such as hay fever and urticaria. Administration is oral.

✚▲ Side-effects/warning: See ANTIHISTAMINES. It may increase appetite and cause weight gain. Because of its sedative properties, the performance of skilled tasks, such as driving, may be impaired.

✪ Related entry: Primalan.

Merbentyl

(Merrell) is a proprietary, prescription-only preparation of the ANTICHOLINERGIC drug dicyclomine hydrochloride. It can be used as an ANTISPASMODIC for the symptomatic relief of smooth muscle spasm in the gastrointestinal tract, and is available as tablets and a syrup. (There are preparations available without prescription, but they are subject to certain limitations.)

✚▲ Side-effects/warning: See DICYCLOMINE HYDROCHLORIDE.

Merbentyl 20

(Merrell) is a proprietary, prescription-only preparation of the ANTICHOLINERGIC drug dicyclomine hydrochloride. It can be used as an ANTISPASMODIC for the symptomatic relief of muscle spasm in the gastrointestinal tract, and is available as tablets.

✚▲ Side-effects/warning: See DICYCLOMINE HYDROCHLORIDE.

mercaptopurine

is a CYTOTOXIC drug which is used as an ANTICANCER treatment of acute leukaemias. It works by preventing cell replication. Administration is oral.

✚▲ Side-effects/warning: See CYTOTOXICS. Avoid its use in patients with porphyria.

✪ Related entry: Puri-Nethol.

Mercilon

(Organon) is a proprietary, prescription-only COMPOUND PREPARATION which can be used as a (*monophasic*) ORAL

M

CONTRACEPTIVE (and also for certain
menstrual problems) of the type that
combines an OESTROGEN and a PROGESTOGEN,
in this case ethinyloestradiol and
desogestrel. It is available as tablets.

✚▲ Side-effects/warning: See DESOGESTREL;
ETHINYLOESTRADIOL.

Merocaine Lozenges

(Merrell) is a proprietary, non-prescription
COMPOUND PREPARATION of the ANTISEPTIC
agent CETYLPYRIDINIUM CHLORIDE and the
LOCAL ANAESTHETIC benzocaine. It can be
used for the temporary relief of the pain
and discomfort of a sore throat and
superficial, minor mouth infections. It is
available as lozenges and is not normally
given to children under 12 years, except on
medical advice.

✚▲ Side-effects/warning: See BENZOCAINE.

Merocets
Gargle/Mouthwash

(Marion Merrell Dow) is a proprietary,
non-prescription preparation of the
ANTISEPTIC agent CETYLPYRIDINIUM CHLORIDE.
It can be used for the symptomatic relief
of sore throat and minor irritations of
the throat and mouth. It is available as an
oral solution for use as a gargle or
mouthwash.

Merocets Lozenges

(Marion Merrell Dow) is a proprietary,
non-prescription preparation of the
ANTISEPTIC agent CETYLPYRIDINIUM CHLORIDE.
It can be used for the symptomatic relief
of sore throat and minor irritations of
the throat and mouth, and is available
as lozenges.

Meronem

(Zeneca) is a proprietary, prescription-only
COMPOUND PREPARATION of the ANTIBACTERIAL
and (BETA-LACTAM) ANTIBIOTIC drug
meropenem. It can be used to treat a
range of infections, and is available in a
form for injection.

✚▲ Side-effects/warning: See MEROPENEM.

meropenem

is a recently introduced ANTIBACTERIAL and
ANTIBIOTIC drug. It is a new sort of BETA-
LACTAM (a carbapenem) with a broad-
spectrum of activity against many Gram-
positive and Gram-negative bacteria. Unlike
its earlier analogue imipenem, it is not
degraded by an enzyme in the kidney. It
can be used to treat meningitis, infections
in the periphery (ie the body), such as the
urethra and cervix, and for infections
acquired in hospitals. Administration is by
injection.

✚ Side-effects: Nausea, vomiting,
diarrhoea, abdominal pain; upset liver
function; blood dyscrasias (neutropenia,
eosinophilia, thrombocytopenia); headache,
loss of sensation in the extremities; rash,
pruritus and urticaria; convulsions have
been reported, and there may be local
reactions, including pain, at the injection
site.

▲ Warning: Administer with caution to
patients with liver or kidney impairment, or
who are pregnant or breast-feeding. Do not
use if there is known hypersensitivity to
meropenem, and administer with care to
those with hypersensitivity to penicillins and
other beta-lactams.

✪ Related entry: Meronem.

Merothol Lozenges

(Marion Merrell Dow) is a proprietary,
non-prescription COMPOUND PREPARATION of
the ANTISEPTIC agent CETYLPYRIDINIUM
CHLORIDE and the DECONGESTANTS CINEOLE and
MENTHOL. It can be used for the
symptomatic relief of sore throat and nasal
congestion, and is available as lozenges.

Merovit Lozenges

(Marion Merrell Dow) is a proprietary,
non-prescription preparation of the
ANTISEPTIC agent CETYLPYRIDINIUM CHLORIDE
(with vitamin C). It can be used for the
symptomatic relief of a minor sore throat
due to a cold, and is available as lozenges.
It is not normally given to children under
six years, except on medical advice.

M

mersalyl
is a DIURETIC which is now almost never administered, except when all other methods of treating fluid retention have not been successful or are not tolerated. It is toxic and can be administered only by intramuscular injection: an intravenous injection may cause a severe fall in blood pressure.

✚ Side-effects: There may be gastrointestinal disturbances; some patients experience allergic reactions. This drug is very toxic to the renal system.

▲ Warning: It should not be administered to patients with certain kidney disorders or who are pregnant; and with caution to those who have recently had a heart attack, or who suffer from certain heartbeat irregularities.

mesalazine
is an AMINOSALICYLATE which can be used in the treatment of ulcerative colitis, particularly in patients sensitive to the sulphonamide content of sulphasalazine. Administration can be either oral or by suppositories or a foam enema.

✚ Side-effects: Nausea, diarrhoea, abdominal pain, headache, exacerbated colitis symptoms, kidney, liver and pancreas problems and blood disorders.

▲ Warning: It should not be administered to patients who have kidney impairment, or who are allergic to aspirin or other salicylates; it should be administered with caution to those who are pregnant or breast-feeding.

✪ Related entries: Asacol; Pentasa; Salofalk.

mesna
is a synthetic drug which has the property of combating the haemorrhagic cystitis that is a toxic complication caused by CYTOTOXIC drugs (eg CYCLOPHOSPHAMIDE and IFOSFAMIDE). It works by reacting with a toxic metabolite (breakdown product) produced by the cytotoxic drugs and which is the cause of the haemorrhagic cystitis. Mesna is therefore used as an adjunct in the treatment of certain forms of cancer. Administration is either oral or by injection.

✚ Side-effects: Overdosage may cause gastrointestinal disturbances, headache, tiredness, pain in the limbs, depression, irritability, rash and lack of energy.

✪ Related entry: Uromitexan.

mesterolone
is an ANDROGEN, a male SEX HORMONE, produced mainly in the testes and which, along with other androgens, promotes the development of the secondary male sexual characteristics. Therapeutically, it may be administered to treat hormonal deficiency, for instance, for delayed puberty in boys. Administration is oral.

✚▲ Side-effects/warning: See ANDROGENS; but there is no effect on sperm production.

✪ Related entry: Pro-Viron.

Mestinon
(Roche) is a proprietary, prescription-only preparation of the ANTICHOLINESTERASE and PARASYMPATHOMIMETIC pyridostigmine (as bromide). It can be used to treat myasthenia gravis and also to stimulate intestinal activity, and is available as tablets and in a form for injection.

✚▲ Side-effects/warning: See PYRIDOSTIGMINE.

mestranol
is a synthetic OESTROGEN, a female SEX HORMONE, which is a constituent in several *combined* ORAL CONTRACEPTIVES and is also used in HRT. Administration is oral as tablets in a calendar pack.

✚▲ Side-effects/warning: See OESTROGENS.

✪ Related entries: Norinyl-1; Ortho-Novin 1/50; Syntex Menophase.

Metalpha
(Ashbourne) is a proprietary, prescription-only preparation of the ANTISYMPATHETIC drug methyldopa. It can be administered as an ANTIHYPERTENSIVE, and is available as tablets.

✚▲ Side-effects/warning: See METHYLDOPA.

Metamucil

(Procter & Gamble) is a proprietary, non-prescription preparation of the (*bulking-agent*) LAXATIVE ispaghula husk. It can be used for the relief of constipation, and is available as a powder. It is not normally used for children under six years, except on medical advice.

✚▲ Side-effects/warning: See ISPAGHULA HUSK.

Metanium

(Bengué) is a proprietary, non-prescription preparation of the white pigment TITANIUM DIOXIDE (and other titanium salts) in a silicone base. It can be administered as a BARRIER CREAM for nappy rash and related skin conditions, and is available as an ointment.

metaraminol

is a SYMPATHOMIMETIC and VASOCONSTRICTOR drug which can be used to treat cases of acute hypotension, particularly in emergency situations as a temporary measure while preparations are made for a blood transfusion. Administration is by injection or infusion.

✚▲ Side-effects/warning: See NORADRENALINE.

○ Related entry: Aramine.

Metenix 5

(Hoechst) is a proprietary, prescription-only preparation of the (THIAZIDE-like) DIURETIC metolazone. It can be used, either alone or in conjunction with other drugs, in the treatment of oedema and as an ANTIHYPERTENSIVE, and is available as tablets.

✚▲ Side-effects/warning: See METOLAZONE.

Meterfolic

(Sinclair) is a proprietary, non-prescription COMPOUND PREPARATION of ferrous fumarate and folic acid. It can be used as an IRON and folic acid supplement during pregnancy, and is available as tablets.

✚▲ Side-effects/warning: See FERROUS FUMARATE; FOLIC ACID.

metformin hydrochloride

is a BIGUANIDE drug which is used in DIABETIC TREATMENT of Type II diabetes (non-insulin-dependent diabetes mellitus; NIDDM; maturity-onset diabetes), particularly in patients who are not totally dependent on additional supplies of INSULIN. It works by increasing the utilization and decreasing the formation of glucose, to make up for the reduction in insulin available from the pancreas. Administration is oral.

✚ Side-effects: There may be nausea and vomiting, with diarrhoea and weight loss. Body uptake of CYANOCOBALAMIN (vitamin B_{12}) or its analogues may be reduced.

▲ Warning: It should not be administered to patients with certain heart, liver or kidney disorders, who are dehydrated, alcoholics, have severe infection, trauma or are pregnant or breast-feeding.

○ Related entry: Glucophage.

methadone hydrochloride

is an (OPIOID) NARCOTIC ANALGESIC drug and on the Controlled Drugs List. It is used primarily for the relief of severe pain, but is less effective and less SEDATIVE than morphine and acts for a longer time. It is also used as a substitute for addictive opioids in detoxification therapy. Administration can be either oral or by injection.

✚▲ Side-effects/warning: See OPIOIDS.

○ Related entries: Methadose; Physeptone.

Methadose

(Rosemont) is a proprietary, prescription-only preparation of the (OPIOID) NARCOTIC ANALGESIC methadone hydrochloride, which is on the Controlled Drugs List. It is used for drug-dependent persons, and is available as an oral solution diluted with *Methadose Dilutent*.

✚▲ Side-effects/warning: See METHADONE HYDROCHLORIDE.

methenamine hippurate

see HEXAMINE HIPPURATE

M

355

M

methicillin

is an ANTIBACTERIAL and *(penicillin)* ANTIBIOTIC. It was the first of its type to be resistant to the penicillinase enzyme secreted by penicillin-resistant strains of *Staphylococcus aureus*. It has since been superseded, however, by orally active, penicillinase-resistant penicillins (for example, FLUCLOXACILLIN) and is no longer administered. In recent years the occurrence of methicillin-resistant strains of *Staphylococcus* has created major problems in hospitals throughout the world. The similar antibiotic PIVMECILLINAM HYDROCHLORIDE is present in some COMPOUND PREPARATIONS.

methionine

is an ANTIDOTE to poisoning caused by an overdose of the NON-NARCOTIC ANALGESIC paracetamol. The initial symptoms of paracetamol poisoning more often than not settle within 24 hours, but are followed by an extremely serious toxic effect on the liver that takes several days to develop. The purpose of administering methionine is to prevent these latter effects and it is essential that treatment must commence immediately or as soon as possible after the overdose has been taken. Methionine is used until the drug ACETYLCYSTEINE can be given by intravenous infusion. Administration is oral.
○ Related entries: Methionine Tablets; Pameton.

Methionine Tablets

(Evans) is a proprietary, prescription-only preparation of the ANTIDOTE methionine. It can be used for the emergency treatment of overdose poisoning by the NON-NARCOTIC ANALGESIC paracetamol, and is available as tablets.

methocarbamol

is a SKELETAL MUSCLE RELAXANT drug which is administered for the symptomatic relief of muscle spasm and works by an action on the central nervous system.

Administration is either oral or by injection.
✚ Side-effects: There may be light-headedness, lassitude, dizziness, confusion, restlessness, anxiety, drowsiness, nausea, allergic rash, angio-oedema and convulsions.
▲ Warning: It should not be administered to patients with brain damage, epilepsy or myasthenia gravis. Administer with caution to those with impaired liver or kidney function. Drowsiness may impair the performance of skilled tasks, such as driving; avoid alcohol as its effects are enhanced.
○ Related entries: Robaxin; Robaxisal Forte.

methohexital

see METHOHEXITONE SODIUM

methohexitone sodium

(methohexital) is a BARBITURATE which can be used as a GENERAL ANAESTHETIC for induction and maintenance of anaesthia during short operations. Administration is by injection.
✚▲ Side-effects/warning: See BARBITURATES.
○ Related entry: Brietal Sodium.

methotrexate

is a CYTOTOXIC drug which is used primarily as an ANTICANCER treatment of childhood acute lymphoblastic leukaemia, but also to treat other lymphomas, choriocarcinoma and some solid tumours. It works by inhibiting the activity of an enzyme essential to the DNA metabolism in cells. It is also used as an IMMUNOSUPPRESSANT to treat rheumatoid arthritis and (under specialist supervision) severe resistant psoriasis. Administration is either oral or by injection.
✚▲ Side-effects/warning: See CYTOTOXICS. It should not be given to patients with severe kidney impairment; and avoid its use in those with porphyria.
○ Related entries: Matrex; Methotrexate.

Methotrexate

(Lederle) is a proprietary, prescription-only

preparation of the IMMUNOSUPPRESSANT and CYTOTOXIC methotrexate. It can be used to treat rheumatoid arthritis and as an ANTICANCER drug for lymphoblastic leukaemia, other lymphomas and some solid tumours. It is available as tablets and in forms for injection.

+▲ Side-effects/warning: See METHOTREXATE.

methotrimeprazine

(levomepromazine) is chemically a PHENOTHIAZINE. It is administered as an ANTIPSYCHOTIC drug in order to tranquillize patients who are suffering from psychotic disorders, such as schizophrenia, and also to calm and soothe patients with a terminal illness. Administration can be either oral or by injection.

+▲ Side-effects/warning: See CHLORPROMAZINE HYDROCHLORIDE; but there is more of a sedative effect and a risk of postural hypotension.

✪ Related entry: Nozinan.

methoxamine hydrochloride

is a SYMPATHOMIMETIC and VASOCONSTRICTOR drug which is used primarily to raise lowered blood pressure caused by the induction of anaesthesia. Administration is by infusion or injection.

+▲ Side-effects/warning: See NORADRENALINE. It is not used in patients with severe cardiovascular disease; there may be hypertension.

✪ Related entry: Vasoxine.

methyl cysteine hydrochloride

(mecyteine hydrochloride) is a MUCOLYTIC drug which is administered to reduce the viscosity of sputum and so acts as an EXPECTORANT in patients with disorders of the upper respiratory tract (eg chronic asthma or bronchitis). Administration is oral.

✪ Related entry: Visclair.

methyl nicotinate

is a drug with mild, local pain-relieving properties, which are principally due to its COUNTER-IRRITANT, or RUBEFACIENT, action. It can be administered to the mouth or ears in order to relieve the pain of teething, ulcers or minor scratches. Administration is by topical application.

✪ Related entries: Algipan Rub; Cremalgin Balm; Deep Heat Spray; Dubam; PR Spray; Ralgex Cream; Ralgex Heat Spray; Transvasin Heat Spray.

methyl salicylate

is used as a COUNTER-IRRITANT, or RUBEFACIENT, for local pain-relief of underlying muscle or joint pains (though how it acts is not clear). It is administered topically to the skin, and is available as a non-proprietary liniment and ointment and in several proprietary preparations as a cream or a balsam.

+ Side-effects: On topical administration there may be local irritation. It should not be used on broken skin or mucous membranes.

▲ Warning: It should not be used on broken or inflamed skin. It can cause sensitivity to bright sunlight; systemic side-effects may occur with prolonged or excessive use.

✪ Related entries: Algipan Rub; Aspellin; Balmosa Cream; Bengué's Balsam; Deep Heat Massage Liniment; Deep Heat Maximum Strength; Deep Heat Spray; Dubam; Germoline Ointment; Monphytol; PR Heat Spray; Radian B Muscle Rub; Ralgex Stick.

methyl valerate

is a constituent of a proprietary COMPOUND PREPARATION that contains several aromatic substances and which is used during withdrawal from smoking tobacco products. Administration is oral.

✪ Related entry: Nicobrevin.

methyl violet

see CRYSTAL VIOLET

M

methylcellulose

is a *bulking-agent* LAXATIVE which works by increasing the overall mass of faeces and also retaining a lot of water and so stimulating bowel movement. However, the full effect may not be achieved for many hours. It can be used in patients who cannot tolerate bran when treating a range of bowel conditions, including diverticular disease and irritable bowel syndrome. Administration is oral.

✚▲ Side-effects/warning: See ISPAGHULA HUSK.

❍ Related entry: Celevac.

methyldopa

is an ANTISYMPATHETIC drug which acts in the brain to reduce the activity of the sympathetic nervous system. It can be administered as an ANTIHYPERTENSIVE (commonly in combination with a DIURETIC) of moderate to severe hypertension. Administration can be either oral or by injection or infusion.

✚ Side-effects: There may be dry mouth, drowsiness, fluid retention, diarrhoea; sedation, depression, impaired liver function, skin and blood disorders and nasal stuffiness; parkinsonian symptoms and failure to ejaculate.

▲ Warning: It should not be administered to patients with certain blood or liver disorders, phaeochromocytoma or a history of depression. Administer with care to those with kidney damage. Regular blood counts and tests on liver function are necessary during treatment. Methyldopa may cause drowsiness and impair the performance of skilled tasks, such as driving or operating machinery; and the effects of alcohol may be enhanced.

❍ Related entries: Aldomet; Dopamet; Metalpha.

methyldopate hydrochloride

is the form of the ANTIHYPERTENSIVE drug methyldopa that is used for injection.

✚▲ Side-effects/warning: See METHYLDOPA.

methylphenidate hydrochloride

is a drug that is used to treat hyperkinesis (hyperactivity) or attention-deficit hyperactivity disorder in children. In contrast, in adults it acts as a weak STIMULANT. Administration is oral.

✚▲ Side-effects/warning: See DEXAMPHETAMINE SULPHATE; also rash, urticaria and dermatitis, fever and blood changes (requiring monitoring).

❍ Related entry: Ritalin.

methylphenobarbitone

(methyphenobarbital) is a BARBITURATE which is administered as an ANTICONVULSANT and ANTI-EPILEPTIC to treat all forms of epilepsy (except absence seizures). It is largely converted in the liver to PHENOBARBITONE and therefore has similar actions and effects. Administration is oral. Preparations containing methylphenobarbitone are on the Controlled Drugs List.

✚▲ Side-effects/warning: See BARBITURATES.

❍ Related entry: Prominal.

methylprednisolone

is a CORTICOSTEROID with ANTI-INFLAMMATORY properties. It is used to relieve the inflammation of allergic reaction, to treat cerebral oedema (fluid retention in the brain), shock, rheumatic disease and inflammatory skin disorders, such as eczema. Administration (as methylprednisolone, methylprednisolone acetate or methylprednisolone sodium succinate) can be oral, by topical application or by injection or intravenous infusion.

✚▲ Side-effects/warning: See CORTICOSTEROIDS.

❍ Related entries: Depo-Medrone; Depo-Medrone with Lidocaine; Medrone; Solu-Medrone.

methylrosanilium chloride

see CRYSTAL VIOLET

methyphenobarbital

see METHYLPHENOBARBITONE

methysergide

is a potentially dangerous drug that is used, under strict medical supervision in hospital, as an ANTIMIGRAINE treatment to prevent severe recurrent attacks and similar headaches in patients for whom other forms of treatment have failed. Administration is oral.

✚ Side-effects: Nausea, vomiting, abdominal discomfort, heartburn, insomnia, weight gain, rashes, mental disturbences, hair loss, cramps, effects on the cardiovascular system, drowsiness and dizziness.

▲ Warning: It is not to be used in patients with certain kidney, lung, liver or cardiovascular disorders; severe hypertension, urinary tract disorders, collagen disease or cellulitis; or who are pregnant or breast-feeding. Administer with caution to those with peptic ulcer. Withdrawal of treatment should be gradual.

○ Related entry: Deseril.

metipranolol

is a BETA-BLOCKER which can be used as a GLAUCOMA TREATMENT for chronic simple glaucoma. It is thought to work by slowing the rate of production of the aqueous humour in the eye. Administration is topical.

✚ Side-effects: There may be some systemic absorption after using eye-drops, so some of the side-effects listed under PROPRANOLOL HYDROCHLORIDE may be seen. Dry eyes and some local allergic reactions, including conjunctivitis of the eyelids, may also occur. Its preparation does not contain the preservative benzalkonium chloride, found in several eye-drops for glaucoma, so it can be used by patients who are allergic to this preservative and those wearing soft contact lenses.

▲ Warning: In view of possible absorption, dangerous side-effects should be borne in mind, particularly the danger of

bronchospasm in asthmatics and interactions with calcium-channel blockers.

○ Related entry: Minims Metipranolol.

metirosine

is an ANTISYMPATHETIC drug which inhibits the enzymes that produce NORADRENALINE and is used in the preoperative treatment of phaeochromocytoma. Administration is oral as capsules.

✚ Side-effects: Sedation, severe diarrhoea, sensitivity reactions and extrapyramidal symptoms.

▲ Warning: Increased fluid intake during treatment is essential. Regular checks on overall blood volume are advisable. Sedation may effect the ability to drive or operate machinery.

○ Related entry: Demser.

metoclopramide hydrochloride

is an effective ANTI-EMETIC and ANTINAUSEANT drug with useful MOTILITY STIMULANT properties. It can be used to prevent vomiting caused by gastrointestinal disorders or by chemotherapy or radiotherapy (in the treatment of cancer). It works both by a direct action on the vomiting centre of the brain (where it is an ANTAGONIST of dopamine) and by actions within the intestine. It enhances the strength of oesophageal sphincter contraction (preventing the passage of stomach contents up into the gullet), stimulates emptying of the stomach and increases the rate at which food is moved along the intestine. These last actions lead to its use in non-ulcer dyspepsia, for gastric stasis and to prevent reflux oesophagitis. Administration is either oral or by injection.

✚ Side-effects: There may be extrapyramidal effects, especially in the young and elderly; tardive dyskinesia (involuntary motor movements), raised levels of the hormone prolactin in the blood. Drowsiness, restlessness, depression and diarrhoea have been reported.

▲ Warning: It should be administered with

caution to patients with impaired kidney or liver function; porphyria; who are pregnant, breast-feeding or under 20 years old.

○ Related entries: Gastrobid Continus; Gastroflux; Gastromax; Maxolon; Migravess; Paramax; Parmid; Primperan.

metolazone

is one of the THIAZIDE class of DIURETICS. It can be used as an ANTIHYPERTENSIVE, either alone or in conjunction with other types of drugs, and also in the treatment of oedema associated with congestive heart failure. Administration is oral.

+▲ Side-effects/warning: See BENDROFLUAZIDE. There can be marked diuresis (urine production) when given with frusemide.

○ Related entry: Metenix 5.

Metopirone

(Ciba) is a proprietary, prescription-only preparation of the ENZYME INHIBITOR metyrapone. It can be used to treat conditions that result from the excessive secretion of corticosteroids into the bloodstream (eg Cushing's syndrome) and also to treat postmenopausal breast cancer. It is available as capsules.

+▲ Side-effects/warning: See METYRAPONE.

metoprolol tartrate

is a BETA-BLOCKER which can be used as an ANTIHYPERTENSIVE for raised blood pressure, as an ANTI-ANGINA treatment to relieve symptoms and improve exercise tolerance, as an ANTI-ARRHYTHMIC to regularize heartbeat and to treat myocardial infarction, as an ANTIMIGRAINE treatment to prevent migraine attacks and as an ANTITHYROID drug for short-term treatment of thyrotoxicosis. Administration is either oral or by injection. It is also available for use as an antihypertensive treatment in the form of COMPOUND PREPARATIONS with DIURETICS.

+▲ Side-effects/warning: See PROPRANOLOL HYDROCHLORIDE.

○ Related entries: Arbralene; Betaloc;

Betaloc-SA; Co-Betaloc; Co-Betaloc SA; Lopresor; Lopresor SR; Mepranix.

Metosyn

(Zeneca) is a proprietary, prescription-only preparation of the CORTICOSTEROID and ANTI-INFLAMMATORY fluocinonide. It can be used to treat severe, acute inflammatory skin disorders, such as eczema, that are unresponsive to less powerful drugs and also psoriasis. It is available as a cream, ointment or scalp lotion.

+▲ Side-effects/warning: See FLUOCINONIDE.

metriphonate

is an organophosphorus ANTHELMINTIC compound that destroys the blood fluke *Schistosoma haematobium*, which causes a form of bilharzia that is common in North Africa and the Middle East. The disease is contracted by bathing in water contaminated by fluke larvae. Adult flukes then infest the veins of the bladder, ureter and other pelvic organs, causing severe inflammation. Metriphonate has largely been superseded by PRAZIQUANTEL. Administration is oral, and it is not available in the UK.

Metrodin High Purity

(Serono) is a proprietary, prescription-only preparation of urofollitrophin, which is a form of the pituitary HORMONE, follicle-stimulating hormone (FSH), and is prepared from human menopausal urine that contains FSH. It can be used primarily to treat women suffering from specific hormonal deficiencies in infertility treatment and in assisted conception (eg in *in vitro* fertilization; IVF). It is available in a form for injection.

+▲ Side-effects/warning: See UROFOLLITROPHIN.

Metrogel

(Sandoz) is a proprietary, prescription-only preparation of the ANTIMICROBIAL metronidazole, which has ANTIBACTERIAL and

ANTIPROTOZOAL actions. It can be applied topically as a gel to treat acute acne rosacea outbreaks.

+▲ Side-effects/warning: See METRONIDAZOLE.

Metrolyl

(Lagap) is a proprietary, prescription-only preparation of the ANTIMICROBIAL metronidazole, which has ANTIBACTERIAL and ANTIPROTOZOAL actions. It can be used to treat bacterial infections, such as vaginitis, dental infections, and infections that can occur after surgery. Its antiprotozoal activity is effective against the organisms that cause amoebic dysentery, giardiasis and trichomoniasis. It is available as tablets.

+▲ Side-effects/warning: See METRONIDAZOLE.

metronidazole

is an (AZOLE) ANTIMICROBIAL drug with ANTIBACTERIAL and ANTIPROTOZOAL actions. As an antibacterial agent its spectrum is narrow, being limited to activity against anaerobic bacteria, including bacterial vaginal infections caused by *Gardnerella vaginalis*, dental infections, leg ulcers, pressure sores and during surgery. It acts by interfering with bacterial DNA replication. As an antiprotozoal it is specifically active against the protozoa *Entamoeba histolytica* (which causes dysentery), *Giardia lamblia* (giardiasis; an infection of the small intestine) and *Trichomonas vaginalis* (vaginitis). It is also used to treat outbreaks of acne rosacea and to deodorize fungating, malodorous tumours. Additionally, it has been used to treat guinea worms (*Dracunculus medinensis*). Administration can be oral as tablets or a suspension (as metronidazole benzoate), topical in the form of anal suppositories or vaginal pessaries or by injection or infusion.

+ Side-effects: These include nausea and vomiting with drowsiness, headache, rashes and itching. Some patients experience a discolouration of the urine. Prolonged treatment may eventually cause neuromuscular disorders or seizures.

▲ Warning: It should be administered with caution to patients with impaired liver function or who are pregnant or breast-feeding. During treatment patients must avoid alcohol, which would cause very unpleasant side-effects.

✪ Related entries: Anabact; Dentomycin; Elyzol; Flagyl; Flagyl Compak; Flagyl S; Metrogel; Metrolyl; Metrotop; Vaginyl; Zadstat.

Metrotop

(Pharmacia) is a proprietary, prescription-only preparation of the ANTIMICROBIAL metronidazole, which has both ANTIPROTOZOAL and ANTIBACTERIAL properties. It can be used to deodorize and treat fungating, malodorous tumours, and is available as a gel for topical application.

+▲ Side-effects/warning: See METRONIDAZOLE.

metyrapone

is an ENZYME INHIBITOR that inhibits the production of both *glucocorticoid* and *mineralocorticoid* CORTICOSTEROIDS by the adrenal glands. It can therefore be used to treat conditions that result from the excessive secretion of corticosteroids into the bloodstream (such as Cushing's syndrome). It can also be used as an ANTICANCER treatment of postmenopausal breast cancer. Administration is oral.

+ Side-effects: Occasional nausea and vomiting, dizziness, headache, hypotension and allergic reactions.

▲ Warning: It is not to be used in patients with adrenal insufficiency; or who are pregnant or breast-feeding. Administer with care to those with hypopituitary function.

✪ Related entry: Metopirone.

mexiletine hydrochloride

is an ANTI-ARRHYTHMIC drug which is used to reduce heartbeat irregularities, particularly after a heart attack. Administration is either oral or by injection or infusion.

M

✚ Side-effects: Slowing of the heart and low blood pressure; nausea and vomiting; constipation; tremor, eye-twitch, confusion; jaundice and hepatitis; blood disorders.

▲ Warning: It should not be administered to patients who have a slow heart rate or heart block; and use with care in those with certain liver disorders.

○ Related entries: Mexitil; Mexitil PL.

Mexitil

(Boehringer Ingelheim) is a proprietary, prescription-only preparation of the ANTI-ARRHYTHMIC drug mexiletine hydrochloride. It can be used to treat irregularities of the heartbeat, and is available as capsules and in a form for injection or infusion.

✚▲ Side-effects/warning: See MEXILETINE HYDROCHLORIDE.

Mexitil PL

(Boehringer Ingelheim) is a proprietary, prescription-only preparation of the ANTI-ARRHYTHMIC drug mexiletine hydrochloride. It can be used to treat irregularities of the heartbeat, and is available as modified-release capsules (*Perlongets*).

✚▲ Side-effects/warning: See MEXILETINE HYDROCHLORIDE.

Miacalcic

(Sandoz) is a proprietary, prescription-only preparation of the THYROID HORMONE calcitonin, in the form of salcatonin. It can be used to lower blood levels of calcium when they are abnormally high (hypercalcaemia) and to treat Paget's disease of the bone. It is available in a form for subcutaneous, intramuscular or intravenous injection.

✚▲ Side-effects/warning: See SALCATONIN.

mianserin hydrochloride

is a TRICYCLIC-related ANTIDEPRESSANT which is used to treat depressive illness, especially in cases where a degree of SEDATION may be useful. Administration is oral.

✚▲ Side-effects/warning: See AMITRIPTYLINE HYDROCHLORIDE; but

potentially serious blood disorders may be seen (a regular full blood count is necessary). Flu-like symptoms may occur with painful joints and jaundice.

Micanol

(Evans) is a proprietary, non-prescription preparation of dithranol. It can be used to treat subacute and chronic psoriasis, and is available as a cream.

✚▲ Side-effects/warning: See DITHRANOL.

Micolette Micro-enema

(Cusi) is a proprietary, non-prescription preparation of sodium citrate, sodium alkylsulphoacetate, sorbic acid and GLYCEROL. It can be used as a LAXATIVE, and is administered as an enema.

✚▲ Side-effects/warning: See SODIUM CITRATE.

miconazole

is an (AZOLE) ANTIFUNGAL drug which can be used to treat and prevent many forms of fungal infection, including athlete's foot, oropharyngial infections such as aspergillosis, candidiasis, acne and intestinal infection. In solution, the drug can be used for irrigation of the bladder. Administration can be oral, by topical application or by injection (for systemic infections).

✚ Side-effects: Nausea and vomiting, pruritus and rashes. The injection form contains a derivative of castor oil that may cause sensitivity reactions.

▲ Warning: It is not to be used in patients with porphyria; administer with care to those who are pregnant.

○ Related entries: Acnidazil; Benoxyl 5 Cream; Benoxyl 10 Lotion; Daktacort; Daktarin; Daktarin Cream; Daktarin Oral Gel; Daktarin Powder; Daktarin Spray Powder; Femeron; Femeron Soft Pessary; Gyno-Daktarin; Nericur.

Micralax Micro-enema

(Evans) is a proprietary, non-prescription preparation of sodium citrate, sodium alkylsulphoacetate and sorbic acid. It can be used as a LAXATIVE, and is available as an enema.

✚▲ Side-effects/warning: See SODIUM CITRATE.

Microgynon 30

(Schering) is a proprietary, prescription-only COMPOUND PREPARATION which can be used as a (*monophasic*) ORAL CONTRACEPTIVE (and also for certain menstrual problems) of the type that combines an OESTROGEN and a PROGESTOGEN, in this case ethinyloestradiol and levonorgestrel. It is available as tablets in a calendar pack.

✚▲ Side-effects/warning: See ETHINYLOESTRADIOL; LEVONORGESTREL.

Micronor

(Ortho) is a proprietary, prescription-only preparation which can be used as an ORAL CONTRACEPTIVE of the PROGESTOGEN-only pill (POP) type and contains norethisterone. It is available as tablets in a calendar pack.

✚▲ Side-effects/warning: See NORETHISTERONE.

Micronor HRT

(Cilag) is a proprietary, prescription-only preparation of the PROGESTOGEN norethisterone. It can be used in HRT, and is available as tablets.

✚▲ Side-effects/warning: See NORETHISTERONE.

Microval

(Wyeth) is a proprietary, prescription-only preparation which can be used as an ORAL CONTRACEPTIVE of the PROGESTOGEN-only pill (POP) type and contains levonorgestrel. It is available as tablets in a calendar pack.

✚▲ Side-effects/warning: See LEVONORGESTREL.

Mictral

(Sanofi Winthrop) is a proprietary, prescription-only preparation of the ANTIBACTERIAL and (QUINOLONE) ANTIBIOTIC nalidixic acid. It can be used to treat infections, particularly of the urinary tract and including cystitis, and is available as granules.

✚▲ Side-effects/warning: See NALIDIXIC ACID.

midazolam

is a BENZODIAZEPINE which can be used as an ANXIOLYTIC and SEDATIVE in preoperative medication, because its ability to cause amnesia means that the patient forgets the unpleasant procedure. Administration is by injection.

✚▲ Side-effects/warning: See BENZODIAZEPINES; but the incidence of side-effects is lower than in some other benzodiazepines; it may cause respiratory depression after injection.

✪ Related entry: Hypnovel.

Midrid

(Shire) is a proprietary, non-prescription COMPOUND PREPARATION of the SYMPATHOMIMETIC and VASOCONSTRICTOR isometheptene mucate and the NON-NARCOTIC ANALGESIC paracetamol. It can be used to relieve acute migraine attacks and other headaches, and is available as capsules; it is not to be given to children.

✚▲ Side-effects/warning: See ISOMETHEPTENE MUCATE; PARACETAMOL.

Mifegyne

(Roussel) is a proprietary, prescription-only preparation of the uterine stimulant mifepristone. It is used as an ABORTIFACIENT for termination of pregnancy at up to 63 days of gestation, and is available as tablets.

✚▲ Side-effects/warning: See MIFEPRISTONE.

mifepristone

is a progestogen HORMONE ANTAGONIST which is used as an ABORTIFACIENT for termination of uterine pregnancy at up to 63 days of gestation. It is taken by mouth as tablets and under medical supervision with monitoring and followed, if necessary, with

M a PROSTAGLANDIN (eg GEMEPROST or DINOPROSTONE).

✚ Side-effects: Vaginal bleeding (which can be severe), uterine pain, nausea and vomiting, faintness, hypotension, rashes; infections of the uterus and urinary tract.

▲ Warning: To be used to terminate ectopic pregnancy; not to be used with certain adrenal gland disorders, certain blood disorders or by smokers over 35 years old. Administer with caution to patients with certain cardiovascular diseases, asthma, liver or kidney disorders, with a history of heart infection (endocarditis) or who have artificial heart valves.

⊘ Related entry: Mifegyne.

Migraleve

(Pfizer) is a proprietary, non-prescription COMPOUND PREPARATION which is used for acute migraine attacks, not for preventing them (prophylactically). It is available in the form of two types of tablets wrapped in different colours: a pink pack (1) containing the ANTIHISTAMINE buclizine hydrochloride, the NON-NARCOTIC ANALGESIC paracetamol and the (OPIOID) NARCOTIC ANALGESIC codeine phosphate; and a yellow pack (2), containing tablets without buclizine hydrochloride. There is a further form called *Migraleve Duo* which contains both types (1 and 2). The preparations are not normally given to children under ten years, except on medical advice.

✚▲ Side-effects/warning: See BUCLIZINE HYDROCHLORIDE; CODEINE PHOSPHATE; PARACETAMOL.

Migravess

(Bayer) is a proprietary, prescription-only COMPOUND PREPARATION of the ANTI-EMETIC and ANTINAUSEANT metoclopramide hydrochloride and the (NSAID) NON-NARCOTIC ANALGESIC aspirin. It can be used as an ANTIMIGRAINE treatment for acute migraine attacks. It is available as effervescent tablets and also as a stronger preparation called *Migravess Forte*.

✚▲ Side-effects/warning: See ASPIRIN;

METOCLOPRAMIDE HYDROCHLORIDE. Note the side-effects of metoclopramide hydrochloride in young people.

Migril

(Wellcome) is a proprietary, prescription-only COMPOUND PREPARATION of the ergot VASOCONSTRICTOR ergotamine tartrate, the ANTINAUSEANT cyclizine (as hydrochloride) and the STIMULANT caffeine (as hydrate). It can be used as an ANTIMIGRAINE treatment and also for some other vascular headaches, and is available as tablets.

✚▲ Side-effects/warning: See CAFFEINE; CYCLIZINE; ERGOTAMINE TARTRATE.

Mil-Par

(SmithKline Beecham) is a proprietary, non-prescription COMPOUND PREPARATION of the LAXATIVES liquid paraffin and magnesium hydroxide. It can be used for the temporary relief of constipation, and is available as a liquid suspension.

✚▲ Side-effects/warning: See LIQUID PARAFFIN; MAGNESIUM HYDROXIDE.

Mildison

(Yamanouchi) is a proprietary, prescription-only preparation of the CORTICOSTEROID and ANTI-INFLAMMATORY hydrocortisone. It can be used to treat mild inflammatory skin conditions, such as eczema, and is available as a cream.

✚▲ Side-effects/warning: See HYDROCORTISONE.

Milk of Magnesia Liquid

(SmithKline Beecham) is a proprietary, non-prescription preparation of the ANTACID magnesium hydroxide. It can be used for the relief of stomach discomfort, indigestion, hyperacidity, heartburn, flatulence and constipation. It is available as a suspension (and also as *Raspberry Milkshake Flavour*) and is not normally given to children under one year, except on medical advice.

✚▲ Side-effects/warning: See MAGNESIUM HYDROXIDE.

Milk of Magnesia Tablets

(SmithKline Beecham) is a proprietary, non-prescription preparation of the ANTACID magnesium hydroxide. It can be used for the relief of indigestion, nausea, biliousness, acid stomach, heartburn and flatulence. It is available as tablets and is not normally given to children under one year, except on medical advice.

+▲ Side-effects/warning: See MAGNESIUM HYDROXIDE.

milrinone

is a PHOSPHODIESTERASE INHIBITOR which is used, in the short term, in congestive HEART FAILURE TREATMENT (especially where other drugs have been unsuccessful) and in acute heart failure. Administration is by injection.

+▲ Side-effects/warning: See ENOXIMONE. Blood potassium should be controlled and kidney function monitored. It may cause chest pain.

✪ Related entry: Primacor.

Min-I-Jet Adrenaline

(IMS) is a proprietary, prescription-only preparation of the natural HORMONE adrenaline (as adrenaline hydrochloride). It is used as a SYMPATHOMIMETIC drug to treat acute and severe bronchial asthma attacks, in the emergency treatment of acute allergic reactions and for angio-oedema and cardiopulmonary resuscitation. It is available in a form for intramuscular, subcutaneous or intravenous injection.

+▲ Side-effects/warning: See ADRENALINE.

Min-I-Jet Aminophylline

(IMS) is a proprietary, prescription-only preparation of the BRONCHODILATOR aminophylline. It can be used to treat severe acute asthma attacks, and is available in a form for injection.

+▲ Side-effects/warning: See AMINOPHYLLINE.

Min-I-Jet Bretylate Tosylate

(IMS) is a proprietary, prescription-only preparation of the ADRENERGIC-NEURONE BLOCKER bretylium tosylate. It can be used in resuscitation and as an ANTI-ARRHYTHMIC treatment of ventricular arrhythmias where other treatments have not been successful. It is available in a form for injection.

+▲ Side-effects/warning: See BRETYLIUM TOSYLATE.

Min-I-Jet Frusemide

(IMS) is a proprietary, prescription-only preparation of the (*loop*) DIURETIC frusemide. It can be used to treat oedema, particularly pulmonary (lung) oedema in patients with chronic heart failure, and low urine production due to kidney failure (oliguria). It is available in a form for injection or infusion.

+▲ Side-effects/warning: See FRUSEMIDE.

Min-I-Jet Isoprenaline

(IMS) is a proprietary, prescription-only preparation of the BETA-RECEPTOR STIMULANT and SYMPATHOMIMETIC isoprenaline (as isoprenaline hydrochloride). It can be used as a CARDIAC STIMULANT to treat acute heart block and severe bradycardia, and is available in a form for intravenous injection.

+▲ Side-effects/warning: See ISOPRENALINE.

Min-I-Jet Lignocaine

(IMS) is a proprietary, prescription-only preparation of the LOCAL ANAESTHETIC lignocaine hydrochloride. It can be used as an ANTI-ARRHYTHMIC drug to treat irregularities in the heartbeat, especially after a heart attack, and is available in a form for injection.

+▲ Side-effects/warning: See LIGNOCAINE HYDROCHLORIDE.

Min-I-Jet Lignocaine Hydrochloride with Adrenaline

(IMS) is a proprietary, prescription-only COMPOUND PREPARATION of the LOCAL ANAESTHETIC lignocaine hydrochloride and adrenaline. It can be used for dental

365

M anaesthesia and a variety of surgical procedures after local injection. It is available in a form for injection.
+▲ Side-effects/warning: See ADRENALINE; LIGNOCAINE HYDROCHLORIDE.

Min-I-Jet Mannitol (25%)

(IMS) is a proprietary, prescription-only preparation of the (*osmotic*) DIURETIC mannitol. It can be used in GLAUCOMA TREATMENT and to treat oedema, and is available as a 25% solution for intravenous infusion.
+▲ Side-effects/warning: See MANNITOL.

Min-I-Jet Morphine Sulphate

(IMS) is a proprietary, prescription-only preparation of the (OPIOID) NARCOTIC ANALGESIC morphine sulphate, and is on the Controlled Drugs List. It can be used to treat severe pain, for example, in patients who have a terminally illness, and is available in disposable syringes ready for use.
+▲ Side-effects/warning: See MORPHINE SULPHATE.

Min-I-Jet Naloxone

(IMS) is a proprietary, prescription-only preparation of the OPIOID ANTAGONIST drug naloxone hydrochloride. It can be used to treat patients who have taken an overdose of opioids and also postoperative respiratory depression (which has been caused by opioid analgesia during operations), and is available in syringes ready for use.
+▲ Side-effects/warning: See NALOXONE HYDROCHLORIDE.

Min-I-Jet Sodium Bicarbonate

(IMS) is a proprietary, prescription-only preparation of sodium bicarbonate. It can be used to treat metabolic acidosis, and is available in a form for injection.
+▲ Side-effects/warning: See SODIUM BICARBONATE.

mineral supplements 🔢

are formulations of some of the salts of essential (required in the diet) dietary minerals, which may be taken, usually by mouth, to make up deficiencies in the diet, or where there are problems with absorption of the minerals into the body from normal foodstuffs. Examples include: CALCIUM, IRON, phosphorus, potassium, sodium and zinc.

Minihep

(Leo) is a proprietary, prescription-only preparation of the ANTICOAGULANT heparin (as heparin sodium). It can be used to treat various forms of thrombosis, and is available in a form for injection.
+▲ Side-effects/warning: See HEPARIN.

Minihep Calcium

(Leo) is a proprietary, prescription-only preparation of the ANTICOAGULANT heparin (as heparin calcium). It can be used to treat various forms of thrombosis, and is available in a form for injection.
+▲ Side-effects/warning: See HEPARIN.

Minims Amethocaine Hydrochloride

(Chauvin) is a proprietary, prescription-only preparation of the LOCAL ANAESTHETIC amethocaine hydrochloride. It can be used by topical application for ophthalmic procedures, and is available as eye-drops.
+▲ Side-effects/warning: See AMETHOCAINE HYDROCHLORIDE.

Minims Artificial Tears

(Chauvin) is a proprietary, non-prescription preparation of HYDROXYETHYLCELLULOSE. It is used as artificial tears where there is dryness of the eyes due to disease, and is available as eye-drops.

Minims Atropine Sulphate

(Chauvin) is a proprietary, prescription-only preparation of the ANTICHOLINERGIC drug atropine sulphate. It can be used to

dilate the pupils and so facilitate inspection of the eyes, and is available as eye-drops.
+▲ Side-effects/warning: See ATROPINE SULPHATE.

Minims Benoxinate (Oxybuprocaine) Hydrochloride

(Chauvin) is a proprietary, prescription-only preparation of the LOCAL ANAESTHETIC oxybuprocaine hydrochloride. It can be used by topical application for ophthalmic procedures, and is available as eye-drops.
+▲ Side-effects/warning: See OXYBUPROCAINE HYDROCHLORIDE.

Minims Chloramphenicol

(Chauvin) is a proprietary, prescription-only preparation of the ANTIBACTERIAL and ANTIBIOTIC chloramphenicol. It can be used to treat bacterial infections in the eye, and is available as eye-drops.
+▲ Side-effects/warning: See CHLORAMPHENICOL.

Minims Cyclopentolate

(Chauvin) is a proprietary, prescription-only preparation of the ANTICHOLINERGIC drug cyclopentolate hydrochloride. It can be used to dilate the pupil and paralyse focusing and so facilitate inspection of the eyes, and is available as eye-drops.
+▲ Side-effects/warning: See CYCLOPENTOLATE HYDROCHLORIDE.

Minims Fluorescein Sodium

(Chauvin) is a proprietary, non-prescription preparation of the dye FLUORESCEIN SODIUM. It can be used on the surface of the eye in order to carry out ophthalmic diagnostic procedures, and is available as eye-drops.

Minims Gentamicin

(Chauvin) is a proprietary, prescription-only preparation of the ANTIBACTERIAL and (AMINOGLYCOSIDE) ANTIBIOTIC gentamicin (as sulphate). It can be used to treat an extensive range of infection, particularly

serious infections caused by Gram-negative bacteria, and is available as an eye ointment.
+▲ Side-effects/warning: See GENTAMICIN.

Minims Homatropine Hydrobromide

(Chauvin) is a proprietary, prescription-only preparation of the ANTICHOLINERGIC drug homatropine hydrobromide. It can be used to dilate the pupils and paralyse certain eye muscles in order to carry out ophthalmic examination, and is available as eye-drops.
+▲ Side-effects/warning: See HOMATROPINE HYDROBROMIDE.

Minims Lignocaine and Fluorescein

(Chauvin) is a proprietary, prescription-only preparation of the LOCAL ANAESTHETIC lignocaine hydrochloride (with the diagnostic dye fluorescein). It is used in ophthalmic diagnostic procedures, and is available as eye-drops.
+▲ Side-effects/warning: See LIGNOCAINE HYDROCHLORIDE.

Minims Metipranolol

(Chauvin) is a proprietary, prescription-only preparation of the BETA-BLOCKER metipranolol. It can be used for GLAUCOMA TREATMENT, and is available as eye-drops.
+▲ Side-effects/warning: See METIPRANOLOL. It is used by patients allergic to the preservative benzalkonium chloride, which is found in several other similar eye-drops, and can be used by those wearing soft contact lenses.

Minims Neomycin Sulphate

(Chauvin) is a proprietary, prescription-only preparation of the ANTIBACTERIAL and (AMINOGLYCOSIDE) ANTIBIOTIC neomycin sulphate. It can be used to treat bacterial infections in the eye, and is available as eye-drops.
+▲ Side-effects/warning: See NEOMYCIN SULPHATE.

M

Minims Phenylephrine Hydrochloride

(Chauvin) is a proprietary, non-prescription preparation of the SYMPATHOMIMETIC drug phenylephrine hydrochloride. It can be used to dilate the pupils for ophthalmic examination, and is available as eye-drops.
✚▲ Side-effects/warning: See PHENYLEPHRINE HYDROCHLORIDE.

Minims Pilocarpine Nitrate

(Chauvin) is a proprietary, prescription-only preparation of the PARASYMPATHOMIMETIC pilocarpine. It can be used to constrict the pupil and in GLAUCOMA TREATMENT, and is available as eye-drops.
✚▲ Side-effects/warning: See PILOCARPINE.

Minims Prednisolone

(Chauvin) is a proprietary, prescription-only preparation of the CORTICOSTEROID and ANTI-INFLAMMATORY prednisolone (as sodium phosphate). It can be used to treat conditions in and around the eye, and is available as eye-drops.
✚▲ Side-effects/warning: See PREDNISOLONE.

Minims Proxymetacaine Hydrochloride

(Chauvin) is a proprietary, prescription-only preparation of the LOCAL ANAESTHETIC proxymetacaine (as hydrochloride). It can be used during ophthalmic procedures, and is available as eye-drops.
✚▲ Side-effects/warning: See PROXYMETACAINE.

Minims Rose Bengal

(Chauvin) is a proprietary, non-prescription preparation of the dye ROSE BENGAL. It can be used on the surface of the eye for ophthalmic diagnostic procedures, and is available as eye-drops.

Minims Sodium Chloride

(Chauvin) is a proprietary, non-prescription preparation of saline solution (sodium chloride). It can be used for the irrigation of the eyes and to facilitate the removal of harmful substances, and is available as eye-drops.
✚▲ Side-effects/warning: See SODIUM CHLORIDE.

Minims Tropicamide

(Chauvin) is a proprietary, prescription-only preparation of tropicamide. It can be used to dilate the pupils to facilitate inspection of the eyes, and is available as eye-drops.
✚▲ Side-effects/warning: See TROPICAMIDE.

Minitran

(3M) is a proprietary, non-prescription preparation of the VASODILATOR and ANTI-ANGINA drug glyceryl trinitrate. It can be used to treat and prevent angina pectoris. It is available as a self-adhesive dressing (patch) from which, when placed on the chest wall, it is absorbed through the skin and helps to give lasting relief.
✚▲ Side-effects/warning: See GLYCERYL TRINITRATE.

Minocin

(Lederle) is a proprietary, prescription-only preparation of the ANTIBACTERIAL and (TETRACYCLINE) ANTIBIOTIC minocycline. It can be used to treat a wide range of infections, and is available as tablets.
✚▲ Side-effects/warning: See MINOCYCLINE.

Minocin MR

(Lederle) is a proprietary, prescription-only preparation of the ANTIBACTERIAL and (TETRACYCLINE) ANTIBIOTIC minocycline. It can be used to treat a wide range of infections (including acne), and is available as capsules.
✚▲ Side-effects/warning: See MINOCYCLINE.

minocycline

is a broad-spectrum ANTIBACTERIAL and (TETRACYCLINE) ANTIBIOTIC. It has a wider range of action than most other tetracyclines, because it is also effective in preventing certain forms of meningitis (caused by *Neisseria meningitidis*). Administration is oral.

✚▲ Side-effects/warning: See TETRACYCLINE. It may cause dizziness and vertigo, rashes and pigmentation. There have been reports of liver damage. It can be used in patients with impaired kidney function.

○ Related entries: Aknemin; Blemix; Minocin; Minocin MR.

Minodiab

(Pharmacia) is a proprietary, prescription-only preparation of the SULPHONYLUREA glipizide. It is used in DIABETIC TREATMENT of Type II diabetes (non-insulin-dependent diabetes mellitus; NIDDM; maturity-onset diabetes), and is available as tablets.

✚▲ Side-effects/warning: See GLIPIZIDE.

minor tranquillizer

see ANXIOLYTICS

minoxidil

is a VASODILATOR which can be used as an ANTIHYPERTENSIVE (often combined with a DIURETIC or BETA-BLOCKER). Administration is oral. It can also be used, as a lotion, to treat male-pattern baldness (in men and women).

✚ Side-effects: There are gastrointestinal disturbances and weight gain; there may also be fluid retention, a rise in the heart rate and breast tenderness. When used topically to the scalp, there may be itching and dermatitis.

▲ Warning: It should not be administered to patients with phaeochromocytoma or porphyria. Administer with care to those who are pregnant or have certain heart disorders. When used as a lotion, avoid contact with the eyes and mucous membranes.

○ Related entries: Loniten; Regaine.

Mintec

(Monmouth) is a proprietary, non-prescription preparation of the ANTISPASMODIC peppermint oil. It can be used to relieve the discomfort of abdominal colic and distension, particularly in irritable bowel syndrome, and is available as capsules.

✚▲ Side-effects/warning: See PEPPERMINT OIL.

Mintezol

(Merck Sharp & Dohme) is a proprietary, non-prescription preparation of the ANTHELMINTIC drug thiabendazole. It can be used to treat intestinal infestations, especially by the *Strongyloides* species, and to assist in the treatment of resistant infections by hookworm, whipworm and roundworm. It is available as chewable tablets.

✚▲ Side-effects/warning: See THIABENDAZOLE.

Minulet

(Wyeth) is a proprietary, prescription-only COMPOUND PREPARATION that can be used as a (*monophasic*) ORAL CONTRACEPTIVE (and also for certain menstrual problems) of the type that combines an OESTROGEN and a PROGESTOGEN, in this case ethinyloestradiol and gestodene. It is available as tablets in a calendar pack.

✚▲ Side-effects/warning: See DESOGESTREL; GESTODENE.

Miochol

(Ciba Vision) is a proprietary, prescription-only preparation of the PARASYMPATHOMIMETIC acetylcholine chloride. It is used mainly to contract the pupils prior to surgery on the iris, the cornea or other sections of the exterior of the eye. It is available as a solution for intraocular irrigation.

✚▲ Side-effects/warning: See ACETYLCHOLINE CHLORIDE.

Mirena

(Pharmacia-Leiras) is a proprietary, prescription-only CONTRACEPTIVE device that releases the PROGESTOGEN levonorgestrel. It is available in the form of an intrauterine system, a T-shaped plastic frame with a drug reservoir and threads attached to the base.

✚▲ Side-effects/warning: See LEVONORGESTREL.

misoprostol

is a synthetic analogue of the PROSTAGLANDIN E₁ (ALPROSTADIL). It can be used as an ULCER-HEALING DRUG, because it inhibits acid secretion and promotes protective blood flow to the mucosal layer of the intestine. It cannot be used to treat dyspepsia, but can be very useful in protecting against ulcers caused by non-steroidal anti-inflammatory drugs (NSAIDS) and for this reason is now available in combination with some (NSAID) non-narcotic analgesic AND ANTIRHEUMATIC drugs (eg *Arthrotec* and *Napratec*) in the treatment of rheumatic disease. Administration is oral.

✚ Side-effects: Diarrhoea (which may be severe), nausea, flatulence and vomiting, abdominal pain, dyspepsia, abnormal vaginal bleeding, dizziness and rashes.

▲ Warning: It should not be administered to women who are pregnant or planning pregnancy; and used with caution in patients with severe hypotension.

✪ Related entries: Arthrotec; Cytotec; Napratec.

mitomycin

is a CYTOTOXIC drug (of ANTIBIOTIC origin), which is used as an ANTICANCER treatment of cancers of the upper gastrointestinal tract, recurrent superficial bladder tumours and breast tumours. Administration is by injection or bladder instillation.

✚▲ Side-effects/warning: See CYTOTOXICS. It can cause lung fibrosis and kidney damage.

✪ Related entry: Mitomycin C Kyowa.

Mitomycin C Kyowa

(Kyowa Hakko) is a proprietary, prescription-only preparation of the (CYTOTOXIC) ANTICANCER drug mitomycin.

It can be used in the treatment of upper gastrointestinal cancer, breast cancer and some superficial bladder tumours. It is available in forms for injection and for bladder instillation.

✚▲ Side-effects/warning: See MITOMYCIN.

Mitoxana

(ASTA Medica) is a proprietary, prescription-only preparation of the (CYTOTOXIC) ANTICANCER drug ifosfamide, which can be used in the treatment of cancer. It is available in a form for injection.

✚▲ Side-effects/warning: See IFOSFAMIDE.

mitoxantrone

see MITOZANTRONE

mitozantrone

(mitoxantrone) is a CYTOTOXIC drug that is chemically related to doxorubicin. It is administered as an ANTICANCER treatment for several types of cancer, for example, breast cancer. Administration is by intravenous infusion.

✚▲ Side-effects/warning: See CYTOTOXICS; there are also effects on the heart.

✪ Related entry: Novantrone.

Mivacron

(Wellcome) is a proprietary, prescription-only preparation of the (*non-depolarizing*) SKELETAL MUSCLE RELAXANT mivacurium chloride. It can be used to induce muscle paralysis during surgery, and is available in a form for injection.

✚▲ Side-effects/warning: See MIVACURIUM CHLORIDE.

mivacurium chloride

is a (*non-depolarizing*) SKELETAL MUSCLE RELAXANT which is used to induce muscle paralysis during surgery. Administration is by injection.

✚▲ Side-effects/warning: See TUBOCURARINE CHLORIDE. It may cause the release of histamine.

✪ Related entry: Mivacron.

M

Mixtard 30/70

(Novo Nordisk, Wellcome) is a proprietary, non-prescription preparation of (mixed) BIPHASIC ISOPHANE INSULIN, highly purified porcine insulins. It is used as a DIABETIC TREATMENT to treat and maintain diabetic patients. It is a preparation of both neutral (30%) and isophane (70%) insulins, and is available in vials for injection and has an intermediate duration of action. HUMAN MIXTARD 30/70 is also available.

✚▲ Side-effects/warning: See INSULIN.

MMR

(District Health Authorities) is a proprietary, prescription-only preparation of a VACCINE that can be used for the prevention of measles, mumps and rubella (German measles) in children. It is available in a form for injection.

✚▲ Side-effects/warning: See MMR VACCINE.

MMR II

(Merck Sharp & Dohme) is a proprietary, prescription-only preparation of a VACCINE that can be used for the prevention of measles, mumps and rubella (German measles) in children. It is available in a form for injection.

✚▲ Side-effects/warning: See MMR VACCINE.

MMR vaccine

is a combined VACCINE used for IMMUNIZATION against measles, mumps and rubella. It uses live but weakened (attenuated) strains of the viruses and was introduced with the objective of eliminating rubella (German measles) through universal vaccination of children before they began school. The vaccine is available from District Health Authorities under a number of names that include 'MMR II'.

✚▲ Side-effects/warning: See VACCINES. There may be fever, malaise and/or rash about a week after administration; there may be a swelling of the parotid gland (salivary gland in the jaw) after two to three weeks.

◯ Related entries: MMR; MMR II.

Mobic

(Boehringer Ingelheim) is a proprietary, prescription-only preparation of the (NSAID) NON-NARCOTIC ANALGESIC and ANTIRHEUMATIC meloxicam. It can be used to treat pain and inflammation in rheumatoid arthritis, and for short-term exacerbation of osteoarthritis. It is available as tablets and suppositories.

✚▲ Side-effects/warning: See MELOXICAM.

Mobiflex

(Roche) is a proprietary, prescription-only preparation of the (NSAID) NON-NARCOTIC ANALGESIC and ANTIRHEUMATIC tenoxicam. It can be used to treat the pain and inflammation of rheumatism and other musculoskeletal disorders. It is available as tablets or in a form for injection.

✚▲ Side-effects/warning: See TENOXICAM.

Mobilan

(Galen) is a proprietary, prescription-only preparation of the (NSAID) NON-NARCOTIC ANALGESIC and ANTIRHEUMATIC indomethacin. It can be used to treat the pain and inflammation of rheumatism and other musculoskeletal disorders, and is available as capsules.

✚▲ Side-effects/warning: See INDOMETHACIN.

moclobemide

is a recently introduced type of MONOAMINE-OXIDASE INHIBITOR (MAOI) ANTIDEPRESSANT which is used to treat major depressive illness. It is a reversible inhibitor of the monoamine oxidase type A (therefore termed RIMA) and reported to show less potentiation of dangerous side-effects of tyramine found in foodstuffs (a common side-effect of other MAOIs). Interactions with other medicines is also claimed to be less. It should not be used in conjunction with conventional MAO inhibitors, but in view of its short duration of action the switch to other forms of antidepressant may be quicker than is usual. However, there may be a more STIMULANT action than with

M

most other MAOIs, making it less suitable for agitated patients. Administration is oral.
✚ Side-effects: There is some stimulation resulting in restlessness, agitation, sleep disturbances; also dizziness, nausea, confusion, changes in liver enzymes and lowered blood sodium.
▲ Warning: Avoid its use in patients who are agitated or confused; those with severe liver disorders, thyroid imbalance or phaeochromocytoma; or who are pregnant or breast-feeding.
❍ Related entry: Manerix.

Modalim

(Sanofi Winthrop) is a proprietary, prescription-only preparation of the LIPID-LOWERING DRUG ciprofibrate. It can be used in hyperlipidaemia to reduce the levels, or change the proportions, of various lipids in the bloodstream, and is available as tablets.
✚▲ Side-effects/warning: See CIPROFIBRATE.

Modecate

(Sanofi Winthrop) is a proprietary, prescription-only preparation of the ANTIPSYCHOTIC drug fluphenazine decanoate. It can be used in the long-term maintenance of tranquillization for patients with psychotic disorders (including schizophrenia). It is available in two strengths for depot deep intramuscular injection; the stronger preparation is called *Modecate Concentrate*.
✚▲ Side-effects/warning: See FLUPHENAZINE DECANOATE.

Moditen

(Sanofi Winthrop) is a proprietary, prescription-only preparation of the ANTIPSYCHOTIC drug fluphenazine. It can be used in the long-term maintenance of tranquillization for patients suffering from psychotic disorders (including schizophrenia) and for the short-term control of severe manic or violent agitated states. It is available as tablets (as

fluphenazine hydrochloride) and in a form for depot deep intramuscular injection (as fluphenazine decanoate).
✚▲ Side-effects/warning: See FLUPHENAZINE HYDROCHLORIDE.

Modrasone

(Schering-Plough) is a proprietary, prescription-only preparation of the CORTICOSTEROID and ANTI-INFLAMMATORY alclometasone dipropionate. It can be used to treat inflammatory skin conditions, such as eczema, and is available as a cream and an ointment for topical application.
✚▲ Side-effects/warning: See ALCLOMETASONE DIPROPIONATE.

Modrenal

(Sterling) is a proprietary, prescription-only preparation of the ENZYME INHIBITOR trilostane. It can be used to treat conditions that result from the excessive secretion of corticosteroids into the bloodstream (eg Cushing's syndrome). It can also be used in the ANTICANCER treatment of postmenopausal breast cancer. It is available as capsules.
✚▲ Side-effects/warning: See TRILOSTANE.

Moducren

(Morson) is a proprietary, prescription-only COMPOUND PREPARATION of the BETA-BLOCKER timolol maleate and the DIURETICS hydrochlorothiazide and amiloride hydrochloride. It can be used as an ANTIHYPERTENSIVE for raised blood pressure, and is available as capsules.
✚▲ Side-effects/warning: See AMILORIDE HYDROCHLORIDE; HYDROCHLOROTHIAZIDE; TIMOLOL MALEATE.

Moduret-25

(Du Pont) is a proprietary, prescription-only COMPOUND PREPARATION of the (*potassium-sparing*) DIURETIC amiloride hydrochloride and the (THIAZIDE) diuretic hydrochlorothiazide (a combination called co-amilozide 2.5/25). It can be used to treat oedema and as an ANTIHYPERTENSIVE, and is available as tablets.

+▲ Side-effects/warning: See AMILORIDE HYDROCHLORIDE; HYDROCHLOROTHIAZIDE.

Moduretic

(Du Pont) is a proprietary, prescription-only COMPOUND PREPARATION of the (*potassium-sparing*) DIURETIC amiloride hydrochloride and the (THIAZIDE) diuretic hydrochlorothiazide (a combination called co-amilozide 5/50). It can be used to treat oedema and as an ANTIHYPERTENSIVE, and is available as tablets and an oral solution.

+▲ Side-effects/warning: See AMILORIDE HYDROCHLORIDE; HYDROCHLOROTHIAZIDE.

moexipril hydrochloride

is an ACE INHIBITOR and acts as a VASODILATOR. It can be used as an ANTIHYPERTENSIVE and in HEART FAILURE TREATMENT, and is often used in conjunction with other classes of drugs, particularly (THIAZIDE) DIURETICS or CALCIUM-CHANNEL BLOCKERS. Administration is oral.

+▲ Side-effects/warning: See CAPTOPRIL.
❂ Related entry: Perdix.

Mogadon

(Roche) is a proprietary, prescription-only preparation of the BENZODIAZEPINE nitrazepam. It can be used as a fairly long-acting HYPNOTIC for short-term treatment of insomnia (where some daytime sedation is acceptable). It is available as tablets.

+▲ Side-effects/warning: See NITRAZEPAM.

Moisture-eyes

(Co-Pharma) is a proprietary, non-prescription preparation of HYPROMELLOSE. It can be used as artificial tears to treat dryness of the eyes due to disease, and is available as eye-drops.

Molcer

(Wallace) is a proprietary, non-prescription preparation of docusate sodium. It can be used for the dissolution and removal of earwax, and is available as ear-drops.

+▲ Side-effects/warning: See DOCUSATE SODIUM.

Molipaxin

(Roussel) is a proprietary, prescription-only preparation of the (TRICYCLIC-related) ANTIDEPRESSANT trazodone hydrochloride. It can be used to treat depressive illness, especially in anxious patients where a degree of sedation may be useful, and is available as tablets, capsules and a sugar-free liquid.

+▲ Side-effects/warning: See TRAZODONE HYDROCHLORIDE.

Monit

(Lorex) is a proprietary, non-prescription preparation of the VASODILATOR and ANTI-ANGINA drug isosorbide mononitrate. It can be used for HEART FAILURE TREATMENT and to treat and prevent angina pectoris. It is available as tablets.

+▲ Side-effects/warning: See ISOSORBIDE MONONITRATE.

Monit SR

(Lorex) is a proprietary, non-prescription preparation of the VASODILATOR and ANTI-ANGINA drug isosorbide mononitrate. It can be used to treat and prevent angina pectoris, and is available as modified-release tablets.

+▲ Side-effects/warning: See ISOSORBIDE MONONITRATE.

Mono-Cedocard

(Pharmacia) is a proprietary, non-prescription preparation of the VASODILATOR and ANTI-ANGINA drug isosorbide mononitrate. It can be used for HEART FAILURE TREATMENT and to treat and prevent angina pectoris. It is available as tablets.

+▲ Side-effects/warning: See ISOSORBIDE MONONITRATE.

Mono-Cedocard Retard-50

see MCR-50

monoamine-oxidase inhibitors ▣

or MAOIs, are ENZYME-INHIBITORS and constitute one of the three major classes of

M

ANTIDEPRESSANT drugs that are used to relieve the symptoms of depressive illness. Chemically, they are usually hydrazine derivatives and include ISOCARBOXAZID, PHENELZINE and TRANYLCYPROMINE. Although they are well established, having been used for many years, they are nowadays used much less often than the TRICYCLIC antidepressants, largely because of the dangers of interactions with foodstuffs and other drugs. However, they may be used when other classes of antidepressant have not proved useful, or for some reason cannot be used. Their action is said to be better suited for use in patients with hypochondria, phobias or hysterical episodes. Treatment often takes some weeks to show maximal beneficial effects.

If a monoamine-oxidase inhibitor is used after certain other antidepressants, including tricyclics and SSRIs (or vice versa), a suitably long wash-out period must be allowed for to minimize interactions.

MAOIs work by inhibiting the enzyme that metabolizes monoamines (including noradrenaline and serotonin), which, in the brain, results in a change in mood. However, this same enzyme detoxifies the amine tyramine in the body, so when certain foodstuffs that contain this amine (eg cheese, fermented soya bean products, meat or yeast extracts and some alcoholic beverages) are ingested, or medicines that contain sympathomimetic amines are taken (eg cough and cold 'cures' that contain ephedrine hydrochloride or pseudoephedrine hydrochloride) the outcome may be a hypertensive crisis. A patient-guidance treatment card is provided and should be carried at all times. See PHENELZINE for actions and side-effects.

Monoclate-P

(Armour) is a proprietary, prescription-only preparation of dried human factor VIII fraction, which acts as a HAEMOSTATIC drug to reduce or stop bleeding in the treatment of disorders in which bleeding is prolonged and potentially dangerous (mainly haemophilia A). It is available in a form for infusion or injection.

+▲ Side-effects/warning: See FACTOR VIII FRACTION, DRIED.

Monocor

(Cyanamid) is a proprietary, prescription-only preparation of the BETA-BLOCKER bisoprolol fumarate. It can be used as an ANTIHYPERTENSIVE for raised blood pressure and as an ANTI-ANGINA treatment to relieve symptoms and improve exercise tolerance. It is available as tablets.

+▲ Side-effects/warning: See BISOPROLOL FUMARATE.

monoethanolamine oleate

see ETHANOLAMINE OLEATE

Mononine

(Armour) is a recently introduced, proprietary, prescription-only preparation of factor IX fraction, dried, prepared from human blood plasma. It can be used to treat patients with a deficiency in factor IX (haemophilia B), and is available in a form for infusion.

+▲ Side-effects/warning: See FACTOR IX FRACTION, DRIED.

Monoparin

(CP) is a proprietary, prescription-only preparation of the ANTICOAGULANT heparin (as heparin sodium). It can be used to treat various forms of thrombosis, and is available in a form for injection.

+▲ Side-effects/warning: See HEPARIN.

Monoparin Calcium

(CP) is a proprietary, prescription-only preparation of the ANTICOAGULANT heparin (as heparin calcium). It can be used to treat various forms of thrombosis, and is available in a form for injection.

+▲ Side-effects/warning: See HEPARIN.

Monotrim

(Duphar) is a proprietary, prescription-

only preparation of the ANTIBACTERIAL trimethoprim. It can be used to treat infections of the upper respiratory tract and the urinary tract, and is available as tablets, a sugar-free suspension and in a form for injection.
+▲ Side-effects/warning: See TRIMETHOPRIM.

Monovent

(Lagap) is a proprietary, prescription-only preparation of the BETA-RECEPTOR STIMULANT terbutaline sulphate. It can be used as a BRONCHODILATOR in reversible obstructive airways disease, as an ANTI-ASTHMATIC treatment in severe acute asthma and for the alleviation of symptoms of chronic bronchitis and emphysema. It may also be used to prevent premature labour. It is available as a syrup.
+▲ Side-effects/warning: See TERBUTALINE SULPHATE.

Monozide 10

(Lederle) is a proprietary, prescription-only COMPOUND PREPARATION of the BETA-BLOCKER bisoprolol fumarate and the (THIAZIDE) DIURETIC hydrochlorothiazide. It can be used as an ANTIHYPERTENSIVE for raised blood pressure, and is available as tablets.
+▲ Side-effects/warning: See BISOPROLOL FUMARATE; HYDROCHLOROTHIAZIDE.

Monphytol

(LAB) is a proprietary, non-prescription COMPOUND PREPARATION of a number of ANTISEPTIC and KERATOLYTIC agents, including methyl undecenoate, methyl salicylate, salicylic acid, propyl salicylate and chlorbutol. It can be used to treat skin infections, particularly of the nails, caused by *Tinea* fungi (eg athlete's foot). It is available as a paint for topical application.
+▲ Side-effects/warning: See METHYL SALICYLATE; SALICYLIC ACID.

Monuril

(Pharmax) is a proprietary, prescription-only preparation the ANTIBACTERIAL and ANTIBIOTIC fosfomycin. It can be used to treat urinary tract infections, including uncomplicated lower urinary-tract infections, and is available in the form of oral granules.
+▲ Side-effects/warning: See FOSFOMYCIN.

moracizine hydrochloride

is an ANTI-ARRHYTHMIC drug which can be used to reduce certain heartbeat irregularities, particularly after a heart attack. Administration is oral.
+ Side-effects: Gastrointestinal disturbances; headache, fatigue, palpitations; heart failure; jaundice; blood disorders, dizziness, chest pain and changes in liver function.
▲ Warning: It should be avoided in a wide variety of heart disturbances; in patients with certain kidney or liver disorders; or who are pregnant or breast-feeding.
✪ Related entry: Ethmozine.

Morcap SR

(Sanofi Winthrop) is a proprietary, prescription-only preparation of the (OPIOID) NARCOTIC ANALGESIC morphine sulphate, and is on the Controlled Drugs List. It can be used primarily to relieve pain following surgery and the pain experienced during the final stages of a terminal malignant disease. It is available as modified-release capsules.
+▲ Side-effects/warning: See MORPHINE SULPHATE.

Morhulin Ointment

(Seton) is a proprietary, non-prescription COMPOUND PREPARATION of ZINC OXIDE and COD-LIVER OIL. It can be used as an EMOLLIENT for minor wounds, pressure sores, skin ulcers, eczema and nappy rash, and is available as a cream.

morphine hydrochloride

see MORPHINE SULPHATE

morphine sulphate

is a powerful (OPIOID) NARCOTIC ANALGESIC

M

and is the principal alkaloid of opium. It is widely administered to treat severe pain and to relieve the associated stress and anxiety. It is used during operations as an analgesic and to enhance the actions of GENERAL ANAESTHETICS; to relieve cough in the terminally ill; as an ANTITUSSIVE (though it may cause nausea and vomiting); and for reducing secretion and peristalsis in the intestine, which means that it has a powerful ANTIDIARRHOEAL and antimotility action and is therefore used in some antidiarrhoeal mixtures. Tolerance occurs extremely readily and dependence (addiction) may follow.

Administration may be oral as granules for dissolving, as oral solutions or as tablets, or by suppositories or injection (morphine is more active when given by injection). Proprietary preparations that contain morphine (in the form of morphine tartrate, morphine hydrochloride or morphine sulphate) are all on the Controlled Drugs List. It is sometimes available as a COMPOUND PREPARATION with atropine (when used in general anaesthesia) and with an ANTI-EMETIC, such as CYCLIZINE.

+▲ Side-effects/warning: See OPIOIDS. It may also cause itching and a rash.

✪ Related entries: Aspav; Cyclimorph; Diocalm; Enterosan; Ipecacuanha and Morphine Mixture, BP; J Collis Browne's Mixture; J Collis Browne's Tablets; Kaolin and Morphine Mixture, BP; Min-I-Jet Morphine Sulphate; Morcap SR; Morphine Sulphate Rapiject; MST Continus; MXL; Oramorph; Papaveretum; Sevredol.

Morphine Sulphate Rapiject

(IMS) is a proprietary, prescription-only preparation of the (OPIOID) NARCOTIC ANALGESIC morphine sulphate, and is on the Controlled Drugs List. It can be used to treat severe pain, for example, in the terminally ill, and is available in disposable syringes ready for use.

+▲ Side-effects/warning: See MORPHINE SULPHATE.

Motens

(Boehringer Ingelheim) is a proprietary, prescription-only preparation of the CALCIUM-CHANNEL BLOCKER lacidipine. It can be used as an ANTIHYPERTENSIVE, and is available as tablets.

+▲ Side-effects/warning: See LACIDIPINE.

Motifene 75 mg

(Panpharma) is a proprietary, prescription-only preparation of the (NSAID) NON-NARCOTIC ANALGESIC and ANTIRHEUMATIC diclofenac sodium. It can be used to treat the pain and inflammation of arthritis and rheumatism and other musculoskeletal disorders, including juvenile arthritis. It is available as modified-release capsules.

+▲ Side-effects/warning: See DICLOFENAC SODIUM.

motility stimulants 🗓

are a class of drugs that stimulate stomach emptying and the rate of passage of food along the intestine. They can also enhance closure of the oesophageal sphincter, thereby reducing reflux passage of stomach contents up into the oesophagus and may have ANTI-EMETIC properties. Older drugs of this class (eg METOCLOPRAMIDE HYDROCHLORIDE) have undesirable effects on the brain. Some recently introduced motility stimulants, such as CISAPRIDE, do not have this action and are thought to work by acting at receptors for 5-HT (serotonin) to cause release of acetylcholine (see NEUROTRANSMITTER) from nerves within the gut wall.

Motilium

(Sanofi Winthrop) is a proprietary, prescription-only preparation of the ANTINAUSEANT and ANTI-EMETIC domperidone. It can be used to treat drug-induced nausea and vomiting, especially during treatment with cytotoxic drugs, and for Parkinson's disease. It is available as tablets, a sugar-free suspension and as suppositories.

+▲ Side-effects/warning: See DOMPERIDONE.

Motipress

(Sanofi Winthrop) is a proprietary, prescription-only COMPOUND PREPARATION of the ANTIPSYCHOTIC drug fluphenazine hydrochloride and the (TRICYCLIC) ANTIDEPRESSANT nortriptyline hydrochloride; in the ratio 1:20. It can be used to treat depressive illness with anxiety, and is available as tablets.

+▲ Side-effects/warning: See FLUPHENAZINE HYDROCHLORIDE; NORTRIPTYLINE HYDROCHLORIDE.

Motival

(Sanofi Winthrop) is a proprietary, prescription-only COMPOUND PREPARATION of the ANTIPSYCHOTIC drug fluphenazine hydrochloride and the (TRICYCLIC) ANTIDEPRESSANT nortriptyline hydrochloride; in the ratio 1:20. It can be used to treat depressive illness with anxiety, and is available as tablets.

+▲ Side-effects/warning: See FLUPHENAZINE HYDROCHLORIDE; NORTRIPTYLINE HYDROCHLORIDE.

Motrin

(Upjohn) is a proprietary, prescription-only preparation of the (NSAID) NON-NARCOTIC ANALGESIC and ANTIRHEUMATIC ibuprofen. It can be used to relieve pain, particularly the pain and inflammation of rheumatic disease and other musculoskeletal disorders, and is available as tablets.

+▲ Side-effects/warning: See IBUPROFEN.

Movelat Relief Cream

(Panpharma) is a proprietary, non-prescription COMPOUND PREPARATION of salicylic acid and heparinoid (mucopolysaccharide polysulphate), which both have COUNTER-IRRITANT, or RUBEFACIENT, actions. It can be applied to the skin for symptomatic relief of underlying muscle or joint pain. It is available as a cream and a gel and is not normally used for children, except on medical advice.

+▲ Side-effects/warning: See HEPARINOID; SALICYLIC ACID.

Movicol

(Norgine) is proprietary, non-prescription preparation of macrogol (polyethylene glycol) with sodium and potassium salts. It can be used as a LAXATIVE in the short-term treatment of chronic constipation. It is available as a powder to make up in water.

+▲ Side-effects/warning: See BOWEL-CLEANSING SOLUTIONS.

moxisylyte

see THYMOXAMINE

moxonidine

is a recently introduced ANTIHYPERTENSIVE which can be used to treat mild to moderate essential hypertension. It has a site of action within the central nervous system. Administration is oral.

+ Side-effects: Dry mouth; tiredness, headache, sedation, dizziness, nausea, insomnia and vasodilatation.

▲ Warning: It should not be used in those with a history of angio-edema; various heart disorders; severe heart failure; severe coronary artery disease, unstable angina; severe liver disease or renal impairment; also possibly a number of other disorders; or in pregnancy and breast-feeding. Administer with care to those with kidney impairment; Withdrawal of treatment should be gradual.

✪ Related entry: Physiotens.

MR vaccine

is a combined VACCINE for IMMUNIZATION against measles and rubella. It uses live but weakened (attenuated) strains of the viruses and is intended to eliminate rubella (German measles) through universal vaccination of children prior to school. The aim is to immunize all children irrespective of previous vaccinations and this policy will allow discontinuation of the previous single-antigen rubella immunization programme. MR vaccine is available from District Health Authorities under a number of names, including Eolarix MR Vaccine and Mérieux MR Vaccine.

+▲ Side-effects/warning: See VACCINES.

M

MST Continus

(Napp) is a proprietary, prescription-only preparation of the (OPIOID) NARCOTIC ANALGESIC morphine sulphate, and is on the Controlled Drugs List. It can be used primarily to relieve pain following surgery and the pain experienced during the final stages of a terminal malignant disease. It is available as modified-release tablets and as an oral suspension.

✚▲ Side-effects/warning: See MORPHINE SULPHATE.

Mu-Cron Syrup, Junior

(Zyma) is a proprietary, non-prescription COMPOUND PREPARATION of the DECONGESTANT phenylpropanolamine hydrochloride. It can be used for the symptomatic relief of chesty coughs, nasal congestion (including hay fever), colds and flu. It is available as a syrup and is not normally given to children under two years, except on medical advice.

✚▲ Side-effects/warning: See PHENYLPROPANOLAMINE HYDROCHLORIDE.

Mu-Cron Tablets

(Zyma) is a proprietary, non-prescription, COMPOUND PREPARATION of the NON-NARCOTIC ANALGESIC paracetamol and the SYMPATHOMIMETIC and DECONGESTANT phenylpropanolamine hydrochloride. It can be used for the symptomatic relief of sinus pain, nasal congestion (including hay fever), colds and flu. It is available as capsules and is not normally given to children, except on medical advice.

✚▲ Side-effects/warning: See PARACETAMOL; PHENYLPROPANOLAMINE HYDROCHLORIDE.

Mucaine

(Wyeth) is a proprietary, prescription-only COMPOUND PREPARATION of the ANTACIDS aluminium hydroxide and magnesium hydroxide and the LOCAL ANAESTHETIC drug OXETHAZAINE. It can be used to relieve reflux oesophagitis and hiatus hernia, and is available as an oral suspension.

✚▲ Side-effects/warning: See ALUMINIUM HYDROXIDE; MAGNESIUM HYDROXIDE.

Mucodyne

(Rhône-Poulenc Rorer) is a proprietary, prescription-only preparation of the MUCOLYTIC and EXPECTORANT carbocisteine. It can be used to reduce the viscosity of sputum and thus facilitate expectoration in patients with chronic asthma or bronchitis. It is available as capsules and a syrup.

✚▲ Side-effects/warning: See CARBOCISTEINE.

Mucogel Suspension

(Pharmax) is a proprietary, non-prescription COMPOUND PREPARATION of the ANTACIDS aluminium hydroxide and magnesium hydroxide. It can be used to relieve indigestion, dyspepsia, heartburn, reflux oesophagitis and hiatus hernia, and is available as an oral suspension.

✚▲ Side-effects/warning: See ALUMINIUM HYDROXIDE; MAGNESIUM HYDROXIDE.

mucolytics ▨

are drugs that dissolve, or break down, mucus. They are generally used in an effort to reduce the viscosity of sputum in the upper airways and thus facilitate expectoration (coughing up sputum) and so they may also be regarded as EXPECTORANTS. It is not clear how they work, though mucolytic agents are commonly prescribed to treat such conditions as asthma and chronic bronchitis. They can also be used to increase tear secretion (lacrimation) in chronic conditions where this is reduced, causing sore, dry eyes. The best-known and most-used mucolytics are ACETYLCYSTEINE, CARBOCISTEINE and METHYL CYSTEINE HYDROCHLORIDE.

mucopolysaccharide polysulphate

see HEPARINOID

Multiparin

(CP) is a proprietary, prescription-only preparation of the ANTICOAGULANT heparin (as heparin sodium). It can be used to treat various forms of thrombosis, and is

available in a form for injection.
+▲ Side-effects/warning: See HEPARIN.

multivitamin 🔢

preparations contain a selection of various
VITAMINS. There are a large number of such
preparations available and are mostly used
as dietary supplements and for making up
vitamin deficiencies. The choice of a
particular multivitamin depends on its
content. They are not normally available
through the National Health Service, except
when used in infusion solutions. However,
Children's Vitamin Drops (vitamins A, C
and D) is recommended by the Department
of Health for routine supplement to the diet
of young children, and is available without
prescription direct to families under the
Welfare Food Scheme.
○ Related entry: Children's Vitamin Drops.

mumps vaccine

is a VACCINE used for IMMUNIZATION and is
made from a suspension of live, attenuated
mumps viruses cultured in chick embryo
tissue. Administration is by injection.
(Combined with measles and rubella
vaccine, it constitutes MMR VACCINE).
+▲ Side-effects/warning: See VACCINES. As
these vaccines are prepared from virus
strains grown in chicken embryos, they
should be used with caution in individuals
known to be sensitive to eggs.
○ Related entry: Mumpsvax.

Mumpsvax

(Morson) is a proprietary, prescription-
only preparation of a VACCINE (Jeryl Lynn
strain, made from live, attenuated viruses).
It can be used for IMMUNIZATION against
mumps, and is available in a form for
injection.
+▲ Side-effects/warning: See MUMPS
VACCINE.

mupirocin

is an ANTIBACTERIAL and ANTIBIOTIC drug
which is unrelated to any other antibiotic. It
can be used to treat bacterial skin infection

and is of value in treating infections caused
by bacteria resistant to other antibacterials,
for instance, in and around the nostrils (eg
methoxycillin-resistant *Staphylococcus
aureus*). Administration is by topical
application.
+ Side-effects: It may sting at the site of
application.
▲ Warning: It is not to be used on patients
with known hypersensitivity to mupirocin
(or any of the constituents of the ointment
preparation).
**○ Related entries: Bactroban; Bactroban
Nasal.**

Mustine hydrochloride

(Boots) is a proprietary, prescription-only
preparation of the (CYTOTOXIC) ANTICANCER
drug mustine hydrochloride. It can be used
in the treatment of Hodgkin's disease, and
is available in a form for intravenous
infusion.
+▲ Side-effects/warning: See MUSTINE
HYDROCHLORIDE.

mustine hydrochloride

(chlormethine hydrochloride) is a
CYTOTOXIC drug which is used as an
ANTICANCER drug in the treatment of the
lymphatic cancer Hodgkin's disease.
Administration is by intravenous infusion.
+▲ Side-effects/warning: See CYTOTOXICS.
○ Related entry: Mustine Hydrochloride.

MXL

(Napp) is a proprietary, prescription-only
preparation of the (OPIOID) NARCOTIC
ANALGESIC morphine sulphate, and is on the
Controlled Drugs List. It can be used
primarily to relieve severe pain following
surgery and the pain experienced during
the final stages of a terminal malignant
disease. It is available as capsules.
+▲ Side-effects/warning: See MORPHINE
SULPHATE.

Myambutol

(Lederle) is a proprietary, prescription-only
preparation of the ANTIBACTERIAL ethambutol

M

hydrochloride. It can be used as an ANTITUBERCULAR treatment, and is available as tablets.

✚▲ Side-effects/warning: See ETHAMBUTOL HYDROCHLORIDE.

Mycardol

(Sanofi Winthrop) is a proprietary, non-prescription preparation of the VASODILATOR and ANTI-ANGINA drug pentaerythritol tetranitrate. It can be used to prevent angina pectoris, and is available as tablets.

✚▲ Side-effects/warning: See PENTAERYTHRITOL TETRANITRATE.

Mycifradin

(Upjohn) is a proprietary, prescription-only preparation of the ANTIBACTERIAL and (AMINOGLYCOSIDE) ANTIBIOTIC neomycin sulphate. It can be used to reduce bacterial levels in the intestines before surgery, and is available as tablets.

✚▲ Side-effects/warning: See NEOMYCIN SULPHATE.

Mycil Athlete's Foot Ointment

(Crookes) is a proprietary, non-prescription preparation of the ANTIFUNGAL drug tolnaftate. It can be used to treat fungal infections responsible for athlete's foot (tinea pedis), dhobie itch (tinea cruris) and prickly heat (miliaria). It is available as an ointment.

✚▲ Side-effects/warning: See TOLNAFTATE.

Mycil Athlete's Foot Spray

(Crookes) is a proprietary, non-prescription preparation of the ANTIFUNGAL drug tolnaftate. It can be used to treat fungal infections responsible for athlete's foot (tinea pedis), dhobie itch (tinea cruris) and prickly heat (miliaria). It is available as a spray for topical application.

✚▲ Side-effects/warning: See TOLNAFTATE.

Mycil Powder

(Crookes) is a proprietary, non-prescription COMPOUND PREPARATION of the ANTIFUNGAL drug tolnaftate and the ANTISEPTIC chlorhexidine (as hydrochloride). It can be used to treat fungal infections responsible for athlete's foot (tinea pedis), dhobie itch (tinea cruris) and prickly heat (miliaria). It is available as a powder for topical application.

✚▲ Side-effects/warning: See CHLORHEXIDINE; TOLNAFTATE.

Mycobutin

(Pharmacia) is a proprietary, prescription-only preparation of the ANTIBACTERIAL, ANTITUBERCULAR and ANTIBIOTIC rifabutin. It can be used in the prevention of *Mycobacterium avium* infection in immunocompromised patients and for the treatment of pulmonary tuberculosis and mycobacterial disease. It is available as capsules.

✚▲ Side-effects/warning: See RIFABUTIN.

mycophenolate mofetil

is a newly introduced CYTOTOXIC and IMMUNOSUPPRESSANT drug. It is mainly used to reduce tissue rejection in transplant patients as prophylaxis of acute renal transplant rejection (in combination with corticosteroids and cyclosporin) in specialist use. Administration is oral.

✚ Side-effects: Nausea and vomiting, diarrhoea or constipation, abdominal pain; hypertension, oedema, chest pain; shortness of breath, cough; insomnia, headache, dizziness and tremor; succeptibility to infections (including cytomegalovirus, herpes simplex, aspergillosis, candidiasis, urinary-tract infection and pneumonia); various blood dyscrasias, electrolyte disturbances, hyperglycaemia, and a number of other reported effects.

▲ Warning: It is not to be given to patients who are, or plan shortly to become, pregnant or breast-feeding; monitoring is required throughout treatment with blood count check; cautions in serious gastrointestinal disease (risk of haemorrhage).

✪ Related entry: CellCept.

Mycota Cream

(Seton) is a proprietary, non-prescription, preparation of the ANTIFUNGAL agents zinc undecenoate and UNDECENOIC ACID. It can be used to treat athlete's foot, and is available as a cream for topical application.

Mycota Powder

(Seton) is a proprietary, non-prescription preparation of the ANTIFUNGAL agents zinc undecenoate and UNDECENOIC ACID. It can be used to treat athlete's foot, and is available as a dusting powder for topical application.

Mycota Spray

(Seton) is a proprietary, non-prescription preparation of the ANTIFUNGAL agents zinc undecenoate and UNDECENOIC ACID. It can be used to treat athlete's foot, and is available as a spray for topical application.

Mydriacyl

(Alcon) is a proprietary, prescription-only preparation of the ANTICHOLINERGIC drug tropicamide. It can be used to dilate the pupil to facilitate inspection of the eyes, and is available as eye-drops.
✚▲ Side-effects/warning: See TROPICAMIDE.

Mydrilate

(Boehringer Ingelheim) is a proprietary, prescription-only preparation of the ANTICHOLINERGIC drug cyclopentolate hydrochloride. It can be used to dilate the pupils and paralyse focusing of the eye to allow ophthalmic examination, and is available as eye-drops.
✚▲ Side-effects/warning: See CYCLOPENTOLATE HYDROCHLORIDE.

Myleran

(Wellcome) is a proprietary, prescription-only preparation of the (CYTOTOXIC) ANTICANCER drug busulphan. It can be administered in the treatment of chronic myeloid leukaemias, and is available as tablets.
✚▲ Side-effects/warning: See BUSULPHAN.

Myocrisin

(Rhône-Poulenc Rorer) is a proprietary, prescription-only preparation of the ANTI-INFLAMMATORY and ANTIRHEUMATIC sodium aurothiomalate. It can be used to treat rheumatoid arthritis and juvenile arthritis, and is available in a form for injection.
✚▲ Side-effects/warning: See SODIUM AUROTHIOMALATE.

Myotonine

(Glenwood) is a proprietary, prescription-only preparation of the PARASYMPATHOMIMETIC bethanechol chloride. It can be used to stimulate motility in the intestines or to treat urinary retention, particularly following surgery, and is available as tablets.
✚▲ Side-effects/warning: See BETHANECHOL CHLORIDE.

Mysoline

(Zeneca) is a proprietary, prescription-only preparation of the ANTICONVULSANT and ANTI-EPILEPTIC primidone. It can be used in the treatment of all forms of epilepsy (except absence seizures) and of essential tremor. It is available as tablets and as an oral suspension.
✚▲ Side-effects/warning: See PRIMIDONE.

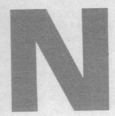

N

nabilone

is a synthetic cannabinoid (a drug derived from cannabis). It is used as an ANTI-EMETIC and ANTINAUSEANT to relieve toxic side-effects, particularly the nausea and vomiting associated with chemotherapy. However, it too has significant side-effects. Administration is oral.

✚ Side-effects: Euphoria, drowsiness, vertigo, dry mouth, visual and sleep disturbances, difficulty in concentrating, nausea, headache, confusion, psychosis, depression, movement disorders, decreased appetite and abdominal pain.

▲ Warning: Administer with care to patients with severe liver impairment, heart disease, hypertension or psychiatric disorders. The effect of alcohol may be enhanced and it may impair the performance of skilled tasks, such as driving.

○ Related entry: Cesamet.

nabumetone

is a (NSAID) NON-NARCOTIC ANALGESIC and ANTIRHEUMATIC drug. It is used primarily to relieve pain and inflammation, particularly in osteoarthritis and rheumatoid arthritis. Administration is oral.

✚▲ Side-effects/warning: See NSAID.
○ Related entry: Relifex.

Nacton

(Pharmark) is a proprietary, prescription-only preparation of the ANTICHOLINERGIC drug poldine methylsulphate. It can be used as an ANTISPASMODIC for the symptomatic relief of smooth muscle spasm in the gastrointestinal tract, and is available as tablets.

✚▲ Side-effects/warning: See POLDINE METHYLSULPHATE.

nadolol

is a BETA-BLOCKER which can be used as an ANTIHYPERTENSIVE for raised blood pressure, as an ANTI-ANGINA treatment to relieve symptoms and improve exercise tolerance and as an ANTI-ARRHYTHMIC to regularize heartbeat and to treat myocardial infarction. It can also be used as an ANTITHYROID drug for short-term treatment of thyrotoxicosis and as an ANTIMIGRAINE treatment to prevent attacks. Administration is oral. It is also available, as an antihypertensive treatment, in the form of COMPOUND PREPARATIONS with DIURETICS.

✚▲ Side-effects/warning: See PROPRANOLOL HYDROCHLORIDE.
○ Related entries: Corgard; Corgaretic 40; Corgaretic 80.

nafarelin

is an analogue of the hypothalamic HORMONE GONADORELIN (gonadotrophin-releasing hormone; GnRH). It reduces the secretion of gonadotrophin by the pituitary gland, which results in the reduced secretion of SEX HORMONES by the ovaries. It is used to treat endometriosis (a growth of the lining of the uterus at inappropriate sites) and for pituitary desensitization before induction of ovulation for *in vitro* fertilization. Administration is by topical application as a nasal spray (it is absorbed into the systemic circulation from the nasal mucosa).

✚▲ Side-effects/warning: See BUSERELIN.
○ Related entry: Synarel.

naftidrofuryl oxalate

is a VASODILATOR which dilates the blood vessels of the extremities and so can be used to treat peripheral vascular disease (Raynaud's phenomenon). Administration is either oral or by infusion.

✚ Side-effects: There may be nausea and pain in the abdomen.
▲ Warning: It should be administered with care to patients with certain heart, kidney or liver disorders.
⊘ Related entry: Praxilene.

nalbuphine hydrochloride

is a NARCOTIC ANALGESIC, an OPIOID, that is very similar to morphine in relieving pain, but with fewer side-effects and possibly less abuse potential. Like morphine, it is used primarily to relieve moderate to severe pain, especially during or after surgery. Administration is by injection.
✚▲ Side-effects/warning: See OPIOIDS; it is reported to cause less nausea and vomiting than morphine.
⊘ Related entry: Nubain.

Nalcrom

(Fisons) is a proprietary, prescription-only preparation of the ANTI-ALLERGIC drug sodium cromoglycate. It can be used to treat allergy to certain foodstuffs, and is available as capsules.
✚▲ Side-effects/warning: See SODIUM CROMOGLYCATE.

nalidixic acid

is an ANTIBACTERIAL and ANTIBIOTIC drug, one of the original members of the QUINOLONE family. It is used primarily to treat Gram-negative infections of the urinary tract and works by inhibiting DNA replication in the bacterial cell. Administration is oral.
✚▲ Side-effects/warning: See QUINOLONES. It is not to be used by patients with porphyria or a history of convulsive disorders. Avoid strong sunlight. Additional side-effects include certain psychoses, weakness and tingling in the extremities.
⊘ Related entries: Mictral; Negram; Uriben.

Nalorex

(Du Pont) is a proprietary, prescription-only preparation of the OPIOID ANTAGONIST naltrexone hydrochloride. It can be used to reverse the effects of (OPIOID) NARCOTIC ANALGESICS. Pharmacologically, it is an opioid and is used in detoxification therapy for formerly opioid-dependent individuals to help prevent relapse. It is available as tablets.
✚▲ Side-effects/warning: See NALTREXONE HYDROCHLORIDE.

naloxone hydrochloride

is a powerful OPIOID ANTAGONIST which is used primarily as an antidote to an overdose of (OPIOID) NARCOTIC ANALGESICS. It is quick but short-acting and effectively reverses the respiratory depression, coma or convulsions that follow overdosage of opioids. Administration is by intramuscular or intravenous injection and may be repeated at short intervals until there is some response. It is also used at the end of operations to reverse respiratory depression caused by (opioid) narcotic analgesics, and in newborn babies where mothers have been administered large amounts of opioid (such as pethidine) for pain-relief during labour. Administration is by injection.
▲ Warning: It should not be administered to patients who are physically dependent on narcotics.
⊘ Related entries: Min-I-Jet Naloxone; Narcan.

naltrexone hydrochloride

is an OPIOID ANTAGONIST of (OPIOID) NARCOTIC ANALGESICS. It is used in detoxification treatment for formerly opioid-dependent individuals to help prevent relapse. Since it is an antagonist of dependence-forming opioids (such as heroin), it will precipitate withdrawal symptoms in those already taking opioids. During naltrexone treatment, the euphoric effects of habit-forming opioids are blocked, so helping prevent re-addiction. It should only be used in specialist clinics. (For overdose with opioids the related drug naloxone is normally used.) Administration is oral.
✚ Side-effects: There may be nausea, vomiting, abdominal pain, anxiety,

nervousness, difficulty in sleeping, headache and pain in the joints and muscles. There may also be diarrhoea or constipation, sweating, dizziness, chills, irritability, rash, lethargy and decreased sexual potency. There have been reports of liver and blood abnormalities.

▲ Warning: Administer with care to patients with certain kidney or liver disorders (function tests before and during treatment are advisable).

○ Related entry: Nalorex.

nandrolone

is an *anabolic* STEROID which has similar actions to the male SEX HORMONE TESTOSTERONE (though it has far fewer masculinizing effects). It can be used to treat osteoporosis and aplastic anaemia. Administration (in the form of nandrolone decanoate or nandrolone phenylpropionate) is by injection.

✚ Side-effects: Acne, sodium retention with oedema, virilization (voice changes in women, with amenorrhoea), inhibition of sperm production, effects on the bones and liver function.

▲ Warning: It is not to be administered to patients with severe liver function disorders, cancer of the prostate gland, male breast cancer or porphyria; or who are pregnant. Administer with caution to those with impaired heart or kidney or liver function, hypertension, diabetes, epilepsy or migraine. When treating young patients, bone growth should be monitored.

○ Related entry: Deca-Durabolin.

naphazoline hydrochloride

is a SYMPATHOMIMETIC and VASOCONSTRICTOR drug which is used for the symptomatic relief of conjunctivitis. Administration is by topical application as eye-drops.

✚▲ Side-effects/warning: See XYLOMETAZOLINE HYDROCHLORIDE.

○ Related entry: Clearine Eye Drops.

Napratec

(Searle) is a proprietary, prescription-only COMPOUND PREPARATION of the powerful (NSAID) NON-NARCOTIC ANALGESIC and ANTIRHEUMATIC naproxen and the ULCER-HEALING DRUG the PROSTAGLANDIN misoprostol. It is administered to treat the pain and inflammation of rheumatoid and osteoarthritis. This combined preparation represents a somewhat novel approach to minimizing the gastrointestinal side-effects of the NSAID by supplementing the local hormone whose production has been inhibited and which is necessary for the unimpaired circulation of blood in the gastrointestinal lining. It is available as tablets.

✚▲ Side-effects/warning: See MISOPROSTOL; NAPROXEN.

Naprosyn

(Syntex) is a proprietary, prescription-only preparation of the (NSAID) NON-NARCOTIC ANALGESIC and ANTIRHEUMATIC drug naproxen. It can be used to relieve pain and inflammation, particularly rheumatic and arthritic pain, acute gout and other musculoskeletal disorders. It is available as tablets, enteric-coated tablets (under the name *Naprosyn EC*), modified-release tablets (under the name *Naprosyn S/R*), an oral suspension, granules for oral solution and as suppositories.

✚▲ Side-effects/warning: See NAPROXEN.

naproxen

is a (NSAID) NON-NARCOTIC ANALGESIC and ANTIRHEUMATIC drug. It is used to relieve pain and inflammation, particularly rheumatic and arthritic pain, gout, juvenile arthritis and other musculoskeletal disorders and period pain. Administration (either as naproxen or naproxen sodium) can be oral or by suppositories.

✚▲ Side-effects/warning: See NSAID. The risk of gastrointestinal side-effects is intermediate for this group. Suppositories may cause rectal irritation and bleeding.

○ Related entries: Arthrosin; Arthroxen; Laraflex; Napratec; Naprosyn; Nycopren; Prosaid; Synflex; Timpron; Valrox.

Narcan

(Du Pont) is a proprietary, prescription-only preparation of the OPIOID ANTAGONIST naloxone hydrochloride, which is used to treat acute overdosage of (OPIOID) NARCOTIC ANALGESICS, such as morphine. It is available in ampoules for injection and as a weaker form (*Narcan Neonatal*) for the treatment of respiratory depression in babies born to mothers who have been given narcotic analgesics during labour or who are drug addicts.

+▲ Side-effects/warning: See NALOXONE HYDROCHLORIDE.

narcotic analgesics ⏏

are OPIOIDS, such as MORPHINE SULPHATE, and have powerful actions on the central nervous system and alter the perception of pain. Because of their numerous possible side-effects, the most important of which is drug dependence (habituation, or addiction), this class is usually used under strict medical supervision and normally the drugs are only available on prescription. Other notable side-effects include depression of respiration, nausea and vomiting, sometimes hypotension, constipation (therefore they can be used as ANTIDIARRHOEAL drugs), inhibition of coughing (ANTITUSSIVE) and constriction of the pupils (miosis).

Other narcotic analgesics are CODEINE PHOSPHATE, DIAMORPHINE HYDROCHLORIDE (heroin), METHADONE HYDROCHLORIDE, PENTAZOCINE and PETHIDINE HYDROCHLORIDE. Narcotic analgesics are used for different types and severities of pain. For example, pethidine is used during labour, since it produces prompt, short-lasting analgesia and causes less respiratory depression to the baby.

It is now recognized that the characteristic pharmacology of the narcotic analgesics follows from their acting as mimics of natural opioid neurotransmitters (enkephalins, endorphins, dynorphins) in the brain. Most effects of the opioid narcotic analgesics (eg respiratory depression) may be reversed with an OPIOID ANTAGONIST (eg naloxone hydrochloride). See also NON-NARCOTIC ANALGESIC; NSAID.

narcotic antagonists

see OPIOID ANTAGONISTS

narcotics ⏏

are agents that induce stupor and insensibility. Commonly, the term is applied to the OPIOIDS (such as MORPHINE SULPHATE and DIAMORPHINE HYDROCHLORIDE), but it can also be used to describe SEDATIVES, HYPNOTICS and ALCOHOL, which act directly on the brain centres to depress their functioning. In law, certainly in the USA, the term tends to be used to describe any *addictive* drug that is used illegally and is the subject of abuse, even if it is a stimulant (eg cocaine or amphetamine). See also NARCOTIC ANALGESICS.

Nardil

(Parke-Davis) is a proprietary, prescription-only preparation of the (MONOAMINE-OXIDASE INHIBITOR) ANTIDEPRESSANT phenelzine. It can be used to treat depressive illness, and is available as tablets.

+▲ Side-effects/warning: See PHENELZINE.

Narphen

(Napp) is a proprietary, prescription-only preparation of the (OPIOID) NARCOTIC ANALGESIC phenazocine hydrobromide, and is on the Controlled Drugs List. It can be used to relieve severe pain or biliary pain, and is available as tablets.

+▲ Side-effects/warning: See PHENAZOCINE HYDROBROMIDE.

nasal decongestants ⏏

are drugs that relieve or reduce the symptoms of congestion of the nose. They are generally, and most safely, administered in the form of nose-drops or as a nasal spray, which avoids the tendency of such drugs to cause side-effects like raised blood pressure, though some are administered

N

orally. Most nasal decongestants are SYMPATHOMIMETICS, which work by constricting blood vessels in general, including those within the mucous membranes of the nasal cavity, so reducing the thickness of the membranes, improving drainage and possibly also decreasing mucous and fluid secretions. However, rhinitis (inflammation of the mucous membrane of the nose), especially when caused by allergy (eg hay fever), is usually dealt with by using ANTIHISTAMINES, which inhibit the detrimental and congestive effects of histamine released by the allergic response, or by drugs which inhibit the allergic response itself, and so effectively reduce inflammation (eg CORTICOSTEROIDS and SODIUM CROMOGLYCATE). Nasal decongestants are often included in COMPOUND PREPARATIONS intended for the relief of cold symptoms.

Naseptin

(Zeneca) is a proprietary, prescription-only COMPOUND PREPARATION of the ANTIBACTERIAL and (AMINOGLYCOSIDE) ANTIBIOTIC neomycin sulphate and the ANTISEPTIC chlorhexidine (as hydrochloride). It can be used to treat staphylococcal infections in and around the nostrils, and is available as a cream for topical application.

➕▲ Side-effects/warning: See CHLORHEXIDINE; NEOMYCIN SULPHATE.

Natrilix

(Servier) is a proprietary, prescription-only preparation of the (THIAZIDE-like) DIURETIC indapamide. It can be used, either alone or in conjunction with other drugs, as an ANTIHYPERTENSIVE, and is available as tablets (also in a modified-release version called *Natrilix SR*).

➕▲ Side-effects/warning: See INDAPAMIDE.

Natulan

(Roche) is a proprietary, prescription-only preparation of the (CYTOTOXIC) ANTICANCER drug procarbazine. It can be used in the treatment of the lymphatic cancer

Hodgkin's disease, and is available as capsules.

➕▲ Side-effects/warning: See PROCARBAZINE.

Navidrex

(Ciba) is a proprietary, prescription-only preparation of the (THIAZIDE) DIURETIC cyclopenthiazide. It can be used to treat oedema and as an ANTIHYPERTENSIVE, and is available as tablets.

➕▲ Side-effects/warning: See CYCLOPENTHIAZIDE.

Navispare

(Ciba) is a proprietary, prescription-only COMPOUND PREPARATION of the (*potassium-sparing*) DIURETIC amiloride hydrochloride and the (THIAZIDE) diuretic cyclopenthiazide. It can be used as an ANTIHYPERTENSIVE, and is available as tablets.

➕▲ Side-effects/warning: See AMILORIDE HYDROCHLORIDE; CYCLOPENTHIAZIDE.

Navoban

(Sandoz) is a proprietary, prescription-only preparation of the ANTI-EMETIC and ANTINAUSEANT tropisetron. It can be used to give relief from nausea and vomiting, especially in patients receiving radiotherapy or chemotherapy and where other drugs are ineffective. It is available as capsules or in a form for injection.

➕▲ Side-effects/warning: See TROPISETRON.

Nebcin

(Lilly) is a proprietary, prescription-only preparation of the ANTIBACTERIAL and (AMINOGLYCOSIDE) ANTIBIOTIC tobramycin. It can be used to treat a range of serious bacterial infections, and is available in a form for injection.

➕▲ Side-effects/warning: See TOBRAMYCIN.

nedocromil sodium

is used as an ANTI-ALLERGIC drug to prevent recurrent attacks of asthma or, when applied topically, for allergic rhinitis of the nose and allergic vernal

keratoconjunctivitis in the eye.
Administration is by inhalation from an
aerosol, as a nose spray or eye-drops.
✚ Side-effects: If absorbed, there may be
nausea, headache, vomiting, dyspepsia and
abdominal pain.
⊘ Related entries: Rapitil; Tilade; Tilarin.

nefazodone

is an ANTIDEPRESSANT of the SSRI group. It is
used to treat depressive illness and has the
advantage over some other antidepressants
because it has relatively less SEDATIVE and
ANTICHOLINERGIC side-effects. Also, it both
inhibits re-uptake of 5-HT and blocks 5-HT
receptors and so differs somewhat from
other SSRIs. The onset of action may take
some weeks to reach full effect and offset
on discontinuation is also slow.
Administration is oral.
✚ Side-effects: Weakness, dry mouth,
nausea, sleepiness, dizziness; less frequently,
chills, fever, hypotension on standing,
constipation, light-headedness, loss of
sensation in the extremities, confusion,
unsteady gait and minor visual problems.
▲ Warning: It is not to be used by patients
who are breast-feeding. Use with care in
epilepsy, a history of mania, who are elderly,
with liver and kidney impairment, and
pregnancy. It may impair performance of
skilled tasks, such as driving.
⊘ Related entry: Dutonin.

nefopam hydrochloride

is a NON-NARCOTIC ANALGESIC which is used to
treat moderate pain. Administration is
either oral or by injection.
✚ Side-effects: There may be nausea,
nervous agitation, dizziness, headache,
insomnia or drowsiness; dry mouth,
difficulty in urination, blurred vision,
increased heart rate and sweating.
Confusion and hallucinations have been
reported and it may colour the urine pink.
▲ Warning: It should not be administered
to patients who suffer from convulsive
disorders.
⊘ Related entry: Acupan.

Negram

(Sanofi Winthrop) is a proprietary,
prescription-only preparation of the
ANTIBACTERIAL and (QUINOLONE) ANTIBIOTIC
nalidixic acid. It can be used to treat
various infections, particularly those of the
urinary tract, and is available as tablets and
an oral suspension.
✚▲ Side-effects/warning: See NALIDIXIC
ACID.

Neo-Cortef

(Cusi) is a proprietary, prescription-only
COMPOUND PREPARATION of the ANTI-
INFLAMMATORY and CORTICOSTEROID drug
hydrocortisone (as acetate) and the
ANTIBACTERIAL and (AMINOGLYCOSIDE)
ANTIBIOTIC neomycin sulphate. It can be
used to treat bacterial infections in the
outer ear and inflammation in the eye, and
is available as ear-drops, eye-drops and an
ointment.
✚▲ Side-effects/warning: See
HYDROCORTISONE; NEOMYCIN SULPHATE.

Neo-Cytamen

(Evans) is a proprietary, prescription-only
preparation of the VITAMIN
hydroxocobalamin. It can be used to
correct diagnosed clinical deficiency of
vitamin B_{12}, including pernicious anaemia,
and is available in a form for injection.
✚▲ Side-effects/warning: See
HYDROXOCOBALAMIN.

Neo-Mercazole

(Roche) is a proprietary, prescription-only
preparation of carbimazole. It can be used
to treat the effects of an excess of thyroid
hormones in the bloodstream
(thyrotoxicosis), and is available as tablets.
✚▲ Side-effects/warning: See CARBIMAZOLE.

Neo-NaClex

(Goldshield) is a proprietary, prescription-
only preparation of the (THIAZIDE) DIURETIC
bendrofluazide. It can be used in HEART
FAILURE TREATMENT, as an ANTIHYPERTENSIVE to
treat oedema. It is available as tablets.

N ✚▲ Side-effects/warning: See BENDROFLUAZIDE.

Neo-NaClex-K

(Goldshield) is a proprietary, prescription-only COMPOUND PREPARATION of the (THIAZIDE) DIURETIC bendrofluazide and the potassium supplement POTASSIUM CHLORIDE. It can be used in HEART FAILURE TREATMENT, as an ANTIHYPERTENSIVE treatment and to treat oedema. It is available as tablets, which should be swallowed whole with plenty of fluid at mealtimes or when in an upright posture.

✚▲ Side-effects/warning: See BENDROFLUAZIDE.

Neogest

(Schering) is a proprietary, prescription-only preparation which can be used as an ORAL CONTRACEPTIVE of the PROGESTOGEN-only pill (POP) type and contains norgestrel. It is available as tablets in a calendar pack.

✚▲ Side-effects/warning: See NORGESTREL.

neomycin sulphate

is a broad-spectrum ANTIBACTERIAL and ANTIBIOTIC drug, and an original member of the AMINOGLYCOSIDE family. It is effective in treating some superficial bacterial infections and has quite a widespread use when used topically (in the eyes, ears or on the skin). However, it is too toxic to be administered by intravenous or intramuscular injection. It is occasionally administered orally in order to reduce the levels of bacteria in the colon prior to intestinal surgery or examination, or in liver failure. When administered orally it is not absorbed from the gastrointestinal tract. Administration can be either oral or topical

✚▲ Side-effects/warning: See GENTAMICIN. Prolonged or widespread topical application may eventually lead to sensitivity reactions.

⊙ Related entries: Adcortyl with Graneodin; Audicort; Betnesol-N; Betnovate-N; Cicatrin; Dermovate-NN; Dexa-Rhinaspray; Eumovate-N; FML-Neo; Graneodin; Gregoderm; Maxitrol; Minims Neomycin

Sulphate; Mycifradin; Naseptin; Neo-Cortef; Neosporin; Nivemycin; Otomize; Otosporin; Predsol-N; Synalar N; Tri-Adcortyl.

Neoral

(Sandoz) is a proprietary, prescription-only preparation of the IMMUNOSUPPRESSANT cyclosporin. It can be used to prevent tissue rejection in transplant patients, to treat severe, active rheumatoid arthritis and certain severe, resistant skin conditions (under specialist supervision). It is available as capsules.

✚▲ Side-effects/warning: See CYCLOSPORIN.

Neosporin

(Cusi) is a proprietary, prescription-only COMPOUND PREPARATION of the ANTIBACTERIAL and ANTIBIOTIC neomycin sulphate, the antibacterial and (*polymyxin*) antibiotic polymyxin B sulphate and gramicidin. It can be used to treat infections and inflammation of the eye, and is available as eye-drops.

✚▲ Side-effects/warning: See GRAMICIDIN; NEOMYCIN SULPHATE; POLYMYXIN B SULPHATE.

neostigmine

is an ANTICHOLINESTERASE drug which enhances the effects of the NEUROTRANSMITTER acetylcholine (and of certain cholinergic drugs). Because of this property, it has PARASYMPATHOMIMETIC actions and can be used to stimulate the bladder to treat urinary retention and the intestine to treat paralytic ileus. It can also be used to treat the neuromuscular transmission disorder myasthenia gravis. Administration is either oral (as neostigmine bromide) or by injection (as neostigmine methylsulphate).

✚ Side-effects: Nausea and vomiting, increased salivation, diarrhoea and abdominal cramps.

▲ Warning: It should not be administered to patients with intestinal or urinary blockage; it should be administered with caution to those with asthma, epilepsy, myocardial infarction, peptic ulcer, parkinsonism, hypotension, slow heart rate

or who are pregnant or breast-feeding.
✪ Related entry: Robinul-Neostigmine.

Neotigason
(Roche) is a proprietary, prescription-only
preparation of acitretin. It can be used as a
systemic treatment of long-term, severe
psoriasis and certain other skin disorders,
and is available as a capsules.
✚▲ Side-effects/warning: See ACITRETIN.

Nephril
(Pfizer) is a proprietary, prescription-only
preparation of the (THIAZIDE) DIURETIC
polythiazide. It can be used, either alone or
in conjunction with other drugs, in the
treatment of oedema and as an
ANTIHYPERTENSIVE. It is available as tablets.
✚▲ Side-effects/warning: See POLYTHIAZIDE.

Nericur
(Schering) is a proprietary, non-
prescription COMPOUND PREPARATION of the
ANTIFUNGAL miconazole (as nitrate) and the
KERATOLYTIC and ANTIMICROBIAL benzoyl
peroxide. It can be used in the treatment of
acne, and is available as a gel for topical
application.
✚▲ Side-effects/warning: See BENZOYL
PEROXIDE; MICONAZOLE.

Nerisone
(Schering) is a proprietary, prescription-
only preparation of the CORTICOSTEROID and
ANTI-INFLAMMATORY diflucortolone valerate. It
can be used to treat severe, acute
inflammatory skin disorders, such as
eczema and psoriasis. It is available as a
cream and an ointment for topical
application (a stronger preparation,
Nerisone Forte, is also available).
✚▲ Side-effects/warning: See
DIFLUCORTOLONE VALERATE.

Netillin
(Schering-Plough) is a proprietary,
prescription-only preparation of the
ANTIBACTERIAL and (AMINOGLYCOSIDE)
ANTIBIOTIC netilmicin (as sulphate). It can

be used to treat a range of serious bacterial
infections, and is available in a form for
injection.
✚▲ Side-effects/warning: See NETILMICIN.

netilmicin
is a broad-spectrum (AMINOGLYCOSIDE)
ANTIBIOTIC which can be used, alone or in
combination with other antibiotics, to treat
serious bacterial infections caused by
Gram-negative bacteria, especially those
that are resistant to the more commonly
used aminoglycoside gentamicin.
Administration is by injection.
✚▲ Side-effects/warning: See GENTAMICIN.
✪ Related entry: Netillin.

Neulactil
(Rhône-Poulenc Rorer) is a proprietary,
prescription-only preparation of the
ANTIPSYCHOTIC drug pericyazine. It can be
used to treat psychotic disorders, such as
schizophrenia, and also severe anxiety in
the short term. It is available as tablets and
a syrup.
✚▲ Side-effects/warning: See PERICYAZINE.

neuroleptics
see ANTIPSYCHOTICS

Neurontin
(Parke-Davis) is a proprietary,
prescription-only preparation of the
ANTICONVULSANT and ANTI-EPILEPTIC
gabapentin. It can be used to assist in the
control of seizures that have not responded
to other drugs, and is available as capsules.
✚▲ Side-effects/warning: See GABAPENTIN.

neurotransmitters 🖩
are chemical messengers, which on release
from a nerve ending act near to where they
are released to excite or inhibit either other
nerves or the cells within organs innervated
by the nerves (such as the heart, intestine,
skeletal muscle and glands).
Neurotransmitters are therefore rather
similar to HORMONES, however, unlike the
latter they act locally rather than reaching

N

their target tissue via the blood. Such mediators work by interacting with specific recognition sites on cells, which are called RECEPTORS, that 'recognize' only that mediator (or chemically similar analogues). They may be blocked by drugs called receptor antagonists (see BETA-BLOCKERS and ALPHA-ADRENOCEPTOR BLOCKERS). Examples of neurotransmitters include acetylcholine (see ACETYLCHOLINE CHLORIDE), DOPAMINE, NORADRENALINE and SEROTONIN (5-HT).

neutral insulin
see SOLUBLE INSULIN

Neutrexin
(Speywood) is a proprietary, prescription-only preparation of the ANTIPROTOZOAL trimetrexate. It can be used to treat pneumonia caused by the protozoan micro-organism *Pneumocystis carinii* in patients whose immune system has been suppressed, for instance, in AIDS. It is available in a form for injection.
✚▲ Side-effects/warning: See TRIMETREXATE.

Neutrogena Dermatological Cream
(Neutrogena) is a proprietary, non-prescription EMOLLIENT preparation of GLYCEROL. It can be used for dry skin, and is available as a cream.

niacin
is another name for NICOTINIC ACID, which is a form of VITAMIN B.

Nicabate
(Merrell) is a proprietary, non-prescription preparation of the ALKALOID nicotine. It can be used to help alleviate the withdrawal symptoms experienced when giving up smoking tobacco products. It is available in the form of a skin patch for transdermal delivery (that is, absorbed through the skin).
✚▲ Side-effects/warning: See NICOTINE.

nicardipine hydrochloride
is a CALCIUM-CHANNEL BLOCKER which can be used as an ANTI-ANGINA drug to treat and prevent attacks and also as an ANTIHYPERTENSIVE. Administration is oral.
✚ Side-effects: There may be nausea and headache; dizziness, flushing, palpitations and increased heart rate; drowsiness or insomnia; hypotension, oedema, gastrointestinal disturbances; increased salivation; rashes; increased frequency of urination; blood upsets.
▲ Warning: Administer with care to those with certain heart, aortic, kidney or liver disorders, and who are elderly. Do not use in pregnancy. Treatment should be stopped if ischaemic heart pain occurs.
❂ Related entries: Cardene; Cardene SR.

niclosamide
is a synthetic ANTHELMINTIC drug which is used to treat infestation by tapeworms. Administration is oral.
✚ Side-effects: There may be gastrointestinal disturbances (nausea, retching and abdominal pain), light-headedness and itchy skin.
❂ Related entry: Yomesan.

Nicobrevin
(Intercare) is a proprietary, non-prescription COMPOUND PREPARATION of METHYL VALERATE, quinine and CAMPHOR (with eucalyptus oil). It can be used to alleviate the withdrawal symptoms experienced when giving up smoking tobacco products, and is available as a chewing gum (which must be kept out of the reach of children).
✚▲ Side-effects/warning: See QUININE.

Niconil
(Elan) is a proprietary, non-prescription preparation of the ALKALOID nicotine. It can be used to alleviate the withdrawal symptoms experienced when giving up smoking tobacco products. It is available in the form of a skin patch for transdermal delivery (absorbed through the skin).
✚▲ Side-effects/warning: See NICOTINE.

nicorandil

is a POTASSIUM-CHANNEL ACTIVATOR and VASODILATOR drug which can be used as an ANTI-ANGINA treatment to prevent and treat angina pectoris. Administration is oral.

✚ Side-effects: Headache (especially on first taking the drug, but usually transitory); cutaneous vasodilatation with flushing; nausea, vomiting, dizziness and weakness have also been reported. At high dosage, there may be effects on heart rate and blood pressure.

▲ Warning: It should not be used in patients with hypotension or certain heart disorders. Administer with care to those who are pregnant or breast-feeding, with low blood pressure, pulmonary oedema or myocardial infarction. It may impair the performance of skilled tasks, such as driving and operating machinery.

○ Related entry: Ikorel.

Nicorette

(Pharmacia) is a proprietary, non-prescription preparation of the ALKALOID nicotine (as resin). It can be used to alleviate the withdrawal symptoms experienced when giving up smoking tobacco products. It is available as a chewing gum (the nicotine is absorbed from the mucosal lining of the mouth) which must be kept out of the reach of children.

✚▲ Side-effects/warning: See NICOTINE.

Nicorette Nasal Spray

(Pharmacia) is a proprietary, prescription-only preparation of the ALKALOID nicotine. It can be used to alleviate the withdrawal symptoms experienced when giving up smoking tobacco products. It is available as a metered nasal spray (the nicotine is absorbed into the systemic circulation from the nasal mucosa).

✚▲ Side-effects/warning: See NICOTINE.

Nicorette Patch

(Pharmacia) is a proprietary, non-prescription preparation of the ALKALOID nicotine. It can be used to alleviate the withdrawal symptoms experienced when giving up smoking tobacco products. It is available (in strengths of 5, 10 and 15 mg) in the form of a skin patch for transdermal delivery (absorbed through the skin).

✚▲ Side-effects/warning: See NICOTINE.

Nicorette Plus

(Pharmacia) is a proprietary, non-prescription preparation of the ALKALOID nicotine (as resin). It can be used to alleviate the withdrawal symptoms experienced when giving up smoking tobacco products, and is available as a chewing gum (the nicotine is absorbed from the mucosal lining of the mouth). Keep it out of the reach of children.

✚▲ Side-effects/warning: See NICOTINE.

nicotinamide

is a derivative (the amide) of the B complex vitamin NICOTINIC ACID. It is used primarily as a constituent in vitamin supplements, especially in cases where a large dose is required because it does not have as great a VASODILATOR effect as nicotinic acid. It is also used in some topical skin preparations for the treatment of acne (when it is used as a gel).

✚ Side-effects: If administered topically, dryness of skin; also pruritus, erythema, burning and irritation.

▲ Warning: If used topically, avoid contact with eyes and mucous membranes (including nose and mouth); reduce frequency of application if excessive dryness, irritation or peeling.

○ Related entry: Papulex.

nicotine

is an ALKALOID found in tobacco products and is absorbed into the body whether the tobacco is smoked or chewed. It causes a SYMPATHOMIMETIC effect on the cardiovascular system with a rise in blood pressure and heart rate and stimulation of the central nervous system. Like many habituating drugs there is tolerance to its

N

action, so bigger doses are required on continued usage and there is a marked psychological and physical withdrawal syndrome if an individual abruptly stops using it, in other words drug-dependence becomes established. It is available in various replacement forms to help those trying to give it up, including as chewing gum (it is absorbed into the systemic circulation from the lining of the mouth) and skin patches for transdermal delivery (absorbed through the skin).

✚ Side-effects: Cold and flu-like symptoms, with headache, nausea, dizziness, insomnia, dreaming, muscle ache, swelling of tongue, palpitations, acid stomach and skin reaction (with patches).

▲ Warning: Do not use when pregnant or breast-feeding; use with care if there is cardiovascular disease, hyperthyroidism, diabetes, liver or kidney impairment, phaeochromocytoma, gastric ulcers or skin disorders (with patches). Patients should not smoke or use other nicotine products while receiving any kind of treatment.

✪ Related entries: Nicabate; Niconil; Nicorette; Nicorette Nasal Spray; Nicorette Patch; Nicorette Plus; Nicotinell Original Chewing Gum; Nicotinell TTS.

Nicotinell Original Chewing Gum

(Zyma) is a proprietary, non-prescription preparation of the ALKALOID nicotine. It can be used to alleviate the withdrawal symptoms experienced when giving up smoking tobacco products. It is available in the form of chewing gum (2 mg) (the nicotine is absorbed into the systemic circulation from the mucosal lining of the mouth). Keep it out of the reach of children.

✚▲ Side-effects/warning: See NICOTINE.

Nicotinell TTS

(Zyma) is a proprietary, non-prescription preparation of the ALKALOID nicotine. It can be used to alleviate the withdrawal symptoms experienced when giving up

smoking tobacco products. It is available in the form of a skin patch for transdermal delivery (absorbed through the skin).

✚▲ Side-effects/warning: See NICOTINE.

nicotinic acid

or niacin, is a B complex VITAMIN. It is a derivative of pyridine and is required in the diet, but is also synthesized in the body to a small degree from the amino acid tryptophan. Dietary deficiency results in the disease pellagra, but deficiency is rare. Good food sources include meat, cereals and yeast extract. Nicotinic acid may be administered therapeutically as a vitamin supplement (as tablets), but its effect as a VASODILATOR precludes high dosage. It is, indeed, commonly used as a vasodilator, especially in symptomatic relief of peripheral vascular disease (Raynaud's phenomenon). It is also used as a LIPID-LOWERING DRUG because it reduces blood levels of lipids by inhibiting their synthesis in the liver. Derivatives such as inositol nicotinate and nicotinyl alcohol (both for oral administration) are mainly used for their vasodilator actions and nicotinamide (as tablets) for vitamin actions.

✚ Side-effects: There may be nausea and vomiting, flushing, dizziness and headache; palpitations. Itching, rashes and some other side-effects may be reduced by taking with food. Sensitivity reactions and actions on the liver may occur.

▲ Warning: It should not be administered to patients who are pregnant or breast-feeding; and administered with caution to those with diabetes, certain liver disorders, peptic ulcers or gout.

nicotinyl alcohol

is a VASODILATOR drug which can be used to help improve blood circulation to the hands and feet when this is impaired, for example, in peripheral vascular disease (Raynaud's phenomenon). Administration is oral.

✚▲ Side-effects/warning: See NICOTINIC ACID.

✪ Related entry: Ronicol.

nicoumalone

(acenocoumarol) is a synthetic
ANTICOAGULANT which can be used to prevent
the formation of clots in heart disease, after
heart surgery (especially after implantation
of prosthetic heart valves) and to prevent
venous thrombosis and pulmonary
embolism. Administration is oral.

✚▲ Side-effects/warning: See WARFARIN
SODIUM.

✪ Related entry: Sinthrome.

nifedipine

is a CALCIUM-CHANNEL BLOCKER which is
administered as an ANTI-ANGINA drug to
prevent attacks, as an ANTIHYPERTENSIVE and
as a VASODILATOR in peripheral vascular
disease (Raynaud's phenomenon).
Administration is oral as capsules or tablets
(several in modified-release formulations).

✚ Side-effects: There may be nausea and
headache; dizziness, flushing, palpitations;
drowsiness, lethargy and insomnia;
hypotension, oedema; gastrointestinal
disturbances; increased salivation; rashes;
increased frequency of urination; blood
upsets; depression and excessive growth of
gums have been reported.

▲ Warning: Administer with care to those
with certain heart, aortic, kidney or liver
disorders, in cardiac shock, or who are
breast-feeding. Do not use in patients who
are pregnant or have porphyria. Treatment
should be stopped if heart pain occurs.

✪ Related entries: Adalat; Adalat LA; Adalat
Retard: Angiopine; Beta-Adalat; Calcilat;
Cardilate MR; Coracten; Nifensar XL; Tenif.

Nifelease

(Lennon) is a proprietary, prescription-only
preparation of the CALCIUM-CHANNEL BLOCKER
nifedipine. It can be used as an ANTI-ANGINA
drug in the prevention of attacks and as an
ANTIHYPERTENSIVE. It is available as tablets.

✚▲ Side-effects/warning: See NIFEDIPINE.

Nifensar XL

(Rhône-Poulenc Rorer) is a proprietary,
prescription-only preparation of the

CALCIUM-CHANNEL BLOCKER nifedipine. It can
be used as an ANTIHYPERTENSIVE, and is
available as tablets.

✚▲ Side-effects/warning: See NIFEDIPINE.

Night Cold Comfort Capsules

(Boots) is a proprietary, non-prescription
COMPOUND PREPARATION of the
SYMPATHOMIMETIC and VASOCONSTRICTOR
pseudoephedrine hydrochloride, the NON-
NARCOTIC ANALGESIC and ANTIPYRETIC
paracetamol, the ANTITUSSIVE pholcodine
and the ANTIHISTAMINE diphenhydramine
hydrochloride. It can be used to relieve
nasal congestion during colds and flu,
aches, cough and fever. It is available as
capsules and is not normally given to
children under 12 years, except on medical
advice.

✚▲ Side-effects/warning: See
DIPHENHYDRAMINE HYDROCHLORIDE;
PARACETAMOL.; PHOLCODINE; PSEUDOEPHEDRINE
HYDROCHLORIDE.

Night Nurse Capsules

(SmithKline Beecham) is a proprietary,
non-prescription COMPOUND PREPARATION of
the NON-NARCOTIC ANALGESIC and ANTIPYRETIC
paracetamol, the ANTITUSSIVE
dextromethorphan hydrobromide and the
SEDATIVE and ANTIHISTAMINE promethazine
hydrochloridethe. It can be used for the
symptomatic relief of colds, chills and flu at
night. It is available as capsules and is not
normally given to children under six years,
except on medical advice.

✚▲ Side-effects/warning: See
DEXTROMETHORPHAN HYDROBROMIDE;
PARACETAMOL; PROMETHAZINE HYDROCHLORIDE.

Night Nurse Liquid

(SmithKline Beecham) is a proprietary,
non-prescription COMPOUND PREPARATION of
the NON-NARCOTIC ANALGESIC and ANTIPYRETIC
paracetamol, the ANTITUSSIVE
dextromethorphan hydrobromide and the
SEDATIVE and ANTIHISTAMINE drug
promethazine hydrochloride. It can be

N

N

used for the symptomatic relief of colds, chills and flu during the night, and is available as a liquid. It is not normally given to children under six years, except on medical advice.

✚▲ Side-effects/warning: See DEXTROMETHORPHAN HYDROBROMIDE; PARACETAMOL; PROMETHAZINE HYDROCHLORIDE.

Nimbex

(GlaxoWellcome) is a proprietary, prescription-only preparation of the (*non-depolarizing*) SKELETAL MUSCLE RELAXANT cisatracurium (as besylate). It can be used to induce muscle paralysis of medium duration during surgery, and is available in a form for injection (and also in a form called *Nimbex Forte*).

✚▲ Side-effects/warning: See CISATRACURIUM.

nimodipine

is a CALCIUM-CHANNEL BLOCKER which is administered to treat and prevent ischaemic damage following subarachnoid haemorrhage. Administration can be either oral or by intravenous infusion.

✚ Side-effects: Changes in heart rate; hypotension, headaches, gastrointestinal disorders, flushes, nausea, feeling of warmth, blood disorders and changes in liver enzymes.

▲ Warning: Administer with caution because of cerebral oedema and greatly increased intracranial pressure; and with caution also to those patients who have impaired kidney function, or who are pregnant.

✪ Related entry: Nimotop.

Nimotop

(Bayer) is a proprietary, prescription-only preparation of the CALCIUM-CHANNEL BLOCKER nimodipine. It can be used to treat and prevent ischaemic damage following subarachnoid haemorrhage, and is available as tablets and in a form for infusion.

✚▲ Side-effects/warning: See NIMODIPINE.

Nirolex for Chesty Coughs

(Boots) is a proprietary, non-prescription COMPOUND PREPARATION of the EXPECTORANT agent GUAIPHENESIN, the SYMPATHOMIMETIC and DECONGESTANT ephedrine hydrochloride, glycerin, sucrose and menthol. It can be used for the symptomatic relief of chesty coughs, and is available as a liquid. It is not normally given to children under five years, except on medical advice.

✚▲ Side-effects/warning: See EPHEDRINE HYDROCHLORIDE.

Nirolex Lozenges

(Boots) is a proprietary, non-prescription preparation of the (OPIOID) NARCOTIC ANALGESIC and ANTITUSSIVE dextromethorphan hydrobromide. It can be used for the symptomatic relief of dry and ticklish coughs, and is available as lozenges. It is not normally given to children under six years.

✚▲ Side-effects/warning: See DEXTROMETHORPHAN HYDROBROMIDE.

nisoldipine

is a CALCIUM-CHANNEL BLOCKER which can be used as an ANTI-ANGINA drug to prevent attacks and as an ANTIHYPERTENSIVE. Administration is oral.

✚ Side-effects: Oedema in the lower extremities; headache; dizziness, flushing, hypotension, gastrointestinal disturbances, nausea, constipation, allergic skin reactions; increased frequency of urination; liver function disturbances.

▲ Warning: Administer with care to those with certain heart, aortic, kidney or liver disorders, and who are elderly. Do not use in pregnancy or breast feeding. Avoid eating grapefruit or drinking grapefruit juice, as this may affect the metabolism of the drug.

✪ Related entry: Syscor MR.

Nitoman

(Roche) is a proprietary, prescription-only preparation of the tetrabenazine. It can be used to assist a patient to regain voluntary control of movement in Huntington's chorea and related disorders. It is available as tablets.

+▲ Side-effects/warning: See
TETRABENAZINE.

nitrates

are powerful SMOOTH MUSCLE RELAXANTS. They are mainly used as VASODILATORS to relax the walls of blood vessels in the treatment or prevention of angina pectoris (heart pain) and in HEART FAILURE TREATMENT. The best-known and most-used nitrates include GLYCERYL TRINITRATE, ISOSORBIDE DINITRATE, ISOSORBIDE MONONITRATE and PENTAERYTHRITOL TETRANITRATE.
Administration is commonly as tablets to be held under the tongue (sublingual) until dissolved, but aerosol sprays (directed into the mouth) are also used. Other preparations available are modified-release tablets, impregnated dressings, ointment for topical application on the chest and in a form for injection.

nitrazepam

is a BENZODIAZEPINE which is used as a relatively long-acting HYPNOTIC for the short-term treatment of insomnia. Administration is oral.

+▲ Side-effects/warning: See
BENZODIAZEPINES.

✪ Related entries: Mogadon; Remnos; Somnite; Unisomnia.

Nitro-Dur

(Schering-Plough) is a proprietary, non-prescription preparation of the VASODILATOR and ANTI-ANGINA drug glyceryl trinitrate. It can be used to treat and prevent angina pectoris. It is available on a self-adhesive dressing (patch) and, when placed on the chest wall, is absorbed through the skin and helps to give lasting relief.

+▲ Side-effects/warning: See GLYCERYL TRINITRATE.

Nitrocine

(Schwarz) is a proprietary, prescription-only preparation of the VASODILATOR and

ANTI-ANGINA drug glyceryl trinitrate. It can be used in HEART FAILURE TREATMENT and to treat and prevent angina pectoris. It is available in a form for injection.

+▲ Side-effects/warning: See GLYCERYL TRINITRATE.

nitrofurantoin

is an ANTIBACTERIAL drug which is used, in particular, to treat infections of the urinary tract and to prevent infection during surgery on the genitourinary tract. It is especially useful in treating kidney infections that prove to be resistant to other forms of therapy. Administration is oral.

+ Side-effects: There may be loss of appetite, nausea, vomiting and diarrhoea; impaired lung function; peripheral neuropathy, causing tingling and other sensory disorders in the fingers and toes (patients should report such symptoms). Rarely, there is liver damage, allergic skin reactions and blood disorders.

▲ Warning: It should not be administered to patients with impaired kidney function, porphyria or with G6PD deficiency. Administer with caution to those with diabetes, anaemia and certain lung and kidney disorders. Lung, liver and peripheral nerve function should be monitored in long-term treatment. Urine may be coloured yellow or brown.

✪ Related entries: Furadantin; Macrobid; Macrodantin.

Nitrolingual Pumpspray

(Lipha) is a proprietary, non-prescription preparation of the VASODILATOR and ANTI-ANGINA drug glyceryl trinitrate. It can be used to treat and prevent angina pectoris, and is available as an aerosol spray used in metered doses under the tongue.

+▲ Side-effects/warning: See GLYCERYL TRINITRATE.

Nitrolingual Spray

(Lipha) is a proprietary, non-prescription preparation of the VASODILATOR and ANTI-ANGINA drug glyceryl trinitrate. It can be

N

used to treat and prevent angina pectoris, and is available as an aerosol spray used in metered doses under the tongue.
✚▲ Side-effects/warning: See GLYCERYL TRINITRATE.

Nitromin

(Dominion) is a proprietary, non-prescription preparation of the VASODILATOR and ANTI-ANGINA drug glyceryl trinitrate. It can be used to treat and prevent angina pectoris and in HEART FAILURE TREATMENT. It is available in the form of a sublingual aerosol spray in metered doses.
✚▲ Side-effects/warning: See GLYCERYL TRINITRATE.

Nitronal

(Lipha) is a proprietary, prescription-only preparation of the VASODILATOR and ANTI-ANGINA drug glyceryl trinitrate. It can be used in HEART FAILURE TREATMENT and to treat and prevent angina pectoris. It is available in a form for injection.
✚▲ Side-effects/warning: See GLYCERYL TRINITRATE.

nitrous oxide

is a gas that is used as an inhalant GENERAL ANAESTHETIC for both induction and maintenance of general anaesthesia. It also has analgesic properties and is used in subanaesthetic concentrations, for instance, in childbirth. Administration is by inhalation.
✚ Side-effects: Nausea and vomiting and effects on the blood.

Nivaquine

(Rhône-Poulenc Rorer) is a proprietary, prescription-only preparation of the ANTIMALARIAL drug chloroquine (as sulphate). It can be used to prevent or suppress certain forms of malaria and also as an ANTIRHEUMATIC to treat rheumatoid disease. It is available as tablets, a syrup and in a form for injection. (This product also appears in a non-prescription preparation, as tablets or a syrup, labelled for use in the prevention of malaria.)
✚▲ Side-effects/warning: See CHLOROQUINE.

Nivemycin

(Boots) is a proprietary, prescription-only preparation of the ANTIBACTERIAL and (AMINOGLYCOSIDE) ANTIBIOTIC neomycin sulphate. It can be used to reduce bacterial levels in the intestines before surgery, and is available as tablets and an elixir.
✚▲ Side-effects/warning: See NEOMYCIN SULPHATE.

nizatidine

is a H_2-ANTAGONIST and ULCER-HEALING DRUG. It can be used to assist in the treatment of benign peptic (gastric and duodenal) ulcers, to relieve heartburn in cases of reflux oesophagitis (caused by regurgitation of acid and enzymes into the oesophagus), Zollinger-Ellison syndrome and a variety of conditions where reduction of acidity is beneficial. It works by reducing the secretion of gastric acid (by acting as a histamine receptor H_2-receptor antagonist), so reducing erosion and bleeding from peptic ulcers and allowing them a chance to heal. However, nizatidine should not be used until a full diagnosis of gastric bleeding or serious pain has been made, because its action in restricting gastric secretions may possibly mask the presence of stomach cancer. Administration is either oral or by intravenous injection or infusion.
✚▲ Side-effects/warning: See CIMETIDINE; but it does not significantly inhibit microsomal drug-metabolizing enzymes.
✪ Related entry: Axid.

Nizoral

(Janssen) is a proprietary, prescription-only preparation of the (IMIDAZOLE) ANTIFUNGAL drug ketoconazole. It can be used to treat serious systemic and skin-surface fungal infections, and is available as tablets, an oral suspension and a cream for topical application. It is also available as a non-prescription shampoo called *Nizoral*

Dandruff Shampoo for scalp conditions, sebhorroeic dermatitis and dandruff.

+▲ Side-effects/warning: See KETOCONAZOLE.

NODS Tropicamide

(Smith & Nephew) is a proprietary, prescription-only preparation of the ANTICHOLINERGIC drug tropicamide. It can be used to dilate pupils and facilitate inspection of the eyes, and is available as ophthalmic applicator strips.

+▲ Side-effects/warning: See TROPICAMIDE.

Noltam

(Lederle) is a proprietary, prescription-only preparation of the sex HORMONE ANTAGONIST tamoxifen, which, because it inhibits the effect of OESTROGENS, is used primarily as an ANTICANCER treatment for cancers that depend on the presence of oestrogen in women, particularly breast cancer. It can also be used to treat certain conditions of infertility. It is available as tablets.

+▲ Side-effects/warning: See TAMOXIFEN.

Nolvadex

(Zeneca) is a proprietary, prescription-only preparation of the sex HORMONE ANTAGONIST tamoxifen, which, because it inhibits the effect of OESTROGENS, is used primarily as an ANTICANCER treatment for cancers that depend on the presence of oestrogen in women, particularly breast cancer. It can also be used to treat certain conditions of infertility. It is available as tablets in three strengths (the stronger ones under the trade names *Nolvadex-D* and *Nolvadex-Forte*).

+▲ Side-effects/warning: See TAMOXIFEN.

non-narcotic analgesics 🔃

are certain drugs that relieve pain. The term non-narcotic distinguishes them from the NARCOTIC ANALGESCIS, though they are referred to by many names, including *weak analgesics* and, in medical circles, a very large number are referred to as *non-steroidal anti-inflammatory drugs* or NSAIDS. The latter term refers to the valuable ANTI-INFLAMMATORY action of some members of the class. Non-narcotic analgesics are drugs that have no tendency to produce dependence (addiction), but are by no means free of side-effects. For example, ASPIRIN-like drugs can cause gastrointestinal upsets ranging from dyspepsia to serious haemorrhage. However, they can be used for a wide variety of purposes, from mild aches and pains (at a lower range of dosage) to the treatment of rheumatoid arthritis (at higher dosages: see ANTIRHEUMATIC). PARACETAMOL does not have strong anti-inflammatory actions, but is non-narcotic and, as do other non-narcotic analgesics, has valuable ANTIPYRETIC action. These drugs work by altering the synthesis of prostaglandins (natural LOCAL HORMONES within the body) that induce pain. Often drugs in this class are used in combination with other ANALGESICS (eg codeine) or with drugs of other classes (eg caffeine). See also IBUPROFEN and INDOMETHACIN.

non-steroidal anti-inflammatory drugs

See NSAID

nonoxinol

is a SPERMICIDAL drug that is used to assist barrier methods of contraception (such as the condom). Administration is by topical application as a jelly.

✪ Related entries: C-Film; Delfen; Double Check; Duracreme; Duragel; Gynol II; Ortho-Creme; Orthoforms.

nootropic agents 🔃

are cognition enhancers (memory enhancers or *smart drugs*) that allegedly enhance mental performance. No drugs have been absolutely proved to have this action, but the term was coined to define drugs chemically resembling PIRACETAM (*Nootropil*), which were reported to improve mental function in tests. The main putative use for such drugs would be in the treatment of Alzheimer's disease (presenile dementia) and similar neurodegenerative diseases, though drug trials do not so far offer much encouragement. Several ways have been proposed for how these may work. Cerebral vasodilators are believed to increase blood supply to areas of the brain that are supposed to have a defective blood supply. Such drugs include PAPAVERINE, BETA-ADRENOCEPTOR STIMULANTS (eg ISOXSUPRINE), CALCIUM-CHANNEL BLOCKERS (eg NIMODIPINE) and certain ERGOT ALKALOIDS with ALPHA-ADRENOCEPTOR BLOCKING actions (eg CO-DERGOCRINE MESYLATE).

Defective function of neurones (cholinergic neurones) in the central nervous system that release the NEUROTRANSMITTER, ACETYLCHOLINE, has for some considerable time been thought to have an important role in Alzheimer's disease, so ANTICHOLINESTERASES, (eg the atypical agent tacrine) have been administered to enhance cholinergic nerve function (though at the price of extensive side-effects). Clearly, there is a great deal still to be discovered and understood about memory processes.

Nootropil

(UCB Pharma) is a proprietary, prescription-only preparation of the recently introduced ANTI-EPILEPTIC drug piracetam. It can be used in the treatment of cortical myoclonus (involuntary spasmic contractions of muscles of the body), and is available as tablets and an oral solution.

+▲ Side-effects/warning: See PIRACETAM.

noradrenaline

is both a HORMONE and a NEUROTRANSMITTER and is chemically a catecholamine. (In the USA, it is called *norepinephrine* or *levarterenol*.) It is produced and secreted (along with the closely related substance ADRENALINE) as a hormone into the bloodstream by the adrenal gland (from the region called the medulla, which is the central core of the adrenal gland – hence the term *adrenomedullary hormone*). The adrenal gland constitutes an important part

of the sympathetic nervous system. Noradrenaline also acts as a neurotransmitter. It is released from nerve endings by electrical signals travelling from the central nervous system via nerves in the body, in order to either activate or inhibit a wide variety of muscles, glands and metabolic processes. The responses of the body to stimulation of the sympathetic nervous system are primarily concerned with reactions to stress. In the face of stress, or the need for exertion, the body uses adrenaline and noradrenaline to cause constriction of some blood vessels while dilating others, with the net effect of the two catecholamines increasing blood flow to the skeletal muscles and heart. The heart rate is raised and there is relaxation of the smooth muscles of the intestine and bronchioles. There is also a rise in concentration of energy supplying glucose and free fatty-acids in the bloodstream. The actions of noradrenaline and adrenaline are similar, though noradrenaline causes a more marked rise in blood pressure, whereas adrenaline stimulates the heart more. In order to bring about one or sometimes several of these responses SYMPATHOMIMETIC drugs that mimic certain of these actions (eg adrenaline, ISOPRENALINE and PHENYLEPHRINE HYDROCHLORIDE) are administered therapeutically. Noradrenaline itself is not extensively used, however, because its actions in the body are so widespread. But in emergencies it may be administered as a vasoconstrictor in acute hypotension and cardiac arrest (when it is injected in the form of noradrenaline acid tartrate).

+ Side-effects: There may be palpitation of the heart with slowed and irregular heartbeat; and headache.

▲ Warning: It should not be administered to patients who are undergoing a myocardial infarction, or who are pregnant. Leakage of the hormone into the tissues at the site of injection may cause tissue damage.

✿ Related entry: Levophed.

noradrenaline acid tartrate

is the chemical form used in medicine of the naturally occurring NORADRENALINE.

Norcuron

(Organon-Teknika) is a proprietary, prescription-only preparation of the (*non-depolarizing*) SKELETAL MUSCLE RELAXANT vecuronium bromide. It can be used to induce muscle paralysis during surgery, and is available in a form for injection.
+▲ Side-effects/warning: See VECURONIUM BROMIDE.

Norditropin

(Novo Nordisk) is a proprietary, prescription-only preparation of somatropin (the biosynthetic form of the pituitary HORMONE human growth hormone). It can be used to treat hormonal deficiency and associated symptoms (in particular, short stature). It is available in various forms for injection.
+▲ Side-effects/warning: See SOMATROPIN.

norepinephrine

see NORADRENALINE

norethisterone

is a PROGESTOGEN. It is used primarily as a constituent in ORAL CONTRACEPTIVES that combine an OESTROGEN with a progestogen, in implant contraception, in HRT (hormone replacement therapy) and as an ANTICANCER drug to assist in the treatment of sex-hormone linked cancers (eg breast cancer). Administration is either oral or topical as skin patches.
+▲ Side-effects/warning: See PROGESTOGEN.
✪ Related entries: BiNovum; Brevinor; Climagest; Climesse; Elleste-Duet; Estracombi; Estrapak 50; Evorel Pak; Kliofem; Loestrin 20; Loestrin 30; Menzol; Micronor; Micronor HRT; Noriday; Norimin; Norinyl-1; Noristerat; Ortho-Novin 1/50; Ovysmen; Primolut N; Synphase; Syntex Menophase; TriNovum; TriNovum ED; Trisequens; Utovlan.

Norflex

(3M) is a proprietary, prescription-only preparation of the SKELETAL MUSCLE RELAXANT orphenadrine citrate. It can be used for short-term, symptomatic relief of skeletal muscle spasm, and is available in a form for injection.
+▲ Side-effects/warning: See ORPHENADRINE CITRATE.

norfloxacin

is an ANTIBACTERIAL and (QUINOLONE) ANTIBIOTIC drug which can be given to patients who are allergic to penicillin, or whose strain of bacterium is resistant to more commonly used antibacterials. Administration can be either oral or topical.
+▲ Side-effects/warning: See QUINOLONES; but it may also include depression, anorexia and tinnitus.
✪ Related entry: Utinor.

Norgalex Micro-enema

(Norgine) is a proprietary, non-prescription preparation of the (*stimulant*) LAXATIVE docusate sodium. It can be used to relieve constipation and also to evacuate the rectum prior to abdominal procedures. It is available as an enema.
+▲ Side-effects/warning: See DOCUSATE SODIUM.

norgestimate

is a PROGESTOGEN used as a constituent of the *combined* ORAL CONTRACEPTIVES that contain an OESTROGEN and a PROGESTOGEN. Administration is oral.
+▲ Side-effects/warning: See PROGESTOGEN.
✪ Related entry: Cilest.

Norgeston

(Schering) is a proprietary, prescription-only preparation which can be used as an ORAL CONTRACEPTIVE of the PROGESTOGEN-only pill (POP) type and contains levonorgestrel. It is available as tablets in a calendar pack.
+▲ Side-effects/warning: See LEVONORGESTREL.

norgestrel

is a female SEX HORMONE, a PROGESTOGEN, which is used in *progesterone-only* ORAL CONTRACEPTIVES and also, in combination with OESTROGEN, in HRT (hormone replacement therapy). Administration is oral. (LEVONORGESTREL is a stronger form of norgestrel.)

✚▲ Side-effects/warning: See PROGESTOGEN.

✪ Related entries: Cyclo-Progynova; Neogest; Prempak-C.

Noriday

(Syntex) is a proprietary, prescription-only preparation which can be used as an ORAL CONTRACEPTIVE of the PROGESTOGEN-only pill (POP) type and contains levonorgestrel. It is available as tablets in a calendar pack.

✚▲ Side-effects/warning: See NORETHISTERONE.

Norimin

(Syntex) is a proprietary, prescription-only COMPOUND PREPARATION which can be used as a (*monophasic*) ORAL CONTRACEPTIVE (and also for certain menstrual problems) of the type that combines an OESTROGEN and a PROGESTOGEN, in this case ethinyloestradiol and norethisterone. It is available as tablets in a calendar pack.

✚▲ Side-effects/warning: See ETHINYLOESTRADIOL; NORETHISTERONE.

Norinyl-1

(Syntex) is a proprietary, prescription-only COMPOUND PREPARATION which can be used as a (*monophasic*) ORAL CONTRACEPTIVE (and also for certain menstrual problems) of the type that combines an OESTROGEN and a PROGESTOGEN, in this case mestranol and norethisterone. It is available as tablets in a calendar pack.

✚▲ Side-effects/warning: See MESTRANOL; NORETHISTERONE.

Noristerat

(Schering) is a proprietary, prescription-only preparation which can be used as a parenteral CONTRACEPTIVE of the PROGESTOGEN-only pill type and contains norethisterone (as enanthate). It is available in a form for intramuscular depot implant injection.

✚▲ Side-effects/warning: See NORETHISTERONE.

Normacol

(Norgine) is a proprietary, non-prescription preparation of the (*bulking-agent*) LAXATIVE sterculia. It can be used to relieve constipation, and is available as a powder. It is not normally given to children under six years, except on medical advice.

✚▲ Side-effects/warning: See STERCULIA.

Normacol Plus

(Norgine) is a proprietary, non-prescription preparation of the (*bulking-agent*) LAXATIVE sterculia (with added frangula bark). It can be used to relieve constipation, and is available as a powder.

✚▲ Side-effects/warning: See STERCULIA.

normal immunoglobulin

(gamma globulin; human normal immunoglobulin; HNIG) is used in IMMUNIZATION to give *passive immunity* by the injection of immunoglobulin prepared from the pooled blood plasma donated by individuals with antibodies to viruses prevalent in the general population, including hepatitis A virus, rubeola (measles) and rubella (German measles). It is commonly given to patients at risk, such as infants who cannot tolerate vaccines that incorporate live (though weakened) viruses (*active immunity*). Administration is normally by intramuscular injection. (There are also special forms for intravenous infusion, including formulations for patients undergoing a bone-marrow transplant, or patients with certain congenital blood component deficiencies, eg agammaglobulinaemia, hypogammaglobulinaemia, idiopathic thrombocytopenic purpurea and Kawasaki syndrome.)

+▲ Side-effects/warning: See
IMMUNIZATION.
✪ Related entries: Gammabulin;
Kabiglobulin.

Normax

(Evans) is a proprietary, prescription-only
preparation of co-danthramer 50/60, which
is a (*stimulant*) LAXATIVE based on
danthron and docusate sodium. It can be
used to relieve constipation and to prepare
patients for abdominal procedures. It is
available as capsules.
+▲ Side-effects/warning: See DANTHRON;
DOCUSATE SODIUM.

Normegon

(Organon) is a proprietary, prescription-
only HORMONE preparation of a form of the
human menopausal gonadotrophins, which
contains FOLLICLE-STIMULATING HORMONE
(FSH) and LUTEINISING HORMONE (LH). It can
be administered to treat infertile women
who have proven hypopituitarism and who
do not respond to CLOMIPHENE CITRATE
(which is another drug that is commonly
used to treat infertility) and also in
superovulation treatment in assisted
conception (as with *in vitro* fertilization).
It is available in a form for intramuscular
injection.
+▲ Side-effects/warning: See HUMAN
MENOPAUSAL GONADOTROPHINS.

Norplant

(Roussel) is a proprietary, prescription-
only preparation which can be used as a
parenteral CONTRACEPTIVE of the
PROGESTOGEN-only type and contains
levonorgestrel. It is available as capsules
for implantation.
+▲ Side-effects/warning: See
LEVONORGESTREL. Prolonged bleeding and
amenorrhagia is common.

Norprolac

(Sandoz) is a recently introduced
proprietary, prescription-only preparation
of the drug quinagolide. It can be

administered to treat HORMONE disorders
(hyperprolactinaemia), and is available as
tablets.
+▲ Side-effects/warning: See QUINAGOLIDE.

nortriptyline hydrochloride

is an ANTIDEPRESSANT of the TRICYCLIC group.
It has mild SEDATIVE properties and is
administered primarily to treat depressive
illness. As with several other drugs of its
type, nortriptyline may also be used to
prevent bed-wetting by children.
Administration is oral.
+▲ Side-effects/warning: See
AMITRIPTYLINE HYDROCHLORIDE; but is less
sedating.
✪ Related entries: Allegron; Motipress;
Motival.

Norvir

(Abbott) is a proprietary, prescription-only
preparation of the ANTIVIRAL drug ritonavir.
It can be used in the treatment of AIDS, and
is available as capsules and as an oral
solution.
+▲ Side-effects/warning: See RITONAVIR.

Novantrone

(Lederle) is a proprietary, prescription-only
preparation of the (CYTOTOXIC) ANTICANCER
drug mitozantrone. It can be used in the
treatment of certain types of cancer,
including breast cancer, and is available in
a form for intravenous infusion.
+▲ Side-effects/warning: See
MITOZANTRONE.

NovoSeven

(Novo Nordisk) is a proprietary,
prescription-only preparation of
recombinant human antihaemophilic factor
VII, which acts as a HAEMOSTATIC drug to
reduce or stop bleeding. It can be
administered in the treatment of certain
disorders in which bleeding is prolonged
and potentially dangerous, which usually
means patients with inhibitors to factors
VIII and IX. It is available in a form for
infusion or injection.

N

N

Nozinan

(Link) is a proprietary, prescription-only preparation of the ANTIPSYCHOTIC drug methotrimeprazine (as hydrochloride). It can be used to tranquillize patients with psychotic disorders, such as schizophrenia, and to calm and soothe those with terminal illness. It is available as tablets or in a form for injection.

+▲ Side-effects/warning: See METHOTRIMEPRAZINE.

NSAID ?

is an abbreviation for *non-steroidal anti-inflammatory drug*, which is used to describe a large group of drugs, of which ASPIRIN is an original member. Although they are all acidic compounds of different chemical structures, they have several important actions in common. They can be used as ANTI-INFLAMMATORY drugs (to the extent that some may be used as ANTIRHEUMATIC treatments), as NON-NARCOTIC ANALGESICS (particularly when the pain is associated with inflammation) and as ANTIPYRETICS (with the added advantage that they lower body temperature only when it is raised in fever). Additionally, some NSAIDs may be used as ANTIPLATELET drugs, because they can be used to beneficially reduce platelet aggregation. All these actions are thought to be due to the ability of NSAIDs to change the synthesis and metabolism of the natural LOCAL HORMONES the PROSTAGLANDINS. In practice, the side-effects of NSAIDs are so extensive that the use of individual members depends on the ability of individual patients to tolerate their side-effects. Some with the least side-effects are regarded as safe enough for non-prescription, over-the-counter sale, such as aspirin and IBUPROFEN. Although PARACETAMOL shares some of the NSAIDs' properties, it is only very weakly anti-inflammatory and is not necessarily classified with them. See also ANALGESIC.

+ Side-effects: Gastrointestinal upsets, dyspepsia, nausea, diarrhoea, bleeding and ulceration. There may be hypersensitivity reactions, including rash, bronchospasm, oedema, headache, blood disorders, ringing in the ears, dizziness and fluid retention. Reversible kidney failure, particularly in renal impairment. Liver damage is rare. The gastrointestinal upsets may be minimized by taking the drug with milk or food.

▲ Warning: Use with care in patients with allergic disorders (especially asthma and skin conditions), in the elderly and where there are certain liver or kidney disorders. They should not be used where there is a tendency to, or active, peptic ulceration; but different NSAIDs vary in the severity of their gastrointestinal side-effects (eg azapropazone is high-risk, whereas ibuprofen has a lower risk). NSAIDs should not be taken by those who are pregnant and some are best avoided when breast-feeding (eg aspirin). See ACEMETACIN; AZAPROPAZONE; BENORYLATE; DICLOFENAC SODIUM; DIFLUNISAL; ETODOLAC; FENBUFEN; FENOPROFEN; FLURBIPROFEN; INDOMETHACIN; KETOPROFEN; MEFENAMIC ACID; NABUMETONE; NAPROXEN; PHENYLBUTAZONE; PIROXICAM; SALICYLATE; SULINDAC; TENOXICAM; TIAPROFENIC ACID; TOLMETIN.

Nu-Seals Aspirin

(Lilly) is a proprietary, non-prescription preparation of the (NSAID) NON-NARCOTIC ANALGESIC and ANTIRHEUMATIC aspirin. It can be used to treat chronic pain, such as that of arthritis and rheumatism, and also as an ANTIPLATELET aggregation (antithrombotic) drug. It is available as tablets.

+▲ Side-effects/warning: See ASPIRIN.

Nubain

(Du Pont) is a proprietary, prescription-only preparation of the (OPIOID) NARCOTIC ANALGESIC nalbuphine hydrochloride. It can be used to treat moderate to severe pain, particularly the pain experienced during or following surgical procedures or a heart attack, and is available in a form for injection.

+▲ Side-effects/warning: See NALBUPHINE HYDROCHLORIDE.

N

Nuelin

(3M) is a proprietary, non-prescription preparation of the BRONCHODILATOR theophylline. It can be used as an ANTI-ASTHMATIC (including for the treatment of severe acute asthma) and to treat chronic bronchitis. It is available as tablets and as a liquid.

✚▲ Side-effects/warning: See THEOPHYLLINE.

Nuelin SA

(3M) is a proprietary, non-prescription preparation of the BRONCHODILATOR theophylline. It can be used as an ANTI-ASTHMATIC (including for the treatment of severe acute asthma) and to treat chronic bronchitis. It is available as tablets and modified-release tablets (including *Nuelin SA 250*).

✚▲ Side-effects/warning: See THEOPHYLLINE.

Nulacin Tablets

(Goldshield) is a proprietary, non-prescription COMPOUND PREPARATION of the ANTACID agents calcium carbonate, magnesium carbonate, magnesium oxide and magnesium trisilicate. It can be used to relieve the pain and discomfort of indigestion, heartburn, acid indigestion and hiatus hernia. It is available as tablets and is not normally given to children, except on medical advice.

✚▲ Side-effects/warning: See CALCIUM CARBONATE; MAGNESIUM CARBONATE; MAGNESIUM TRISILICATE.

Nurofen

(Crookes) is a proprietary, non-prescription preparation of the (NSAID) NON-NARCOTIC ANALGESIC, ANTIRHEUMATIC and ANTIPYRETIC ibuprofen. It can be used for the relief of headache, period pain, muscular pain, dental pain and feverishness. It is available as tablets and is not normally given to children under 12 years, except on medical advice.

✚▲ Side-effects/warning: See IBUPROFEN.

Nurofen 400

(Crookes) is a proprietary, non-prescription preparation of the (NSAID) NON-NARCOTIC ANALGESIC, ANTIRHEUMATIC and ANTIPYRETIC ibuprofen. It can be used for the relief of headache, period pain, muscular pain, dental pain and feverishness. It is available as tablets (high dose) and is not normally given to children, except on medical advice.

✚▲ Side-effects/warning: See IBUPROFEN.

Nurofen Cold & Flu

(Crookes) is a proprietary, non-prescription COMPOUND PREPARATION of the (NSAID) NON-NARCOTIC ANALGESIC and ANTI-RHEUMATIC ibuprofen, and the DECONGESTANT pseudoephedrine hydrochloride. It can be used to relieve cold and flu symptoms, and is available as tablets. It is not normally given to children under 12 years, except on medical advice.

✚▲ Side-effects/warning: See IBUPROFEN; PSEUDOEPHEDRINE HYDROCHLORIDE.

Nurofen Micro-granules

(Crookes) is a proprietary, non-prescription preparation of the (NSAID) NON-NARCOTIC ANALGESIC, ANTIRHEUMATIC and ANTIPYRETIC ibuprofen. It can be used for the relief of headache, period pain, muscular pain, dental pain and feverishness. It is available as effervescent granules in sachets (high dose) and is not normally given to children, except on medical advice.

✚▲ Side-effects/warning: See IBUPROFEN.

Nurofen Plus

(Crookes) is a proprietary, non-prescription COMPOUND PREPARATION of the (NSAID) NON-NARCOTIC ANALGESIC and ANTI-RHEUMATIC ibuprofen, and the (OPIOID) NARCOTIC ANALGESIC codeine phosphate. It can be used for headache, migraine and period, muscular, dental or rheumatic pain. It is available as tablets and is not normally given to children, except on medical advice.

✚▲ Side-effects/warning: See IBUPROFEN; CODEINE PHOSPHATE.

Nurofen Soluble

(Crookes) is a proprietary, non-prescription preparation of the (NSAID) NON-NARCOTIC ANALGESIC, ANTIRHEUMATIC and ANTIPYRETIC ibuprofen. It can be used for the relief of pain, including headache, period pain, muscular pain, dental pain and feverishness, and is available as soluble tablets.

+▲ Side-effects/warning: See IBUPROFEN.

Nurse Sykes Powders

(Waterhouse) is a proprietary, non-prescription COMPOUND PREPARATION of the (NSAID) NON-NARCOTIC ANALGESIC and ANTIRHEUMATIC aspirin, the non-narcotic analgesic paracetamol and the STIMULANT caffeine. It can be used to relieve cold and flu symptoms, mild to moderate pain and aches and pains. It is available as a powder and is not normally given to children under 12 years, except on medical advice.

+▲ Side-effects/warning: See ASPIRIN; CAFFEINE; PARACETAMOL.

Nutraplus

(Novex) is a proprietary, non-prescription preparation of the HYDRATING AGENT urea. It can be used to treat dry, scaling and itching skin, and is available as a cream.

nutritional preparations ⓔ

(nutritional supplements) are primarily used in medicine for the nutrition of patients who cannot tolerate normal foods for some reason. Their use is only seen as essential under certain circumstances, such as after major bowel surgery, serious stomach and intestinal disorders, for those allergic to certain food products, such as cows' milk or gluten (gluten-intolerance), and for those unable to metabolize certain sugars and amino acids (eg phenylketonuria).

Nutrizym 10

(Merck) is a proprietary, non-prescription preparation of the digestive ENZYME pancreatin. It can be used to treat

deficiencies of digestive juices that are normally supplied by the pancreas. It is available as capsules.

+▲ Side-effects/warning: See PANCREATIN.

Nutrizym 22

(Merck) is a proprietary, non-prescription preparation of the digestive ENZYME pancreatin. It can be used to treat deficiencies of digestive juices that are normally supplied by the pancreas. It is available as capsules, which are at a higher strength than *Nutrizym 10*.

+▲ Side-effects/warning: See PANCREATIN.

Nutrizym GR

(Merck) is a proprietary, non-prescription preparation of the digestive ENZYME pancreatin. It can be used to treat deficiencies of digestive juices that are normally supplied by the pancreas, and is available as capsules.

+▲ Side-effects/warning: See PANCREATIN.

Nuvelle

(Schering) is a proprietary, prescription-only COMPOUND PREPARATION of the female SEX HORMONES oestradiol (as valerate; an OESTROGEN) and levonorgestrel (a PROGESTOGEN). It can be used to treat menopausal problems in HRT, and is available as tablets.

+▲ Side-effects/warning: See LEVONORGESTREL; OESTRADIOL.

Nycopren

(Nycomed) is a proprietary, prescription-only preparation of the (NSAID) NON-NARCOTIC ANALGESIC and ANTIRHEUMATIC naproxen. It can be used to relieve pain and inflammation, particularly rheumatic and arthritic pain, acute gout and to treat other musculoskeletal disorders. It is available as tablets.

+▲ Side-effects/warning: See NAPROXEN.

Nylax Tablets

(Crookes) is a proprietary, non-prescription COMPOUND PREPARATION of the

(*stimulant*) LAXATIVES bisacodyl, phenolphthalein and senna. It can be used for the short-term relief of constipation, and is available as tablets. It is not normally given to children, except on medical advice.
➕▲ Side-effects/warning: See BISACODYL; PHENOLPHTHALEIN; SENNA.

Nystadermal

(Squibb) is a proprietary, prescription-only COMPOUND PREPARATION of the ANTIFUNGAL and ANTIBIOTIC nystatin and the CORTICOSTEROID triamcinolone acetonide. It can be used to treat serious fungal infections with inflammation, and is available as a cream for topical application.
➕▲ Side-effects/warning: See NYSTATIN; TRIAMCINOLONE ACETONIDE.

Nystaform

(Bayer) is a proprietary, prescription-only COMPOUND PREPARATION of the ANTIFUNGAL and ANTIBIOTIC nystatin and the ANTISEPTIC chlorhexidine. It can be used to treat *Candida* fungal infections of the skin, and is available as a cream for topical application.
➕▲ Side-effects/warning: See CHLORHEXIDINE; NYSTATIN.

Nystaform-HC

(Bayer) is a proprietary, prescription-only COMPOUND PREPARATION of the ANTIFUNGAL and ANTIBIOTIC nystatin and the ANTI-INFLAMMATORY and CORTICOSTEROID hydrocortisone. It can be used to treat fungal infections with inflammation of the skin, such as nappy rash, and is available as a cream for topical application.
➕▲ Side-effects/warning: See HYDROCORTISONE; NYSTATIN.

Nystan

(Squibb) is a range of proprietary, prescription-only preparations of the ANTIFUNGAL and ANTIBIOTIC nystatin. They can be used to treat fungal infections (eg candidiasis; thrush) and are available in a variety of forms. Preparations for oral

administration include tablets, a suspension, a gluten-, lactose- and sugar-free suspension, granules for solution and pastilles (for treating mouth infections). For vaginal and vulval infections there is a vaginal cream, a gel and pessaries (vaginal inserts). A cream, a gel, an ointment and dusting powder are available for topical application.
➕▲ Side-effects/warning: See NYSTATIN.

nystatin

is a (*polyene*) ANTIBIOTIC with ANTIFUNGAL properties. It is effective when administered topically or orally. When taken orally, it is not absorbed into the blood and its antifungal action is restricted to the mouth and gastrointestinal tract. Nystatin is primarily used to treat the yeast infection candidiasis (thrush) of the skin, mucous membranes and intestinal tract. Administration can be either oral or topical in a variety of forms.
➕ Side-effects: There may be nausea, vomiting or diarrhoea, local irritation, sensitization of the mouth and a rash.
✪ Related entries: Dermovate-NN; Flagyl Compak; Gregoderm; Nystadermal; Nystaform; Nystaform-HC; Nystan; Nystatin-Dome; Terra-Cortril Nystatin; Timodine; Tinaderm-M; Tri-Adcortyl; Tri-Adcortyl Otic; Trimovate.

Nystatin-Dome

(Lagap) is a proprietary, prescription-only preparation of the ANTIFUNGAL and ANTIBIOTIC nystatin. It can be used to treat intestinal candidiasis (thrush) and oral infections, and is available as a suspension.
➕▲ Side-effects/warning: See NYSTATIN.

Nytol

(Stafford Miller) is a proprietary, non-prescription preparation of the ANTIHISTAMINE diphenhydramine hydrochloride, which has marked SEDATIVE properties. It can be used to help induce sleep in the treatment of temporary sleep disturbances, and is available as tablets. It

N

is not normally given to children under 16 years, except on medical advice.
✚▲ Side-effects/warning: See DIPHENHYDRAMINE HYDROCHLORIDE.

Nytol One-a-Night
(Stafford Miller) is a proprietary, non-prescription preparation of the ANTIHISTAMINE diphenhydramine hydrochloride, which has marked SEDATIVE properties. It can be used to help induce sleep in the treatment of temporary sleep disturbances, and is available as tablets. It is not normally given to children under 16 years, except on medical advice.
✚▲ Side-effects/warning: See DIPHENHYDRAMINE HYDROCHLORIDE.

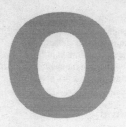

Occlusal
(Euroderma) is a proprietary, non-prescription preparation of the KERATOLYTIC agent salicylic acid (with lactic acid). It can be used to remove warts and hard skin, and is available as a liquid paint.
✚▲ Side-effects/warning: See SALICYLIC ACID.

octreotide
is a long-lasting analogue of the hypothalamic HORMONE somatostatin (hypothalamic release-inhibiting hormone). It is used as an ANTICANCER treatment for the relief of the symptoms that are caused by the release of hormones from carcinoid tumours of the endocrine system, including VIPomas and glucagonomas. It can also be used for the short-term treatment of acromegaly. Administration is by subcutaneous or intravenous injection.
✚ Side-effects: There may be gastrointestinal upsets, including nausea and vomiting, anorexia, bloating, pain, flatulence, fatty faeces and diarrhoea. Kidney dysfunction, gallstone formation and pain at injection site have also been reported.
▲ Warning: It should not be administered to patients who are pregnant or breast-feeding. In patients with diabetes there may be a reduction in antidiabetic drug requirement. Gall bladder and thyroid function should be monitored. Withdrawal of treatment should be gradual.
✪ Related entry: Sandostatin.

O

Ocufen

(Allergan) is a proprietary, prescription-only preparation of the (NSAID) NON-NARCOTIC ANALGESIC flurbiprofen (with polyvinyl alcohol). It can be used by topical application to inhibit constriction of the pupil during an operation on the eye, and is available as eye-drops.

+▲ Side-effects/warning: See FLURBIPROFEN.

Ocusert Pilo

(Rhône-Poulenc Rorer) is a proprietary, prescription-only preparation of the PARASYMPATHOMIMETIC pilocarpine. It can be used to constrict the pupil and treat glaucoma, and is available as plastic inserts (*Pilo-20* and *Pilo-40*) that are placed under the eyelid.

+▲ Side-effects/warning: See PILOCARPINE.

Odrik

(Roussel) is a proprietary, prescription-only preparation of the ACE INHIBITOR trandolapril. It can be used as an ANTIHYPERTENSIVE in conjunction with other classes of drug, and is available as capsules.

+▲ Side-effects/warning: See TRANDOLAPRIL.

oestradiol

is the main female SEX HORMONE produced and secreted by the ovaries. It is an OESTROGEN and is used therapeutically to make up hormonal deficiencies, for instance, in HRT (hormone replacement therapy). Administration can be oral, by injection or implants.

+▲ Side-effects/warning: See OESTROGENS.
✪ Related entries: Climagest; Climaval; Climesse; Cyclo-Progynova; Estracombi; Estraderm MX; Estraderm TTS; Estrapak 50; Elleste-Duet; Elleste-Solo; Estring; Evorel; Evorel Pak; Femoston; Femapak 80; Fematrix; FemSeven; Hormonin; Menorest; Nuvelle; Oestradiol Implants; Oestrogel; Progynova; Progynova TS; Trisequens; Vagifem; Zumenon.

Oestradiol Implants

(Organon) is a proprietary, prescription-only preparation of the OESTROGEN oestradiol. It can be used in HRT, and is available in the form of an implant.

+▲ Side-effects/warning: See OESTRADIOL.

Oestrifen

(Ashbourne) is a proprietary, prescription-only preparation of the sex HORMONE ANTAGONIST tamoxifen, which, because it inhibits the effect of OESTROGENS, is used primarily as an ANTICANCER treatment for cancers that depend on the presence of oestrogen in women, particularly breast cancer. Additionally, it can be used to treat certain conditions of infertility. It is available as of tablets.

+▲ Side-effects/warning: See TAMOXIFEN.

oestriol

is a female SEX HORMONE, an OESTROGEN, produced and secreted by the ovary. It is used therapeutically to make up hormonal deficiencies (sometimes in combination with a PROGESTOGEN) and to treat menstrual, menopausal or other gynaecological problems (such as infertility). Administration is either oral or by topical application.

+▲ Side-effects/warning: See OESTROGENS.
✪ Related entries: Hormonin; Ortho-Gynest; Ovestin; Trisequens.

Oestrogel

(Hoechst, Roussel) is a proprietary, prescription-only preparation of the OESTROGEN oestradiol. It can be used in HRT, and is available in the form of a gel for topical application.

+▲ Side-effects/warning: See OESTRADIOL.

oestrogens

is the name given to the group of (STEROID) SEX HORMONES that promote the growth and functioning of the female sex organs and the development of female sexual characteristics. In their natural forms, they are produced and secreted mainly by the

O

ovary (and to a small extent the placenta of
pregnant women, the adrenal cortex, and –
in men – the testes). Natural and
synthesized oestrogens are used
therapeutically, sometimes in combination
with PROGESTOGENS, to treat menstrual,
menopausal (HRT) or other gynaecological
problems, and as ORAL CONTRACEPTIVES (in
combination with progesterones). Some
synthetic oestrogens are also used to treat
certain cancers (eg prostate and breast
cancer). The best-known and most-used
oestrogens are ETHINYLOESTRADIOL,
MESTRANOL, OESTRADIOL, OESTRIOL and
STILBOESTROL.

✚ Side-effects: Depending on the dose,
route of administration and the particular
preparation used; there may be nausea,
vomiting, weight gain and oedema, tender
and enlarged breasts, premenstrual
syndrome-like symptoms, headache,
depression; sometimes rash and changes in
liver function.

▲ Warning: They should not be
administered to patients with certain
oestrogen-dependent cancers, a history of
thrombosis, inflamed endometrial lining of
the uterus or impaired liver function.
Prolonged treatment (without oestrogen)
increases the risk of cancer of the
endometrium. Administer with caution to
patients who have diabetes or suffer from
epilepsy, have certain heart or kidney
disorders, multiple sclerosis, porphyria, who
are pregnant or breast-feeding or who have
hypertension or migraine.

ofloxacin

is a broad-spectrum ANTIBACTERIAL and
(QUINOLONE) ANTIBIOTIC drug. It is
administered to treat infections in those
patients who are unable to take penicillin
because they are allergic to it, or for
patients who have infections resistant to
more the commonly used antibacterials. It
can be used to treat infections of the
genitourinary tract, including both
gonorrhoea and non-gonorrhoeal
infections, some respiratory infections,

infections of the cervix and septicaemia.
Administration can be either oral or by
intravenous infusion.

✚▲ Side-effects/warning: See QUINOLONES.
Administer with caution to patients with a
history of psychiatric illness or G6PD
deficiency. It should not be used in
epileptics. Other possible side-effects can
include inflamed tendons, anxiety, unsteady
gait, tremor, tingling in the extremities,
psychotic reactions and effects on the blood
and cardiovascular system.

✪ Related entries: Exocin; Tarivid.

Oilatum

(Stiefel) is a proprietary, non-prescription
preparation of the EMOLLIENT arachis oil. It
can be used to soften skin, and is available
as an ointment, a shower emollient and a
bath emulsion.

✚▲ Side-effects/warning: See ARACHIS OIL.

olanzapine

is a recently introduced ANTIPSYCHOTIC drug
which can be used to tranquillize patients
suffering from schizophrenia.
Administration is oral.

✚▲ Side-effects/warning: See
CHLORPROMAZINE HYDROCHLORIDE; but less
sedation and extrapyramidal symptoms;
oedema; dizziness.

✪ Related entry: Zyprexa.

Olbetam

(Pharmacia) is a proprietary, prescription-
only preparation of the LIPID-LOWERING DRUG
acipimox. It can be used in hyperlipidaemia
to reduce the levels, or change the
proportions, of various lipids (eg
cholesterol and LDL) in the bloodstream. It
is available as capsules.

✚▲ Side-effects/warning: See ACIPIMOX.

olive oil

can be used therapeutically to soften
earwax prior to syringing the ears, or to
treat the yellow-brown, flaking skin that
commonly appears on the heads of young
infants (cradle cap) prior to shampooing.

olsalazine sodium

is an AMINOSALICYLATE which is used primarily to induce and maintain remission of the symptoms of ulcerative colitis – often in patients who are sensitive to the more commonly prescribed sulphasalazine. Administration is oral.

✚ Side-effects: Nausea, watery diarrhoea, abdominal cramps, headaches, dyspepsia, joint pain and rashes.

▲ Warning: It should not be administered to patients who are allergic to aspirin or other salicylates, or where there is impaired kidney function; administer with caution to those who are pregnant or breast-feeding.

✪ Related entry: Dipentum.

omega-3 marine triglycerides

are derived from fish oils and used as LIPID-LOWERING DRUGS in hyperlipidaemia to reduce the levels, or change the proportions, of various lipids (eg cholesterol and LDL) in the bloodstream. Administration is oral.

✚▲ Side-effects/warning: There may be belching and nausea.

✪ Related entry: Maxepa.

omeprazole

is an ULCER-HEALING DRUG. It works by being a PROTON-PUMP INHIBITOR and so interferes with the secretion of gastric acid from the parietal (acid-producing) cells of the stomach lining. It is used for the treatment of benign gastric and duodenal ulcers (including those that complicate NSAID therapy), Zollinger-Ellison syndrome and reflux oesophagitis (inflammation of the oesophagus caused by regurgitation of acid and enzymes). It can also be used in conjunction with antibiotics to treat gastric *Helicobacter pylori* infection. Omeptazole may be tried in cases where there has been a poor response to conventional therapies, especially H_2-ANTAGONISTS. Administration is oral.

✚ Side-effects: These include diarrhoea or constipation, nausea, flatulence; dizziness, headaches, sleep disorders, disturbances of vision, oedema, hair loss, liver dysfunction, gynaecomasia and sometimes impotence in males, blood, skin and mood disorders (some of these last side-effects occur only in the very ill).

▲ Warning: Administer only when the ulcer has been established to be benign; avoid its use in patients who are pregnant or breast-feeding.

✪ Related entry: Losec.

Omnopon

see PAPAVERETUM

Oncovin

(Lilly) is a proprietary, prescription-only preparation of the (CYTOTOXIC) ANTICANCER drug vincristine sulphate. It can be used in the treatment of acute leukaemias, lymphomas and certain solid tumours, and is available in a form for injection.

✚▲ Side-effects/warning: See VINCRISTINE SULPHATE.

ondansetron

is a recently introduced ANTI-EMETIC and ANTINAUSEANT which gives relief from nausea and vomiting, especially in patients receiving radiotherapy or chemotherapy and where other drugs are ineffective. It acts by blocking the action of the naturally occurring mediator SEROTONIN. Administration is either oral or by injection or infusion.

✚ Side-effects: Headache, constipation, warmth or flushing in the head and over stomach. Hypersensitivity reactions, effects on liver enzymes and chest pain have been reported.

▲ Warning: Administer with caution to patients with liver impairment, or who are pregnant or breast-feeding.

✪ Related entry: Zofran.

One-Alpha

(Leo) is a proprietary, prescription-only preparation of the VITAMIN D analogue alfacalcidol. It can be used to treat a

O

deficiency of vitamin D, and is available as capsules, a solution and in a form for injection.

+▲ Side-effects/warning: See ALFACALCIDOL.

Operidine

(Janssen) is a proprietary, prescription-only preparation of the (OPIOID) NARCOTIC ANALGESIC phenoperidine hydrochloride, and is on the Controlled Drugs List. It is used primarily during surgery, and is available in a form for injection.

+▲ Side-effects/warning: See PHENOPERIDINE HYDROCHLORIDE.

Ophthaine

(Squibb) is a proprietary, prescription-only preparation of the LOCAL ANAESTHETIC proxymetacaine (as hydrochloride). It can be used during ophthalmic procedures, and is available as eye-drops.

+▲ Side-effects/warning: See PROXYMETACAINE.

Ophthalin

(CIBA Vision) is a proprietary, prescription-only preparation of sodium hyaluronate, which is a visco-elastic polymer normally present in the aqueous and vitreous humour of the eye. It can be used during surgical procedures on the eye, and is available in a form for injection.

+▲ Side-effects/warning: See SODIUM HYALURONATE.

opiates ▣

are members of a group of drugs that chemically are ALKALOIDS, and are closely related to the natural constituents of opium (eg MORPHINE). They powerfully influence certain functions of the central nervous system, and because of this property they can be used as NARCOTIC ANALGESICS to relieve pain. They also have two other actions: they can be used as ANTITUSSIVES to reduce coughing and, because of an antimotility action, as powerful ANTIDIARRHOEAL drugs. Therapeutically, the most important opiate is probably

morphine. They are all potentially habituating (addictive), especially the synthetic derivative of heroin, diamorphine. Today, the term OPIOID is increasingly used to embrace all drugs irrespective of chemical structure, including naturally occuring peptide NEUROTRANSMITTERS, that share this common pharmacology.

Opilon

(Parke-Davis) is a proprietary, prescription-only preparation of the ALPHA-ADRENOCEPTOR BLOCKER thymoxamine, which has VASODILATOR properties. It can be used to treat peripheral vascular disease (primary Raynaud's phenomenon), and is available as tablets.

+▲ Side-effects/warning: See THYMOXAMINE.

opioid antagonists ▣

are drugs that oppose the actions of OPIOIDS, which are used for a number of purposes, including as NARCOTIC ANALGESICS for pain-relief, ANTITUSSIVES and as ANTIDIARRHOEAL or antimotility treatments. It is now recognized that opioids achieve their characteristic actions by mimicking naturally occurring peptide NEUROTRANSMITTERS (enkephalins, endorphins and dynorphins), so now the term opioid is used to describe any chemical, synthetic or natural, that acts on *opioid* RECEPTORS.

Opioid antagonists occupy these receptors without stimulating them and so can reverse the actions of a wide range of opioid drugs. This is a potentially beneficial action, because an opioid antagonist, such as NALOXONE HYDROCHLORIDE, can effectively reverse the respiratory depression, coma or convulsions that result from an overdose of opioids. Administration of naloxone hydrochloride is by intramuscular or intravenous injection and may be repeated at short intervals until there is some response. It is also used at the end of operations to reverse respiratory depression caused by narcotic analgesics, and in newborn babies where mothers have been given large amounts of opioid (such as pethidine) for pain-relief during labour. It is also very effective in reviving individuals who have overdosed on heroin.

NALTREXONE HYDROCHLORIDE, another opioid antagonist, is used in detoxification therapy to help prevent relapse of formerly opioid-dependent patients. It is able to do this because as an antagonist of dependence-forming opioids (such as heroin), it will precipitate withdrawal symptoms in those already taking opioids.

opioids ☐

is a term that has superseded OPIATES and includes polypeptide agents. Opioids influence the central nervous system and so they can be used as NARCOTIC ANALGESICS to relieve pain. They can also be used therapeutically for their ANTITUSSIVE and ANTIDIARRHOEAL, or antimotility, actions. It is now recognized that the characteristic actions of opioids are due to their ability to mimic natural NEUROTRANSMITTERS (enkephalins, endorphins, dynorphins) and because of this the term opioid is used for any chemical (synthetic or natural) that acts on opioid RECEPTORS.

Opioid drugs have similar pharmacological actions and potential side-effects. But the severity of these effects, and the strength of their analgesic and other therapeutic actions, varies with individual drugs, the dose and route of administration. The risk of habituation (addiction) is also much greater with the stronger drugs (eg morphine and diamorphine) than with the weaker ones (eg dextromethorphan, codeine and dihydrocodeine). See ALFENTANIL; BUPRENORPHINE; CO-CODAMOL; CO-DYDRAMOL; CO-PHENOTROPE; CO-PRAXAMOL; CODEINE PHOSPHATE; DEXTROMETHORPHAN HYDROBROMIDE; DEXTROMORAMIDE; DEXTROPROPOXYPHENE HYDROCHLORIDE; DIAMORPHINE HYDROCHLORIDE; DIPIPANONE; FENTANYL; LOPERAMIDE HYDROCHLORIDE; MEPTAZINOL; METHADONE HYDROCHLORIDE; MORPHINE SULPHATE; NALBUPHINE HYDROCHLORIDE; NALOXONE HYDROCHLORIDE; NALTREXONE HYDROCHLORIDE; PAPAVERETUM; PENTAZOCINE; PETHIDINE HYDROCHLORIDE; PHENAZOCINE HYDROBROMIDE; PHENOPERIDINE HYDROCHLORIDE; PHOLCODINE; TRAMADOL HYDROCHLORIDE.

✚ Side-effects: There may be nausea and vomiting, loss of appetite, urinary retention and constipation. There is commonly sedation and euphoria, which may lead to a state of mental detachment or confusion. Also, there may be a dry mouth, flushing of the face, sweating, headache, palpitations, slowed heart rate, postural hypotension (a lowering of blood pressure on standing, causing dizziness), miosis (pupil constriction), mood change and hallucinations.

▲ Warning: Opioids (even the weaker examples) should not be administered to patients with depressed breathing or asthma, who have raised intracranial pressure or a head injury. They should always be administered with caution to those with hypotension, certain liver or kidney disorders, or hypothyroidism (under-activity of the thyroid gland); or who are pregnant or breast-feeding. Dosage should be reduced for the elderly or debilitated. Treatment by injection may cause some pain and tissue damage at the site of the injection.

Opticrom

(Fisons) is a proprietary, prescription-only preparation of the ANTI-ALLERGIC drug sodium cromoglycate. It can be used to treat allergic conjunctivitis, and is available as eye-drops (called *Opticrom Aqueous*) and an eye ointment. It is also available without a prescription subject to certain conditions of quantity and use.

✚▲ Side-effects/warning: See sodium CROMOGLYCATE.

Opticrom Allergy Eye Drops

(Fisons) is a proprietary, non-prescription preparation of the ANTI-ALLERGIC drug sodium cromoglycate. It can be used to

O

treat allergic conjunctivitis, and is available as eye-drops.

✚▲ Side-effects/warning: See SODIUM CROMOGLYCATE.

Optimax

(Merck) is a proprietary, prescription-only preparation of the ANTIDEPRESSANT tryptophan. It can be used to treat long-standing depressive illness in cases where no other treatment is suitable. It is available as tablets.

✚▲ Side-effects/warning: See TRYPTOPHAN.

Optimine

(Schering-Plough) is a proprietary, non-prescription preparation of the ANTIHISTAMINE azatadine maleate. It can be used to relieve the symptoms of allergic reactions, such as hay fever and urticaria, and is available as tablets and a syrup.

✚▲ Side-effects/warning: See AZATADINE MALEATE.

Optrex Hayfever Allergy Eye Drops

(Crookes) is a proprietary, non-prescription preparation of the ANTI-ALLERGIC drug sodium cromoglycate. It can be used to treat allergic conjunctivitis, and is available as eye-drops.

✚▲ Side-effects/warning: See SODIUM CROMOGLYCATE.

Orabase

(ConvaTec) is a proprietary, non-prescription preparation of CARMELLOSE SODIUM (with pectin and gelatin). It can be used for the mechanical protection of oral and perioral lesions, and is available as an oral paste .

Orahesive

(ConvaTec) is a proprietary, non-prescription preparation of CARMELLOSE SODIUM (with pectin and gelatin). It can be used for the mechanical protection of oral and perioral lesions, and is available as a powder.

oral contraceptives ▣

are prophylactic (preventive) SEX HORMONE preparations, which are taken by women to prevent conception following sexual intercourse and are commonly referred to as the *pill*. The majority of oral contraceptives contain both an OESTROGEN and a PROGESTOGEN. The oestrogen inhibits the release of FOLLICLE-STIMULATING HORMONE (FSH) and prevents egg development; the progestogen inhibits release of LUTEINISING HORMONE (LH), prevents ovulation and makes the cervix mucus unsuitable for sperm. Their combined action is to alter the uterine lining (endometrium) and prevent any fertilized eggs from implanting. This type of preparation is known as the *combined oral contraceptive* (COC), or *combined pill*, and is taken daily for three weeks and stopped for one week during which menstruation occurs (*phased monophasic* form).

Two further forms of the combined pill (the phased formulations) are the biphasic and triphasic pills. In these the hormonal content varies according to the time of the month at which each pill is to be taken (and are produced in a 'calendar pack') and the dose is reduced to the bare minimum. Another type of pill is the progestogen-only pill (POP) and this is thought to work by making the cervical mucus inhospitable to sperm and by preventing implantation. This form has the advantage that it can be used by breast-feeding women.

An alternative to the progesterone-only pill is to administer the progestogen as an injection or an implant (which is renewed every three months). Post-coital contraception is also available in an emergency and involves the use of a high-dose combined preparation – the morning-after pill. All the oral contraceptive preparations produce side-effects and a form that is suited to each patient requires expert advice. Various oral contraceptive preparations are also used in the treatment of certain menstrual problems.

✚▲ Side-effects/warning: See OESTROGENS; PROGESTOGEN. Adverse effects are more pronounced with the combined pill; thrombo-embolism, weight gain, nausea, flushing, irritability, depression, dizziness, increased blood pressure, impaired liver function and glucose tolerance, amenorrhoea after coming off the pill. Slight changes in cervical and breast cancer rates (depending on dose and preparation).

oral hypoglycaemics ▣

are drugs, usually synthetic agents, taken by mouth to reduce the levels of glucose (sugar) in the bloodstream and are used mainly in the treatment of Type II diabetes (non-insulin-dependent diabetes mellitus; NIDDM; maturity-onset diabetes) when there is some residual capacity in the pancreas to produce the HORMONE insulin. The main type of oral hypoglycaemic is the SULPHONYLUREA group (eg CHLORPROPAMIDE and GLIBENCLAMIDE), but the (BIGUANIDE) METFORMIN HYDROCHLORIDE and ACARBOSE are also effective. Additionally, GUAR GUM can be administered in the diet. However, INSULIN, which is mainly used in Type I diabetes (insulin-dependent diabetes mellitus; IDDM; juvenile-onset diabetes), can not be taken by mouth and must be injected.

Oralcer

(Vitabiotics) is a proprietary, non-prescription preparation of the ANTIMICROBIAL drug clioquinol (and vitamin C). It can be used to treat infections and ulcers in the mouth, and is available as lozenges.
✚▲ Side-effects/warning: See CLIOQUINOL.

Oraldene

(Warner Wellcome) is a proprietary, non-prescription preparation of the ANTISEPTIC hexetidine. It can be used to treat minor mouth infections, including thrush and sores and ulcers in the mouth. It is available as a mouthwash.
✚▲ Side-effects/warning: See HEXETIDINE.

Oramorph

(Boehringer Ingelheim) is a proprietary, prescription-only preparation of the (OPIOID) NARCOTIC ANALGESIC morphine sulphate. It can be used primarily to relieve pain following surgery, or the pain experienced during the final stages of terminal malignant disease. It is available as oral solutions, oral unit-dose vials and as modified-release tablets called *Oramorph SR*. The more concentrated unit-dose vials and the SR tablets are on the Controlled Drugs List, and the SR tablets are not administered to children.
✚▲ Side-effects/warning: See MORPHINE SULPHATE.

Orap

(Janssen) is a proprietary, prescription-only preparation of the ANTIPSYCHOTIC drug pimozide. It can be used (with care) to treat and tranquillize patients with psychotic disorders, particularly those with schizophrenia, and also to treat Gilles de la Tourette syndrome. It is available as tablets.
✚▲ Side-effects/warning: See PIMOZIDE.

Orbenin

(Forley) is a proprietary, prescription-only preparation of the ANTIBACTERIAL and (PENICILLIN) ANTIBIOTIC cloxacillin. It can be used to treat bacterial infections, particularly staphylococcal infections that prove to be resistant to penicillin. It is available as capsules and in a form for injection.
✚▲ Side-effects/warning: See CLOXACILLIN.

orciprenaline sulphate

is a SYMPATHOMIMETIC and BETA-RECEPTOR STIMULANT which has some beta$_2$-receptor selectivity (though much less than SALBUTAMOL and is therefore more likely to cause side-effects). It is mainly used as a BRONCHODILATOR in reversible obstructive airways disease and as an ANTI-ASTHMATIC treatment in severe acute asthma. It can also be used for the alleviation of symptoms of chronic bronchitis and emphysema.

O

Administration is by aerosol.
✚▲ Side-effects/warning: See SALBUTAMOL; but it is more likely to cause cardiac problems such as arrhythmias.
○ Related entry: Alupent.

Orelox

(Roussel) is a proprietary, prescription-only preparation of the ANTIBACTERIAL and (CEPHALOSPORIN) ANTIBIOTIC cefpodoxime. It can be used to treat infections of the respiratory tract (including bronchitis and pneumonia) and tonsillitis, and is usually reserved for infections that are recurrent, chronic or resistant to other drugs. It is available as tablets.
✚▲ Side-effects/warning: See CEFPODOXIME.

Orgafol

(Organon) is a proprietary, prescription-only preparation of a pituitary HORMONE called urofollitrophin, which is prepared from human menopausal urine containing FOLLICLE-STIMULATING HORMONE (FSH). It is used primarily as an infertility treatment for women suffering from specific hormonal deficiencies. It is available in a form for injection.
✚▲ Side-effects/warning: See UROFOLLITROPHIN.

Orgaran

(Durbon) is a proprietary, prescription-only preparation of the heparinoid, danaparoid sodium. It can be used as an ANTICOAGULANT for the prevention of deep vein thrombosis, and is available in a form for injection.
✚▲ Side-effects/warning: See DANAPAROID SODIUM.

Original Andrews Salts

(SmithKline Beecham) is a proprietary, non-prescription COMPOUND PREPARATION of the ANTACID calcium bicarbonate and the LAXATIVE magnesium sulphate (and citric acid). It can be used for the relief of upset stomach, indigestion, symptoms of over indulgence and constipation. It is available as an effervescent powder and is not normally used for children under 3 years, except on medical advice.
✚▲ Side-effects/warning: See CALCIUM CARBONATE; MAGNESIUM SULPHATE.

Orimeten

(Ciba) is a proprietary, prescription-only preparation of the sex HORMONE ANTAGONIST aminoglutethimide. It can be used as an ANTICANCER treatment for Cushing's syndrome caused by cancer of the thyroid gland, and is available as tablets.
✚▲ Side-effects/warning: See AMINOGLUTETHIMIDE.

Orlept

(CP) is a proprietary, prescription-only preparation of the ANTICONVULSANT and ANTI-EPILEPTIC sodium valproate. It can be used to treat all forms of epilepsy, and is available as tablets and a liquid.
✚▲ Side-effects/warning: See SODIUM VALPROATE.

orphenadrine citrate

is an ANTICHOLINERGIC drug which is also used as a SKELETAL MUSCLE RELAXANT for short-term, symptomatic relief of skeletal muscle spasm. It works by an action on the central nervous system, and is administered by injection. See also ORPHENADRINE HYDROCHLORIDE.
✚▲ Side-effects/warning: See BENZHEXOL HYDROCHLORIDE. Avoid its use in patients with porphyria.
○ Related entry: Norflex.

orphenadrine hydrochloride

is an ANTICHOLINERGIC drug which is used in the treatment of some types of parkinsonism (see ANTIPARKINSONISM). It increases mobility and decreases rigidity and tremor, but has only a limited effect on bradykinesia, and also the tendency to produce an excess of saliva is reduced. It is thought to work by correcting the over-effectiveness of the NEUROTRANSMITTER ACETYLCHOLINE (cholinergic excess), which is caused by the deficiency of dopamine that occurs in parkinsonism. It also has the capacity to treat these conditions, in some cases, where they are produced by drugs. Administration is oral.

+▲ Side-effects/warning: See BENZHEXOL HYDROCHLORIDE; but it is more euphoric and may cause insomnia. Avoid its use in patients with porphyria.

✪ Related entries: Biorphen; Disipal.

Ortho Dienoestrol

(Cilag) is a proprietary, prescription-only preparation of the OESTROGEN dienoestrol, which is a SEX HORMONE. It can be used to treat infection and irritation of the membranous surface of the vagina, including vaginal atrophy in HRT (hormone-replacement therapy), and is available as a vaginal cream.

+▲ Side-effects/warning: See DIENOESTROL.

Ortho-Creme

(Ortho) is a proprietary, non-prescription SPERMICIDAL CONTRACEPTIVE for use in combination with barrier methods of contraception (such as a condom). It is available as a cream containing nonoxinol in a water-soluble basis.

+▲ Side-effects/warning: See NONOXINOL.

Ortho-Gynest

(Cilag) is a proprietary, prescription-only preparation of the OESTROGEN oestriol, a SEX HORMONE, which can be used to treat infection and irritation of the membranous surface of the vagina, including vaginal atrophy in HRT. It is available as an intravaginal cream and pessaries.

+▲ Side-effects/warning: See OESTRIOL.

Ortho-Novin 1/50

(Cilag) is a proprietary, prescription-only COMPOUND PREPARATION which can be used as a (*monophasic*) ORAL CONTRACEPTIVE (and also for certain menstrual problems) of the type that combines an OESTROGEN and a

PROGESTOGEN, in this case mestranol and norethisterone. It is available in as tablets in a calendar pack.

+▲ Side-effects/warning: See MESTRANOL; NORETHISTERONE.

Orthoforms

(Ortho) is a proprietary, non-prescription SPERMICIDAL CONTRACEPTIVE for use in combination with barrier methods of contraception (such as a condom). It is available as a pessary containing nonoxinol.

+▲ Side-effects/warning: See NONOXINOL.

Orudis

(Rhône-Poulenc Rorer) is a proprietary, prescription-only preparation of the (NSAID) NON-NARCOTIC ANALGESIC and ANTIRHEUMATIC ketoprofen. It can be used to relieve arthritic and rheumatic pain and inflammation, to treat other musculoskeletal disorders, pain and inflammation following orthopaedic surgery and period pain. It is available as capsules and suppositories.

+▲ Side-effects/warning: See KETOPROFEN.

Oruvail Gel 2.5%

(Rhône-Poulenc Rorer) is a proprietary, prescription-only preparation of the (NSAID) NON-NARCOTIC ANALGESIC and ANTIRHEUMATIC ketoprofen, which also has COUNTER-IRRITANT, or RUBEFACIENT, actions. It can be applied to the skin for symptomatic relief of underlying muscle or joint pain. It is available as a gel for topical application to the skin and is not normally used for children, except on medical advice.

+▲ Side-effects/warning: See KETOPROFEN; but adverse effects on topical application are limited.

Osmolax

(Ashbourne) is a proprietary, non-prescription preparation of the (*osmotic*) LAXATIVE lactulose. It can be used to relieve constipation, and is available as an oral solution.

+▲ Side-effects/warning: See LACTULOSE.

O

Ossopan

(Sanofi Winthrop) is a proprietary, non-prescription preparation of calcium carbonate. It can be used as a MINERAL SUPPLEMENT for calcium in cases of calcium deficiency. It is available as tablets and granules to be taken by mouth.

+▲ Side-effects/warning: See CALCIUM CARBONATE.

Otex Ear Drops

(DDD) is a proprietary, non-prescription preparation of the ANTISEPTIC and ANTIFUNGAL agent HYDROGEN PEROXIDE in a complex with UREA in GLYCEROL. It can be used to dissolve and wash out earwax, and is available as ear-drops.

Otomize

(Stafford-Miller) is a proprietary, prescription-only COMPOUND PREPARATION of the CORTICOSTEROID dexamethasone and the ANTIBACTERIAL and (AMINOGLYCOSIDE) ANTIBIOTIC neomycin sulphate (and acetic acid). It can be used to treat bacterial infections in the outer ear, and is available as an ear-spray.

+▲ Side-effects/warning: See DEXAMETHASONE; NEOMYCIN SULPHATE.

Otosporin

(Wellcome) is a proprietary, prescription-only COMPOUND PREPARATION of the CORTICOSTEROID hydrocortisone, the ANTIBACTERIAL and (AMINOGLYCOSIDE) ANTIBIOTIC neomycin sulphate and the antibacterial and (POLYMYXIN) antibiotic polymyxin B sulphate. It can be used to treat infections and inflammation in the outer ear, and is available as ear-drops.

+▲ Side-effects/warning: See HYDROCORTISONE; NEOMYCIN SULPHATE; POLYMYXIN B SULPHATE.

Otrivine Adult Formula Drops

(Zyma) is a proprietary, non-prescription preparation of the SYMPATHOMIMETIC and VASOCONSTRICTOR xylometazoline hydrochloride. It can be used as a NASAL DECONGESTANT for the symptomatic relief of nasal congestion, allergic and other forms of rhinitis (including hay fever) and sinusitis. It is available as drops and is not normally given to children under 12 years, except on medical advice.

+▲ Side-effects/warning: See XYLOMETAZOLINE HYDROCHLORIDE.

Otrivine Adult Formula Spray

(Zyma) is a proprietary, non-prescription preparation of the SYMPATHOMIMETIC and VASOCONSTRICTOR xylometazoline hydrochloride. It can be used as a NASAL DECONGESTANT for the symptomatic relief of nasal congestion, allergic and other forms of rhinitis (including hay fever) and sinusitis. It is available as a spray and is not normally given to children under 12 years, except on medical advice.

+▲ Side-effects/warning: See XYLOMETAZOLINE HYDROCHLORIDE.

Otrivine Children's Formula Drops

(Zyma) is a proprietary, non-prescription preparation of the SYMPATHOMIMETIC and VASOCONSTRICTOR xylometazoline hydrochloride. It can be used as a NASAL DECONGESTANT for the symptomatic relief of nasal congestion, allergic and other forms of rhinitis (including hay fever) and sinusitis. It is available as a spray and is not normally given to children under two years, except on medical advice.

+▲ Side-effects/warning: See XYLOMETAZOLINE HYDROCHLORIDE.

Otrivine Menthol Nasal Spray

(Zyma) is a proprietary, non-prescription preparation of the SYMPATHOMIMETIC and VASOCONSTRICTOR xylometazoline hydrochloride. It can be used as a NASAL DECONGESTANT for the symptomatic relief of nasal congestion, allergic and other forms of rhinitis (including hay fever) and

sinusitis. It is available as a nasal spray and is not normally given to children under 12 years, except on medical advice.
+▲ Side-effects/warning: See XYLOMETAZOLINE HYDROCHLORIDE.

Otrivine Metered Dose Sinusitis Spray

(Zyma) is a proprietary, non-prescription preparation of the SYMPATHOMIMETIC and VASOCONSTRICTOR xylometazoline hydrochloride. It can be used as a NASAL DECONGESTANT for the symptomatic relief of nasal congestion, allergic and other forms of rhinitis (including hay fever) and sinusitis. It is available as a nasal spray and is not normally given to children under 12 years, except on medical advice.
+▲ Side-effects/warning: See XYLOMETAZOLINE HYDROCHLORIDE.

Otrivine-Antistin

(Ciba-Vision) is a proprietary, non-prescription of the ANTIHISTAMINE antazoline (as sulphate) and the SYMPATHOMIMETIC and VASOCONSTRICTOR xylometazoline hydrochloride. It can be used as an eye treatment for the relief of conjunctivitis, and is available as eye-drops.
+▲ Side-effects/warning: See ANTAZOLINE; XYLOMETAZOLINE HYDROCHLORIDE.

Ovestin

(Organon) is a proprietary, prescription-only preparation of the OESTROGEN oestriol. It can be used in HRT, and is available as tablets.
+▲ Side-effects/warning: See OESTRIOL.

Ovex Tablets

(Johnson & Johnson) is a proprietary, non-prescription preparation of the ANTHELMINTIC mebendazole. It can be used to treat infection by threadworms, and is available as chewable tablets. It is not normally given to children under two years, except on medical advice.
+▲ Side-effects/warning: See MEBENDAZOLE.

Ovran

(Wyeth) is a proprietary, prescription-only COMPOUND PREPARATION which can be used as a (*monophasic*) ORAL CONTRACEPTIVE (and also for certain menstrual problems) of the type that combines an OESTROGEN and a PROGESTOGEN, in this case ethinyloestradiol and levonorgestrel. It is available as tablets contained in a calendar pack.
+▲ Side-effects/warning: See ETHINYLOESTRADIOL; LEVONORGESTREL.

Ovran 30

(Wyeth) is a proprietary, prescription-only COMPOUND PREPARATION which can be used as a (*monophasic*) ORAL CONTRACEPTIVE (and also for certain menstrual problems) of the type that combines an OESTROGEN and a PROGESTOGEN, in this case ethinyloestradiol and levonorgestrel. It is available as tablets contained in a calendar pack.
+▲ Side-effects/warning: See ETHINYLOESTRADIOL; LEVONORGESTREL.

Ovranette

(Wyeth) is proprietary, prescription-only COMPOUND PREPARATION which can be used as a (*monophasic*) ORAL CONTRACEPTIVE (and also for certain menstrual problems) of the type that combines an OESTROGEN and a PROGESTOGEN, in this instance ethinyloestradiol and levonorgestrel. It is available as tablets contained in a calendar pack.
+▲ Side-effects/warning: See ETHINYLOESTRADIOL; LEVONORGESTREL.

Ovysmen

(Ortho) is a proprietary, prescription-only COMPOUND PREPARATION which can be used as a (*monophasic*) ORAL CONTRACEPTIVE (and also for certain menstrual problems) of the type that combines an OESTROGEN and a PROGESTOGEN, in this instance ethinyloestradiol and norethisterone. It is available as tablets contained in a calendar pack.
+▲ Side-effects/warning: See ETHINYLOESTRADIOL; NORETHISTERONE.

O

Owbridge's for Dry Tickly and Allergy Coughs

(Chefaro) is a proprietary, non-prescription preparation of the (OPIOID) NARCOTIC ANALGESIC and ANTITUSSIVE dextromethorphan hydrobromide with glycerine. It can be used for the symptomatic relief of dry, ticklish unproductive coughs, and is available as an oral liquid. It is not normally given to children, except on medical advice.

✚▲ Side-effects/warning: See DEXTROMETHORPHAN HYDROBROMIDE.

oxazepam

is a BENZODIAZEPINE which is used as an ANXIOLYTIC in the short-term treatment of anxiety. Administration is oral.

✚▲ Side-effects/warning: See BENZODIAZEPINES.

oxerutins

are mixtures of RUTOSIDES that are thought to reduce the fragility and the permeability of capillary blood vessels. They are used to treat disorders of the veins, for example, cramp in the legs, and for oedema. Administration is oral.

✚ Side-effects: Flushing, headache, rashes and gastrointestinal disturbances.

❂ Related entry: Paroven.

oxethazaine

is a LOCAL ANAESTHETIC which is used by topical application for the relief of local pain. It is a constituent of a proprietary ANTACID which is administered as an oral suspension.

❂ Related entry: Mucaine.

oxitropium bromide

is an ANTICHOLINERGIC drug that has the properties of a BRONCHODILATOR. It is primarily used to treat chronic bronchitis, but it can also be used as an ANTI-ASTHMATIC. Administration is by aerosol.

✚▲ Side-effects/warning: See IPRATROPIUM BROMIDE. There may be blurring of vision.

❂ Related entry: Oxivent.

Oxivent

(Boehringer Ingelheim) is a proprietary, prescription-only preparation of the ANTICHOLINERGIC drug oxitropium bromide, which also has BRONCHODILATOR properties. It can be used to treat chronic bronchitis and other disorders of the upper respiratory tract. It is available as an aerosol spray administered from a breath-activated *Autohaler* and as a metered aerosol.

✚▲ Side-effects/warning: See OXITROPIUM BROMIDE.

oxpentifylline

(pentoxifylline) is a VASODILATOR drug which dilates the blood vessels of the extremities and can be used to treat peripheral vascular disease (Raynaud's phenomenon). Administration is oral.

✚ Side effects: Gastrointestinal disturbances; headache, dizziness; there may be flushing and a speeding of the heart.

▲ Warning: It should not be used in patients with brain haemorrhage, or with certain heart disorders.

❂ Related entry: Trental.

oxprenolol hydrochloride

is a BETA-BLOCKER which can be used as an ANTIHYPERTENSIVE for raised blood pressure, as an ANTI-ANGINA treatment to relieve symptoms and improve exercise tolerance and as an ANTI-ARRHYTHMIC to regularize heartbeat and to treat myocardial infarction. It can also be used as an ANXIOLYTIC, particularly for symptomatic relief of tremor and palpitations. Administration is oral. It is also available, as an antihypertensive, in the form of COMPOUND PREPARATIONS with a DIURETIC.

✚▲ Side-effects/warning: See PROPRANOLOL HYDROCHLORIDE.

❂ Related entries: Apsolox; Slow-Trasicor; Trasicor; Trasidrex.

Oxy 10 Lotion

(SK&F) is a proprietary, non-prescription preparation of the KERATOLYTIC and

ANTIMICROBIAL drug benzoyl peroxide
(10%). It can be used for the treatment of
acne and spots, and is available as a lotion
for topical application.

➕▲ Side-effects/warning: See BENZOYL
PEROXIDE.

Oxy 5 Lotion

(SK&F) is a proprietary, non-prescription
preparation of the KERATOLYTIC and
ANTIMICROBIAL drug benzoyl peroxide (5%).
It can be used for the treatment of acne and
spots, and is available as a lotion for topical
application.

➕▲ Side-effects/warning: See BENZOYL
PEROXIDE.

oxybuprocaine hydrochloride

(benoxinate) is a LOCAL ANAESTHETIC which is
used by topical application in ophthalmic
procedures. Aministration is by topical
application.

➕ Side-effects: There may be initial stinging
on application.

⊙ Related entry: Minims Benoxinate
(Oxybuprocaine) Hydrochloride.

oxybutynin hydrochloride

is an ANTICHOLINERGIC drug which can be
administered as an ANTISPASMODIC to treat
urinary frequency, incontinence and
bladder spasms. Administration is oral.

➕ Side-effects: These include dry mouth,
blurred vision, constipation, nausea,
abdominal discomfort, difficulty in
urination, flushing of the face, headache,
dizziness, diarrhoea, dry skin and heart
irregularities.

▲ Warning: It should not be administered
to patients with intestinal obstruction, severe
ulcerative colitis, toxic megacolon,
glaucoma, or bladder obstruction. Use with
care in those patients with certain heart,
liver or kidney disorders, hyperthyroidism,
prostatic hypertrophy, hiatus hernia with
reflux oesophagitis or porphyria; or who are
pregnant or breast-feeding.

⊙ Related entries: Cystrin; Ditropan.

oxymetazoline hydrochloride

is a SYMPATHOMIMETIC, an alpha-
adrenoreceptor stimulant, which is
generally used for its VASOCONSTRICTOR
properties that make it an effective NASAL
DECONGESTANT. It is applied topically to the
nasal passages where it constricts the blood
vessels of the nose, reducing congestion in
the nasal mucous membranes and possibly
also reducing secretions. Administration is
in the form of nose-drops or a nasal spray.

➕▲ Side-effects/warning: See
XYLOMETAZOLINE HYDROCHLORIDE.

⊙ Related entries: Afrazine; Dristan Nasal
Spray; Sudafed Nasal Spray; Vicks Sinex
Decongestant Nasal Spray.

oxymetholone

is an (*anabolic*) STEROID which is used to
treat aplastic anaemia. Administration is
oral.

➕ Side-effects: Nausea, vomiting,
diarrhoea, sleeplessness, excitement, muscle
cramps, chills, acne, jaundice and liver
toxicity, pruritus, oedema, congestive heart
failure, effects on bones; with high doses,
masculinization in women and children,
amenorrhoea, changes in fertility, raised
blood calcium and changes in blood lipids.

▲ Warning: It is not to be administered to
patients with severe impairment of liver
function, certain cancers, who are pregnant
or have porphyria. Administer with caution
to those with heart, kidney or liver disorders,
hypertension, diabetes, epilepsy or migraine.
Bone growth should be monitored when
treating young people or children.

⊙ Related entry: Anapolon 50.

Oxymycin

(DDSA Pharmaceuticals) is a proprietary,
prescription-only preparation of the
ANTIBACTERIAL and (TETRACYCLINE) ANTIBIOTIC
oxytetracycline. It can be used to treat a
wide range of infections, and is available as
tablets.

➕▲ Side-effects/warning: See
OXYTETRACYCLINE.

O

O

oxypertine

is an ANTIPSYCHOTIC drug which is
administered to treat and tranquillize
patients suffering from psychotic disorders,
for example, schizophrenia. The drug may
also be used, but in the short-term only, in
the treatment of severe anxiety.
Administration is oral.

✚▲ Side-effects/warning: See
CHLORPROMAZINE HYDROCHLORIDE; however,
there are usually fewer extrapyramidal
symptoms (muscle tremor and rigidity) and
occasional photophobia. There may also be
some excitation or sedation, depending on
the strength of the dose administered.
✿ Related entry: Oxypertine.

Oxypertine

(Sterwin) is a proprietary, prescription-only
preparation of the ANTIPSYCHOTIC drug
oxypertine. It can be used to treat and
tranquillize patients with psychotic
disorders, such as schizophrenia. It can
also be used for the short-term treatment
of severe anxiety. It is available as tablets
and capsules.

✚▲ Side-effects/warning: See OXYPERTINE.

oxyphenisatin

(oxyphenisatine) is a (*stimulant*) LAXATIVE
which is used to promote defecation and so
relieve constipation. It would seem, though
it is not certain, to achieve its action by
stimulating motility in the intestine. It can
also be administered to evacuate the colon
prior to rectal examination or surgery.
Administration is topical as an enema.

✚ Side-effects: Abdominal cramps.

▲ Warning: It is best to avoid repeated use
because it can damage the liver. It must not
be administered to patients with with
intestinal obstruction.
✿ Related entry: Veripaque.

oxyphenisatine

see OXYPHENISATIN

oxytetracycline

is a broad-spectrum ANTIBACTERIAL and

(TETRACYCLINE) ANTIBIOTIC which can be
administered to treat quite an extensive
range of serious infections, particularly
those of the urinogenital and respiratory
tracts and of the skin (for example, acne).
Administration is oral.

✚▲ Side-effects/warning: See
TETRACYCLINE. It should not be administered
to patients with porphyria.
✿ Related entries: Berkmycen; Oxymycin;
Oxytetramix; Terra-Cortril; Terra-Cortril
Nystatin; Terramycin; Trimovate.

Oxytetramix

(Ashbourne) is a proprietary, prescription-
only preparation of the ANTIBACTERIAL and
(TETRACYCLINE) ANTIBIOTIC drug
oxytetracycline. It can be used to treat a
wide range of infections, and is available as
tablets.

✚▲ Side-effects/warning: See
OXYTETRACYCLINE.

oxytocin

is a natural pituitary HORMONE produced
and secreted by the posterior pituitary
gland. It increases the contractions of the
uterus during normal labour and also
stimulates lactation. Therapeutically,
oxytocin may be administered by injection
or infusion to induce or assist labour (or
abortion), to speed up the third stage of
labour (delivery of the placenta) and it is
also used in conjunction with the
VASOCONSTRICTOR drug ERGOMETRINE MALEATE
to help stop bleeding following childbirth
and abortion.

✚ Side-effects: High doses may lead to
violent contractions of the uterus, which
may result in a rupture of the uterine wall
and/or cause foetal distress. In the mother,
there may be hypertension, haemorrhage in
the subarachnoid space, water retention,
oedema of the lungs and pain.

▲ Warning: It should not be administered
to patients who suffer from certain
abnormalities of the uterus; who have a
mechanical obstruction to delivery; where
the foetus is in evident distress; in placenta

praevia; or where there is a risk of embolism. It should be administered with caution to those patients who suffer from hypertension and certain other cardiovascular disorders; who are about to undergo a multiple birth; or who have previously had a Caesarean section.
☉ Related entries: Syntocinon; Syntometrine.

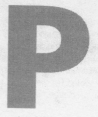

Pacifene
(Sussex) is a proprietary, non-prescription preparation of the (NSAID) NON-NARCOTIC ANALGESIC, ANTIRHEUMATIC and ANTIPYRETIC drug ibuprofen. It can be used for the relief of pain, including headache, period pain, muscular pain, dental pain and feverishness, and also for the symptomatic relief of cold and flu. It is available as tablets and is not normally given to children under 12 years, except on medical advice.
＋▲ Side-effects/warning: See IBUPROFEN.

Pacifene Maximum Strength
(Sussex) is a proprietary, non-prescription preparation of the (NSAID) NON-NARCOTIC ANALGESIC, ANTIRHEUMATIC and ANTIPYRETIC drug ibuprofen. It can be used for the relief of pain, including headache, period pain, muscular pain, dental pain and feverishness, and also for the symptomatic relief of cold and flu. It is available as tablets and is not normally given to children under 12 years, except on medical advice.
＋▲ Side-effects/warning: See IBUPROFEN.

paclitaxel
is a CYTOTOXIC drug, the first of a new group of drugs termed the *taxanes*. It is used as an ANTICANCER drug in the treatment of ovarian and breast cancer. Administration is by intravenous infusion.
＋▲ Side-effects/warning: See CYTOTOXICS.
☉ Related entry: Taxol.

Paldesic

(RP) is a proprietary, non-prescription preparation of the NON-NARCOTIC ANALGESIC and ANTIPYRETIC paracetamol. It is available as a paediatric oral solution, which, on medical advice, can be used to reduce fever in infants over three months (or temperature following vaccination at two months).

+▲ Side-effects/warning: See PARACETAMOL.

Palfium

(Boehringer Mannheim) is a proprietary, prescription-only preparation of the (OPIOID) NARCOTIC ANALGESIC dextromoramide, and is on the Controlled Drugs List. It can be used to relieve severe pain, especially during the final stages of terminal malignant disease, and is available as tablets and suppositories.

+▲ Side-effects/warning: See DEXTROMORAMIDE.

Paludrine

(Zeneca) is a proprietary, non-prescription preparation of the ANTIMALARIAL proguanil hydrochloride. It can be used in the prevention of malaria, and is available as tablets.

+▲ Side-effects/warning: See PROGUANIL HYDROCHLORIDE.

Pamergan P100

(Martindale) is a proprietary, prescription-only COMPOUND PREPARATION of the (OPIOID) NARCOTIC ANALGESIC pethidine hydrochloride and the SEDATIVE and HYPNOTIC (and ANTIHISTAMINE) promethazine hydrochloride, and is on the Controlled Drugs List. It can be used to relieve pain, especially during childbirth, and is available in a form for injection.

+▲ Side-effects/warning: See PETHIDINE HYDROCHLORIDE; PROMETHAZINE HYDROCHLORIDE.

Pameton

(SmithKline Beecham) is a proprietary, non-prescription COMPOUND PREPARATION of the NON-NARCOTIC ANALGESIC and ANTIPYRETIC paracetamol and the amino acid METHIONINE (an antidote to paracetamol overdose). It can be used to provide relief from painful and feverish conditions, such as period pain, toothache, cold and flu symptoms, and to reduce high body temperature (especially for patients likely to overdose). It is available as capsule-shaped tablets (*Caplets*) and is not normally given to children under six years, except on medical advice.

+▲ Side-effects/warning: See PARACETAMOL.

Panadeine Tablets

(SmithKline Beecham) is a proprietary, non-prescription COMPOUND ANALGESIC preparation of the NON-NARCOTIC ANALGESIC and ANTIPYRETIC paracetamol and the NARCOTIC ANALGESIC codeine phosphate (a combination known as co-codamol 8/500). It can be used to treat pain, such as toothache, sore throat, period pain, arthritis and rheumatic pain, and to reduce high body temperature. It is available as tablets and is not normally given to children under seven years, except on medical advice.

+▲ Side-effects/warning: See CODEINE PHOSPHATE; PARACETAMOL.

Panadol Baby and Infant Suspension

(SmithKline Beecham) is a proprietary, non-prescription preparation of the NON-NARCOTIC ANALGESIC and ANTIPYRETIC paracetamol. It can be used to relieve pain, such as teething pain and toothache, to reduce high body temperature and fever in babies and infants with colds, flu or childhood infections (eg chicken pox). It is available as a suspension and should not be given to babies under two months.

+▲ Side-effects/warning: See PARACETAMOL.

Panadol Capsules

(SmithKline Beecham) is a proprietary, non-prescription preparation of the NON-NARCOTIC ANALGESIC and ANTIPYRETIC paracetamol. It can be used to treat mild pain and to reduce high body temperature, such as musculoskeletal pain, toothache, period pain and to relieve cold and flu symptoms. It is available as capsules and is not normally given to children under 12 years, except on medical advice.

✚▲ Side-effects/warning: See PARACETAMOL.

Panadol Extra Soluble Tablets

(SmithKline Beecham) is a proprietary, non-prescription COMPOUND PREPARATION of the NON-NARCOTIC ANALGESIC and ANTIPYRETIC paracetamol and the STIMULANT caffeine. It can be used to treat mild pain and to reduce high body temperature, such as musculoskeletal pain, toothache, period pain and to relieve cold and flu symptoms. It is available as soluble tablets and is not normally given to children under 12 years, except on medical advice.

✚▲ Side-effects/warning: See CAFFEINE; PARACETAMOL.

Panadol Extra Tablets

(SmithKline Beecham) is a proprietary, non-prescription COMPOUND PREPARATION of the NON-NARCOTIC ANALGESIC and ANTIPYRETIC paracetamol and the STIMULANT caffeine. It can be used to treat mild pain, such as musculoskeletal pain, toothache and period pain, to reduce high body temperature and to relieve cold and flu symptoms. It is available as tablets and is not normally given to children under 12 years, except on medical advice.

✚▲ Side-effects/warning: See CAFFEINE; PARACETAMOL.

Panadol Junior

(SmithKline Beecham) is a proprietary, non-prescription preparation of the NON-NARCOTIC ANALGESIC and ANTIPYRETIC paracetamol. It can be used to treat pain, reduce high body temperature and to relieve cold and flu symptoms, sore throat, headache and toothache. It is available as an orange powder in sachets and is not

normally given to children under three years, except on medical advice.

✚▲ Side-effects/warning: See PARACETAMOL.

Panadol Soluble

(SmithKline Beecham) is a proprietary, non-prescription preparation of the NON-NARCOTIC ANALGESIC and ANTIPYRETIC paracetamol. It can be used to treat pain such as musculoskeletal pain, toothache and period pain, to reduce high body temperature and to relieve cold and flu symptoms. It is available as effervescent tablets and is not normally given to children under six years, except on medical advice.

✚▲ Side-effects/warning: See PARACETAMOL.

Panadol Tablets

(SmithKline Beecham) is a proprietary, non-prescription preparation of the NON-NARCOTIC ANALGESIC and ANTIPYRETIC paracetamol. It can be used to treat pain, such as musculoskeletal pain, toothache and period pain, to reduce high body temperature and to relieve cold and flu symptoms. It is available as effervescent tablets and is not normally given to children under six years, except on medical advice.

✚▲ Side-effects/warning: See PARACETAMOL.

Panadol Ultra

(SmithKline Beecham) is a proprietary, non-prescription COMPOUND PREPARATION of the NON-NARCOTIC ANALGESIC and ANTIPYRETIC paracetamol and the OPIOID NARCOTIC ANALGESIC codeine phosphate. It can be used to treat pain, such as musculoskeletal pain, sciatica, strains, toothache and period pain, to reduce high body temperature and to relieve cold and flu symptoms and sore throat. It is available as tablets and is not to be given to children, except on medical advice.

✚▲ Side-effects/warning: See CODEINE PHOSPHATE; PARACETAMOL.

Pancrease

(Cilag) is a proprietary, non-prescription preparation of the digestive ENZYME

P

pancreatin. It can be used to treat a deficiency of the digestive juices that are normally supplied by the pancreas, and is available as capsules.

✚▲ Side-effects/warning: See PANCREATIN.

Pancrease HL

(Cilag) is a proprietary, non-prescription preparation of the digestive ENZYME pancreatin. It can be used to treat a deficiency of the digestive juices that are normally supplied by the pancreas, and is available as capsules (at a higher strength than *Pancrease*).

✚▲ Side-effects/warning: See PANCREATIN.

pancreatin

is the term used to describe extracts of the pancreas that contain pancreatic ENZYME. It can be given by mouth to treat deficiencies due to impaired natural secretion by the pancreas, such as in cystic fibrosis, and also following operations involving removal of pancreatic tissue, such as panreatectomy and gastrectomy. The enzymes are inactivated by the acid in the stomach and so preparations should be taken with food or with certain other drugs, such as H_2-ANTAGONISTS, that reduce acid secretion. Alternatively, pancreatin is available as enteric-coated capsules, which overcome some of these problems, but are destroyed by heat and should be mixed with food after its preparation. The majority of pancreatin preparations are of porcine origin and administered as capsules or granules.

✚ Side-effects: Irritation of the skin around the mouth and anus; there may be gastrointestinal upsets, including nausea, vomiting and abdominal discomfort; and at high dose there may be raised uric acid levels in the blood and urine.

▲ Warning: There may be hypersensitivity reactions in those that handle the powder. There are particular problems (fibrotic structures in the bowel) that seem to be associated with high-dose preparations and these should only be taken with specialist advice.

⊙ Related entries: Creon; Creon 25 000; Nutrizym 10; Nutrizym 22; Nutrizym GR; Pancrease; Pancrease HL; Pancrex; Pancrex V.

Pancrex

(Paines & Byrne) is a proprietary, non-prescription preparation of the digestive ENZYME pancreatin. It can be used to treat a deficiency of the digestive juices that are normally supplied by the pancreas, and is available as granules.

✚▲ Side-effects/warning: See PANCREATIN.

Pancrex V

(Paines & Byrne) is a proprietary, non-prescription preparation of the digestive ENZYME pancreatin. It can be used to treat a deficiency of the digestive juices that are normally supplied by the pancreas, and is available as capsules (one preparation is called *Pancrex V 125*), tablets and a powder.

✚▲ Side-effects/warning: See PANCREATIN.

pancuronium bromide

is a *non-depolarizing* SKELETAL MUSCLE RELAXANT which is used to induce muscle paralysis during surgery. Administration is by injection.

✚▲ Side-effects/warning: See TUBOCURARINE CHLORIDE.

⊙ Related entry: Pavulon.

Panda Baby Cream & Castor Oil Cream with Lanolin

(Thornton & Ross) is a proprietary, non-prescription COMPOUND PREPARATION of ZINC OXIDE, castor oil, wool fat (lanolin) and several other minor constituents. It can be used as an EMOLLIENT and a BARRIER CREAM for nappy rash and to protect chapped skin.

✚▲ Side-effects/warning: See CASTOR OIL; WOOL FAT.

PanOxyl 10 Gel

(Stiefel) is a proprietary, non-prescription preparation of the KERATOLYTIC and ANTIMICROBIAL benzoyl peroxide (10%). It can be used to treat acne, and is available as a gel for topical application. It is not normally used on children, except on medical advice.

+▲ Side-effects/warning: See BENZOYL PEROXIDE.

PanOxyl 5 Gel

(Stiefel) is a proprietary, non-prescription preparation of the KERATOLYTIC and ANTIMICROBIAL benzoyl peroxide (5%). It can be used to treat acne, and is available as a gel for topical application. It is not normally used on children, except on medical advice.

+▲ Side-effects/warning: See BENZOYL PEROXIDE.

PanOxyl Aquagel 10

(Stiefel) is a proprietary, non-prescription preparation of the KERATOLYTIC and ANTIMICROBIAL benzoyl peroxide (10%). It can be used to treat acne, and is available as a gel for topical application.

+▲ Side-effects/warning: See BENZOYL PEROXIDE.

PanOxyl Aquagel 25

(Stiefel) is a proprietary, non-prescription preparation of the KERATOLYTIC and ANTIMICROBIAL benzoyl peroxide (5%). It can be used to treat acne, and is available as a gel for topical application.

+▲ Side-effects/warning: See BENZOYL PEROXIDE.

PanOxyl Aquagel 5

(Stiefel) is a proprietary, non-prescription preparation of the KERATOLYTIC and ANTIMICROBIAL benzoyl peroxide (2.5%). It can be used to treat acne, and is available as a gel for topical application.

+▲ Side-effects/warning: See BENZOYL PEROXIDE.

PanOxyl Wash

(Stiefel) is a proprietary, non-prescription preparation of the KERATOLYTIC and ANTIMICROBIAL benzoyl peroxide (10%). It can be used to treat acne, and is available

as a lotion for topical application. It is not normally used on children, except on medical advice.

+▲ Side-effects/warning: See BENZOYL PEROXIDE.

pantoprazole

is an ULCER-HEALING DRUG which works as an inhibitor of gastric acid secretion in the parietal (acid-producing) cells of the stomach lining by acting as a PROTON-PUMP INHIBITOR. It is used for the treatment of benign gastric and duodenal ulcers (including those complicating NSAID therapy) and reflux oesophagitis. Administration is oral.

+▲ Side-effects/warning: See OMEPRAZOLE. Special care is necessary in liver impairment.

✪ Related entry: Protium.

Papaveretum

is a non-proprietary, prescription-only COMPOUND PREPARATION of alkaloids of opium, most of which is made up of morphine with the rest largely consisting of codeine and papaverine. It is used as an (OPIOID) NARCOTIC ANALGESIC primarily during or following surgery, but can also be used as a sedative prior to an operation. Administration is either oral as tablets or by injection. (A proprietary preparation of papaveretum called *Omnopon* was formerly available). Preparations containing papaveretum are on the Controlled Drugs List because the drug is potentially addictive.

+▲ Side-effects/warning: See MORPHINE SULPHATE.

papaverine

is a SMOOTH MUSCLE RELAXANT which is rarely used any more, though it is included in a proprietary pain remedy. There have been some recent trials of its use for impotence by direct injection into the corpus cavernosum. Administration is either oral or by injection.

+ Side-effects: Local burning pain and

P haematoma (swelling) at the site of injection.

▲ Warning: It should be administered with care to patients with certain cardiovascular disorders.

○ Related entry: Aspav.

Papulex

(Euroderma) is a proprietary, non-prescription preparation of nicotinamide. It can be used to treat acne, and is available as a gel.

+▲ Side-effects/warning: See NICOTINAMIDE.

paracetamol

(called acetaminophen in the USA) is a NON-NARCOTIC ANALGESIC which can be used to treat all forms of mild to moderate pain. It also has ANTIPYRETIC properties and can be used to reduce fever and raised body temperature. In many ways it is similar to aspirin, except that it does not cause gastric irritation or relieve inflammation. Many proprietary preparations are COMPOUND ANALGESICS that combine paracetamol and aspirin. Administration can be oral or as suppositories.

+ Side-effects: There are few side-effects if dosage is low, though there may be rashes, acute pancreatitis and blood disorders; high overdosage or prolonged use may result in liver dysfunction.

▲ Warning: It should be administered with caution to patients with impaired liver function or who suffer from alcoholism (which causes liver damage).

○ Related entries: Actron; Anadin Extra; Anadin Extra Soluble Tablets; Anadin Paracetamol Tablets; Beechams All-In-One; Beechams Flu-Plus Hot Lemon; Beechams Hot Blackcurrant; Beechams Hot Lemon; Beechams Hot Lemon and Honey; Beechams Powders Capsules; Benylin Day and Night; Benylin Four Flu Liquid; Benylin Four Flu Tablets; Calpol Infant Suspension; Calpol Infant Suspension, Sugar-Free; Calpol Six Plus Suspension; Catarrh-Ex; co-codamol; Codanin Tablets; Cold Relief Capsules; Coldrex Tablets; Cool Lemon Lemsip; Cosalgesic; Cupanol Over 6 Paracetamol Oral Suspension; Cupanol Under 6 Paracetamol Oral Suspension; Day Cold Comfort Capsules; Day Nurse Capsules; Day Nurse Liquid; Disprin Extra; Disprol Junior; Disprol Paracetamol Suspension; Distalgesic; Doan's Backache Pills; Feminax; Fennings Children's Cooling Powders; Flurex Cold/Flu Capsules with Cough Suppressant; Flurex Tablets; Fortagesic; Fynnon Calcium Aspirin; Galake; Hedex Headcold Cherry Menthol Powders; Hedex Extra Tablets; Hedex Tablets; Infadrops; Kapake; Lemsip Cold Relief Capsules; Lemsip Flu Strength Pseudoephedrine Formula; Lemsip Night-time; Lemsip Maximum Strength; Lemsip Menthol Extra; Lemsip Original; Lobak; Medinol Over 6; Medinol Under 6; Medised; Midrid; Migraleve; Mu-Cron Syrup, Junior; Mu-Cron Tablets; Night Cold Comfort Capsules; Night Nurse Capsules; Night Nurse Liquid; Nurse Sykes Powders; Paldesic; Pameton; Panadeine Tablets; Panadol Baby and Infant Suspension; Panadol Capsules; Panadol Extra Soluble Tablets; Panadol Extra Tablets; Panadol Junior; Panadol Soluble; Panadol Tablets; Panadol Ultra; Paracets; Paracets Capsules; Paracodol Capsules; Paraclear; Paracodol Tablets; Paradote; Parake; Paramax; Paramol Tablets; Powerin Analgesic Tablets; Propain Tablets; Remedeine; Resolve; Salzone; Sinutab Tablets; Solpadeine Capsules; Solpadeine Soluble Tablets; Solpadeine Tablets; Solpadol; Sudafed-Co Tablets; Syndol; Tramil 500 Analgesic Capsules; Triogesic Tablets; Tylex; Veganin Tablets; Vicks Mednite.

Paracets

(Sussex) is a proprietary, non-prescription preparation of the NON-NARCOTIC ANALGESIC and ANTIPYRETIC paracetamol. It can be used to treat mild to moderate pain, such as toothache and period pain, to reduce high body temperature and to relieve cold and flu symptoms. It is available as tablets and is not normally given to children under six years, except on medical advice.

+▲ Side-effects/warning: See PARACETAMOL.

Paracets Capsules

(Sussex) is a proprietary, non-prescription preparation of the NON-NARCOTIC ANALGESIC and ANTIPYRETIC paracetamol. It can be used to treat mild to moderate pain, such as toothache and period pain, to reduce high body temperature and to relieve cold and flu symptoms. It is available as capsules and is not normally given to children under six years, except on medical advice.

+▲ Side-effects/warning: See PARACETAMOL.

Paraclear

(Roche) is a proprietary, non-prescription preparation of the NON-NARCOTIC ANALGESIC and ANTIPYRETIC paracetamol. It can be used to treat mild to moderate pain, such as toothache and period pain, to reduce high body temperature and to relieve cold and flu symptoms. It is available as effervescent tablets and is not normally given to children under six years, except on medical advice.

+▲ Side-effects/warning: See PARACETAMOL.

Paraclear Extra Strength

(Roche) is a proprietary, non-prescription COMPOUND PREPARATION of the NON-NARCOTIC ANALGESIC and ANTIPYRETIC paracetamol and the STIMULANT caffeine. It can be used to treat mild to moderate pain, such as toothache and period pain, to reduce high body temperature and to relieve cold and flu symptoms. It is available as tablets and is not normally given to children under six years, except on medical advice.

+▲ Side-effects/warning: See CAFFEINE; PARACETAMOL.

Paracodol Capsules

(Roche) is a proprietary, non-prescription COMPOUND PREPARATION of the NON-NARCOTIC ANALGESIC and ANTIPYRETIC paracetamol and the (OPIOID) NARCOTIC ANALGESIC codeine phosphate (a combination known as co-codamol 8/500). It can be used to treat mild to moderate pain and to reduce high body temperature. It is available as tablets

and is not normally given to children under 12 years, except on medical advice.
+▲ Side-effects/warning: See CODEINE PHOSPHATE; PARACETAMOL.

Paracodol Tablets

(Roche) is a proprietary, non-prescription COMPOUND ANALGESIC preparation of the NON-NARCOTIC ANALGESIC and ANTIPYRETIC paracetamol and the (OPIOID) NARCOTIC ANALGESIC codeine phosphate (a combination known as co-codamol 8/500). It can be used to relieve mild to moderate pain and to reduce high body temperature. It is available as tablets and is not normally given to children under six years, except on medical advice.

+▲ Side-effects/warning: See CODEINE PHOSPHATE; PARACETAMOL.

Paradote

(Penn) is a proprietary, non-prescription COMPOUND PREPARATION of the (NSAID) NON-NARCOTIC ANALGESIC and ANTIPYRETIC paracetamol and the amino acid METHIONINE (an antidote to paracetamol overdose). It can be used to provide relief from painful and feverish conditions, such as period pain, toothache and cold and flu symptoms, and to reduce high body temperature (especially for patients likely to overdose). It is available as tablets.

+▲ Side-effects/warning: See PARACETAMOL.

paraffin

is a hydrocarbon derived from petroleum. Its main therapeutic use is as a base for ointments such as either YELLOW SOFT PARAFFIN or WHITE SOFT PARAFFIN. As a mineral oil, LIQUID PARAFFIN is used as a LAXATIVE and is also incorporated into many preparations as an EMOLLIENT.

Parake

(Galen) is a proprietary, non-prescription COMPOUND ANALGESIC preparation of the NON-NARCOTIC ANALGESIC and ANTIPYRETIC paracetamol and the (OPIOID) NARCOTIC ANALGESIC codeine phosphate (a

P

combination known as co-codamol 8/500).
It can be used to relieve pain and to reduce
high body temperature. It is available as
tablets and is not normally given to children
under seven years, except on medical
advice.
✚▲ Side-effects/warning: See CODEINE
PHOSPHATE; PARACETAMOL.

paraldehyde

is a drug that is used mainly as an
ANTICONVULSANT and ANTI-EPILEPTIC in the
treatment of status epilepticus (severe and
continuous epileptic seizures).
Administration is by injection or enema.
✚ Side-effects: Rash, pain and abscess after
injections, rectal irritation after enema.
▲ Warning: Administer with caution to
patients with lung disease or impaired liver
function.

Paramax

(Lorex) is a proprietary, prescription-only
COMPOUND PREPARATION of the ANTI-EMETIC
and ANTINAUSEANT metoclopramide
hydrochloride and the NON-NARCOTIC
ANALGESIC paracetamol. It can be used as an
ANTIMIGRAINE treatment for acute migraine
attacks, and is available as tablets and an
effervescent powder.
✚▲ Side-effects/warning: See
METOCLOPRAMIDE HYDROCHLORIDE;
PARACETAMOL. Note the side-effects in young
people.

Paramol Tablets

(Seton) is a proprietary non-prescription
COMPOUND ANALGESIC preparation of the NON-
NARCOTIC ANALGESIC paracetamol and the
(OPIOID) NARCOTIC ANALGESIC and ANTITUSSIVE
dihydrocodeine tartrate. It can be used for
general pain-relief, including period pains,
headache, toothache and muscular aches,
and for cough relief. It is available as
tablets and is not normally given to children
under 12 years, except on medical advice.
(The proprietary name *Paramol* was
formerly used for a prescription-only
combination known as co-dydramol.)

✚▲ Side-effects/warning: See
DIHYDROCODEINE TARTRATE; PARACETAMOL.

Paraplatin

(Bristol-Myers) is a proprietary,
prescription-only preparation of the
(CYTOTOXIC) ANTICANCER drug carboplatin. It
can be used specifically in the treatment of
ovarian cancer, and is available in a form
for injection.
✚▲ Side-effects/warning: See CARBOPLATIN.

parasympathomimetics ▣

are drugs that have effects similar to those
of the parasympathetic nervous system.
They work by mimicking the actions of the
natural neurotransmitter acetylcholine (eg
CARBACHOL and PILOCARPINE). The
ANTICHOLINESTERASE drugs (eg NEOSTIGMINE)
are *indirect parasympathomimetics*
because they prolong the duration of action
of the naturally released acetylcholine.
Direct parasympathomimetics act at
(so-called 'muscarinic') receptors for
acetylcholine. Important
parasympathomimetic actions include
slowing of the heart, vasodilation,
constriction of the bronchioles of the lung,
stimulation of the muscles of the intestine
and bladder and constriction of the pupil
and altered focusing of the eye.
ANTICHOLINERGIC drugs oppose some of these
actions.

parathormone

see CALCITONIN

parathyroid hormone

see CALCITONIN

Parlodel

(Sandoz) is a proprietary, prescription-only
preparation of bromocriptine. It is used
primarily to treat parkinsonism, but not the
parkinsonian symptoms caused by certain
drug therapies (see ANTIPARKINSONISM). It
can also be used to treat a number of other
hormonal disorders, and is available as
tablets and capsules.

+▲ Side-effects/warning: See
BROMOCRIPTINE.

Parmid

(Lagap) is a proprietary, prescription-only
preparation of the ANTI-EMETIC and
ANTINAUSEANT metoclopramide
hydrochloride. It can be used for the
treatment of nausea and vomiting,
particularly when associated with
gastrointestinal disorders and after
treatment with radiation or cytotoxic drugs.
It also has gastric MOTILITY STIMULANT
actions and can be used in the treatment of
non-ulcer dyspepsia, gastric stasis and for
prevention of reflux oesophagitis. It is
available as tablets and an oral solution.
+▲ Side-effects/warning: See
METOCLOPRAMIDE HYDROCHLORIDE. Note the
side-effects in young people.

Parnate

(SK&F) is a proprietary, prescription-only
preparation of the MONOAMINE-OXIDASE
INHIBITOR (MAOI) ANTIDEPRESSANT
tranylcypromine. It is available as tablets.
+▲ Side-effects/warning: See
TRANYLCYPROMINE.

Paroven

(Zyma) is a proprietary, non-prescription
preparation of oxerutins. It can be used to
treat cramp and other manifestations of
poor circulation in the veins, such as
oedema, and is available as capsules.
+▲ Side-effects/warning: See OXERUTINS.

paroxetine

is an ANTIDEPRESSANT of the recently
developed SSRI group. It can be used to
treat depressive illness and has the
advantage over some other antidepressants
because it has less sedative and
ANTICHOLINERGIC side-effects. Administration
is oral.
+▲ Side-effects/warning: See FLUOXETINE.
There may be spasm of facial muscles and
withdrawal symptoms may be marked.
✪ **Related entry: Seroxat.**

Parstelin

(SK&F) is a proprietary, prescription-only
COMPOUND PREPARATION of the MONOAMINE-
OXIDASE INHIBITOR (MAOI) ANTIDEPRESSANT
tranylcypromine and the ANTIPSYCHOTIC drug
trifluoperazine. It can be used to treat
depressive illness, particularly in
association with anxiety, and is available as
tablets.
+▲ Side-effects/warning: See
TRANYLCYPROMINE; TRIFLUOPERAZINE.

Partobulin

(Immuno) is a proprietary, prescription-
only preparation of anti-D Rh_0
immunoglobulin. It can be used to prevent
rhesus-negative mothers from making
antibodies against foetal rhesus-positive
cells that may pass into the mother's
circulation during childbirth, so protecting
a future child from haemolytic disease of
the newborn. It should be injected within a
few days of birth.
+▲ Side-effects/warning: See ANTI-D (RH_0)
IMMUNOGLOBULIN.

Parvolex

(Evans) is a proprietary, prescription-only
preparation of the ANTIDOTE acetylcysteine.
It can be used to treat overdose poisoning
by the NON-NARCOTIC ANALGESIC paracetamol,
and is available in a form for injection.
+▲ Side-effects/warning: See
ACETYLCYSTEINE.

Pavacol-D

(Boehringer Ingelheim) is a proprietary,
non-prescription preparation of the
(OPIOID) ANTITUSSIVE pholcodine. It can be
used for dry or painful coughs, and is
available as a linctus.
+▲ Side-effects/warning: See PHOLCODINE.

Pavulon

(Organon-Teknika) is a proprietary,
prescription-only preparation of the
(*non-depolarizing*) SKELETAL MUSCLE
RELAXANT pancuronium bromide. It can be
used to induce muscle paralysis during

P

429

P

surgery, and is available in a form for injection.
+▲ Side-effects/warning: See PANCURONIUM BROMIDE.

Pecram

(Zyma) is a proprietary, non-prescription preparation of the BRONCHODILATOR aminophylline (as aminophylline hydrate). It can be used as an ANTI-ASTHMATIC and in bronchitis treatment, and is available as modified-release tablets.
+▲ Side-effects/warning: See AMINOPHYLLINE.

pediculicidals ☒

are drugs used to kill lice of the genus *Pediculus*, which infest either the body or the scalp, or both, and cause intense itching. Scratching tends to damage the skin surface and may eventually cause weeping lesions with bacterial infection as well. The best-known and most-used pediculicides include MALATHION and CARBARYL. LINDANE, which was once commonly administered, is now no longer used for lice on the scalp because resistant strains of lice have developed. Administration is topical, usually as a lotion, and contact between the drug and the skin should be as long as possible (at least 12 hours or overnight) and repeated after seven days.

pemoline

is used to treat hyperkinesis (hyperactivity) in children, but, in contrast, in adults it acts as a weak STIMULANT. Administration is oral.
+▲ Side-effects/warning: See DEXAMPHETAMINE SULPHATE; but also mania, depression, muscle twitches and movement disorders, blood changes and liver abnormalities.
✪ Related entry: Volital.

Penbritin

(Beecham) is a proprietary, prescription-only preparation of the broad-spectrum ANTIBACTERIAL and (PENICILLIN) ANTIBIOTIC ampicillin. It can be used to treat systemic bacterial infections, infections of the upper respiratory tract, the ear, nose and throat and of the urinogenital tracts. It is available as capsules, a syrup, a paediatric suspension and in a form for injection.
+▲ Side-effects/warning: See AMPICILLIN.

penciclovir

is an ANTIVIRAL drug that is similar to ACYCLOVIR. It is used to treat labial herpes simplex infection. Administration is topical.
+▲ Side-effects/warning: See acyclovir.
✪ Related entry: Vectavir.

Pendramine

(ASTA Medica) is a proprietary, prescription-only preparation of the CHELATING AGENT penicillamine. It can be used as an ANTIDOTE to copper or lead poisoning, to reduce copper levels in Wilson's disease and as a long-term treatment for rheumatoid arthritis. It is available as tablets.
+▲ Side-effects/warning: See PENICILLAMINE.

Penetrol Catarrh Inhalant

(Seton) is a proprietary, non-prescription COMPOUND PREPARATION of the aromatic oils MENTHOL and peppermint. It can be used for the symptomatic relief of nasal congestion associated with catarrh, hay fever and colds. It is available as an inhalant and is not normally given to children under ten years, except on medical advice.
+▲ Side-effects/warning: See PEPPERMINT OIL.

Penetrol Inhalant

(Seton) is a proprietary, non-prescription preparation of MENTHOL and peppermint oil. It can be used for the symptomatic relief of catarrh, hay fever and nasal congestion, and is available as an inhalant. It is not normally given to children under three months, except on medical advice.
+▲ Side-effects/warning: See PEPPERMINT OIL.

penicillamine

is a derivative of penicillin and is an
extremely effective CHELATING AGENT. It binds
various metal ions within the body, so
facilitating their excretion (elimination
from the body). It can be used as an
ANTIDOTE to various types of metallic
poisoning (eg copper and lead) and to
reduce copper levels in Wilson's disease. It
is also used in the long-term treatment of
severe rheumatoid arthritis or juvenile
chronic arthritis, where it has ANTI-
INFLAMMATORY and ANTIRHEUMATIC actions.
Administration is oral.

✚ Side-effects: Nausea, anorexia, fever,
rashes, taste impairment, blood and kidney
disturbances, lupus-like syndrome or
muscle weakness.

▲ Warning: It should not be used in
patients known to have sensitivity to
penicillins or with lupus erythematus.
Administer with care to those with kidney
impairment, who are pregnant and with
known sensitivity to certain other drugs.
Regular monitoring of body functions is
required.

✪ Related entries: Distamine; Pendramine.

penicillin G

see BENZYLPENICILLIN

penicillin V

see PHENOXYMETHYLPENICILLIN

penicillinase inhibitors ⬚

are drugs used to inhibit ENZYMES that are
produced by certain (*penicillin-resistant*)
bacteria, which break down some of the
PENICILLIN class of ANTIBIOTICS, effectively
rendering the latter useless. Consequently,
treatment of infections caused by such
bacteria has normally necessitated the
administration of either *penicillinase-
resistant penicillins*, such as
FLUCLOXACILLIN, or entirely different classes
of antibiotic. However, some antibiotic
preparations combine a *penicillinase-
sensitive* drug with an inhibitor of the
penicillinase enzyme, which then artificially

gives that antibiotic penicillinase-resistance
(for example CLAVULANIC ACID and
TAZOBACTAM are inhibtors of penicillinase
(beta-lactamase).

penicillins ⬚

are ANTIBACTERIAL and ANTIBIOTIC drugs
which work by interfering with the synthesis
of bacterial cell walls. The early penicillins
were mainly effective against Gram-positive
bacteria, though they could be used against
the Gram-negative organisms that caused
gonorrhoea and meningitis, as well as the
organism causing syphilis. Later penicillins
(eg AMPICILLIN and PIPERACILLIN) expanded
the spectrum to include a greater range of
Gram-negative organisms. They are
absorbed rapidly by most (but not all) body
tissues and fluids and are excreted in the
urine. One great disadvantage of penicillins
is that many patients are allergic to them –
allergy to one, means allergy to all of them
– and may have reactions that range from a
minor rash right up to anaphylactic shock,
which occasionally can be fatal. Otherwise
they are remarkably non-toxic. Rarely, very
high dosage may cause convulsions,
haemolytic anaemia or abnormally high
levels of sodium or potassium in the body
with consequent symptoms. Those taken
orally tend to cause diarrhoea and there is
also a risk with broad-spectrum penicillins
of allowing a superinfection to develop. The
best-known and most-used penicillins
include BENZYLPENICILLIN (penicillin G; the
first of the penicillins),
PHENOXYMETHYLPENICILLIN (penicillin V),
FLUCLOXACILLIN, AMPICILLIN and AMOXYCILLIN.
See also AZLOCILLIN; BACAMPICILLIN
HYDROXIDE; CARBENICILLIN; CLOXACILLIN;
METHICILLIN; PHENOXYMETHYLPENICILLIN;
PIVAMPICILLIN; PROCAINE PENICILLIN;
TEMOCILLIN; TICARILLIN.

PenMix 10/90

(Novo Nordisk) is a proprietary, non-
prescription preparation of human BIPHASIC
ISOPHANE INSULIN (10% soluble/90%
isophane). It is used as a DIABETIC

TREATMENT to treat and maintain diabetic patients, and is available in cartridges for injection with *Novopen* devices and in prefilled, disposable injectors. It has an intermediate duration of action.

✛▲ Side-effects/warning: See INSULIN.

PenMix 20/80

(Novo Nordisk) is a proprietary, non-prescription preparation of human BIPHASIC ISOPHANE INSULIN (20% soluble/80% isophane). It is used as a DIABETIC TREATMENT to treat and maintain diabetic patients, and is available in cartridges (*Penfill*) for injection with *Novopen* devices and as prefilled, disposable injectors. It has an intermediate duration of action.

✛▲ Side-effects/warning: See INSULIN.

PenMix 30/70

(Novo Nordisk) is a proprietary, non-prescription preparation of human BIPHASIC ISOPHANE INSULIN (30% soluble/70% isophane). It is used as a DIABETIC TREATMENT to treat and maintain diabetic patients, and is available in cartridges (*Penfill*) for injection with *Novopen* devices and as prefilled, disposable injectors. It has an intermediate duration of action.

✛▲ Side-effects/warning: See INSULIN.

PenMix 40/60

(Novo Nordisk) is a proprietary, non-prescription preparation of human BIPHASIC ISOPHANE INSULIN (40% soluble/60% isophane). It is used as a DIABETIC TREATMENT to treat and maintain diabetic patients, and is available in cartridges (*Penfill*) for injection with *Novopen* devices and as prefilled, disposable injectors. It has an intermediate duration of action.

✛▲ Side-effects/warning: See INSULIN.

PenMix 50/50

(Novo Nordisk) is a proprietary, non-prescription preparation of human BIPHASIC

ISOPHANE INSULIN (50% soluble/50% isophane). It is used as a DIABETIC TREATMENT to treat and maintain diabetic patients, and is available in cartridges (*Penfill*) for injection with *Novopen* devices and as prefilled, disposable injectors. It has an intermediate duration of action.

✛▲ Side-effects/warning: See INSULIN.

Pentacarinat

(Rhône-Poulenc Rorer) is a proprietary, prescription-only preparation of the ANTIPROTOZOAL drug pentamidine isethionate. It can be used to treat pneumonia caused by the protozoan micro-organism *Pneumocystis carinii* in patients whose immune system has been suppressed (either following transplant surgery or because of a condition such as AIDS). It is available only for specialist use and is administered either by injection or inhalation.

✛▲ Side-effects/warning: See PENTAMIDINE ISETHIONATE.

pentaerythritol tetranitrate

is a short-acting VASODILATOR and ANTI-ANGINA drug which is used to prevent attacks of angina pectoris (ischaemic heart pain) when it is taken before exercise. It works by dilating the blood vessels returning blood to the heart and so reducing the heart's workload. Administration is oral.

✛▲ Side-effects/warning: See GLYCERYL TRINITRATE.

✪ Related entry: Mycardol.

pentamidine isethionate

(pentamidine isetionate) is an ANTIPROTOZOAL drug which is used to treat pneumonia caused by the protozoan micro-organism *Pneumocystis carinii* in patients whose immune system has been suppressed (either following transplant surgery or because of a condition such as AIDS). It has also been used as an antiprotozoal to treat a form of leishmaniasis. It is available only for specialist use and is administered either by injection or inhalation.

✚ Side-effects: It can cause severe hypotension while being administered or immediately after. There may also be serious pancreatitis, hypoglycaemia, arrhythmias, blood disorders, kidney failure and various other potentially serious side-effects.

▲ Warning: Administer with care to patients with certain liver, kidney and blood disorders. Careful monitoring is required.

◯ Related entry: Pentacarinat.

pentamidine isetionate

see PENTAMIDINE ISETHIONATE

Pentasa

(Yamanouchi) is a proprietary, prescription-only preparation of the AMINOSALICYLATE mesalazine. It can be used to treat patients who suffer from ulcerative colitis, and is available as modified-release tablets, suppositories and as a retention enema.

✚▲ Side-effects/warning: See MESALAZINE.

pentazocine

is a powerful NARCOTIC ANALGESIC which can be used to treat moderate to severe pain. It is an OPIOID and is like morphine sulphate in effect and action, but is less likely to cause dependence. However, it can precipitate withdrawal symptoms if used in patients dependent on opioids. Administration can be oral, topical or by injection. The proprietary forms are on the Controlled Drugs List. It is also available as COMPOUND PREPARATIONS in combination with PARACETAMOL.

✚▲ Side-effects/warning: See OPIOIDS. Disturbances and hallucinations are thought to occur. It is not suitable for use in patients with certain heart complications and should be avoided in patients with porphyria.

◯ Related entries: Fortagesic; Fortral.

Pentostam

(Wellcome) is a proprietary, prescription-only preparation of sodium stibogluconate, which has ANTIPROTOZOAL properties. It can be used to treat skin infections by protozoal micro-organisms of the genus *Leishmania* (eg leishmaniasis). It is available in a form for injection.

✚▲ Side-effects/warning: See SODIUM STIBOGLUCONATE.

pentoxifylline

see OXPENTIFYLLINE

Pentran

(Berk) is a proprietary, prescription-only preparation of the ANTICONVULSANT and ANTI-EPILEPTIC drug phenytoin. It can be administered to treat and prevent most forms of seizure and also trigeminal (facial) neuralgia. It is available as tablets.

✚▲ Side-effects/warning: See PHENYTOIN.

Pentrax

(Euroderma) is a proprietary, non-prescription preparation of coal tar. It can be used to treat skin conditions, such as dandruff (seborrhoeic dermatitis) and psoriasis of the scalp, and is available as a liquid scalp preparation.

✚▲ Side-effects/warning: See COAL TAR.

Pepcid

(Morson) is a proprietary, prescription-only preparation of the H_2-ANTAGONIST famotidine. It can be used as an ULCER-HEALING DRUG for benign peptic ulcers (in the stomach or duodenum), gastro-oesophagial reflux, dyspepsia and associated conditions. It is available as tablets.

✚▲ Side-effects/warning: See FAMOTIDINE.

Pepcid AC

(Johnson & Johnson) is a proprietary, non-prescription preparation of the H_2-ANTAGONIST famotidine. It can be used for the acute relief of the pain and discomfort of heartburn, dyspepsia and excess stomach acid, and is available as tablets for short-term use only.

✚▲ Side-effects/warning: See FAMOTIDINE.

P

peppermint oil

is used to relieve the discomfort of abdominal colic and distension, particularly in irritable bowel syndrome. It is thought to act as an ANTISPASMODIC by directly relaxing the smooth muscle of the intestinal walls. It is also incorporated into preparations for the relief of catarrh and nasal congestion. Administration is oral.

✚ Side-effects: There may be heartburn and rarely allergic reactions, such as rash, headache, muscle tremor, slowing of the heart and unsteady gait.

✪ Related entries: Colpermin; J Collis Browne's Mixture; KLN Suspension; Mintec; Penetrol Catarrh Inhalant.

Peptimax

(Ashbourne) is a proprietary preparation of the H₂-ANTAGONIST cimetidine. It is available on prescription or without a prescription in a limited amount and for short-term uses only. It can be used as an ULCER-HEALING DRUG for benign peptic ulcers (in the stomach or duodenum), gastro-oesophageal reflux, dyspepsia and associated conditions. It is available as tablets.

✚▲ Side-effects/warning: See CIMETIDINE.

Per/Vac

is an abbreviation for PERTUSSIS VACCINE (whooping cough vaccine), which is usually administered in combination with diphtheria and tetanus vaccine (*triple vaccine*) as DTPer/Vac/Ads.

✚▲ Side-effects/warning: See PERTUSSIS VACCINE.

Percutol

(Cusi) is a proprietary, non-prescription preparation of the VASODILATOR and ANTI-ANGINA drug glyceryl trinitrate. It can be used to treat and prevent angina pectoris. It is available in the form of an ointment for use on a dressing secured to the skin surface (on the chest, abdomen or thigh).

✚▲ Side-effects/warning: See GLYCERYL TRINITRATE.

Perdix

(Schwarz) is a proprietary, prescription-only preparation of the ACE INHIBITOR moexipril hydrochloride . It can be used as an ANTIHYPERTENSIVE, and is available as tablets.

✚▲ Side-effects/warning: See MOEXIPRIL HYDROCHLORIDE.

Perfan

(Merrell) is a proprietary, prescription-only preparation of the PHOSPHODIESTERASE INHIBITOR enoximone. It can be used, in the short term, in HEART FAILURE TREATMENT, especially where other drugs have not been successful. It is available in a form for infusion or injection.

✚▲ Side-effects/warning: See ENOXIMONE.

pergolide

is a recently introduced ANTIPARKINSONISM drug which is an ERGOT ALKALOID derivative and is similar to BROMOCRIPTINE in that it is useful in reducing 'off' periods in the disease. Administration is oral.

✚ Side-effects: Hallucinations, confusion, impaired muscle movements, somnolence, nausea and abdominal pain, dyspepsia, double vision, rhinitis, laboured breathing, insomnia, constipation or diarrhoea, hypotension and charges in heart rate or rhythm.

▲ Warning: Administer with care to patients with certain heart disorders, dyskinesias, history of confusion or hallucinations, porphyria; or who are pregnant or breast-feeding.

✪ Related entry: Celance.

Pergonal

(Serono) is a proprietary, prescription-only HORMONE preparation of human menopausal gonadotrophins, which contains FOLLICLE-STIMULATING HORMONE (FSH) and LUTEINISING HORMONE (LH). It can be used in infertility treatment in women with proven hypopituitarism and who do not respond to CLOMIPHENE CITRATE (another drug commonly used to treat infertility) and also in superovulation treatment in assisted conception (as with *in vitro* fertilization; IVF). It is available in a form for intramuscular injection.

✚▲ Side-effects/warning: See HUMAN MENOPAUSAL GONADOTROPHINS.

Periactin

(Merck Sharp & Dohme) is a proprietary, non-prescription preparation of cyproheptadine hydrochloride, which is a drug with ANTIHISTAMINE activity. It can be used for the symptomatic relief of allergic disorders, such as hay fever and urticaria, and is available as tablets and a syrup.

✚▲ Side-effects/warning: See CYPROHEPTADINE HYDROCHLORIDE.

pericyazine

is chemically a PHENOTHIAZINE and is used as an ANTIPSYCHOTIC drug to treat patients suffering from schizophrenia and other psychoses, particularly during behavioural disturbances. It can also be used in the short-term treatment of severe anxiety. Administration is oral.

✚▲ Side-effects/warning: See CHLORPROMAZINE HYDROCHLORIDE; but is more sedating and initially hypotension may occur.

✪ Related entry: Neulactil.

Perinal

(Demal) is a proprietary, prescription-only COMPOUND PREPARATION of the CORTICOSTEROID and ANTI-INFLAMMATORY drug hydrocortisone (as acetate) and the LOCAL ANAESTHETIC lignocaine hydrochloride. It can be used to treat haemorrhoids and inflammation in the anal region, and is available as a spray for topical application.

✚▲ Side-effects/warning: See HYDROCORTISONE; LIGNOCAINE HYDROCHLORIDE.

perindopril

is an ACE INHIBITOR and acts as a VASODILATOR. It can be used as an ANTIHYPERTENSIVE and in HEART FAILURE TREATMENT, and is often used in conjunction with other classes of drugs, particularly (THIAZIDE) DIURETICS. Administration is oral.

✚▲ Side-effects/warning: See CAPTOPRIL.

✪ Related entry: Coversyl.

permethrin

is a PEDICULICIDAL drug which can be used to treat infestations by lice and as a SCABICIDAL to treat skin infestation by mites (scabies). Administration is topical in the form of a cream rinse and a skin cream.

✚ Side-effects: Skin irritation, including itching, reddening and stinging; rarely, there may be swelling and rashes.

▲ Warning: Avoid contact with the eyes and do not use on broken or infected skin. Administer with caution to patients who are pregnant or breast-feeding.

✪ Related entry: Lyclear.

Permitabs

(Bioglan) is a proprietary, non-prescription preparation of the ANTISEPTIC potassium permanganate. It can be used for cleaning and deodorizing suppurating eczematous reactions and wounds. It is available as tablets for solution for topical application.

✚▲ Side-effects/warning: See POTASSIUM PERMANGANATE.

perphenazine

is chemically a PHENOTHIAZINE. It is used as an ANTIPSYCHOTIC drug to treat schizophrenia and other psychoses, in the short-term treatment of severe anxiety and as an ANTINAUSEANT and ANTI-EMETIC to relieve nausea and vomiting. Administration is oral.

✚▲ Side-effects/warning: See CHLORPROMAZINE HYDROCHLORIDE; but is less sedating and extrapyramidal symptoms (muscle tremor and rigidity) are more likely.

✪ Related entries: Fentazin; Triptafen.

Persantin

(Boehringer Ingelheim) is a proprietary, prescription-only preparation of the ANTIPLATELET drug dipyridamole. It can be

P

used to prevent thrombosis, and is available as tablets and in a form for injection.
+▲ Side-effects/warning: See DIPYRIDAMOLE.

Pertofran

(Ciba) is a proprietary, prescription-only preparation of the (TRICYCLIC) ANTIDEPRESSANT desipramine hydrochloride. It is available as tablets.
+▲ Side-effects/warning: See DESIPRAMINE HYDROCHLORIDE.

pertussis vaccine

(whooping-cough) is a VACCINE used for IMMUNIZATION and is a suspension of dead pertussis bacteria *Bordetella pertussis*. When injected, it causes the body's immune system to form antibodies against the bacteria and so provide *active immunity*. Administration of the vaccine is normally by three injections one month apart and is combined with diphtheria and tetanus vaccine (*triple vaccine*) or adsorbed diphtheria, tetanus and pertussis vaccine (DTPer/Vac/Ads).
+▲ Side-effects/warning: See VACCINES. Administer with particular care to children with a history of febrile convulsions, and with caution to children whose relatives have a history of seizures or who appear to have any form of neurological disorder.
◐ Related entries: Adsorbed Diphtheria, Tetanus and Pertussis Vaccine; Trivax-AD.

pethidine hydrochloride

is an (OPIOID) NARCOTIC ANALGESIC which is used primarily for the relief of moderate to severe pain, especially during labour and operations. It is less effective than morphine and not suitable for relieving severe, chronic pain. Its effect is rapid and short-lasting, so its SEDATIVE properties are made use of only as a premedication prior to surgery, or to enhance the effects of other anaesthetic drugs during or following surgery. Administration is either oral or by injection. Its proprietary preparation is on the Controlled Drugs List.

+▲ Side-effects/warning: See OPIOIDS; but, compared to many opioids, it is less likely to cause constipation and there is less depression of respiration in the newborn when used to relieve pain during labour. It should not be used in patients with severe kidney damage. Overdose can cause convulsions.
◐ Related entry: Pamergan P100.

Pevaryl

(Cilag) is a proprietary, non-prescription preparation of the ANTIFUNGAL drug econazole nitrate. It can be used to treat fungal infections on the skin, such as nail infections and in the genital areas, and is available as a cream and a lotion.
+▲ Side-effects/warning: See ECONAZOLE NITRATE; but side-effects are limited with topical application.

Pevaryl TC

(Cilag) is a proprietary, non-prescription COMPOUND PREPARATION of the CORTICOSTEROID triamcinolone and the ANTIFUNGAL econazole nitrate. It can be used to treat fungal infections of the skin, such as nail infections and in the genital areas, and is available as a cream for topical application.
+▲ Side-effects/warning: See ECONAZOLE NITRATE; TRIAMCINOLONE; but side-effects are limited with topical application.

Pharmalgen

(Allerayde) is a proprietary, prescription-only preparation of desensitizing vaccine. It is available in a version for bee venom or for wasp venom and can be used in diagnosing and desensitizing patients who are allergic to one or the other. It is available in a form for injection.
+▲ Side-effects/warning: See DESENSITIZING VACCINES.

Pharmorubicin Rapid Dissolution

(Pharmacia) is a proprietary, prescription-only preparation of the (CYTOTOXIC) ANTICANCER drug epirubicin hydrochloride.

It can be used to treat several types of cancer, including breast cancer, and is available in a form for injection.
+▲ Side-effects/warning: See EPIRUBICIN HYDROCHLORIDE.

Pharmorubicin Solution for Injection

(Pharmacia) is a prescription-only, proprietary preparation of the (CYTOTOXIC) ANTICANCER drug epirubicin hydrochloride. It can be used to treat several types of cancer, including breast cancer, and is available in a form for injection.
+▲ Side-effects/warning: See EPIRUBICIN HYDROCHLORIDE.

Phasal

(Lagap) is a proprietary, prescription-only preparation of the ANTIMANIA drug lithium (as lithium carbonate). It is used to treat acute mania, manic-depressive bouts and recurrent depression, and is available as tablets.
+▲ Side-effects/warning: See LITHIUM.

phenazocine hydrobromide

is an (OPIOID) NARCOTIC ANALGESIC which is used primarily for the relief of severe pain, especially pain arising from disorders of the bile ducts. Administration is oral. Its proprietary preparation is on the Controlled Drugs List.
+▲ Side-effect/warning: See OPIOIDS.
✪ Related entry: Narphen.

phenelzine

is an ANTIDEPRESSANT of the MONOAMINE-OXIDASE INHIBITOR (MAOI) group. It is used particularly when treatment with TRICYCLIC antidepressants (eg AMITRIPTYLINE HYDROCHLORIDE or IMIPRAMINE HYDROCHLORIDE) has failed, and is one of the safer, less STIMULANT MAO inhibitors. However, a suitably long wash-out period is necessary before switching between different groups of antidepressant. Administration (as phenelzine sulphate) is oral. Treatment with the drug requires a strict dietary regime (for example, a patient must avoid eating cheese, meat or yeast extracts, or drinking alcoholic beverages) and extreme care must be taken if using certain other forms of medication.
+ Side-effects: Drowsiness, fatigue, headache; there may be weakness and dizziness, particularly on standing up from lying or sitting (postural hypotension). There may be dry mouth and blurred vision, difficulty in urinating, constipation, sweating, oedema, rash, nervousness and sexual disturbances. There may be changes in appetite and weight gain. Susceptible patients may experience agitation, confusion, hallucinations, tremor or even psychotic episodes. There are rare reports of jaundice and liver disorders, of severely lowered blood sodium and of peripheral nerve disease.
▲ Warning: It should not be administered to patients with certain liver disorders, vascular disease of the brain or abnormal secretion of hormones by the adrenal glands (phaeochromocytoma). Administer with caution to patients with certain cardiovascular diseases, epilepsy, diabetes, blood disorders or who are agitated or elderly. Counselling, or supervision, over diet and any other medication is essential. Withdrawal of treatment should be gradual.
✪ Related entry: Nardil.

Phenergan

(Rhône-Poulenc Rorer) is a proprietary, non-prescription preparation of the ANTIHISTAMINE promethazine hydrochloride. It can be used for the symptomatic relief of allergic conditions of the upper respiratory tract and skin, including hay fever, allergic rhinitis, urticaria and for the treatment of anaphylactic reaction. It has marked SEDATIVE actions and can be used in treating temporary sleep disorders and as an ANTINAUSEANT to prevent motion sickness. It is available as tablets and an elixir (for motion sickness) and is not normally given to children under two years, except on medical advice. It is also available on a

P

P

prescription-only basis in a form for injection.

+▲ Side-effects/warning: See PROMETHAZINE HYDROCHLORIDE.

Phenergan Nitetime

(Rhône-Poulenc Rorer) is a proprietary, non-prescription preparation of the ANTIHISTAMINE promethazine hydrochloride. It has marked SEDATIVE actions and can be used in treating temporary sleep disorders. It is available as tablets and is not normally given to children, except on medical advice.

+▲ Side-effects/warning: See PROMETHAZINE HYDROCHLORIDE.

phenindamine tartrate

is an ANTIHISTAMINE which can be used for the symptomatic relief of allergic symptoms such as hay fever and urticaria. Administration is oral.

+▲ Side-effects/warning: See ANTIHISTAMINES. But it differs from most other antihistamines because it may cause mild stimulation.

✪ Related entry: Thephorin.

phenindione

is an ANTICOAGULANT drug which is effective when taken orally (though it is not as commonly used as warfarin sodium) and is used in the treatment and prevention of thrombosis, such as after insertion of prosthetic heart valves. Administration is oral.

+▲ Side-effects/warning: See WARFARIN SODIUM. There may also be hypersensitivity reactions, including rashes and fever; blood disorders; diarrhoea; kidney and liver damage. Avoid when breast-feeding.

✪ related entry: Dindevan.

pheniramine maleate

is an ANTIHISTAMINE which can be used for the symptomatic relief of allergic symptoms such as hay fever and urticaria. It is also included in several cough and decongestant preparations. Administration is oral.

438 **+▲** Side-effects/warning: See

ANTIHISTAMINES. Because of its sedative property, the performance of skilled tasks, such as driving, may be impaired.

✪ Related entries: Daneral SA; Triominic Tablets.

phenobarbital

see PHENOBARBITONE

phenobarbitone

(phenobarbital) is a BARBITURATE which is used as an ANTICONVULSANT and ANTI-EPILEPTIC in the prevention of most types of recurrent epileptic seizures (except absence seizures). Administration is either oral or by injection. Preparations containing phenobarbitone are on the Controlled Drugs List.

+▲ Side-effects/warning: See BARBITURATES. The doses administered in the prevention of epileptic attacks are calculated to minimize drowsiness and sedation. There may be additional side-effects such as lethargy, drowsiness, unsteady gait, skin reactions, mental depression (or paradoxical excitement, restlessness and confusion – especially in the elderly – or overactivity in children). Administer with care to patients with impaired liver or kidney function, respiratory depression or who are pregnant or breast-feeding. It should not be given to those with porphyria. Withdrawal of treatment should be gradual.

✪ Related entry: Gardenal Sodium.

phenol

or carbolic acid, is a DISINFECTANT and ANTISEPTIC which is used for cleaning wounds or inflammation (such as boils and abscesses), for mouth, throat or ear hygiene and to inject into haemorrhoids. Administration is topical.

+ Side-effects: There may be skin irritation.

▲ Warning: It is toxic and corrosive if swallowed in concentrated form.

✪ Related entries: Blisteze; Chloraseptic; Germoline Cream; Germoline Ointment; Secaderm; TCP Antiseptic Throat Pastilles; TCP Liquid Antiseptic.

phenolphthalein

is a *stimulant* LAXATIVE which works by having an irritant action on the gastrointestinal tract. It is not used quite as much as it once was due to its side-effects and long-lasting action, which may continue for up to several days because the drug is recycled through the liver. Proprietary preparations that contain phenolphthalein usually contain other laxatives as well.

✚▲ Side-effects/warning: The laxative effects may continue for several days; there may be discolouration of the urine and skin rashes.

✪ Related entries: Agarol; Alophen Pills; Bonomint; Brooklax; Carter's Little Pills; Correctol; Ex-Lax Chocolate; Ex-Lax Pills; Nylax Tablets; Reguletts.

phenoperidine hydrochloride

is an (OPIOID) NARCOTIC ANALGESIC which is used to relieve pain during surgery, particularly in combination with a GENERAL ANAESTHETIC to enhance its effects. Its additional property as a respiratory depressant is sometimes made use of in the treatment of patients who undergo prolonged assisted respiration. Administration is by injection.

✚▲ Side-effects/warning: See OPIOIDS.

✪ Related entry: Operidine.

phenothiazines

(or phenothiazine derivatives) are a group of drugs that all have a similar chemical structure. Many of them are used as ANTIPSYCHOTIC drugs (eg CHLORPROMAZINE HYDROCHLORIDE, FLUPHENAZINE HYDROCHLORIDE, PROMAZINE HYDROCHLORIDE, THIORIDAZINE and TRIFLUOPERAZINE) and it is thought that their ability to block DOPAMINE receptors in the brain is the reason for their usefulness in treating psychoses. A number of them are also powerful ANTINAUSEANTS or ANTI-EMETICS and others (eg PIPERAZINE) are ANTHELMINTICS. See also METHOTRIMEPRAZINE; PERICYAZINE; PERPHENAZINE; PIPOTHIAZINE PALMITATE; PROCHLORPERAZINE.

phenothrin

is a PEDICULICIDAL drug which is used to treat infestations by head and pubic lice (crabs). Administration is topical as a lotion.

✚ Side-effects: There may be skin irritation.

▲ Warning: Avoid contact with the eyes and do not use on broken or infected skin. It may cause wheezing in asthmatics.

✪ Related entry: Full Marks Lotion.

phenoxybenzamine hydrochloride

is an ALPHA-ADRENOCEPTOR BLOCKER which is used, in combination with BETA-BLOCKERS, as a short-term ANTIHYPERTENSIVE and for severe hypertensive crises in phaeochromocytoma. It can also be used to manage severe shock that is unresponsive to conventional treatment. Administration is either oral or by injection.

✚ Side-effects: The heart rate increases; there may be postural hypotension (dizziness, particularly on standing up from a lying or sitting position) and lethargy. There is sometimes nasal congestion and contraction of the pupils. There may be gastrointestinal disturbances or a failure to ejaculate.

▲ Warning: It should be administered with caution to patients with certain heart conditions, severe arteriosclerosis, impaired kidney function or who are elderly.

✪ Related entry: Dibenyline.

phenoxymethylpenicillin

(penicillin V) is a widely used ANTIBACTERIAL and ANTIBIOTIC drug. It is particularly effective in treating tonsillitis, infection of the middle ear, certain skin infections and to prevent recurrent streptococcal throat infection, which can lead to episodes of rheumatic fever. Administration is oral.

✚▲ Side-effects/warning: See BENZYLPENICILLIN.

✪ Related entry: Apsin.

P

Phensedyl Plus

(Rhône-Poulenc Rorer) is a proprietary, non-prescription COMPOUND PREPARATION of the ANTIHISTAMINE promethazine hydrochloride, the (OPIOID) ANTITUSSIVE pholcodine and the SYMPATHOMIMETIC pseudoephedrine hydrochloride. It can be used for the symptomatic relief of coughs and colds, and is available as a syrup. It is not normally given to children, except on medical advice.

✚▲ Side-effects/warning: See PHOLCODINE; PROMETHAZINE HYDROCHLORIDE; PSEUDOEPHEDRINE HYDROCHLORIDE.

Phensic

(SmithKline Beecham) is a proprietary, non-prescription COMPOUND PREPARATION of the (NSAID) NON-NARCOTIC ANALGESIC and ANTIRHEUMATIC aspirin and the STIMULANT caffeine. It can be administered to treat mild to moderate pain and to provide relief of mild upper airways infections, such as colds and flu. It is available as capsule-shaped tablets and is not normally given to children under 12 years, except on medical advice.

✚▲ Side-effects/warning: See ASPIRIN; CAFFEINE.

phentermine

is an APPETITE SUPPRESSANT drug which is administered, under medical supervision and on a short-term basis, to aid weight loss in severe obesity. It is a STIMULANT and potentially subject to abuse and so its proprietary preparations are on the Controlled Drugs List. There is growing doubt among experts over the medical value of such treatment. Administration is oral.

✚▲ Side-effects/warning: See FENFLURAMINE HYDROCHLORIDE.

🔾 Related entries: Duromine; Ionamin.

phentolamine mesylate

is an ALPHA-ADRENOCEPTOR BLOCKER which is administered, in combination with BETA-BLOCKERS, as an ANTIHYPERTENSIVE for hypertensive crises in phaeochromocytoma (it is also used in the diagnosis of this condition) and may have some use in the treatment of impotence. Administration is by injection.

✚ Side-effects: Postural hypotension (fall in blood pressure on standing); dizziness; dry mouth and nasal congestion; decreased sweating, gastrointestinal upsets and chest pains in the elderly.

▲ Warning: It should not be used in certain heart disorders. Administer with care to patients with kidney impairment, who are pregnant or have various vascular or blood disorders.

🔾 Related entry: Rogitine.

phenylbutazone

is a (NSAID) NON-NARCOTIC ANALGESIC and ANTIRHEUMATIC which, because of its sometimes severe side-effects, is administered solely in the treatment of ankylosing spondylitis under special conditions of medical supervision in hospitals. Even for that purpose it is used only when all other therapies have failed and treatment may then be prolonged. Administration is oral.

✚ Side-effects: There may be gastrointestinal disturbances, nausea, vomiting and allergic reactions, such as a rash. Less often there is inflammation of the salivary glands of the mouth, throat and neck; and visual disturbances. Rarely, there is severe fluid retention (which in susceptible patients may eventually precipitate heart failure) and serious and potentially dangerous blood disorders.

▲ Warning: It should not be administered to patients with certain cardiovascular diseases, thyroid disease, impaired liver or kidney function; who are pregnant; who have a history of stomach or intestinal haemorrhaging, or who have Sjögren's syndrome (wasting of the salivary glands). Administer with caution to those who are elderly or breast-feeding. Regular and frequent blood counts are essential.

🔾 Related entry: Butacote.

phenylephrine hydrochloride

is a VASOCONSTRICTOR and SYMPATHOMIMETIC drug which is administered by injection or infusion to increase blood pressure (sometimes in emergency situations until it is possible to perform a plasma transfusion). It is also incorporated into a number of proprietary cold cure preparations as a vasoconstrictor and DECONGESTANT and also in eye-drops in order to dilate the pupil to facilitate ophthalmic examination.

✚ Side-effects: Hypertension and headache; changes in heart rate; vomiting, tingling and coolness of the skin.

▲ Warning: See NORADRENALINE. It should not be administered to patients with hyperthyroidism or severe hypertension.

✪ Related entries: Beechams All-In-One; Beechams Flu-Plus Hot Lemon; Beechams Hot Blackcurrant; Beechams Hot Lemon; Beechams Hot Lemon and Honey; Beechams Powders Capsules; Betnovate; Catarrh-Ex; Cold Relief Capsules; Coldrex Tablets; Cool Lemon Lemsip; Dimotapp Elixir; Dimotapp Elixir Paediatric; Dimotapp LA Tablets; Dristan Decongestant Tablets; Fenox Nasal Drops; Fenox Nasal Spray; Flurex Cold/Flu Capsules with Cough Suppressant; Flurex Tablets; Hedex Headcold Cherry Menthol Powders; Isopto Frin; Lemsip Cold Relief Capsules; Lemsip Maximum Strength; Lemsip Menthol Extra; Lemsip Original; Minims Phenylephrine Hydrochloride; Phenylephrine Injection 1%.

Phenylephrine Injection 1%

(Boots) is a proprietary, prescription-only preparation of the SYMPATHOMIMETIC and VASOCONSTRICTOR drug phenylephrine hydrochloride. It can be used to treat cases of acute hypotension, particularly in emergency situations as a temporary measure while preparations are made for blood transfusion. It is available in a form for injection.

✚▲ Side-effects/warning: See PHENYLEPHRINE HYDROCHLORIDE.

phenylpropanolamine hydrochloride

is a SYMPATHOMIMETIC and VASOCONSTRICTOR drug which is used systemically as an upper airways DECONGESTANT in the symptomatic relief of allergic disorders, such as asthma and hay fever (when it is often administered with an ANTIHISTAMINE), and also for the symptomatic relief of colds and flu (often in combination with ANALGESICS).
Administration can be by several routes, including orally in various forms.

✚▲ Side-effects/warning: See EPHEDRINE HYDROCHLORIDE.

✪ Related entries: Aller-eze Plus; Benylin Day and Night; Contac 400; Day Nurse Capsules; Day Nurse Liquid; Dimotapp Elixir; Dimotapp Elixir Paediatric; Dimotapp LA Tablets; Eskornade Capsules; Lemsip Night-Time; Mu-Cron Syrup, Junior; Mu-Cron Tablets; Sinutab Tablets; Triogesic Tablets; Triominic Tablets; Vicks Vaposyrup for Chesty Coughs and Nasal Congestion; Vicks Vaposyrup for Dry Coughs and Nasal Congestion.

phenytoin

is an ANTICONVULSANT and ANTI-EPILEPTIC drug which is used to treat most forms of epilepsy (except absence seizures) and trigeminal (facial) neuralgia. It has also been used as an ANTI-ARRHYTHMIC. Administration (as phenytoin or phenytoin sodium) is either oral or by injection.

✚ Side-effects: Nausea, vomiting, confusion, headache, dizziness, nervousness, insomnia; rarely, movement disorders, peripheral nerve disorders, unsteady gait, slurred speech, eye-flicker and blurred vision, rashes, acne, enlargement of the gums, growth of excess hair and blood disorders.

▲ Warning: Administer with caution to patients with liver impairment or who are pregnant or breast-feeding; avoid its use in those with porphyria. Withdrawal of treatment should be gradual.

✪ Related entries: Epanutin; Epanutin Ready Mixed Parenteral; Pentran.

P

441

P

Phimetin

(BHR) is a proprietary preparation of the H$_2$-ANTAGONIST cimetidine. It is available on prescription or without a prescription in a limited amount and for short-term uses only. It can be used as an ULCER-HEALING DRUG for benign peptic ulcers (in the stomach or duodenum), gastro-oesophageal reflux, dyspepsia and associated conditions. It is available as tablets.

✚▲ Side-effects/warning: See CIMETIDINE.

Phiso-med

(Sanofi Winthrop) is a proprietary, non-prescription preparation of the ANTISEPTIC chlorhexidine (as gluconate). It can be used as a soap or shampoo substitute in acne and seborrhoeic conditions, and for bathing babies in maternity units to prevent cross infection. It is available as a solution.

✚▲ Side-effects/warning: See CHLORHEXIDINE.

pholcodine

is a weak OPIOID which is used as a cough treatment (in preference to stronger opioids of the NARCOTIC ANALGESIC type) and as an ANTITUSSIVE constituent in many cough linctuses or syrups. Although its action resembles that of other opioids, it has no appreciable analgesic effect or addictive liability.

✚▲ Side-effects/warning: See CODEINE PHOSPHATE.

◒ Related entries: Copholco; Copholcoids Cough Pastilles; Day Cold Comfort Capsules; Expulin Children's Cough Linctus – Sugar Free; Expulin Cough Linctus – Sugar Free; Expulin Dry Cough Linctus; Famel Linctus; Galenphol Linctus; Galenphol Linctus, Strong; Galenphol Paediatric Linctus; Night Cold Comfort Capsules; Pavacol-D; Phensedyl Plus; Pholcomed D; Pholcomed Diabetic Forte; Tixylix Cough and Cold; Tixylix Daytime; Tixylix Night-Time.

Pholcomed D

(Medo) is a proprietary, non-prescription preparation of the (OPIOID) ANTITUSSIVE pholcodine. It can be used as a cough treatment for dry or painful coughs, and is available as a sugar-free linctus.

✚▲ Side-effects/warning: See PHOLCODINE.

Pholcomed Diabetic Forte

(Medo) is a proprietary, non-prescription preparation of the (OPIOID) ANTITUSSIVE pholcodine. It can be used as a cough treatment in dry or painful coughs, and is available as a sugar-free linctus.

✚▲ Side-effects/warning: See PHOLCODINE.

PhorPain

(Goldshield) is a proprietary, non-prescription preparation of the (NSAID) NON-NARCOTIC ANALGESIC, ANTIRHEUMATIC and ANTIPYRETIC ibuprofen. It can be used for the relief of headache, backache, muscular pain, dental pain and cold and flu symptoms. It is available as tablets and is not normally given to children under 12 years, except on medical advice.

✚▲ Side-effects/warning: See IBUPROFEN.

PhorPain Double Strength

(Goldshield) is a proprietary, non-prescription preparation of the (NSAID) NON-NARCOTIC ANALGESIC, ANTIRHEUMATIC and ANTIPYRETIC ibuprofen. It can be used for the relief of headache, backache, muscular pain, dental pain and cold and flu symptoms. It is available as tablets and is not normally used in children under 12 years, except on medical advice.

✚▲ Side-effects/warning: See IBUPROFEN.

Phosphate-Sandoz

(Sandoz) is a proprietary, non-prescription COMPOUND PREPARATION of potassium bicarbonate, SODIUM ACID PHOSPHATE and sodium bicarbonate. It can be used as a MINERAL SUPPLEMENT to provide phosphate, which may be required in addition to vitamin D in patients with vitamin D-resistant rickets. It is available as tablets.

✚▲ Side-effects/warning: See SODIUM BICARBONATE.

phosphodiesterase inhibitors ☒

are a relatively new class of drugs which have so far been used in short-term congestive HEART FAILURE TREATMENT, especially where other drugs have been unsuccessful. They work by inhibiting certain enzymes and so effect the heart in ways that mimic SYMPATHOMIMETICS acting at beta-adrenoceptors. Examples of these drugs include ENOXIMONE and MILRINONE.

Phyllocontin Continus

(Napp) is a proprietary, non-prescription preparation of the BRONCHODILATOR aminophylline. It can be used as an ANTI-ASTHMATIC and to treat bronchitis, and is available as modified-release tablets.
➕▲ Side-effects/warning: See AMINOPHYLLINE.

Physeptone

(Wellcome) is a proprietary, prescription-only preparation of the (OPIOID) NARCOTIC ANALGESIC methadone hydrochloride, and is on the Controlled Drugs List. It can be used to treat severe pain, and is available as tablets and in a form for injection.
➕▲ Side-effects/warning: See METHADONE HYDROCHLORIDE.

Physiotens

(Solvay) is a proprietary, prescription-only preparation of the ANTIHYPERTENSIVE moxonidine. It can be used to treat mild to moderate essential hypertension, and is available as tablets.
➕▲ Side-effects/warning: See MOXONIDINE.

physostigmine sulphate

(eserine) is a vegetable ALKALOID and is an ANTICHOLINESTERASE drug that enhances the effects of the NEUROTRANSMITTER acetylcholine (and also of certain cholinergic drugs). Because of this property, it has PARASYMPATHOMIMETIC actions and can be used to stimulate the pupil of the eye in GLAUCOMA TREATMENT (when it is usually given with PILOCARPINE).

Administration is topical.
➕▲ Side-effects/warning: There may be parasympathomimetic side-effects if a sufficient amount is absorbed into the eye (see NEOSTIGMINE).

Phytex

(Pharmax) is a proprietary, non-prescription COMPOUND PREPARATION of several ANTIFUNGAL and KERATOLYTIC drugs, including salicylic acid, tannic acid and boric acid (with ethyl acetate and alcohol). It can be used to treat fungal infections of the skin and nails, and is available as a paint for topical application.
➕▲ Side-effects/warning: See SALICYLIC ACID.

phytomenadione

(vitamin K_1) is a natural form of VITAMIN K and is normally obtained from vegetables and dairy products. Phytomenadione can be used to treat vitamin K deficiency, but not a deficiency caused by malabsorption states (in such cases vitamin K_1 or MENADIOL SODIUM PHOSPHATE, the synthetic form of vitamin K_3, must be used). Administration is either oral or by slow intravenous injection.
➕▲ Side-effects/warning: See VITAMIN K.
✪ Related entry: Konakion.

Picolax

(Nordic) is a proprietary, non-prescription preparation of the (*stimulant*) LAXATIVES sodium picosulphate and magnesium citrate. It can be used to evacuate the bowels before surgery, radiography or endoscopy, and is available as a powder for making into an oral solution.
➕▲ Side-effects/warning: See MAGNESIUM SULPHATE; SODIUM PICOSULPHATE.

pilocarpine

is a PARASYMPATHOMIMETIC drug. It can be applied to the eye to treat glaucoma by improving drainage of aqueous fluid from the eye, and to constrict the pupil of the eye after it has been dilated for ophthalmic examination (administration is as eye-

P

drops). It can be used to alleviate the symptoms of salivary gland hypofunction with dry mouth following irradiation for head and neck cancer (administration is oral).

✚ Side-effects: Impaired focusing of the eye. Systemically, there may be sweating; chills; diarrhoea or constipation, nausea and vomiting, lachrymation, abdominal pain, hypertension, abnormal vision, dizziness, rhinitis, weakness, increased urinary frequency, headache, dyspepsia, vasodilatation, flushing. Other possible side-effects include: respiratory distress, heart function upsets, hypotension, confusion or tremors.

▲ Warning: There can be systemic cholinergic actions when administered as eye-drops if a sufficient amount is absorbed into the body. Systemically, care must be used in asthma and chronic obstructive airways disease (increased bronchial secretions and increased airways resistance); acute iritis, narrow-angle glaucoma; pregnancy and breast-feeding.

✪ Related entries: Isopto Carpine; Minims Pilocarpine Nitrate; Ocusert Pilo; Pilogel; Salagen; Sno Pilo.

Pilogel

(Alcon) is a proprietary, prescription-only preparation of the PARASYMPATHOMIMETIC pilocarpine (with carbomer gel). It can be used in GLAUCOMA TREATMENT and to facilitate inspection of the eye. It is available as an eye gel.

✚▲ Side-effects/warning: See PILOCARPINE.

pimozide

is an ANTIPSYCHOTIC drug which is used to treat patients suffering from psychotic disorders, such as schizophrenia, paranoia and mania. It can also be used to treat Gilles de la Tourette syndrome and in the short-term treatment of severe anxiety. Administration is oral.

✚▲ Side-effects/warning: See CHLORPROMAZINE HYDROCHLORIDE; but is less sedating. It is not to be given to patients who

are breast-feeding or with certain heart arrhythmias.

✪ Related entry: Orap.

pindolol

is a BETA-BLOCKER which can be used as an ANTIHYPERTENSIVE for raised blood pressure and as an ANTI-ANGINA treatment to relieve symptoms and improve exercise tolerance. Administration is oral. It is also available, as an antihypertensive treatment, in COMPOUND PREPARATION with a DIURETIC.

✚▲ Side-effects/warning: See PROPRANOLOL HYDROCHLORIDE.

✪ Related entries: Viskaldix; Visken.

pipenzolate bromide

is an ANTICHOLINERGIC drug which is used to assist in the treatment of gastrointestinal disorders that involve muscle spasm of the intestinal wall. Administration is oral.

✚▲ Side-effects/warning: See ATROPINE SULPHATE.

✪ Related entry: Piptalin.

piperacillin

is a broad-spectrum ANTIBACTERIAL and (PENICILLIN) ANTIBIOTIC which is used to treat many serious or compound forms of bacterial infection, particularly those caused by *Pseudomonas aeruginosa*. Administration is by injection or infusion.

✚▲ Side-effects/warning: See BENZYLPENICILLIN.

✪ Related entries: Pipril; Tazocin.

piperazine

is an ANTHELMINTIC drug (a PHENOTHIAZINE) which is used to treat infestation by roundworm or threadworm. Administration is oral.

✚ Side-effects: There may be nausea and vomiting with diarrhoea; there may also be allergic reactions, such as urticaria. Rarely, there is dizziness, colic and lack of muscular coordination ('worm wobble').

▲ Warning: It should be administered with caution to patients with certain kidney or liver disorders, epilepsy, neurological disease

or who are pregnant.
◐ Related entries: De Witt's Worm Syrup; Expelix; Pripsen Powder; Pripsen Worm Elixir.

piperazine oestrone sulphate

is a female SEX HORMONE, an OESTROGEN, which is used in HRT (hormone replacement therapy). Administration is oral.
+▲ Side-effects/warning: See OESTROGENS.
◐ Related entries: Harmogen; Improvera.

Piportil Depot

(Rhône-Poulenc Rorer) is a proprietary, prescription-only preparation of the ANTIPSYCHOTIC drug pipothiazine palmitate. It can be used in maintenance therapy of patients with psychotic disorders, such as chronic schizophrenia. Administration is by a long-acting depot deep intramuscular injection.
+▲ Side-effects/warning: See PIPOTHIAZINE PALMITATE.

pipothiazine palmitate

(pipotiazine palmitate) is a PHENOTHIAZINE, which is used as an ANTIPSYCHOTIC in maintenance therapy of patients with schizophrenia and other psychoses. Administration is by injection.
+▲ Side-effects/warning: See CHLORPROMAZINE HYDROCHLORIDE. It is not to be administered to patients with parkinsonism or confusional states.
◐ Related entry: Piportil Depot.

pipotiazine palmitate

see PIPOTHIAZINE PALMITATE

Pipril

(Lederle) is a proprietary, prescription-only preparation of the broad-spectrum ANTIBACTERIAL and (PENICILLIN) ANTIBIOTIC piperacillin. It can be used to treat many serious or compound forms of bacterial infection, particularly those caused by *Pseudomonas aeruginosa*, and is available

in a form for injection and infusion.
+▲ Side-effects/warning: See PIPERACILLIN.

Piptalin

(Boehringer Mannheim) is a proprietary, prescription-only COMPOUND PREPARATION of the ANTICHOLINERGIC drug pipenzolate bromide and the ANTIFOAMING AGENT dimethicone. It can be used as an ANTISPASMODIC for the symptomatic relief of smooth muscle spasm in the gastrointestinal tract, and is available as a suspension.
+▲ Side-effects/warning: See DIMETHICONE; PIPENZOLATE BROMIDE.

piracetam

is a recently introduced ANTI-EPILEPTIC drug which is used to treat cortical myoclonus (involuntary spasmic contractions of muscles of the body). There are also unconfirmed reports that it is a NOOTROPIC AGENT, a cognition enhancer that allegedly improves mental performance. Administration is oral.
+▲ Side-effects: Diarrhoea, weight gain, sleepiness, insomnia, depression, rash and overactivity.
▲ Warning: It should not be used in patients with severe liver or kidney impairment, or who are pregnant or breast-feeding. Withdrawal of treatment should be gradual.
◐ Related entry: Nootropil.

pirbuterol

is a SYMPATHOMIMETIC and BETA-RECEPTOR STIMULANT that has beta$_2$-receptor selectivity. It is mainly used as a BRONCHODILATOR in reversible obstructive airways disease and as an ANTI-ASTHMATIC treatment in severe acute asthma. It can also be used for the alleviation of symptoms of chronic bronchitis and emphysema. Administration can be either oral or topical. (Patients should be cautioned not to exceed the stated dose and if a previously effective dose fails to relieve symptoms they should consult their doctor.)

✚▲ Side-effects/warning: See SALBUTAMOL.
❂ Related entry: Exirel.

pirenzepine

is an ANTICHOLINERGIC drug with properties that are different from many others in its class. It can reduce the production of gastric acids and digestive juices from the stomach, so reducing the acidity and without widespread side-effects. It can therefore be used as an ULCER-HEALING DRUG for gastric and duodenal ulcers. Administration is oral.

✚ Side-effects: Rarely, there may be dry mouth and slight visual disturbance. Blood disorders have been reported.

▲ Warning: Do not administer to patients with an enlarged prostate gland, closed-angle glaucoma, paralytic ileus, pyloric stenosis or who are pregnant. Use with care in those with kidney impairment.

Piriton

(Allen & Hanburys) is a proprietary, non-prescription preparation of the ANTIHISTAMINE chlorpheniramine maleate. It can be used to treat allergic conditions, such as hay fever and urticaria, and is available as tablets and a syrup; it is also available on a prescription-only basis in a form for injection.

✚▲ Side-effects/warning: See CHLORPHENIRAMINE MALEATE.

piroxicam

is a (NSAID) NON-NARCOTIC ANALGESIC and ANTIRHEUMATIC drug. It has a long duration of action and is used to treat pain and inflammation in rheumatic disease and other musculoskeletal disorders, including juvenile arthritis and acute gout. Administration can be oral, topical or by injection.

✚▲ Side-effects/warning: See NSAID. It may cause pain at the injection site; it may cause pancreatitis or gastrointestinal disturbances, especially in the elderly.

❂ Related entries: Feldene; Feldene Gel; Flamatrol; Larapam; Pirozip.

Pirozip

(Ashbourne) is a proprietary, prescription-only preparation of the (NSAID) NON-NARCOTIC ANALGESIC and ANTIRHEUMATIC piroxicam. It can be used to treat acute gout, arthritic and rheumatic pain and other musculoskeletal disorders. It is available as capsules.

✚▲ Side-effects/warning: See PIROXICAM.

Pitressin

(Parke-Davis) is a proprietary, prescription-only preparation of the HORMONE vasopressin. It can be administered either for diagnosis or as a DIABETES INSIPIDUS TREATMENT. Alternatively, it can be used to treat the bleeding of varices (varicose veins) in the oesophagus. It is available in a form for injection.

✚▲ Side-effects/warning: See VASOPRESSIN.

pivampicillin

is a more readily absorbed form of the broad-spectrum ANTIBACTERIAL and (PENICILLIN) ANTIBIOTIC ampicillin. It is converted in the body to ampicillin after absorption and has similar actions and uses. Administration is oral.

✚▲ Side-effects/warning: See AMPICILLIN.
❂ Related entry: Pondocillin.

Piz Buin SPF 20 Sun Block Lotion

(Zyma) is a proprietary, non-prescription SUNSCREEN lotion that protects the skin from UVA and UVB ultraviolet radiation (UVB-SPF 20). It is a cream-coloured skin lotion containing the pigment TITANIUM DIOXIDE along with butylmethoxydibenzoyl methane and octyl methoxy-cinnammimate. A patient with a skin condition that requires this sort of protection may be prescribed it at the discretion of his or her doctor.

pizotifen

is an ANTIHISTAMINE and SEROTONIN antagonist which can be used as an ANTIMIGRAINE treatment, particularly for headaches in which blood pressure inside the blood vessels plays a part, such as migraine and cluster headache. Administration is oral.

✚ Side-effects: Anticholinergic effects, drowsiness, increased appetite and weight gain, occaisional nausea and dizziness.

▲ Warning: Administer with care to patients with urinary retention, kidney impairment, closed-angle glaucoma; or who are pregnant or breast-feeding. Drowsiness may impair the performance of skilled tasks, such as driving.

○ Related entry: Sanomigran.

Plaquenil

(Sanofi Winthrop) is a proprietary, prescription-only preparation of hydroxychloroquine sulphate, which has ANTI-INFLAMMATORY and ANTIRHEUMATIC properties. It can be used to treat rheumatoid arthritis (including juvenile arthritis) and lupus erythematosus. It is available as tablets.

✚▲ Side-effects/warning: See HYDROXYCHLOROQUINE SULPHATE.

Platet

(Nicholas) is a proprietary, non-prescription preparation of the (NSAID) NON-NARCOTIC ANALGESIC and ANTIRHEUMATIC aspirin, which can be used as an ANTIPLATELET aggregation (antithrombotic) drug. It can be administered to reduce the formation of blood thrombi (clots), and is available as effervescent tablets.

✚▲ Side-effects/warning: See ASPIRIN.

Plendil

(Schwarz) is a proprietary, prescription-only preparation of the CALCIUM-CHANNEL BLOCKER felodipine. It can be administered as an ANTIHYPERTENSIVE, and is available as tablets.

✚▲ Side-effects/warning: See FELODIPINE.

Plesmet

(Link) is a proprietary, non-prescription preparation of ferrous glycine sulphate. It can be used as an IRON supplement in iron

deficiency ANAEMIA TREATMENT, and is available as a syrup.

✚▲ Side-effects/warning: See FERROUS GLYCINE SULPHATE.

plicamycin

(or mithramycin) is a CYTOTOXIC drug (of ANTIBIOTIC origin). It is used solely as a CALCIUM METABOLISM MODIFIER in the emergency control of calcium metabolism where there are excessive levels of calcium in the blood (hypercalcaemia), which is caused by malignant disease. Administration is by injection.

✚ Side-effects: There may be nausea and vomiting, with hair loss. The blood-cell producing capacity of the bone marrow is reduced.

▲ Warning: Because the drug is toxic the dose should be the minimum that is effective. Regular blood counts are essential during treatment. Administer with great caution to patients with kidney or liver disorders.

pneumococcal vaccine

is a VACCINE used for IMMUNIZATION against pneumonia. It is intended for administration only to those people, such as the elderly, who are at particular risk from infection, for example, from an identified pneumococcal strain prevalent within a community. The duration of protection is considered to be in the region of five years. Administration is by subcutaneous or intramuscular injection.

✚▲ Side-effects/warning: See VACCINES.

○ Related entry: Pneumovax II.

Pneumovax II

(Morson) is a proprietary, prescription-only VACCINE preparation of pneumococcal vaccine. It can be used for prevention of pneumococcal pneumonia in people for whom the risk of contracting the disease is unusually high. It is available in a form for injection.

✚▲ Side-effects/warning: See PNEUMOCOCCAL VACCINE.

P

podophyllum

is a KERATOLYTIC and caustic agent which can be used to treat and dissolve warts and also to reduce the production of new skin cells.

+▲ Side-effects/warning: It may cause considerable irritation (particularly to eyes), avoid face, normal skin and open wounds. Do not use if pregnant or breast-feeding.

✪ Related entries: Condyline; Posalfilin; Warticon; Warticon Fem.

Pol/Vac (Inact)

is an abbreviation for POLIOMYELITIS VACCINE, INACTIVATED.

Pol/Vac (Oral)

is an abbreviation for POLIOMYELITIS VACCINE, LIVE (ORAL).

poldine methylsulphate

(poldine metilsulfate) is an ANTICHOLINERGIC drug which can be used as an ANTISPASMODIC for the symptomatic relief of smooth muscle spasm in the gastrointestinal tract. Administration is oral.

+▲ Side-effects/warning: See ATROPINE SULPHATE.

✪ Related entry: Nacton.

poldine metilsulfate

see POLDINE METHYLSULPHATE

poliomyelitis vaccine

is a VACCINE used for IMMUNIZATION that is available in two types. Poliomyelitis vaccine, inactivated (Salk) is a suspension of dead viruses injected into the body so that the body produces antibodies and becomes immune. Poliomyelitis vaccine live, (oral) (Sabine) is a suspension of live but attenuated polio viruses (of polio virus types 1, 2 and 3) for oral administration. In the UK, the live vaccine is more commonly used and the administration is generally simultaneous with diphtheria-pertussis-tetanus (triple) vaccine during the first year of life with a booster at school-entry age. The inactivated vaccine remains available for those patients who, for some reason,

cannot use the live vaccine.

+▲ Side-effects/warning: See VACCINES.

Poliomyelitis Vaccine, Inactivated

(District Health Authorities) (Pol/Vav – Inact) is a non-proprietary, prescription-only VACCINE preparation of poliomyelitis vaccine inactivated, (Salk). It can be used to provide immunity from infection by polio, and is available in a form for injection.

+▲ Side-effects/warning: See POLIOMYELITIS VACCINE.

Poliomyelitis Vaccine, Live (Oral)

(District Health Authorities) (Pol/Vav – Oral) is a non-proprietary, prescription-only VACCINE preparation of poliomyelitis vaccine live, (oral) (Sabine), which contains 'live' but attenuated polio viruses. It can be used to confer immunity from infection, and is available in a form for oral administration.

+▲ Side-effects/warning: See POLIOMYELITIS VACCINE.

Pollon-Eze

(Johnson & Johnson) is a proprietary, non-prescription preparation of the ANTIHISTAMINE astemizole. It can be used to treat the symptoms of allergic disorders, such as hay fever and urticaria, and is available as tablets.

+▲ Side-effects/warning: See ASTEMIZOLE.

polyestradiol phosphate

is a an analogue of OESTROGEN, a SEX HORMONE, which is used as an ANTICANCER treatment for cancer of the prostate gland. Administration is by intramuscular injection.

+▲ Side-effects/warning: See STILBOESTROL.

✪ Related entry: Estradurin.

Polyfax

(Cusi) is a proprietary, prescription-only

COMPOUND PREPARATION of the ANTIBACTERIAL and ANTIBIOTIC drugs, the (POLYMYXIN) polymyxin B sulphate and bacitracin zinc. It can be used to treat infections of the skin and the eye and is available for topical application as a skin ointment, an eye ointment and as eye-drops.

✚▲ Side-effects/warning: See BACITRACIN ZINC; POLYMYXIN B SULPHATE.

polymyxin B sulphate

is an ANTIBACTERIAL and (POLYMYXIN) ANTIBIOTIC which can be used to treat several forms of bacterial infection, particularly infections caused by Gram-negative bacteria, such as *Pseudomonas aeruginosa*. Its use is restricted because it is very toxic and because of this toxicity it is mainly administered topically.

✚▲ Side-effects/warning: Minimal on topical application.

✪ Related entries: Gregoderm; Maxitrol; Neosporin; Otosporin; Polyfax; Polytrim; Terra-Cortril.

polymyxins ⓘ

are a chemical class of ANTIBIOTICS used for their ANTIBACTERIAL actions. They are active against Gram-negative bacteria, including *Pseudomonas aeruginosa*, and are used to treat skin infections, burns and wounds. The antibiotics of this group can be administered by injection or topical application; although COLISTIN is not absorbed orally it can be used to sterilize the bowel. See also POLYMYXIN B SULPHATE.

polynoxylin

is an ANTIFUNGAL and ANTIBACTERIAL drug which can be used topically as a cream to treat minor skin infections.

✪ Related entry: Anaflex.

polystyrene sulphonate resins

are administered to treat excessively high levels of potassium in the blood (hyperkalaemia), for example, in dialysis patients. Administration is either oral or by

topical application in the form of a retention enema.

✚ Side-effects: Treatment by enemas may cause rectal ulcers.

▲ Warning: Some resins should not be given to patients with hyperparathyroidism, sarcoidosis, multiple myeloma or metastatic cancer; avoid in those patients with congestive heart failure or impaired kidney function. An adequate fluid intake must be maintained.

✪ Related entries: Calcium Resonium; Resonium A.

Polytar Emollient

(Stiefel) is a proprietary, non-prescription preparation of coal tar. It can be used to treat psoriasis, eczema and dermatitis, and is available as a liquid for adding to a bath.

✚▲ Side-effects/warning: See COAL TAR.

polythiazide

is one of the THIAZIDE class of DIURETICS. It can be used as an ANTIHYPERTENSIVE, either alone or in conjunction with other types of drugs, and in the treatment of oedema associated with congestive heart failure. Administration is oral.

✚▲ Side-effects/warning: See BENDROFLUAZIDE.

✪ Related entry: Nephril.

Polytrim

(Cusi) is a proprietary, prescription-only COMPOUND PREPARATION of the ANTIBACTERIAL and ANTIBIOTIC drugs trimethoprim and polymyxin B sulphate. It can be used to treat bacterial infections in the eye, and is available as eye-drops and an eye ointment.

✚▲ Side-effects/warning: See POLYMYXIN B SULPHATE; TRIMETHOPRIM.

polyvinyl alcohol

is a constituent in several preparations that are used as artificial tears to treat dryness of the eye due to disease. Administration is by topical application.

✪ Related entries: Hypotears; Liquifilm Tears; Sno Tears.

P

Ponderax

(Servier) is a proprietary, prescription-only preparation of the APPETITE SUPPRESSANT fenfluramine hydrochloride. It can be used as a short-term, additional treatment in medical therapy for obesity, and is available as modified-release capsules (*Pacaps*).

✚▲ Side-effects/warning: See FENFLURAMINE HYDROCHLORIDE.

Pondocillin

(Leo) is a proprietary, prescription-only preparation of the broad-spectrum ANTIBACTERIAL and (PENICILLIN) ANTIBIOTIC pivampicillin. It can be used to treat systemic bacterial infections, infections of the upper respiratory tract, of the ear, nose and throat and of the urinogenital tracts. It is available as tablets.

✚▲ Side-effects/warning: See PIVAMPICILLIN.

Ponstan

(Parke-Davis) is a proprietary, prescription-only preparation of the (NSAID) NON-NARCOTIC ANALGESIC and ANTIRHEUMATIC mefenamic acid. It can be used to treat pain in rheumatoid arthritis, osteoarthritis and other musculoskeletal disorders and period pain. It is available as capsules, tablets (*Ponstan Forte*) and as a paediatric oral suspension.

✚▲ Side-effects/warning: See MEFENAMIC ACID.

Posalfilin

(Norgine) is a proprietary, non-prescription COMPOUND PREPARATION of the KERATOLYTIC agents salicylic acid and podophyllum (resin). It can be used to treat and remove warts and verrucas (plantar warts), and is available as an ointment for topical application.

✚▲ Side-effects/warning: See PODOPHYLLUM; SALICYLIC ACID.

Posiject

(Boehringer Ingelheim) is a proprietary, prescription-only preparation of the CARDIAC STIMULANT dobutamine hydrochloride, which has SYMPATHOMIMETIC and BETA-RECEPTOR STIMULANT properties. It can be used to treat serious heart disorders, such as cardiogenic shock, septic shock, during heart surgery and in cardiac infarction. It is available in a form for intravenous infusion.

✚▲ Side-effects/warning: See DOBUTAMINE HYDROCHLORIDE.

Potaba

(Glenwood) is a proprietary, non-prescription preparation of potassium aminobenzoate. It can be used to treat scleroderma and Peyronie's disease, and is available as capsules, tablets and as a powder in sachets (called *envules*).

✚▲ Side-effects/warning: See POTASSIUM AMINOBENZOATE.

potassium aminobenzoate

is used in the treatment of disorders associated with excess fibrous tissue, such as scleroderma and Peyronie's disease. There is uncertainty, however, about how it works and how well. Administration is oral.

✚ Side-effects: There may be nausea; anorexia (if so discontinue treatment).

▲ Warning: It should not be administered to patients who are taking sulphonamides and with caution to those with kidney disease.

✪ Related entry: Potaba.

potassium canrenoate

is a mild DIURETIC of the *aldosterone-antagonist* type. It can be used to treat oedema associated with aldosteronism (abnormal production of aldosterone by the adrenal gland), certain heart diseases and liver failure. Administration is by injection.

✚▲ Side-effects/warning: See SPIRONOLACTONE. There may be nausea and vomiting and pain at the injection site.

✪ Related entry: Spiroctan-M.

potassium chloride

is used primarily as a potassium

supplement to correct potassium deficiency, especially due to or following severe loss of body fluids (eg chronic diarrhoea) and treatment with drugs that deplete body reserves (eg some DIURETICS). It may also be used as a substitute for natural salt (SODIUM CHLORIDE) in cases where sodium, for one reason or another, is inadvisable. Administration is either oral or by injection or intravenous infusion.

○ Related entries: Balanced Salt Solution; Burinex K; Diocalm Replenisher; Dioralyte; Diumide-K Continus; Glandosane; Lasikal; Lasix+K; Luborant; Neo-NaClex-K; Sando-K; Slow-K.

potassium citrate

when administered orally has the effect of making the urine alkaline instead of acid, an action that is useful for relieving pain in some infections of the urinary tract or the bladder. Administration is oral.

✚ Side-effects: There may be mild diuresis. Prolonged high dosage may lead to excessively high levels of potassium in the blood.

▲ Warning: It should be administered with caution to patients with heart disease or impaired kidney function.

○ Related entry: Effercitrate.

potassium hydroxyquinoline sulphate

is a drug that has both ANTIBACTERIAL and ANTIFUNGAL properties. It is used mostly as a constituent in anti-inflammatory and antibiotic creams and ointments, for example, in preparations used to treat acne.

✚ Side-effects: Rarely, it may cause sensitivity reactions.

○ Related entries: Quinocort; Quinoderm Cream; Quinoderm Cream 5; Quinoderm Lotio-Gel 5%; Quinoped.

potassium permanganate

is a general ANTISEPTIC agent which can be used in solution for cleaning burns and abrasions, and for maintaining asepsis in wounds that are suppurating or weeping.

✚▲ Side-effects/warning: Avoid contact with mucous membranes, to which it is an irritant. It stains skin and fabric.

○ Related entry: Permitabs.

potassium-channel activators ⚕

are drugs that work by opening pores in cell membranes which allow potassium ions to pass more readily, which has the effect of making these cells electrically less excitable. In blood vessels such drugs have VASODILATOR effects, which cause a reduction of the heart's workload and generally lowers blood pressure. The recently introduced drug of this type is NICORANDIL, which can be used to prevent and treat attacks of angina pectoris.

povidone-iodine

is a complex of iodine on an organic carrier and is used as an ANTISEPTIC. It is topically applied to the skin, especially in sensitive areas (such as the vulva), acne of the scalp and is also used as a mouthwash. It works by slowly releasing the iodine it contains and is available as a gel, an oral solution or vaginal inserts (pessaries).

✚ Side-effects: Rarely, there may be sensitivity reactions.

▲ Warning: These depend on the applications, but it should be used with care by patients with certain kidney diseases, who are pregnant or breast-feeding and on broken skin.

○ Related entries: Betadine; Brush Off Cold Sore Lotion; Savlon Dry; Videne.

Powergel

(Searle) is a proprietary, prescription-only preparation of the (NSAID) NON-NARCOTIC ANALGESIC and ANTIRHEUMATIC ketoprofen, which also has COUNTER-IRRITANT, or RUBEFACIENT, actions. It can be applied to the skin for symptomatic relief of underlying muscle or joint pain, and is available as a gel for topical application to the skin.

✚▲ Side-effects/warning: See KETOPROFEN;

P

but adverse effects on topical application are limited.

Powerin Analgesic Tablets

(Whitehall) is a proprietary, non-prescription COMPOUND PREPARATION of the (NSAID) NON-NARCOTIC ANALGESIC, ANTIRHEUMATIC and ANTIPYRETIC aspirin, the non-narcotic analgesic paracetamol and the STIMULANT caffeine. It can be used to relieve mild to moderate pain, including headache, sore throat, toothache, muscle aches and pains, period pain and to relieve cold and flu symptoms. It is available as tablets and is not normally given to children under 12 years, except on medical advice.

+▲ Side-effects/warning: See ASPIRIN; CAFFEINE; PARACETAMOL.

PR Heat Spray

(Crookes) is a proprietary, non-prescription COMPOUND PREPARATION of methyl salicylate, methyl nicotinate and CAMPHOR, which all have COUNTER-IRRITANT, or RUBEFACIENT, actions. It can be applied to the skin for symptomatic relief of underlying muscle or joint pain, and is available as a spray for topical application. It is not normally used for children under five years, except on medical advice.

+▲ Side-effects/warning: See METHYL SALICYLATE. Avoid inflamed, broken skin and mucous membranes.

Pragmatar

(Bioglan) is a proprietary, non-prescription COMPOUND PREPARATION of coal tar (as cetyl alcohol-coal tar distillate), salicylic acid and sulphur. It can be used for psoriasis and eczema, and is available as a cream.

+▲ Side-effects/warning: COAL TAR; SALICYLIC ACID; SULPHUR.

pralidoxime mesylate

is an ANTIDOTE which is used in conjunction with an ANTICHOLINERGIC drug (usually ATROPINE SULPHATE) to treat poisoning by organophosphorous compounds (eg insecticides). Administration is by injection.

✛ Side-effects: Drowsiness, dizziness, visual disturbances, muscular weakness, nausea, headache, speeding of the heart and breathing, muscle weakness.

▲ Warning: It should not be used to treat poisoning by carbamates or organophosphorous compounds without anticholinesterase activity. Use with caution in patients with myasthenia gravis or impaired kidney function.

pramoxine hydrochloride

is a LOCAL ANAESTHETIC which is included in some proprietary preparations that are used for treating haemorrhoids. Administration is by topical application.
○ Related entries: Anugesic-HC; Proctofoam HC.

pravastatin

is used as a LIPID-LOWERING DRUG in hyperlipidaemia to reduce the levels, or change the proportions, of various lipids in the bloodstream. It is usually administered only to patients in whom a strict and regular dietary regime, alone, or some other therapy is not having the desired effect. Administration is oral.

+▲ Side-effects/warning: See SIMVASTATIN.
○ Related entry: Lipostat.

Praxilene

(Lipha) is a proprietary, non-prescription preparation of the VASODILATOR naftidrofuryl oxalate. It can be used to help improve blood circulation to the hands and feet when this is impaired, for example, in peripheral vascular disease (Raynaud's phenomenon). It is available as tablets and in a form for injection.

+▲ Side-effects/warning: See NAFTIDROFURYL OXALATE.

praziquantel

is an ANTHELMINTIC drug which is the drug of choice (though not available in the UK) in treating infections caused by schistosomes, which are the worms that can colonize the veins of a human host and cause bilharziasis, and is also useful in the treatment of tapeworm infestation. It has a low toxicity and is administered orally.

prazosin hydrochloride

is a selective ALPHA-ADRENOCEPTOR BLOCKER which is used as an ANTIHYPERTENSIVE, often in conjunction with other classes of drug (such as BETA-BLOCKERS or DIURETICS), in congestive HEART FAILURE TREATMENT, in the treatment of urinary retention (eg in benign prostatic hyperplasia) and in peripheral vascular disease (Raynaud's phenomenon). Administration is oral.

✚ Side-effects: Drowsiness and sedation, dizziness and hypotension (particularly on standing); weakness and lack of energy, depression, headache, dry mouth, nausea, urinary frequency and incontinence, palpitations and, rarely, speeding of the heart.

▲ Warning: Initially, it may cause marked postural hypotension, so the patient should lie down when given the drug or it should be taken on retiring to bed. It is not to be used in certain forms of congestive heart failure (eg aortic stenosis). Administer with care to those who are pregnant or breast-feeding or with certain kidney disorders.

❂ Related entries: Alphavase; Hypovase; Hypovase Benign Prostatic Hypertrophy.

Precortisyl

(Roussel) is a proprietary, prescription-only preparation of the CORTICOSTEROID and ANTI-INFLAMMATORY prednisolone. It can be used in the treatment of allergic and rheumatic conditions, particularly those affecting the joints and soft tissues. It is available as tablets in several different forms and strengths (eg *Precortisyl Forte*).

✚▲ Side-effects/warning: See PREDNISOLONE.

Pred Forte

(Allergan) is a proprietary, prescription-only preparation of the CORTICOSTEROID and ANTI-INFLAMMATORY prednisolone (as acetate). It can be used to treat inflammatory conditions in and around the eye, and is available as eye-drops.

✚▲ Side-effects/warning: See PREDNISOLONE.

Predenema

(Pharmax) is a proprietary, prescription-only preparation of the CORTICOSTEROID prednisolone (as sodium metasulphobenzoate). It can be used as an ANTI-INFLAMMATORY treatment for rectal inflammation (eg in ulcerative colitis and Crohn's disease), and is available as a retention enema.

✚▲ Side-effects/warning: See PREDNISOLONE.

Predfoam

(Pharmax) is a proprietary, prescription-only preparation of the CORTICOSTEROID prednisolone (as sodium metasulphobenzoate). It can be used as an ANTI-INFLAMMATORY treatment for inflammation of the rectum (eg in ulcerative colitis and Crohn's disease), and is available as a rectal foam enema.

✚▲ Side-effects/warning: See PREDNISOLONE.

prednisolone

is a synthetic, *glucocorticoid* CORTICOSTEROID with ANTI-INFLAMMATORY properties. It is used in the treatment of a number of rheumatic and allergic conditions (particularly those affecting the joints or the lungs) and collagen disorders. It is also an effective treatment for ulcerative colitis, inflammatory bowel disease, Crohn's disease, rectal or anal inflammation, haemorrhoids and as an IMMUNOSUPPRESSANT in the treatment of myasthenia gravis. It may also be used for systemic corticosteroid therapy. Administration (as prednisolone, prednisolone acetate or prednisolone sodium phosphate) can be oral, by topical application or by injection.

✚▲ Side-effects/warning: See CORTICOSTEROIDS. The type and severity of any side-effects depends on the route of administration.

○ Related entries: Deltacortril Enteric; Deltastab; Minims Prednisolone; Precortisyl; Pred Forte; Predenema; Predfoam; Predsol; Predsol-N; Scheriproct.

prednisone

is a CORTICOSTEROID that is converted in the body to the *glucocorticoid* corticosteroid PREDNISOLONE. It can be used as an ANTI-INFLAMMATORY treatment for a variety of inflammatory and allergic disorders. Administration is oral.

✚▲ Side-effects/warning: See CORTICOSTEROIDS.

○ Related entry: Prednisone.

Prednisone

is a non-proprietary, prescription-only preparation of the CORTICOSTEROID prednisone, which is converted in the body to the *glucocorticoid* corticosteroid. It can be used as an ANTI-INFLAMMATORY treatment for a variety of inflammatory and allergic disorders, and is available as tablets.

✚▲ Side-effects/warning: See PREDNISONE.

Predsol

(Evans) is a proprietary, prescription-only preparation of the CORTICOSTEROID prednisolone (as sodium phosphate). It can be used as an ANTI-INFLAMMATORY treatment for inflammation of the rectum (eg in ulcerative colitis and Crohn's disease) and for non-infected, inflammatory ear and eye conditions. It is available as a retention enema, suppositories and as ear- or eye-drops.

✚▲ Side-effects/warning: See PREDNISOLONE.

Predsol-N

(Evans) is a proprietary, prescription-only COMPOUND PREPARATION of the CORTICOSTEROID prednisolone (as sodium phosphate) and the ANTIBACTERIAL and (AMINOGLYCOSIDE) ANTIBIOTIC neomycin sulphate. It can be used to treat inflammatory ear and eye

conditions, and is available as ear- and eye-drops.

✚▲ Side-effects/warning: See NEOMYCIN SULPHATE; PREDNISOLONE.

Preferid

(Yamanouchi) is a proprietary, prescription-only preparation of the CORTICOSTEROID budesonide. It can be used to treat severe inflammatory skin disorders, such as eczema and psoriasis, and is available as a cream and an ointment.

✚▲ Side-effects/warning: See BUDESONIDE.

Prefil

(Norgine) is a proprietary, non-prescription preparation of the (*bulking-agent*) LAXATIVE sterculia. It can be used in the medical treatment of obesity, where it is intended to make a patient feel full, and is available as granules for solution.

✚▲ Side-effects/warning: See STERCULIA.

Pregaday

(Evans) is a proprietary, non-prescription COMPOUND PREPARATION of ferrous fumarate and folic acid. It can be used as an IRON and folic acid supplement during pregnancy, and is available as tablets.

✚▲ Side-effects/warning: See FERROUS FUMARATE; FOLIC ACID.

Pregnyl

(Organon) is a proprietary, prescription-only preparation of the HORMONE human chorionic gonadotrophin (HCG). It can be used to treat undescended testicles and delayed puberty in boys, and as an infertility treatment in women suffering from specific hormonal deficiency contributing to infertility. It is available in a form for injection.

✚▲ Side-effects/warning: See CHORIONIC GONADOTROPHIN.

Premarin

(Wyeth) is a proprietary, prescription-only preparation of the OESTROGEN conjugated oestrogens. It can be used in HRT, and is

available as tablets in a calendar pack.
+▲ Side-effects/warning: See CONJUGATED
OESTROGENS.

Premique

(Wyeth) is a proprietary, prescription-only
preparation of the OESTROGEN conjugated
oestrogens and medroxyprogesterone
acetate. It can be used in HRT (including for
osteoporosis prophylaxis), and is available
as tablets in a calendar pack.
+▲ Side-effects/warning: See OESTROGENS;
MEDROXYPROGESTERONE ACETATE.

Prempak-C

(Wyeth) is a proprietary, prescription-only
COMPOUND PREPARATION of the female SEX
HORMONES the OESTROGEN conjugated
oestrogens and the PROGESTOGEN norgestrel.
It can be used in HRT, and is available as
tablets in a calendar pack.
+▲ Side-effects/warning: See CONJUGATED
OESTROGENS; NORGESTREL.

Prepadine

(Berk) is a proprietary, prescription-only
preparation of the (TRICYCLIC)
ANTIDEPRESSANT dothiepin hydrochloride. It
can be used to treat depressive illness,
especially in cases where some degree of
sedation is deemed necessary, and is
available as tablets and capsules.
+▲ Side-effects/warning: See DOTHIEPIN
HYDROCHLORIDE.

Prepidil

(Upjohn) is a proprietary, prescription-only
preparation of the PROSTAGLANDIN
dinoprostone. It is used to induce labour,
and is available as a cervical gel for
administration to the cervix.
+▲ Side-effects/warning: See
DINOPROSTONE.

Prepulsid

(Janssen) is a proprietary, prescription-
only preparation of the MOTILITY STIMULANT
cisapride. It can be used to stimulate the
stomach and intestine in a number of

conditions, and is available as tablets and a
suspension.
+▲ Side-effects/warning: See CISAPRIDE.

Prescal

(Ciba) is a proprietary, prescription-only
preparation of the CALCIUM-CHANNEL BLOCKER
isradipine. It can be used as an
ANTIHYPERTENSIVE, and is available as tablets.
+▲ Side-effects/warning: See ISRADIPINE.

Prestim

(Leo) is a proprietary, prescription-only
COMPOUND PREPARATION of the BETA-BLOCKER
timolol maleate and the (THIAZIDE) DIURETIC
bendrofluazide. It can be used as an
ANTIHYPERTENSIVE for raised blood pressure,
and is available as tablets.
+▲ Side-effects/warning: See
BENDROFLUAZIDE; TIMOLOL MALEATE.

Prestim Forte

(Leo) is a proprietary, prescription-only
COMPOUND PREPARATION of the BETA-BLOCKER
timolol maleate and the (THIAZIDE) DIURETIC
bendrofluazide. It can be used as an
ANTIHYPERTENSIVE for raised blood pressure,
and is available as tablets.
+▲ Side-effects/warning: See
BENDROFLUAZIDE; TIMOLOL MALEATE.

Priadel

(Delandale) is a proprietary, prescription-
only preparation of the ANTIMANIA drug
lithium (as lithium carbonate). It can be
used to treat acute mania, manic-depressive
bouts and recurrent depression, and is
available as tablets (a liquid preparation of
lithium citrate is also available).
+▲ Side-effects/warning: See LITHIUM.

prilocaine hydrochloride

is a LOCAL ANAESTHETIC which is used
extensively for relatively minor surgical
procedures, especially by injection in
dentistry and by surface anaesthesia and
nerve block. Administration is by injection
(in several forms) or by topical application.
+▲ Side-effects/warning: See LIGNOCAINE

455

P

HYDROCHLORIDE. It may cause methaemoglobinaemia (an abnormal form of haemoglobin that does not transport oxygen) that may require correction. Avoid its use in those who have anaemia or pre-existing methaemoglobinaemia.
⨁ Related entries: Citanest; Citanest with Octapressin; Emla.

Primacor

(Sanofi Winthrop) is a proprietary, prescription-only preparation of the PHOSPHODIESTERASE INHIBITOR milrinone. It can be used, in the short term, in HEART FAILURE TREATMENT for acute heart failure, especially where other drugs have not been successful. It is available in a form for intravenous infusion or injection.
➕▲ Side-effects/warning: See MILRINONE.

Primalan

(Rhône-Poulenc Rorer) is a proprietary, prescription-only preparation of the ANTIHISTAMINE mequitazine. It can be used to treat the symptoms of allergic disorders, such as hay fever and urticaria, and is available as tablets.
➕▲ Side-effects/warning: See MEQUITAZINE.

primaquine

is an ANTIMALARIAL drug which is used to destroy parasitic forms in the liver that are not destroyed by chloroquine. Administration is oral.
➕ Side-effects: There may be nausea and vomiting, abdominal pain and blood disorders.
▲ Warning: It should be administered with caution to patients who are pregnant or breast-feeding, or who have G6PD deficiency.

Primaxin

(Merck Sharp & Dohme) is a proprietary, prescription-only COMPOUND PREPARATION of the ANTIBACTERIAL and (BETA-LACTAM) ANTIBIOTIC imipenem and the ENZYME INHIBITOR cilastatin, which is a combination known as imipenem with cilastatin. It can be used to treat infections such as those of the urethra and cervix and to prevent infection during operations. It is available in a form for injection or infusion.
➕▲ Side-effects/warning: See IMIPENEM WITH CILASTIN.

primidone

is an ANTICONVULSANT and ANTI-EPILEPTIC drug which is used in the treatment of all forms of epilepsy (except absence seizures) and of essential tremor. It is largely converted in the body to the BARBITURATE drug phenobarbitone and therefore has similar actions and effects. Administration is oral.
➕▲ Side-effects/warning: See PHENOBARBITONE; but there may also be drowsiness, unsteady gait, nausea, rash and disturbances of vision.
⨁ Related entry: Mysoline.

Primolut N

(Schering) is a proprietary, prescription-only preparation of the PROGESTOGEN norethisterone. It can be used to treat uterine bleeding, abnormally heavy menstruation and other menstrual problems, endometriosis and premenstrual tension syndrome. It is available as tablets.
➕▲ Side-effects/warning: See NORETHISTERONE.

Primoteston Depot

(Schering) is a proprietary, prescription-only preparation of the male SEX HORMONE testosterone enanthate, which is an ANDROGEN. It can be used to treat hormonal deficiency in men and as an ANTICANCER treatment for hormone-related cancer in women. It is available in a form for long-acting (depot) injection.
➕▲ Side-effects/warning: See TESTOSTERONE.

Primperan

(Berk) is a proprietary, prescription-only preparation of the ANTI-EMETIC and ANTINAUSEANT metoclopramide hydrochloride. It can be used for the treatment of nausea and vomiting, particularly when associated with gastrointestinal disorders and after treatment with radiation or cytotoxic drugs. It also has gastric MOTILITY STIMULANT actions and can be used in the treatment of non-ulcer dyspepsia, gastric stasis and for prevention of reflux oesophagitis. It is available as tablets, an oral solution and in a form for injection.

+▲ Side-effects/warning: See METOCLOPRAMIDE HYDROCHLORIDE. Note the side-effects in young people in particular.

Prioderm

(Napp) is a proprietary, non-prescription preparation of the SCABICIDAL and PEDICULICIDAL drug malathion. It can be used to treat infestations of the scalp and pubic hair by lice (pediculosis), or of the skin by the itch-mite (scabies). It is available as a cream, a shampoo and a lotion. It is not normally used on children under six months, except on medical advice.

+▲ Side-effects/warning: See MALATHION.

Pripsen Mebendazole

(Seton) is a proprietary, non-prescription preparation of the ANTHELMINTIC drug mebendazole. It can be used to treat infections by threadworm and roundworm, and is available as tablets. It is not normally given to children under two years, except on medical advice.

+▲ Side-effects/warning: See MEBENDAZOLE.

Pripsen Powder

(Seton) is a proprietary, non-prescription COMPOUND PREPARATION of the ANTHELMINTIC drug piperazine (as phosphate) and the *stimulant* LAXATIVE senna. It can be used to treat infections by threadworm and roundworm, and is available as an oral powder. It is not normally given to children under one year, except on medical advice.

+▲ Side-effects/warning: See PIPERAZINE; SENNA.

Pripsen Worm Elixir

(Seton) is a proprietary, non-prescription preparation of the ANTHELMINTIC drug piperazine (as citrate). It can be used to treat infections by threadworm and roundworm, and is available as an oral powder. It is not normally given to children under one year, except on medical advice.

+▲ Side-effects/warning: See PIPERAZINE.

Pro-Banthine

(Baker Norton) is a proprietary, prescription-only preparation of the ANTICHOLINERGIC propantheline bromide. It can be used as an ANTISPASMODIC for gastro-intestinal disorders involving spasm and in the treatment of adult enuresis (urinary incontinence). It is available as tablets.

+▲ Side-effects/warning: See PROPANTHELINE BROMIDE.

Pro-Viron

(Schering) is a proprietary, prescription-only preparation of mesterolone, which has ANDROGEN (male SEX HORMONE) activity. It can be used to make up hormonal deficiency, and is available as tablets.

+▲ Side-effects/warning: See MESTEROLONE.

probenecid

is a drug that alters the transport of chemicals by the kidneys and is used for two main purposes. First, by inhibiting the excretion from the body of certain ANTIBIOTICS (mainly the PENICILLINS and CEPHALOSPORINS), it increases their duration of action. Second, because it increases the excretion of uric acid from the blood, it can be used in the prevention of attacks of chronic gout, which involve high levels of uric acid (hyperuricaemia). Administration is oral as tablets.

+ Side-effects: Infrequently, there may be nausea and vomiting, but usually there is increased urination, headache and flushing, dizziness and rash; rarely, hypersensitivity, liver and kidney changes and blood disorders.

▲ Warning: It is not to be used in patients with blood disorders, certain kidney disorders, porphyria, acute gout or who are using aspirin or other salicylates. When first administering, certain concurrent treatments are required, such as colchicine and a NSAID (not aspirin), and an adequate fluid intake must be maintained. Administer with caution to those with peptic ulcers, renal impairment or G6PD deficiency.
✪ Related entry: Benemid.

procainamide hydrochloride

has LOCAL ANAESTHETIC properties and is used as an ANTI-ARRHYTHMIC to treat heartbeat irregularities, especially after a heart attack. Administration can be either oral or by injection.
✚ Side-effects: There may be nausea, diarrhoea, high temperature, depression, slow heart rate and rashes. There may also be heart failure and/or skin or blood disorders, especially after prolonged treatment.
▲ Warning: It should not be administered to patients with heart failure, heart block, low blood pressure or who are breast-feeding. Administer with caution to those with asthma, the neuromuscular disease myasthenia gravis, lupus, impaired kidney function or who are pregnant.
✪ Related entry: Pronestyl.

procaine

is a LOCAL ANAESTHETIC which, though once popular, is now seldom used because it has been overtaken by local anaesthetics that are longer-lasting and better absorbed through mucous membranes. It cannot be used as a surface anaesthetic because it is poorly absorbed. However, it is still available and can be used for regional anaesthesia or by infiltration, usually in combination with adrenaline. Administration (as procaine hydrochloride) is by injection.
✚ Side-effects: Rarely, there are sensitivity reactions.

procaine penicillin

is an ANTIBACTERIAL and PENICILLIN-type ANTIBIOTIC which is effectively a rather insoluble salt of benzylpenicillin. It is used mainly in long-lasting intramuscular (depot) injections to treat conditions such as syphilis and gonorrhoea, but can also be used to treat the equally serious condition gas gangrene following amputation. Benzylpenicillin is released slowly into the blood over a period of days, therefore avoiding the need for frequent injections. Administration is by injection.
✚▲ Side-effects/warning: See BENZYLPENICILLIN.
✪ Related entry: Bicillin.

procarbazine

is a CYTOTOXIC drug which is used as an ANTICANCER treatment for the lymphatic cancer Hodgkin's disease. Administration is oral.
✚▲ Side-effects/warning: See CYTOTOXICS. There may be a hypersensitivity rash.
✪ Related entry: Natulan.

prochlorperazine

is a PHENOTHIAZINE which is used as an ANTIPSYCHOTIC drug in the treatment of psychotic disorders, such as schizophrenia, as an ANXIOLYTIC in the short-term treatment of anxiety and as an ANTINAUSEANT in the prevention of nausea caused by gastrointestinal disorder, chemotherapy, radiotherapy, motion sickness or by the vertigo that results from infection of the middle or inner ear. Administration (as prochlorperazine maleate or prochlorperazine mesylate) can be oral, topical or by injection.
✚▲ Side-effects/warning: See CHLORPROMAZINE HYDROCHLORIDE; but with less sedation, muscle tremor and rigidity disturbances.
✪ Related entries: Buccastem; Stemetil.

Proctofoam HC

(Stafford-Miller) is a proprietary, prescription-only COMPOUND PREPARATION of the CORTICOSTEROID and ANTI-INFLAMMATORY drug hydrocortisone (as acetate) and the LOCAL ANAESTHETIC drug PRAMOXINE HYDROCHLORIDE. It can be used to treat various painful conditions of the anus and rectum, and is available as a foam in an aerosol.

✚▲ Side-effects/warning: See HYDROCORTISONE.

Proctosedyl

(Roussel) is a proprietary, prescription-only COMPOUND PREPARATION of the CORTICOSTEROID and ANTI-INFLAMMATORY hydrocortisone (as acetate) and the LOCAL ANAESTHETIC cinchocaine hydrochloride. It can be used to treat various painful conditions of the anus and rectum, including haemorrhoids, and is available as an ointment and suppositories.

✚▲ Side-effects/warning: See CINCHOCAINE; HYDROCORTISONE.

procyclidine hydrochloride

is an ANTICHOLINERGIC drug which is used in the treatment of some types of parkinsonism (see ANTIPARKINSONISM). It increases mobility and decreases rigidity and tremor, however, it has only a limited effect on bradykinesia. The tendency to produce an excess of saliva is also reduced. It is thought to work by correcting the over-effectiveness of the NEUROTRANSMITTER ACETYLCHOLINE (cholinergic excess), which is caused by the dopamine deficiency that occurs in parkinsonism. Administration, which may be in conjunction with other drugs used for the relief of parkinsonism, is either oral or by injection.

✚▲ Side-effects/warning: See BENZHEXOL HYDROCHLORIDE.

✪ Related entries: Arpicolin; Kemadrin.

Profasi

(Serono) is a proprietary, prescription-only preparation of the SEX HORMONE human chorionic gonadotrophin (HCG). It can be used to treat undescended testicles and delayed puberty in boys, and as an infertility treatment for women suffering from specific hormonal deficiency. It is available in a form for injection.

✚▲ Side-effects/warning: See CHORIONIC GONADOTROPHIN.

Proflex Pain Relief

(Zyma) is a proprietary, non-prescription preparation of the (NSAID) NON-NARCOTIC ANALGESIC and ANTIRHEUMATIC ibuprofen. It can be used for the symptomatic relief of rheumatic and muscular pain, backache, sprains, strains, lumbago and fibrositis. It is available as a cream for massage into the effected area.

✚▲ Side-effects/warning: See IBUPROFEN.

Proflex Sustained Relief Capsules

(Zyma) is a proprietary, non-prescription preparation of the (NSAID) NON-NARCOTIC ANALGESIC and ANTIRHEUMATIC ibuprofen. It can be used for the relief of muscular pain, rheumatic pain, lumbago and fibrositis. It is available as tablets and is not normally given to children under 12 years, except on medical advice.

✚▲ Side-effects/warning: See IBUPROFEN.

Proflex Tablets

(Zyma) is a proprietary, non-prescription preparation of the (NSAID) NON-NARCOTIC ANALGESIC and ANTIRHEUMATIC ibuprofen. It can be used for the relief of sprains, strains, rheumatic pain, lumbago, backache and fibrositis. It is available as tablets and is not normally given to children under 12 years, except on medical advice.

✚▲ Side-effects/warning: See IBUPROFEN.

Progesic

(Lilly) is a proprietary, prescription-only preparation of the (NSAID) NON-NARCOTIC ANALGESIC and ANTIRHEUMATIC fenoprofen. It can be used to treat and relieve pain, particularly arthritic and rheumatic pain and other musculoskeletal disorders, and is available as tablets.

✚▲ Side-effects/warning: See FENOPROFEN.

P

P

progesterone

is a SEX HORMONE, a PROGESTOGEN, that is found predominantly in women but also in men. In women, it is produced and secreted mainly by the ovaries (and also the placenta of pregnant women and the adrenal glands). It prepares the lining of the uterus (the endometrium) every menstrual cycle to receive a fertilized ovum. Most cycles do not result in fertilization (conception), but if a fertilized ovum does implant in the endometrium the resulting formation of a placenta ensures the continuation of the supply of progesterone and this prevents ovulation. In men, small quantities of progesterone are secreted by the testes and the adrenal glands. Therapeutically, progesterone is administered to women to treat various menstrual and gynaecological disorders. Administration is either by topical application, as anal or vaginal suppositories (pessaries), or by injection.

✚▲ Side-effects/warning: See PROGESTOGEN.

✺ Related entries: Cyclogest; Gestone.

progestogen

is the name of the group of (STEROID) SEX HORMONES formed and released by the ovaries and placenta in women, the adrenal gland and in small amounts by the testes in men. Physiologically, progestogens prepare the lining of the uterus (endometrium) for pregnancy, maintain it throughout pregnancy and prevent the further release of eggs (ovulation). They include the natural progestogen PROGESTERONE and those like it (DYDROGESTERONE, HYDROXYPROGESTERONE HEXANOATE and MEDROXYPROGESTERONE ACETATE) and the analogues of TESTOSTERONE (eg NORGESTREL and NORETHISTERONE; and the recently introduced analogues DESOGESTREL, GESTODENE, LEVONORGESTREL and NORGESTIMATE. All are synthesized for therapeutic use and have many uses, including treatment of menstrual disorders (menorrhagia and severe dysmenorrhoea),

endometriosis (inflammation of the tissues normally lining the uterus), in HRT, in recurrent (habitual) abortion, to relieve the symptoms of premenstrual syndrome and sometimes in the treatment of breast, endometrial and prostate cancers. The most common use is as constituents (with or without OESTROGENS) in ORAL CONTRACEPTIVES. Administration is oral.

✚ Side-effects: Depending on the dose, use and the particular progestogen administered; acne, skin rash, oedema, gastrointestinal disturbances, changes in libido, breast discomfort, premenstrual tension, irregular periods, sleep disturbances or depression.

▲ Warning: It should not be administered to patients with undiagnosed vaginal bleeding, certain cardiovascular disorders, porphyria or certain cancers. Use with care in those with diabetes, heart, liver or kidney disorders, or who are breast-feeding.

Prograf

(Fujisawa) is a proprietary, prescription-only preparation of the IMMUNOSUPPRESSANT tacrolimus. It can be used to prevent tissue rejection in transplant patients, and is available as capsules and in a form for injection.

✚▲ Side-effects/warning: See TACROLIMUS.

proguanil hydrochloride

is an ANTIMALARIAL drug which is used to prevent the contraction of malaria by visitors to tropical countries. Administration is oral.

✚ Side-effects: There may be mild stomach disorders, diarrhoea, occasional skin reactions, mouth ulcers and hair loss.

▲ Warning: It should be administered with caution to patients who suffer from severely impaired kidney function or who are pregnant (folate supplements are required).

✺ Related entry: Paludrine.

Progynova

(Schering Health) is a proprietary, prescription-only preparation of the

OESTROGEN oestradiol (as valerate). It can be used to treat menopausal symptoms, and is available as tablets.

+▲ Side-effects/warning: See OESTRADIOL.

Progynova TS

(Schering Health) is a proprietary, prescription-only preparation of the OESTROGEN oestradiol (as valerate). It can be used to treat menopausal symptoms in HRT, and is available as skin patches.

+▲ Side-effects/warning: See OESTRADIOL.

prolactin

is a HORMONE which is secreted into the bloodstream by the anterior pituitary gland in both men and women. Its main role is in fact the control of lactation, but it also influences several other aspects of body function. Its release is influenced by the hypothalamus through a factor called prolactin-release inhibiting factor (PRIM), which is probably the NEUROTRANSMITTER mediator DOPAMINE. This fact is important, because it explains why the drug BROMOCRIPTINE, which stimulates dopamine RECEPTORS, can be used to suppress prolactin secretion and why, conversely, a dopamine ANTAGONIST increases it. Bromocriptine, when it is clinically necessary, can therefore be administered to prevent or suppress lactation after normal birth or in disease states where there is excessive secretion of prolactin with associated galactorrhea (excessive milk production). The over-production of prolactin can also occur when there is a pituitary tumour or when patients are being treated with (dopamine antagonist) NEUROLEPTIC drugs, METOCLOPRAMIDE HYDROCHLORIDE or METHYLDOPA.

Proleukin

(Chiron) is a proprietary, prescription-only preparation of the IMMUNOMODULATOR aldesleukin, which can be used as an ANTICANCER drug. It can be administered to certain patients in the treatment of metastatic renal cell carcinoma, and is available in a form for injection.

+▲ Side-effects/warning: See ALDESLEUKIN.

Proluton Depot

(Schering) is a proprietary, prescription-only preparation of the PROGESTOGEN (female SEX HORMONE) hydroxyprogesterone hexanoate. It can be used to treat recurrent (habitual) abortion, and is available in a form for long-lasting (depot) injection.

+▲ Side-effects/warning: See HYDROXYPROGESTERONE HEXANOATE.

promazine hydrochloride

is chemically one of the PHENOTHIAZINES. It is used as an ANTIPSYCHOTIC drug to tranquillize agitated and restless patients, especially the elderly. Administration is either oral or by injection.

+▲ Side-effects/warning: See CHLORPROMAZINE HYDROCHLORIDE.

✪ Related entry: Sparine.

promethazine hydrochloride

is an ANTIHISTAMINE, chemically a PHENOTHIAZINE, which also has HYPNOTIC and ANTITUSSIVE properties. It is administered to treat the symptoms of allergic conditions, for instance, hay fever and urticaria, and can also be used in the emergency treatment of anaphylactic shock. It has a SEDATIVE action and can be administered as a preoperative medication, to treat temporary sleep disorders and to sedate children. Administration can be either oral or by injection. See also PROMETHAZINE THEOCLATE.

+▲ Side-effects/warning: See CYCLIZINE; ANTIHISTAMINES. Intramuscular injections may be painful. Avoid its use in patients with porphyria. Because of its sedative side-effects, the performance of skilled tasks, such as driving, may be impaired.

✪ Related entries: Medised; Night Nurse Capsules; Night Nurse Liquid; Pamergan P100; Phenergan; Phenergan Nitetime; Phensedyl Plus; Q-Mazine Syrup; Sominex; Tixylix Night-Time.

P

promethazine teoclate
see PROMETHAZINE THEOCLATE

promethazine theoclate
(promethazine teoclate) is chemically a
PHENOTHIAZINE and is a form of the
ANTIHISTAMINE drug promethazine
hydrochloride, but with a slightly longer
duration of action. It can be administered
as an ANTINAUSEANT to prevent nausea and
vomiting when they are caused by motion
sickness or infection of the ear.
Administration is oral.
✚▲ Side-effects/warning: See
ANTIHISTAMINES. Because of its sedative
property, the performance of skilled tasks,
such as driving, may be impaired.
✪ Related entry: Avomine.

Prominal
(Sanofi Winthrop) is a proprietary,
prescription-only preparation of the
BARBITURATE methylphenobarbitone, and is
on the Controlled Drugs List. It can be used
as an ANTICONVULSANT and ANTI-EPILEPTIC to
treat most forms of epilepsy, and is
available as tablets.
✚▲ Side-effects/warning: See
METHYLPHENOBARBITONE.

Pronestyl
(Squibb) is a proprietary, prescription-only
preparation of the ANTI-ARRHYTHMIC drug
procainamide hydrochloride. It can be used
to treat irregularities in the heartbeat,
especially after a heart attack, and is
available as tablets and in a form for
injection.
✚▲ Side-effects/warning: See
PROCAINAMIDE HYDROCHLORIDE.

Propaderm
(Glaxo) is a proprietary, prescription-only
preparation of the CORTICOSTEROID
beclomethasone dipropionate. It can be
used to treat severe, non-infective skin
inflammation, for example, eczema, and is
available as a cream and an ointment for
topical application.

✚▲ Side-effects/warning: See
BECLOMETHASONE DIPROPIONATE.

propafenone hydrochloride
is an ANTI-ARRHYTHMIC drug which is used to
prevent and treat irregularities of the
heartbeat. Administration is oral as tablets.
✚ Side-effects: Nausea, vomiting, diarrhoea
or constipation; fatigue, headache,
dizziness; rash, postural hypotension
(especially in the elderly), dry mouth,
blurred vision and occasionally heart and
blood disorders.
▲ Warning: It should be administered with
care in the elderly, those who are pregnant
or with certain kidney or liver disorders.
Avoid in patients with severe heart
conditions, electrolyte imbalance and
obstructive lung disease.
✪ Related entry: Arythmol.

Propain Tablets
(Panpharma) is a proprietary,
non-prescription COMPOUND PREPARATION
of the (OPIOID) NARCOTIC ANALGESIC
codeine phosphate, the ANTIHISTAMINE
diphenhydramine hydrochloride, the
NON-NARCOTIC ANALGESIC and ANTIPYRETIC
paracetamol and the STIMULANT caffeine. It
can be used to relieve pain, including
headache, migraine, muscular pain and
period pain, and to relieve cold and flu
symptoms and fever. It is available as
scored tablets and is not normally given to
children under 12 years, except on medical
advice.
✚▲ Side-effects/warning: See CAFFEINE;
CODEINE PHOSPHATE; DIPHENHYDRAMINE
HYDROCHLORIDE; PARACETAMOL.

propamidine isethionate
is an ANTIBACTERIAL which is used
specifically to treat infections of the eyelids
or conjunctiva, including acanthamoeba
keratitis (sometimes in conjunction with
other drugs). Adminisration is by topical
application in the form of eye-drops.
**✪ Related entries: Brolene Eye Drops;
Golden Eye Drops.**

Propanix

(Ashbourne) is a proprietary, prescription-only preparation of the BETA-BLOCKER propranolol hydrochloride. It can be used as an ANTIHYPERTENSIVE for raised blood pressure, as an ANTI-ANGINA drug to relieve symptoms and improve exercise tolerance and as an ANTI-ARRHYTHMIC to regularize heartbeat and treat myocardial infarction. It can also be used as an ANTITHYROID drug for short-term treatment of thyrotoxicosis, as an ANTIMIGRAINE to prevent attacks, as an ANXIOLYTIC, particularly for symptomatic relief of tremor and palpitations, and, with an ALPHA-ADRENOCEPTOR BLOCKER, in the acute treatment of phaeochromocytoma. It is available as modified-release capsules (*Propanix SR*).

+▲ Side-effects/warning: See PROPRANOLOL HYDROCHLORIDE.

propantheline bromide

is an ANTICHOLINERGIC drug which is used in the treatment of gastrointestinal disorders that involve muscle spasm of the intestinal wall, of urinary frequency and adult enuresis (urinary incontinence). Administration is oral as tablets.

+▲ Side-effects/warning: See ATROPINE SULPHATE.

⊘ Related entry: Pro-Banthine.

Propess-RS

(Ferring) is a proprietary, prescription-only preparation of the PROSTAGLANDIN dinoprostone. It can be used to promote cervical ripening and induce labour at term, and is available as a cervical pessary.

+▲ Side-effects/warning: See DINOPROSTONE.

Propine

(Allergan) is a proprietary, prescription-only preparation of the SYMPATHOMIMETIC dipivefrine hydrochloride. It can be used as a GLAUCOMA TREATMENT to reduce intraocular pressure, and is available as eye-drops.

+▲ Side-effects/warning: See DIPIVEFRINE HYDROCHLORIDE.

propofol

is a GENERAL ANAESTHETIC which is used in the induction and maintenance of anaesthesia and for the sedation of patients in intensive care on artificial ventilation. Recovery after treatment is rapid and without any hangover effect. Administration is by injection or infusion.

+ Side-effects: Occasionally, there may be pain on intravenous injection. There may be slowing of the heart. Convulsions, anaphylaxis and delayed recovery have been reported.

▲ Warning: The monitoring of certain body functions is advisable.

⊘ Related entry: Diprivan.

propranolol hydrochloride

is a BETA-BLOCKER which can be used as an ANTIHYPERTENSIVE for raised blood pressure, as an ANTI-ANGINA treatment to relieve symptoms and improve exercise tolerance and as an ANTI-ARRHYTHMIC to regularize heartbeat and to treat and prevent myocardial infarction. It can also be used as an ANTITHYROID drug for short-term treatment of thyrotoxicosis, for the acute treatment of phaeochromocytoma, as an ANTIMIGRAINE treatment to prevent attacks and as an ANXIOLYTIC, particularly for symptomatic relief of tremor and palpitations. Administration is either oral or by injection. It is also available, as an antihypertensive treatment, in the form of COMPOUND PREPARATIONS with DIURETICS.

+ Side-effects: Slowing of the heart rate, asthma-like symptoms and bronchospasm, gastrointestinal disturbances, poor circulation in the extremities, fatigue and sleep-disturbance; heart failure in susceptible patients. There are rare reports of rashes and dry eyes.

▲ Warning: It should not be administered to patients with asthma or any disease of the airways, a history of heart failure, cardiogenic shock or certain abnormal heart rhythms. It should be administered with caution to patients who have certain liver or kidney disorders, are in late

P

pregnancy, who are breast-feeding, diabetics or with myasthenia gravis.

✪ **Related entries:** Angilol; Apsolol; Bedranol SR; Berkolol; Betadur CR; Beta-Prograne; Cardinol; Half-Beta-Prograne; Half-Betadur CR; Half-Inderal LA; Inderal; Inderal-LA; Inderetic; Inderex; Propanix; Sloprolol.

propylthiouracil

is a drug that acts as an indirect HORMONE ANTAGONIST by inhibiting the thyroid gland's production of THYROID HORMONES, and therefore treating an excess of thyroid hormones in the blood and the symptoms that it causes (thyrotoxicosis). Treatment can be on a maintenance basis over a long period (with dosage adjusted to optimum effect), or it can be used just before surgical removal of the thyroid gland. It is administered to patients who are sensitive to the antithyroid drug carbimazole. Administration is oral.

✚▲ Side-effects/warning: See CARBIMAZOLE. Also, it may cause haemorrhage and precipitate lupus syndrome.

Prosaid

(BHR) is a proprietary, prescription-only preparation of the (NSAID) NON-NARCOTIC ANALGESIC and ANTIRHEUMATIC naproxen. It can be used to relieve pain and inflammation, particularly rheumatic and arthritic pain, and to treat other musculoskeletal disorders. It is available as tablets.

✚▲ Side-effects/warning: See NAPROXEN.

Proscar

(Merck Sharp & Dohme) is a proprietary, prescription-only preparation of the ANTI-ANDROGEN finasteride, which is an *indirect* SEX HORMONE ANTAGONIST. It can be used to treat benign prostatic hyperplasia in men, and is available as tablets.

✚▲ Side-effects/warning: See FINASTERIDE.

prostacyclin

see EPOPROSTENOL

prostaglandins

is the name given to members of a family of LOCAL HORMONES (so-called because they exert their effects near to where they are formed), which are produced naturally by many organs and tissues in the body, both normally and in disease states. Naturally occurring members of the family include prostaglandin E_2 (DINOPROSTONE), prostaglandin $F_{2\alpha}$ (DINOPROST) and prostacyclin (EPOPROSTENOL). They are used therapeutically along with synthetic analogues (eg MISOPROSTOL). The uses of the prostaglandins reflect their high potency in causing such bodily actions as contraction of the uterus, softening and dilation of the cervix and dilation of blood vessels. Similarly, the side-effects of these agents used as drugs reflect their other powerful actions; such as stimulating the intestine causing pain, diarrhoea, actions on the brain to cause fever and prolongation of bleeding.

Prostap SR

(Lederle) is a proprietary, prescription-only preparation of leuprorelin acetate, which is an analogue of the hypothalamic HORMONE gonadorelin (gonadothrophin-releasing hormone; GnRH). It can be used as an ANTICANCER drug for cancer of the prostate gland and to treat endometriosis. It is available in a form for subcutaneous or intramuscular injection.

✚▲ Side-effects/warning: See LEUPRORELIN ACETATE.

Prostin E2

(Upjohn) is a proprietary, prescription-only form of the PROSTAGLANDIN dinoprostone. It is used mainly to induce labour, and is available as tablets, vaginal tablets (pessaries), a vaginal gel and in a form for injection.

✚▲ Side-effects/warning: See DINOPROSTONE.

Prostin F2 alpha

(Upjohn) is a proprietary, prescription-only

preparation of the PROSTAGLANDIN $F_{2\alpha}$ dinoprost. It is used mainly to induce therapeutic abortion because of its property of causing uterine contractions. It is available in a form for injection.

+▲ Side-effects/warning: See DINOPROST.

Prostin VR

(Upjohn) is a proprietary, prescription-only form of the PROSTAGLANDIN alprostadil (prostaglandin PGE_1). It is administered to maintain newborn babies with heart defects (to maintain patent ductus arteriosus), while the necessary preparations are being made for corrective surgery in intensive care. It is available in a form for infusion.

+▲ Side-effects/warning: See ALPROSTADIL.

Prosulf

(CP) is a proprietary, prescription-only preparation of protamine sulphate. It can be administered as an ANTIDOTE to heparin overdose, and is available in a form for injection.

+▲ Side-effects/warning: See PROTAMINE SULPHATE.

protamine sulfate

see PROTAMINE SULPHATE

protamine sulphate

(protamine sulfate) can be administered as an ANTIDOTE to treat an overdose of heparin. Administration is by slow intravenous injection.

+▲ Side-effects/warning: Slowing of the heart rate, hypotension and flushing.

✪ Related entry: Prosulf.

protamine zinc insulin

is a form of purified INSULIN, prepared as a sterile complex with protamine and zinc, which is used in DIABETIC TREATMENT to maintain diabetic patients. It is available in vials for injection and has a long duration of action.

+▲ Side-effects/warning: See INSULIN.

✪ Related entry: Hypurin Protamine Zinc.

Prothiaden

(Boots) is a proprietary, prescription-only preparation of the (TRICYCLIC) ANTIDEPRESSANT dothiepin hydrochloride. It can be used to treat depressive illness, especially in cases where some degree of sedation is deemed necessary, and is available as tablets and capsules.

+▲ Side-effects/warning: See DOTHIEPIN HYDROCHLORIDE.

protirelin

(thyrotrophin-releasing hormone; TRH), is a natural hypothalamic HORMONE produced and secreted by the hypothalamus. It in turn acts on the anterior pituitary gland to produce and secrete thyrotrophin (thyroid-stimulating hormone; TRH), a hormone that then causes the production and secretion of yet other hormones in the body. Therapeutically, it is used primarily to assess thyroid function in patients who suffer from under-activity of the pituitary gland (hypopituitarism) or from over-activity of the thyroid gland (hyperthyroidism). Administration is either oral or by injection.

+ Side-effects: There is commonly nausea. Treatment by injection may cause flushing, dizziness, faintness, raised blood pressure and pulse rate, a strange taste in the mouth and a desire to urinate. Occasionally, there may be bronchospasm.

▲ Warning: Administer with caution to patients with severe under-activity of the pituitary gland, myocardial ischaemia, asthma and obstructive airways disease or who are pregnant.

✪ Related entries: Relefact LH-RH/TRH; TRH-Cambridge.

Protium

(Knoll) is a proprietary, prescription-only preparation of the PROTON-PUMP INHIBITOR pantoprazole. It can be used as an ULCER-HEALING DRUG and for associated conditions, and is available as tablets.

+▲ Side-effects/warning: See PANTOPRAZOLE.

P

proton-pump inhibitors ⚡

are a recently introduced type of ULCER-HEALING DRUGS. They work by inhibiting gastric acid secretion in the parietal cells (acid-producing cells) of the stomach lining by interfering with the action of the ion (proton) pump that is responsible for the secretion of acid. They can be used to treat the symptoms of dyspepsia, which is caused by over-production of acid (hyperacidity), chronic problems associated with peptic ulcers (gastric or duodenal) and oesophagitis (inflammation of the oesophagus caused by regurgitation of acid and enzymes). They can also be used as an alternative to treatment with H_2-ANTAGONISTS. Examples of proton-pump inhibitors are LANSOPRAZOLE, OMEPRAZOLE and PANTOPRAZOLE.

protriptyline hydochloride

is an ANTIDEPRESSANT of the TRICYCLIC group. It is used particularly to treat depressive illness in apathetic and withdrawn patients because it has a STIMULANT effect. Administration is oral as tablets.
+▲ Side-effects/warning: See AMITRIPTYLINE HYDROCHLORIDE; but is less sedating, so there may be anxiety, raised heart rate, lowered blood pressure and photosensitive rashes.
○ Related entry: Concordin.

Provera

(Upjohn) is a proprietary, prescription-only preparation of the SEX HORMONE medroxyprogesterone acetate (a synthetic PROGESTOGEN). In women it can be used as an ANTICANCER drug for cancer of the breast or uterine endometrium and as a hormonal supplement for those whose progestogen level requires boosting (eg in endometriosis or dysfunctional uterine bleeding). It is available as tablets.
+▲ Side-effects/warning: See MEDROXYPROGESTERONE ACETATE.

proxymetacaine

is a LOCAL ANAESTHETIC which can be used

(as hydrochloride) by topical application in ophthalmic treatments
+ Side-effects: There may be slight stinging on initial application.
○ Related entries: Minims Proxymetacaine Hydrochloride; Ophthaine.

Prozac

(Dista) is a proprietary, prescription-only preparation of the (SSRI) ANTIDEPRESSANT fluoxetine hydrochloride, which has less SEDATIVE effects than some other antidepressants, and has recently been used to treat bulimia nervosa. It is available as capsules and a liquid.
+▲ Side-effects/warning: See FLUOXETINE.

pseudoephedrine hydrochloride

is a SYMPATHOMIMETIC drug with BRONCHODILATOR, VASOCONSTRICTOR and DECONGESTANT properties. It is sometimes used to treat obstructive airways disease, but is most commonly included in a number of proprietary preparations for treating cold symptoms. Its actions and effects are very similar to those of the closely related drug ephedrine hydrochloride.
+▲ Side-effects/warning: See EPHEDRINE HYDROCHLORIDE.
○ Related entries: Actifed Compound Linctus; Actifed Expectorant; Actifed Syrup; Actifed Tablets; Benylin Cough and Congestion; Benylin Four Flu Liquid; Bronalin Decongestant Elixir; Bronalin Dry Cough Elixir; Day Cold Comfort Capsules; Dimotane Co; Dimotane Co Paediatric; Dimotane Expectorant; Expulin Cough Linctus – Sugar Free; Galpseud; Galpseud Plus; Lemsip Flu Strength Pseudoephedrine Formula; Lemsip Power+; Meltus Dry Cough Elixir, Adult; Meltus Junior Dry Cough Elixir; Night Cold Comfort Capsules; Nurofen Cold & Flu; Phensedyl Plus; Robitussin Chesty Cough with Congestion; Sudafed Co-Tablets; Sudafed Elixir; Sudafed Expectorant; Sudafed Linctus; Sudafed Tablets; Tixylix Cough and Cold; Vicks Medinite.

Psoriderm

(Dermal) is a proprietary, non-prescription COMPOUND PREPARATION of coal tar (with lecithin). It can be used for psoriasis, eczema and dandruff, and is available as a cream, a scalp lotion and a bath emulsion.
+▲ Side-effects/warning: See COAL TAR.

PsoriGel

(Novex) is a proprietary, non-prescription preparation of coal tar. It can be used to treat psoriasis and dermatitis, and is available as a gel.
+▲ Side-effects/warning: See COAL TAR.

Psorin

(Thames) is a proprietary, non-prescription COMPOUND PREPARATION of dithranol, salicylic acid and coal tar. It can be used to treat psoriasis and dermatitis, and is available as an ointment.
+▲ Side-effects/warning: See COAL TAR; DITHRANOL; SALICYLIC ACID.

Pulmadil

(3M) is a proprietary, prescription-only preparation of the BETA-RECEPTOR STIMULANT and SYMPATHOMIMETIC rimiterol hydrobromide. It can be used as a BRONCHODILATOR in reversible obstructive airways disease, as an ANTI-ASTHMATIC treatment in severe acute asthma and for the alleviation of symptoms of chronic bronchitis and emphysema. It is available as an aerosol inhalant.
+▲ Side-effects/warning: See RIMITEROL HYDROBROMIDE.

Pulmicort Inhaler

(Astra) is a proprietary, prescription-only preparation of the CORTICOSTEROID budesonide. It can be used to prevent asthma attacks and is available in inhalers; one preparation, *Pulmicort LS*, is used with the *Nebuhaler* or *Spacer* inhaler devices.
+▲ Side-effects/warning: See BUDESONIDE.

Pulmicort Respules

(Astra) is a proprietary, prescription-only preparation of the CORTICOSTEROID budesonide. It can be used to prevent asthma attacks, and is available in *Respules* for inhalation.
+▲ Side-effects/warning: See BUDESONIDE.

Pulmicort Turbohaler

(Astra) is a proprietary, prescription-only preparation of the CORTICOSTEROID budesonide. It can be used to prevent asthma attacks, and is available as a dry-powder inhaler.
+▲ Side-effects/warning: See BUDESONIDE.

Pump-Hep

(Leo) is a proprietary, prescription-only preparation of the ANTICOAGULANT heparin (as heparin sodium). It can be used to treat various forms of thrombosis, and is available in a form for injection.
+▲ Side-effects/warning: See HEPARIN.

Pur-In Isophane

(CP) is a proprietary, non-prescription preparation of highly purified human ISOPHANE INSULIN. It is used as a DIABETIC TREATMENT to treat and maintain diabetic patients, and is available in vials and cartridges for the *Pur-In Pen* injection device and has an intermediate duration of action.
+▲ Side-effects/warning: See INSULIN.

Pur-In Mix 15/85

(CP) is a proprietary, non-prescription preparation of human BIPHASIC ISOPHANE INSULIN (15% soluble/85% isophane). It is used as a DIABETIC TREATMENT to treat and maintain diabetic patients, and is available in vials and cartridges for the *Pur-In Pen* injection device and has an intermediate duration of action.
+▲ Side-effects/warning: See INSULIN.

Pur-In Mix 25/75

(CP) is a proprietary, non-prescription preparation of human BIPHASIC ISOPHANE INSULIN (25% soluble/75% isophane). It is used as a DIABETIC TREATMENT to treat and

P

P

maintain diabetic patients, and is available
in vials and cartridges for the *Pur-In Pen*
injection device and has an intermediate
duration of action.

✚▲ Side-effects/warning: See INSULIN.

Pur-In Mix 50/50

(CP) is a proprietary, non-prescription
preparation of human BIPHASIC ISOPHANE
INSULIN (50% soluble/50% isophane). It is
used as a DIABETIC TREATMENT to treat and
maintain diabetic patients, and is available
in vials and cartridges for the *Pur-In Pen*
injection device and has an intermediate
duration of action.

✚▲ Side-effects/warning: See INSULIN.

Pur-In Neutral

(CP) is a proprietary, non-prescription
preparation of highly purified human
neutral SOLUBLE INSULIN. It is used as a
DIABETIC TREATMENT to treat and maintain
diabetic patients, and is available in vials
and cartridges for the *Pur-In Pen* injection
device and has a short duration of action.

✚▲ Side-effects/warning: See INSULIN.

Puregon

(Organon) is a proprietary, prescription-
only HORMONE preparation of recombinant
human FOLLICLE-STIMULATING HORMONE
(FSH). It can be used to treat infertile
women with proven hypopituitarism and
who do not respond to CLOMIPHENE CITRATE
(another drug commonly used to treat
infertility) and in superovulation treatment
in assisted conception (as with in vitro
fertilization; IVF). It is available in a form
for injection.

✚▲ Side-effects/warning: See FOLLITROPIN
BETA.

purgatives

see LAXATIVES

Puri-Nethol

(Wellcome) is a proprietary, prescription-
only preparation of the (CYTOTOXIC)
ANTICANCER mercaptopurine. It can be used

in the treatment of acute leukaemias, and is
available as tablets.

✚▲ Side-effects/warning: See
MERCAPTOPURINE.

Pylorid

(Glaxo) is a proprietary, prescription-only
preparation of the H$_2$-ANTAGONIST and ULCER-
HEALING DRUG ranitidine bismuth citrate. It
can be administered to treat benign peptic
ulcers (ie in the stomach or duodenum)
and, in conjunction with ANTIBIOTICS,
duodenal ulceration associated with
Helicobacter pylori infection. It is available
as tablets.

✚▲ Side-effects/warning: See RANITIDINE
BISMUTH CITRATE.

Pyralvex

(Norgine) is a proprietary, non-
prescription preparation of salicylic acid
and rhubarb extract, which have a COUNTER-
IRRITANT, or RUBEFACIENT, action. It can be
applied to the mouth for the symptomatic
relief of the pain and discomfort from
mouth ulcers and denture irritation. It is
available as a cream and a gel for topical
application, and is not normally used for
children, except on medical advice.

✚▲ Side-effects/warning: See SALICYLIC
ACID.

pyrazinamide

is an ANTIBACTERIAL drug and is one of the
major forms of ANTITUBERCULAR treatment.
It is generally administered in combination
with other drugs, for example ISONIAZID and
RIFAMPICIN, in order to cover resistance and
for maximum effect. Because pyrazinamide
is only active against dividing forms of
Mycobacterium tuberculosis, it is most
effective in the early stages of treatment (ie
the first few months). Administration is oral
as tablets.

✚ Side-effects: There may be symptoms of
liver malfunction, including high
temperature, severe weight loss and
jaundice. There may be nausea and
vomiting, and certain sensitivity reactions,

such as urticaria, joint pain and blood disorders.

▲ Warning: It should not be administered to patients with liver damage or porphyria; it should be administered with caution to patients with impaired kidney function, diabetes or gout.

○ Related entry: Rifate.

pyridostigmine

is an ANTICHOLINESTERASE drug which enhances the effects of the NEUROTRANSMITTER acetylcholine (and of certain cholinergic drugs). Because of this property, it has PARASYMPATHOMIMETIC actions and is sometimes used to stimulate the intestine. It is more commonly used to treat the neuromuscular transmission disorder myasthenia gravis. Administration is either oral or by injection.

✚▲ Side-effects/warning: See NEOSTIGMINE; but it has generally weaker parasympathomimetic actions.

○ Related entry: Mestinon.

pyrimethamine

is an ANTIMALARIAL drug which is mainly administered in combination with DAPSONE or SULFADOXINE to prevent or treat malaria. It can also be used, along with a sulphonamide, to treat the protozoal infection toxoplasmosis. Administration is oral as tablets.

✚ Side-effects: There may be rashes, insomnia and blood disorders.

▲ Warning: It should be administered with caution to patients with certain liver or kidney disorders, or who are taking folic acid supplements (eg during pregnancy). A high dosage requires regular blood counts.

○ Related entries: Daraprim; Fansidar; Maloprim.

Pyrogastrone

(Sanofi Winthrop) is a proprietary, prescription-only COMPOUND PREPARATION of the CYTOPROTECTANT drug carbenoxolone sodium, the ANTACIDS aluminium hydroxide, magnesium trisilicate and sodium bicarbonate, and the DEMULCENT agent ALGINIC ACID. It can be used as an ULCER-HEALING DRUG for benign gastric ulceration, and is available as tablets and an oral liquid.

✚▲ Side-effects/warning: See ALUMINIUM HYDROXIDE; CARBENOXOLONE SODIUM; MAGNESIUM TRISILICATE; SODIUM BICARBONATE.

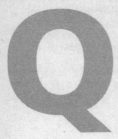

Q

Q-Mazine Syrup

(Seton) is a proprietary, non-prescription preparation of the ANTIHISTAMINE promethazine hydochloride. It can be used as an ANTINAUSEANT for the treatment of motion sickness and also for allergic reactions, such as urticaria. It is available as an oral liquid and is not normally given to children under one year, except on medical advice.

+▲ Side-effects/warning: See PROMETHAZINE HYDOCHLORIDE.

Quellada

(Stafford-Miller) is a proprietary, non-prescription preparation of the SCABICIDAL and PEDICULICIDAL drug lindane. It can be used to treat infestations of the pubic hair by lice (pediculosis) or of the skin by itch-mites (scabies). It is available as a lotion and is not normally used for children under six months, except on medical advice.

+▲ Side-effects/warning: See LINDANE.

Quellada M

(Stafford-Miller) is a proprietary, non-prescription preparation of the SCABICIDAL and PEDICULICIDAL drug malathion. It can be used to treat infestations of the scalp and pubic hair by lice (pediculosis) or of the skin by the itch-mite (scabies), and is available as a liquid and a shampoo.

+▲ Side-effects/warning: See MALATHION.

Questran

(Bristol-Myers) is a proprietary, prescription-only preparation of the LIPID-LOWERING DRUG cholestyramine. It can be used in hyperlipidaemia to reduce the levels, or change the proportions, of lipids in the bloodstream. It has various other uses, including as an ANTIDIARRHOEAL and, in certain circumstances, in biliary disturbances (including pruritus in biliary obstruction or biliary cirrhosis). It is available as a powder to be taken with liquids.

+▲ Side-effects/warning: See CHOLESTYRAMINE.

Questran A

(Bristol-Myers) is a proprietary, prescription-only preparation of the LIPID-LOWERING DRUG cholestyramine. It can be used in hyperlipidaemia to reduce the levels, or change the proportions, of lipids in the bloodstream. It has various other uses, including as an ANTIDIARRHOEAL and in biliary disturbances (including pruritus in biliary obstruction or biliary cirrhosis). It is available as a powder (containing the sweetener aspartame) to be taken with liquids.

+▲ Side-effects/warning: See CHOLESTYRAMINE.

quinagolide

is a recently introduced drug with similar actions to bromocriptine. It can be used to treat HORMONE disorders (hyperprolactinaemia disorders), such as prolactinoma. Administration is oral as tablets.

+▲ Side-effects/warning: See BROMOCRIPTINE. There may also be hypotensive actions, which may be disturbing to some patients, during the first few days of treatment, anorexia, abdominal pain, diarrhoea, insomnia, oedema, flushing and nasal congestion. It is not to be given to patients who are pregnant.

❍ Related entry: Norprolac.

quinalbarbitone sodium

is a BARBITURATE with a rapid onset of action and is used as a HYPNOTIC to promote sleep in conditions of severe, intractable insomnia. Administration is oral. Preparations containing quinalbarbitone sodium are on the Controlled Drugs List.

✚▲ Side-effects/warning: See BARBITURATES.

◎ Related entries: Seconal Sodium; Tuinal.

quinapril

is an ACE INHIBITOR and a powerful VASODILATOR which can be used as an ANTIHYPERTENSIVE and in HEART FAILURE TREATMENT, often when other treatments are not appropriate. It is frequently used in conjunction with other classes of drug, particularly (THIAZIDE) DIURETICS. Administration is oral.

✚▲ Side-effects/warning: See CAPTOPRIL.

◎ Related entries: Accupro; Accuretic; Acezide.

quinidine

is a CINCHONA ALKALOID and is chemically related to QUININE. It is used as an ANTI-ARRHYTHMIC drug to treat heartbeat irregularities. Administration is oral.

✚▲ Side-effects/warning: See PROCAINAMIDE HYDROCHLORIDE. There may also be other heart arrhythmias and a number of blood disorders. It is not to be given to patients with heart block.

◎ Related entry: Kinidin Durules.

quinine

is a CINCHONA ALKALOID and was for a long time the main treatment for malaria. Today, it has largely been replaced by synthetic and less toxic drugs (eg CHLOROQUINE). However, quinine is still used (as quinine sulphate or quinine hydrochloride) against falciparum malaria in cases that prove to be resistant to the newer drugs, or for emergency cases in which large doses are necessary. It can also be used to relieve nocturnal cramps. Administration is either oral or by infusion.

✚ Side-effects: Toxic effects (especially in overdose) – called *cinchonism* – include nausea, headache, abdominal pain, visual

disturbances, tinnitus, a rash and confusion. Some patients may experience visual disturbances and temporary blindness, sensitivity reactions and blood disorders.

▲ Warning: It should not be administered to patients with certain optic nerve disorders or haemoglobinurea. It should be administered with caution to those who suffer from heart block, atrial fibrillation, who have G6PD deficiency or who are pregnant.

◎ Related entry: Nicobrevin.

Quinocort

(Quinoderm) is a proprietary, prescription-only COMPOUND PREPARATION of the ANTI-INFLAMMATORY and CORTICOSTEROID hydrocortisone and the ANTIFUNGAL and ANTIBACTERIAL potassium hydroxyquinoline sulphate. It can be used to treat inflammation, particularly when associated with fungal infections, and is available as a cream for topical application.

✚▲ Side-effects/warning: See HYDROCORTISONE; POTASSIUM HYDROXYQUINOLINE SULPHATE.

Quinoderm Cream

(Quinoderm) is a proprietary, non-prescription COMPOUND PREPARATION of the KERATOLYTIC and ANTIMICROBIAL benzoyl peroxide (10%) and the ANTIFUNGAL and ANTIBACTERIAL potassium hydroxyquinoline sulphate. It can be used to treat acne, and is available as a cream for topical application.

✚▲ Side-effects/warning: See BENZOYL PEROXIDE; POTASSIUM HYDROXYQUINOLINE SULPHATE.

Quinoderm Cream 5

(Quinoderm) is a proprietary, non-prescription COMPOUND PREPARATION of the KERATOLYTIC and ANTIMICROBIAL benzoyl peroxide (5%) and the ANTIFUNGAL and ANTIBACTERIAL potassium hydroxyquinoline sulphate. It can be used to treat acne, and is available as a cream for topical

Q

application.
✚▲ Side-effects/warning: See BENZOYL
PEROXIDE; POTASSIUM HYDROXYQUINOLINE
SULPHATE.

Quinoderm Lotio-Gel 5%
(Quinoderm) is a proprietary, non-
prescription COMPOUND PREPARATION of the
KERATOLYTIC and ANTIMICROBIAL benzoyl
peroxide (5%) and the ANTIFUNGAL and
ANTIBACTERIAL potassium hydroxyquinoline
sulphate. It can be used to treat acne, and
is available as a cream for topical
application.
✚▲ Side-effects/warning: See BENZOYL
PEROXIDE; POTASSIUM HYDROXYQUINOLINE
SULPHATE.

quinolones ▣
(4-quinolones) are ANTIBACTERIAL and
ANTIBIOTIC drugs, which are mainly used to
treat infections in patients who are allergic
to penicillin or whose strain of bacterium is
resistant to standard antibiotics. Although
they are active against a wide range of
infective bacterial organisms, they are
usually more effective against Gram-
negative organisms and also have useful
activity against some Gram-positive
organisms (though not anaerobes). They
work by damaging the internal structure of
bacteria (ie they are *bactericidal*).
Chemically, they are related to NALIDIXIC ACID
and the names of more recently introduced
members end with *-oxacin*. See CINOXACIN;
CIPROFLOXACIN; NORFLOXACIN; OFLOXACIN.
✚ Side-effects: There may be nausea,
diarrhoea, vomiting, abdominal pain;
headache, dizziness, sleep disorders, rash,
pruritis, fever, photosensitivity; increase in
blood creatinine and urea, transient
disturbances in liver enzymes and bilirubin;
joint and muscle pains, blood disorders. Less
frequently, there may be anaphylaxis,
anorexia, confusion, hallucinations and
sensory disturbances.
▲ Warning: Administer with caution to
children or adolescents; to patients with
epilepsy, kidney or liver impairment; or who

are pregnant or breast-feeding. There is a
risk of convulsions being precipitated in
those showing no previous tendencies by
other drugs (eg by NSAIDS).

Quinoped
(Quinoderm) is a proprietary, non-
prescription COMPOUND PREPARATION of the
ANTIFUNGAL drug potassium
hydroxyquinoline sulphate and the
KERATOLYTIC and ANTIMICROBIAL benzoyl
peroxide. It can be used to treat fungal skin
infections, such as athlete's foot, and is
available as a cream.
✚▲ Side-effects/warning: See BENZOYL
PEROXIDE; POTASSIUM HYDROXYQUINOLINE
SULPHATE.

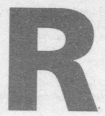

+▲ Side-effects/warning: See VACCINES.
☉ Related entry: Rabies Vaccine BP Pasteur Mérieux.

Rabies Vaccine BP Pasteur Mérieux

(Mérieux) is a proprietary, prescription-only VACCINE preparation which can be used to prevent contracting rabies. It is available in a form for injection.

+▲ Side-effects/warning: See RABIES VACCINE.

Radian B Heat Spray

(Roche) is a proprietary, non-prescription COMPOUND PREPARATION of CAMPHOR, MENTHOL, salicylic acid and ammonium salicylate, which all have COUNTER-IRRITANT, or RUBEFACIENT, actions. It can be applied to the skin for symptomatic relief of muscle and rheumatic pain, sciatica, lumbago, fibrosis and muscle stiffness. It is available as a spray and is not normally used for children, except on medical advice.

+▲ Side-effects/warning: See AMMONIUM SALICYLATE; SALICYLIC ACID.

Radian B Muscle Lotion

(Roche) is a proprietary, non-prescription COMPOUND PREPARATION of CAMPHOR, MENTHOL, the (NSAID) NON-NARCOTIC ANALGESIC and ANTIRHEUMATIC ammonium salicylate and the KERATOLYTIC agent salicylic acid. It is used as a COUNTER-IRRITANT, or RUBEFACIENT, for the symptomatic relief of muscle and rheumatic pain, sciatica, lumbago, fibrosis and muscle stiffness. It is available as a spray for application to the skin and is not normally used for children under six years, except on medical advice.

+▲ Side-effects/warning: See AMMONIUM SALICYLATE; SALICYLIC ACID.

Radian B Muscle Rub

(Roche) is a proprietary, non-prescription COMPOUND PREPARATION of CAMPHOR, MENTHOL, methyl salicylate and capsicum oleoresin. It is used as a COUNTER-IRRITANT, or RUBEFACIENT, for the symptomatic relief of

Rabies Immunoglobulin

(Public Health Laboratory Service) (Antirabies Immunoglobulin Injection) is a non-proprietary, prescription-only preparation of a SPECIFIC IMMUNOGLOBULIN. It can be used in IMMUNIZATION to give immediate immunity against infection by rabies. It is available in a form for intramuscular injection.

+▲ Side-effects/warning: See IMMUNIZATION.

rabies immunoglobulin, human

is a SPECIFIC IMMUNOGLOBULIN which is used in IMMUNIZATION to give immediate *passive immunity* against infection by rabies and can be used in conjunction with RABIES VACCINE. Administration is by intramuscular injection and injection at the site of the bite.

+▲ Side-effects/warning: See IMMUNIZATION.

☉ Related entry: Rabies Immunoglobulin.

rabies vaccine

is a VACCINE used for IMMUNIZATION to prevent contracting rabies (but does not treat people already infected with rabies). It is administered to medical workers and their relatives, who may come into contact with rabid animals or with people who have been bitten by an animal that might be rabid. It can also be administered to people who routinely work with animals (eg vets). The vaccine is of a type known as a *human diploid cell vaccine* and is administered by a course of injections.

R

muscle and rheumatic pain, sciatica, lumbago, fibrosis and muscle stiffness. It is available as an ointment for topical application to the skin and is not normally used for children under six years, except on medical advice.

✚▲ Side-effects/warning: See CAPSICUM OLEORESIN; METHYL SALICYLATE. It should not be used on inflamed or broken skin or mucous membranes.

Ralgex Cream

(Seton) is a proprietary, non-prescription COMPOUND PREPARATION of capsicum oleoresin, glycol salicylate and METHYL NICOTINATE. It is used as a COUNTER-IRRITANT, or RUBEFACIENT, for the symptomatic relief of muscle pain and stiffness, sciatica, lumbago and fibrosis. It is available as a cream for topical application to the skin and is not normally used for children, except on medical advice.

✚▲ Side-effects/warning: See CAPSICUM OLEORESIN; GLYCOL SALICYLATE.

Ralgex Heat Spray

(Seton) is a proprietary, non-prescription COMPOUND PREPARATION of glycol salicylate and METHYL NICOTINATE. It can be used as a COUNTER-IRRITANT, or RUBEFACIENT, for the symptomatic relief of muscle pain and stiffness, sciatica, lumbago and fibrosis. It is available as a spray for topical application to the skin and is not normally used for children under five years, except on medical advice.

✚▲ Side-effects/warning: See GLYCOL SALICYLATE.

Ralgex Stick

(Seton) is a proprietary, non-prescription COMPOUND PREPARATION of MENTHOL, methyl salicylate, glycol salicylate, ethyl salicylate and capsicum oleoresin. It can be used as a COUNTER-IRRITANT, or RUBEFACIENT, for the symptomatic relief of muscle pain and stiffness, sciatica, lumbago and fibrosis. It is available as an embrocation stick for topical application to the skin and is not

normally used for children, except on medical advice.

✚▲ Side-effects/warning: See CAPSICUM OLEORESIN; ETHYL SALICYLATE; GLYCOL SALICYLATE; METHYL SALICYLATE.

raltitrexed

is a CYTOTOXIC drug which is used primarily as an ANTICANCER treatment of colon cancer. Administration is by injection.

✚▲ Side-effects/warning: See CYTOTOXICS.
✪ Related entry: Tomudex.

ramipril

is an ACE INHIBITOR and acts as a VASODILATOR. It can be used as an ANTIHYPERTENSIVE and in HEART FAILURE TREATMENT and sometimes following myocardial infarction (damage to heart muscle, usually after a heart attack). It is often used in conjunction with other classes of drug, particularly (THIAZIDE) DIURETICS. Administration is oral.

✚▲ Side-effects/warning: See CAPTOPRIL.
✪ Related entry: Tritace.

Ramysis

(ISIS) is a proprietary, prescription-only preparation of the ANTIBACTERIAL and (TETRACYCLINE) ANTIBIOTIC doxycycline. It can be used to treat infections of many kinds, and is available as capsules.

✚▲ Side-effects/warning: See DOXYCYCLINE.

ranitidine

is an effective and extensively prescribed H_2-ANTAGONIST and ULCER-HEALING DRUG. It is used in the treatment of benign peptic (gastric and duodenal) ulcers, to relieve heartburn in cases of reflux oesophagitis, Zollinger-Ellison syndrome and a variety of conditions where reduction of acidity is beneficial. It is now also available without prescription – in a limited amount and for short-term uses only – for the relief of heartburn, dyspepsia and hyperacidity. It works by reducing the secretion of gastric acid, so reducing erosion and bleeding from peptic ulcers and allowing them a chance to heal. However, treatment with ranitidine should not start before a full diagnosis of gastric bleeding or serious pain has been made, because its action in restricting gastric secretions may possibly mask the presence of stomach cancer. It can also be used to treat ulceration induced by NSAID treatment. Administration can be either oral or by injection.

+▲ Side-effects/warning: See CIMETIDINE; but it does not significantly inhibit microsomal drug-metabolizing enzymes.
○ Related entries: Zantac; Zantac 75.

ranitidine bismuth citrate

(ranitidine bismutrex) is a compound of the extensively prescribed H₂-ANTAGONIST and ULCER-HEALING DRUG ranitidine, together with bismuth. It can be used in the treatment of benign peptic (gastric or duodenal) ulcers. In the treatment of duodenal ulceration associated with *Helicobacter pylori* infection it is used in conjunction with an ANTIBIOTIC, either AMOXYCILLIN or CLARITHROMYCIN. Ranitidine works by reducing the secretion of gastric acid and (together with the antibiotic) helps to eliminate the bacterium associated with peptic ulceration. Administration is oral.

+▲ Side-effects/warning: See CIMETIDINE (but it does not significantly inhibit microsomal drug-metabolizing enzymes); TRIPOTASSIUM DICITRATOBISMUTHATE. It may cause discoloration of the tongue and faeces. It is not recommended for children.
○ Related entry: Pylorid.

ranitidine bsmutrex

see ranitidine bismuth citrate

Rapifen

(Janssen) is a proprietary, prescription-only preparation of the (OPIOID) NARCOTIC ANALGESIC alfentanil (as hydrochloride), and is on the Controlled Drugs List. It can be used in outpatient surgery, short operational procedures and for the enhancement of anaesthesia. It is available

in a form for injection.
+▲ Side-effects/warning: See ALFENTANIL.

Rapitard MC

(Novo Nordisk) is a proprietary, non-prescription preparation of BIPHASIC INSULIN, highly purified bovine and porcine insulin, and is used in DIABETIC TREATMENT to treat and maintain diabetic patients. It is available in vials for regular injection and has an intermediate duration of action.
+▲ Side-effects/warning: See INSULIN.

Rapitil

(Fisons) is a proprietary, prescription-only preparation of the ANTI-ALLERGIC drug nedocromil sodium. It can be used to treat allergic conjunctivitis in the eye, and is available as eye-drops.
+▲ Side-effects/warning: See NEDOCROMIL SODIUM.

Rastinon

(Hoechst) is a proprietary, prescription-only preparation of the SULPHONYLUREA tolbutamide. It is used in DIABETIC TREATMENT for Type II diabetes (non-insulin-dependent diabetes mellitus; NIDDM; maturity-onset diabetes), and is available as tablets.
+▲ Side-effects/warning: See TOLBUTAMIDE.

razoxane

is a synthetic CYTOTOXIC drug which is used to treat some forms of cancer, including leukaemia. Administration is oral.
+▲ Side-effects/warning: See CYTOTOXICS.
○ Related entry: Razoxin.

Razoxin

(Zeneca) is a proprietary, prescription-only preparation of the (CYTOTOXIC) ANTICANCER drug razoxane. It can be used in the treatment of some cancers, for example, acute leukaemia, and is available as tablets.
+▲ Side-effects/warning: See RAZOXANE.

receptors ▣

are proteins through which many drugs and

R

natural mediators act to exert their effects. Receptors *recognize* and are stimulated by only their own mediators, including neurotransmitters, hormones and local hormones, or drugs that have been designed to mimic these mediators. They are usually situated on the surface membrane of cells and only require tiny amounts of a mediator or other chemical (called agonists) to trigger a reaction that can produce rapid and profound changes in that cell (for instance, biochemical changes or electrical effects). Another class of drug, the ANTAGONISTS, have a different type of action; they can *occupy* (in effect, physically block) the receptor without producing changes in the cell and prevent the agonist type of drug from acting. Examples of receptor types are alpha- and beta-adrenoceptors for ADRENALINE and NORADRENALINE; muscarinic and nicotinic cholinergic receptors for acetylcholine; H_1 and H_2 for histamine; and ANDROGEN or OESTROGEN receptors for SEX HORMONE mediators. In all cases, synthetic drugs have been produced that act, either as agonists or antagonists, at these receptors.

Recombinate

(Baxter) is a proprietary, prescription-only preparation of factor VIII fraction (octocog alfa), which acts as a HAEMOSTATIC drug to reduce or stop bleeding in the treatment of disorders in which bleeding is prolonged and potentially dangerous (mainly haemophilia A). It is available in a form for infusion or injection.

✚▲ Side-effects/warning: see FACTOR VIII FRACTION (DRIED).

Recormon

(Boehringer Mannheim) is a proprietary, prescription-only preparation of epoetin beta (synthesized human erythropoitetin beta). It can be used in ANAEMIA TREATMENT for conditions known to be associated with chronic renal failure in dialysis patients. It is available in a form for injection.

476 ✚▲ Side-effects/warning: See EPOETIN.

sRedoxon

(Roche) is a proprietary, non-prescription preparation of vitamin C (ascorbic acid). It can be used to treat the symptoms of vitamin C deficiency, and is available as tablets and effervescent tablets.

✚▲ Side-effects/warning: See ASCORBIC ACID.

Refolinon

(Pharmacia) is a proprietary, prescription-only preparation of folinic acid. It can be used to counteract the folate-antagonist activity and consequent toxic effects of certain ANTICANCER drugs, especially METHOTREXATE. It is available as tablets and in a form for injection.

✚▲ Side-effects/warning: See FOLINIC ACID.

Regaine

(Upjohn) is a proprietary, non-prescription preparation of the VASODILATOR minoxidil. It can be used to treat male-pattern baldness (in men and women), and is available as a topical solution. It is not usually used for children, except on medical advice.

✚▲ Side-effects/warning: See MINOXIDIL.

Regulan

(Procter & Gamble) is a proprietary, non-prescription preparation of the (*bulking-agent*) LAXATIVE ispaghula husk. It can be used to treat a number of gastrointestinal disorders, including irritable bowel syndrome and diverticular disease. It is available as a (lemon-and-lime flavour) powder for solution in water and is not normally given to children under six years, except on medical advice.

✚▲ Side-effects/warning: See ISPAGHULA HUSK.

Reguletts

(Seton) is a proprietary, non-prescription preparation of the (*stimulant*) LAXATIVE phenolphthalein. It can be used to relieve constipation, and is available as pills. It is not normally given to children, except on medical advice.

+▲ Side-effects/warning: See
PHENOLPHTHALEIN.

Regulose

(Intercare) is a proprietary, non-prescription preparation of the (*osmotic*) LAXATIVE lactulose. It can be used to relieve constipation, and is available as an oral solution.

+▲ Side-effects/warning: See LACTULOSE.

Relaxit Micro-enema

(Pharmacia) is a proprietary, non-prescription preparation of sodium citrate (with sodium lauryl sulphate, sorbic acid, sorbitol and glycerol). It can be used as a LAXATIVE, and is available as an enema.

+▲ Side-effects/warning: See SODIUM CITRATE.

Relaxyl

(Whitehall) is a proprietary, non-prescription preparation of the ANTISPASMODIC drug alverine citrate. It can be used to treat muscle spasm of the gastrointestinal tract, for example, in irritable bowel syndrome, and is available as capsules. It is not normally given to children, except on medical advice.

+▲ Side-effects/warning: See ALVERINE CITRATE.

Relefact LH-RH

(Hoechst) is a proprietary, prescription-only preparation of gonadorelin (gonadotrophin-releasing hormone; GnRH). It can be used as a diagnostic aid in assessing the functioning of the pituitary gland, and is available in a form for intravenous injection.

+▲ Side-effects/warning: See GONADORELIN.

Relefact LH-RH/TRH

(Hoechst) is a proprietary, prescription-only COMPOUND PREPARATION of gonadorelin (gonadotrophin-releasing hormone; GnRH) and protirelin (thyrotrophin-releasing hormone; TRH). It can be used as a diagnostic aid in assessing the functioning of the pituitary gland, and is available in a form for intravenous injection.

+▲ Side-effects/warning: See GONADORELIN; PROTIRELIN.

Relifex

(Bencard) is a proprietary, prescription-only preparation of the (NSAID) NON-NARCOTIC ANALGESIC and ANTIRHEUMATIC nabumetone. It can be used to treat and relieve pain and inflammation, particularly arthritic and rheumatic pain and other musculoskeletal disorders. It is available as tablets and a sugar-free oral suspension.

+▲ Side-effects/warning: See NABUMETONE.

Remedeine

(Napp) is a proprietary, prescription-only COMPOUND ANALGESIC preparation of the NON-NARCOTIC ANALGESIC paracetamol and the (OPIOID) NARCOTIC ANALGESIC dihydrocodeine tartrate, in the ratio 500:20 mg. It can be used as a painkiller, and is available as tablets (and also under the proprietary name *Forte Tablets* in a combination of 500:30 mg).

+▲ Side-effects/warning: See DIHYDROCODEINE TARTRATE; PARACETAMOL.

Remegel Original

(Warner-Wellcome) is a proprietary, non-prescription preparation of the ANTACID calcium carbonate. It can be used for the relief of heartburn, acid indigestion and upset stomach. It is available as chewable tablets and is not normally given to children, except on medical advice.

+▲ Side-effects/warning: See CALCIUM CARBONATE.

remifentanil

is an (OPIOID) NARCOTIC ANALGESIC which is used in the induction of anaesthesia and during surgery to supplement the effect of GENERAL ANAESTHETICS. Administration is by intravenous infusion.

+▲ Side-effects/warning: See OPIOIDS.
✪ Related entry: Ultiva.

R

Remnos

(DDSA) is a proprietary, prescription-only preparation of the BENZODIAZEPINE nitrazepam. It can be used as a relatively long-acting HYPNOTIC for the short-term treatment of insomnia, where a degree of sedation during the daytime is acceptable. It is available as tablets.

✚▲ Side-effects/warning: See NITRAZEPAM.

Rennie Rap-Eze

(Roche) is a proprietary, non-prescription preparation of the ANTACID calcium carbonate. It can be used for the relief of acid indigestion, heartburn, upset stomach, dyspepsia and biliousness. It is available as tablets and is not normally given to children, except on medical advice.

✚▲ Side-effects/warning: See CALCIUM CARBONATE.

Rennie Tablets, Digestif

(Roche) is a proprietary, non-prescription COMPOUND PREPARATION of the ANTACIDS calcium carbonate and magnesium carbonate. It can be used for the relief of acid indigestion, heartburn, upset stomach, dyspepsia, biliousness and overindulgence. It is available as tablets and is not normally given to children under six years, except on medical advice.

✚▲ Side-effects/warning: See CALCIUM CARBONATE; MAGNESIUM CARBONATE.

Replenine

(BPL) is a recently introduced proprietary, prescription-only (heat-treated) preparation of factor IX fraction, dried, which is prepared from human blood plasma. It can be used in treating patients with a deficiency in factor IX (haemophilia B), and is available in a form for infusion.

✚▲ Side-effects/warning: See FACTOR IX FRACTION, DRIED.

reproterol hydrochloride

is a SYMPATHOMIMETIC and BETA-RECEPTOR STIMULANT with beta$_2$-receptor selectivity. It is mainly used as a BRONCHODILATOR in reversible obstructive airways disease and as an ANTI-ASTHMATIC in severe acute asthma. It can also be used for the alleviation of symptoms of chronic bronchitis and emphysema. Administration is by aerosol. (Patients should be cautioned not to exceed the stated dose, and if a previously effective dose fails to relieve symptoms they should consult their doctor.)

✚▲ Side-effects/warning: See SALBUTAMOL.
✪ Related entry: Bronchodil.

Requip

(SmithKline Beecham) is a proprietary, prescription-only preparation of ropinirole (as hydrochloride). It can be used as an ANTIPARKINSONISM drug, and is available as tablets.

✚▲ Side-effects/warning: See ROPINIROLE.

Resiston One

(Fisons) is a proprietary, non-prescription COMPOUND PREPARATION of the ANTI-ALLERGIC drug sodium cromoglycate and the SYMPATHOMIMETIC and DECONGESTANT xylometazoline hydrochloride. It can be used in the prevention of allergic rhinitis, and is available as a nasal aerosol.

✚▲ Side-effects/warning: See SODIUM CROMOGLYCATE; XYLOMETAZOLINE HYDROCHLORIDE.

Resolve

(SmithKline Beecham) is a proprietary, non-prescription preparation of the NON-NARCOTIC ANALGESIC paracetamol, vitamin C and various ANTACID salts. It can be used to treat headache with stomach upset or with nausea (eg migraine). It is available as effervescent granules for dissolving and is not normally given to children under 12 years, except on medical advice.

✚▲ Side-effects/warning: See PARACETAMOL.

Resonium A

(Sanofi Winthrop) is a proprietary, non-prescription preparation of sodium polystyrene sulphonate, which is a resin that can be used to treat high blood potassium levels, particularly in patients who suffer from fluid retention or who undergo kidney dialysis. It is available in the form of a powdered resin for use as a rectal enema or by mouth.

+▲ Side-effects/warning: See POLYSTYRENE SULPHONATE RESINS.

resorcinol

is a KERATOLYTIC agent which, when applied topically, causes skin to peel and relieves itching. It is also used in ointments and lotions for the treatment of acne.

+ Side-effects: There may be local irritation.

▲ Warning: It is not to be used if there are local infections; avoid the eyes, mouth and mucous membranes.

✪ Related entry: Eskamel.

Respacal

(UCB Pharma) is a proprietary, prescription-only preparation of the BETA-RECEPTOR STIMULANT tulobuterol hydrochloride. It can be used as a BRONCHODILATOR in reversible obstructive airways disease, as an ANTI-ASTHMATIC in severe acute asthma and for the alleviation of symptoms of chronic bronchitis and emphysema. It is available as tablets and a syrup.

+▲ Side-effects/warning: See TULOBUTEROL HYDROCHLORIDE.

respiratory stimulants ⏃

(analeptics) are central nervous stimulants that show some degree of selectivity for respiratory stimulation. They have little current use but DOXAPRAM HYDROCHLORIDE is sometimes used to relieve severe respiratory failure in patients who suffer from chronic obstructive airways disease, or who undergo respiratory depression following major surgery, particularly in cases where ventilatory support is not possible. A number of such agents were once used as ANTIDOTES in the event of overdose and poisoning by respiratory depressants, but have been discontinued

because effective doses were close to those causing toxic effects, expecially convulsions. Overdose with respiratory depressants, such as BENZODIAZEPINES and OPIOIDS, is now treated with specific receptor ANTAGONISTS.

Restandol

(Organon) is a proprietary, prescription-only preparation of the ANDROGEN (male SEX HORMONE) testosterone (as undecanoate). It can be used to treat deficiency in men and for breast cancer in women, and is available as capsules.

+▲ Side-effects/warning: See TESTOSTERONE.

Retin-A

(Cilag) is a proprietary, prescription-only preparation of the (retinoid) tretinoin. It can be used to treat severe acne, and is available as a cream, a gel and a lotion.

+▲ Side-effects/warning: See TRETINOIN.

retinol

is the chemical term for vitamin A, which is a fat-soluble vitamin found in meats and milk products and is also synthesized in the body from constituents in green vegetables and carrots. Retinol is essential for growth and the maintenance of mucous surfaces. It is particularly useful in supporting the part of the eye's retina that allows vision in the dark and a deficiency may cause night-blindness and dry eyes. It is administered therapeutically to make up vitamin deficiency (which, however, is rare in Western countries). Administration is usually oral or topically as an emulsion, but it can also be by injection. Derivatives of Vitamin A (retinoids) are used by topical application to treat acne.

+ Side-effects: Massive overdose can cause rough skin, dry hair, an enlarged liver and blood erythrocyte sedimentation rate and enzyme level changes.

▲ Warning: In view of evidence suggesting that high levels of vitamin A may cause birth defects, women who are (or may

R

become) pregnant are advised *not* to take vitamin A supplements (including tablets and fish-liver oil drops), except on the advice of a doctor or an antenatal clinic; nor should they eat liver in any form.

Retrovir

(Wellcome) is a proprietary, prescription-only preparation of the ANTIVIRAL drug zidovudine (azidothymidine; AZT). It can be used in the treatment of AIDS, and is available as capsules, a syrup and in a form for intravenous infusion.

✚▲ Side-effects/warning: See ZIDOVUDINE.

Revanil

(Roche) is a proprietary, prescription-only preparation of the ANTIPARKINSONISM drug lysuride maleate, and is available as tablets.

✚▲ Side-effects/warning: See LYSURIDE MALEATE.

Rheumacin LA

(CP) is a proprietary, prescription-only preparation of the (NSAID) NON-NARCOTIC ANALGESIC and ANTIRHEUMATIC indomethacin. It can be administered to relieve various types of pain and inflammation, particularly rheumatic and arthritic pain and to treat other musculoskeletal disorders (including acute gout and inflammation of joints and tendons). It is available as modified-release capsules.

✚▲ Side-effects/warning: See INDOMETHACIN.

Rheumox

(Wyeth) is a proprietary, prescription-only preparation of the (NSAID) NON-NARCOTIC ANALGESIC and ANTIRHEUMATIC azapropazone. It can be administered to relieve pain and inflammation only of severe rheumatoid arthritis, ankylosing spondylitis and acute gout. It is available as capsules and tablets.

✚▲ Side-effects/warning: See AZAPROPAZONE.

Rhinocort

(Astra) is a proprietary, prescription-only

preparation of the CORTICOSTEROID budesonide. It can be used to treat nasal rhinitis, and is available as a nasal aerosol.

✚▲ Side-effects/warning: See BUDESONIDE.

Rhinocort Aqua

(Astra) is a proprietary, prescription-only preparation of the CORTICOSTEROID budenoside. It can be used to treat nasal rhinitis, and is available as a nasal spray.

✚▲ Side-effects/warning: See BUDESONIDE.

Rhinolast

(ASTA Medica) is proprietary, prescription-only preparation of the ANTIHISTAMINE azelastine hydrochloride. It can be used for the symptomatic relief of allergic rhinitis, and is available as a nasal spray.

✚▲ Side-effects/warning: See AZELASTINE HYDROCHLORIDE.

Rhuaka Herbal Syrup

(Waterhouse) is a proprietary, non-prescription COMPOUND PREPARATION of the (*stimulant*) LAXATIVES senna, RHUBARB and cascara liquid. It can be used to relieve constipation, and is available as a syrup. It is not normally given to children under seven years, except on medical advice.

✚▲ Side-effects/warning: See SENNA.

rhubarb

in a powdered form is sometimes used as a *stimulant* LAXATIVE and is a constituent of some proprietary laxative preparations.

✪ Related entries: Pyralvex; Rhuaka Herbal Syrup.

Rhumalgan

(Lagap) is a non-proprietary, prescription-only version of the (NSAID) NON-NARCOTIC ANALGESIC and ANTIRHEUMATIC drug diclofenac sodium. It can be used to treat arthritic and rheumatic pain and other musculoskeletal disorders. It is available as tablets and modified-release tablets (*Rhumalgan SR*).

✚▲ Side-effects/warning: See DICLOFENAC SODIUM.

ribavirin

see TRIBAVIRIN

Ridaura

(Bencard) is a proprietary, prescription-only preparation of the ANTIRHEUMATIC auranofin. It can be used to treat rheumatoid arthritis, and is available as tablets.

✚▲ Side-effects/warning: See AURANOFIN.

Rideril

(DDSA) is a proprietary, prescription-only preparation of the ANTIPSYCHOTIC thioridazine. It can be used to treat and tranquillize psychotic patients, particularly those experiencing manic forms of behavioural disturbance, and in the short-term treatment of anxiety. It is available as tablets.

✚▲ Side-effects/warning: See THIORIDAZINE.

rifabutin

is an ANTIBACTERIAL, ANTITUBERCULAR and ANTIBIOTIC drug, a recently introduced member of the rifamycin family. It can be used for the prevention of *Mycobacterium avium* infection in immunocompromised patients and for the treatment of pulmonary tuberculosis and mycobacterial disease. Administration is oral.

✚▲ Side-effects/warning: See RIFAMPICIN; there may also be blood and liver disorders, nausea, vomiting and hypersensitivity reactions. Urine, saliva and other bodily secretions may turn orange-red.

✪ Related entry: Mycobutin.

Rifadin

(Merrell) is a proprietary, prescription-only preparation of the ANTIBACTERIAL and ANTIBIOTIC rifampicin. It can be used as an ANTITUBERCULAR drug to treat dapsone-resistant leprosy and other serious infections. It is available as capsules, as a syrup and in a form for intravenous infusion.

✚▲ Side-effects/warning: See RIFAMPICIN.

rifampicin

is an ANTIBACTERIAL, ANTITUBERCULAR and ANTIBIOTIC drug. It is one of the principal drugs used in the treatment of tuberculosis, mainly in combination with other antitubercular drugs, such as ISONIAZID or PYRAZINAMIDE, in order to cover resistance and for maximum effect. It acts against Mycobacterium tuberculosis and sensitive Gram-positive bacteria by inhibiting the bacterial RNA polymerase enzyme. It is also effective in the treatment of leprosy, brucellosis, legionnaires' disease and serious staphylococcal infections. Additionally, it may be used to prevent meningococcal meningitis and *Haemophilus influenzae* (type b) infection. Administration can be either oral or by injection or infusion.

✚ Side-effects: There are many side-effects, including the following: gastrointestinal problems, such as nausea, vomiting, diarrhoea and weight loss; many patients also undergo the symptoms of flu, breathlessness, collapse and shock. Rarely, there is kidney failure, liver dysfunction, jaundice, muscle weakness, alteration in the composition of the blood and/or discolouration of the urine, saliva and other body secretions. Sensitivity reactions, such as a rash or urticaria, and menstrual disturbances.

▲ Warning: It should not be administered to patients with jaundice or porphyria; it should be administered with caution to those with impaired liver function, or who are pregnant or breast-feeding. One other effect of the drug is that soft contact lenses may become discoloured. It may reduce the reliability of the contraceptive pill.

✪ Related entries: Rifadin; Rifater; Rifinah; Rimactane; Rimactazid.

Rifater

(Merrell) is a proprietary, prescription-only COMPOUND PREPARATION of the ANTIBACTERIAL drugs rifampicin, isoniazid and pyrazinamide. It can be used in the ANTITUBERCULAR treatment of pulmonary

R

tuberculosis in the initial, intensive phase, and is available as tablets.
✚▲ Side-effects/warning: See ISONIAZID; PYRAZINAMIDE; RIFAMPICIN.

Rifinah

(Merrell) is a proprietary, prescription-only COMPOUND PREPARATION of the ANTIBACTERIAL drugs rifampicin and isoniazid. It can be used in ANTITUBERCULAR treatment, and is available as tablets in two strengths, *Rifinah 150* and *Rifinah 300*.
✚▲ Side-effects/warning: See ISONIAZID; RIFAMPICIN.

Rilutek

(Rhône-Poulenc Rorer) is a recently introduced proprietary, prescription-only preparation of the specialist drug riluzole, which is used in the treatment of patients with amyotrophic lateral sclerosis. It is available as tablets.
✚▲ Side-effects/warning: See RILUZOLE.

riluzole

is a recently introduced specialist drug which is used in the treatment of patients with amyotrophic lateral sclerosis. Administration is oral.
✚ Side-effects: Nausea, vomiting, weakness, tachycardia, sleepiness, headache, dizziness, vertigo, pain, loss of sensation and alterations in liver function
▲ Warning: It should be administered with care where there is a history of abnormal liver function; there is a risk of neutropenia; dizziness or vertigo may affect performance of skilled tasks, such as driving. It is not to be given to patients who are pregnant or breast-feeding, or who have liver or kidney impairment.
○ Related entry: Rilutek.

Rimacid

(Rima) is a proprietary, prescription-only preparation of the (NSAID) NON-NARCOTIC ANALGESIC and ANTIRHEUMATIC indomethacin. It can be used to treat the pain and inflammation of rheumatic disease and

other musculoskeletal disorders, and is available as capsules.
✚▲ Side-effects/warning: See INDOMETHACIN.

Rimacillin

(Rima) is a proprietary, prescription-only preparation of the broad-spectrum ANTIBACTERIAL and (PENICILLIN) ANTIBIOTIC ampicillin. It can be used to treat systemic bacterial infections, infections of the upper respiratory tract, of the ear, nose and throat and the urinogenital tracts. It is available as capsules and an oral suspension.
✚▲ Side-effects/warning: See AMPICILLIN.

Rimactane

(Ciba) is a proprietary, prescription-only preparation of the ANTIBACTERIAL and ANTIBIOTIC rifampicin. It can be used particularly in ANTITUBERCULAR treatment, but it may also be used to treat other serious infections, and is available as capsules, a syrup and in a form for intravenous infusion.
✚▲ Side-effects/warning: See RIFAMPICIN.

Rimactazid

(Ciba) is a proprietary, prescription-only COMPOUND PREPARATION of the ANTIBACTERIAL drugs rifampicin and isoniazid. It can be used in ANTITUBERCULAR treatment, and is available as tablets in two strengths, *Rimactazid 150* and *Rimactazid 300*.
✚▲ Side-effects/warning: See ISONIAZID; RIFAMPICIN.

Rimafen

(Norton; Rima) is a proprietary, prescription-only preparation of the (NSAID) NON-NARCOTIC ANALGESIC, ANTIRHEUMATIC and ANTIPYRETIC ibuprofen. It can be used to relieve pain, particularly the pain of rheumatic disease and other musculoskeletal disorders, period pain and pain following operations and fever. It is available as tablets.
✚▲ Side-effects/warning: See IBUPROFEN.

Rimapam

(Rima) is a proprietary, prescription-only preparation of the BENZODIAZEPINE diazepam. It can be used as an ANXIOLYTIC in the short-term treatment of anxiety, as a HYPNOTIC to relieve insomnia, as an ANTICONVULSANT and ANTI-EPILEPTIC for status epilepticus, as a SEDATIVE in preoperative medication, as a SKELETAL MUSCLE RELAXANT and to assist in the treatment of alcohol withdrawal symptoms. It is available as tablets.

+▲ Side-effects/warning: See DIAZEPAM.

Rimapurinol

(Rima) is a proprietary, prescription-only preparation of the ENZYME INHIBITOR allopurinol, which is a XANTHINE-OXIDASE INHIBITOR. It can be used to treat excess uric acid in the blood and so prevent renal stones and attacks of gout. It is available as tablets.

+▲ Side-effects/warning: See ALLOPURINOL.

Rimifon

(Cambridge) is a proprietary, prescription-only preparation of the ANTIBACTERIAL drug isoniazid. It can be used in ANTITUBERCULAR treatment, usually in combination with other antitubercular drugs, and is available in a form for injection.

+▲ Side-effects/warning: See ISONIAZID.

rimiterol hydrobromide

is a SYMPATHOMIMETIC, a BETA-RECEPTOR STIMULANT with beta$_2$-receptor selectivity. It is mainly used as a BRONCHODILATOR in reversible obstructive airways disease and as an ANTI-ASTHMATIC treatment in severe acute asthma. It can also be used for the alleviation of symptoms of chronic bronchitis and emphysema. Administration is by aerosol. (Patients should be cautioned not to exceed the stated dose and if a previously effective dose fails to relieve symptoms they should consult their doctor.)

+▲ Side-effects/warning: See SALBUTAMOL; but has a shorter duration of action.

✪ Related entry: Pulmadil.

Rimoxallin

(Rima) is a proprietary, prescription-only preparation of the broad-spectrum ANTIBACTERIAL and (PENICILLIN) ANTIBIOTIC amoxycillin. It can be used to treat systemic bacterial infections, infections of the upper respiratory tract, of the ear, nose and throat and the urinogenital tracts. It is available as capsules and an oral suspension.

+▲ Side-effects/warning: See AMOXYCILLIN.

Rinatec

(Boehringer Ingelheim) is a proprietary, prescription-only preparation of the ANTICHOLINERGIC and BRONCHODILATOR ipratropium bromide. It can be used to treat watery rhinitis, and is available as a metered spray.

+▲ Side-effects/warning: See IPRATROPIUM BROMIDE. Avoid spraying near the eyes.

Rinstead Teething Gel

(Schering-Plough) is a proprietary, non-prescription COMPOUND PREPARATION of the LOCAL ANAESTHETIC lignocaine hydrochloride and the ANTISEPTIC agent CETYLPYRIDINIUM CHLORIDE. It can be used for the temporary relief of pain caused by teething, and is available as a gel for topical application. A similar adult preparation, RINSTEAD ADULT GEL, is also available.

+▲ Side-effects/warning: See LIGNOCAINE HYDROCHLORIDE.

Risperdal

(Janssen; Organon) is a proprietary, prescription-only preparation of the recently introduced ANTIPSYCHOTIC drug risperidone. It can be used to tranquillize patients suffering from schizophrenia and other psychotic disorders, and is available as tablets.

+▲ Side-effects/warning: See RISPERIDONE.

risperidone

is a recently introduced ANTIPSYCHOTIC drug which is used to tranquillize patients suffering from schizophrenia and other acute and chronic psychotic disorders.

R

Administration is oral.

✚▲ Side-effects/warning: See
CHLORPROMAZINE HYDROCHLORIDE; but
agitation may occur more frequently and
there may be nausea, abdominal pain,
dyspepsia, anxiety, concentration
difficulties, headache, dizziness, fatigue and
rhinitis.

✪ Related entry: Risperdal.

Ritalin

(Ciba) is a proprietary, prescription-only
preparation of methylphenidate
hydrochloride, and is on the Controlled
Drugs List. Although a weak STIMULANT in
adults, it can be used to treat hyperkinesis
(hyperactivity) or attention-deficit
hyperactivity disorder in children. It is
available as tablets.

✚▲ Side-effects/warning: See
METHYLPHENIDATE HYDROCHLORIDE.

ritodrine hydrochloride

is a SYMPATHOMIMETIC and BETA-RECEPTOR
STIMULANT drug which can be used in
obstetrics to prevent or delay premature
labour by relaxing the uterus.
Administration is either oral or by injection.

✚ Side-effects: Muscle tremor, nausea,
vomiting, sweating, palpitations and
speeding of the heart, hypotension (low
blood pressure), flushing and dilation of
blood vessels in the extremities. Infusion or
high doses can lead to a lowering of blood
potassium levels, increased uterine bleeding,
oedema of the lungs, chest pains, heart
arrhythmias, enlargement of the salivary
glands and changes in blood picture on
prolonged use.

▲ Warning: Administer with caution to
patients with certain heart disorders,
hypertension, disorders of the thyroid gland,
diabetes and where there are low levels of
blood potassium (hypokalaemia). Care
must be taken with drug interactions. It
should not be used in eclampsia and severe
pre-eclampsia, heart disease, uterine
infections, placenta praevia and other
potential complications. Patient's should be

monitored (pulse rate, pulmonary oedema
and blood pressure).

✪ Related entry: Yutopar.

ritonavir

is a (*protease inhibitor*) ANTIVIRAL drug
which is often used together with other
(*reverse transcriptase*) antivirals, and can
be used in the treatment of progressive or
advanced AIDS. Administration is oral.

✚ Side-effects: Nausea, vomiting,
diarrhoea, abdominal pain; taste
disturbance, throat irritation, dyspepsia and
loss of appetite; vasodilatation; headache,
insomnia and sleep disturbance, dizziness,
muscle weakness and loss of sensation in
the extremities; changes in kidney function,
blood changes, and a number of other
reported symptoms.

▲ Warning: It should not be given to
patients who are breast-feeding or where
there is severely impaired liver function.
Administer with caution to those with
certain kidney disturbances, haemophilia or
who are pregnant.

✪ Related entry: Norvir.

Rivotril

(Roche) is a proprietary, prescription-only
preparation of the BENZODIAZEPINE
clonazepam. It can be used as an
ANTICONVULSANT and ANTI-EPILEPTIC to treat all
forms of epilepsy, especially myoclonus,
status epilepticus. It is available as tablets
and in a form for injection.

✚▲ Side-effects/warning: See CLONAZEPAM.

Roaccutane

(Roche) is a proprietary, prescription-only
preparation of isotretinoin. It can be used
to treat severe acne that proves to be
unresponsive to more common treatments,
and is available as capsules.

✚▲ Side-effects/warning: See
ISOTRETINOIN.

Robaxin

(Shire) is a proprietary, prescription-only
preparation of the SKELETAL MUSCLE RELAXANT

methocarbamol. It can be used to relieve acute muscle spasm, and is available as tablets and in a form for injection.

➕▲ Side-effects/warning: See METHOCARBAMOL.

Robaxisal Forte

(Shire) is a proprietary, prescription-only COMPOUND PREPARATION of the SKELETAL MUSCLE RELAXANT methocarbamol and the (NSAID) NON-NARCOTIC ANALGESIC and ANTIRHEUMATIC aspirin. It can be used primarily in the short-term treatment of rheumatic pain and to relieve the symptoms of other musculoskeletal disorders. It is available as tablets.

➕▲ Side-effects/warning: See ASPIRIN; METHOCARBAMOL.

Robinul

(Wyeth) is a proprietary, prescription-only preparation of the ANTICHOLINERGIC drug glycopyrronium bromide. It can be used before operations for drying up saliva and other secretions, and is available in a form for injection.

➕▲ Side-effects/warning: See GLYCOPYRRONIUM BROMIDE.

Robinul-Neostigmine

(Wyeth) is a proprietary, prescription-only COMPOUND PREPARATION of the ANTICHOLINERGIC drug glycopyrronium bromide and the ANTICHOLINESTERASE neostigmine (as methylsulphate). It can be used at the end of operations to reverse the actions of competitive neuromuscular blocking agents. It is available in a form for injection.

➕▲ Side-effects/warning: See GLYCOPYRRONIUM BROMIDE; NEOSTIGMINE.

Robitussin Chesty Cough Medicine

(Whitehall) is a proprietary, non-prescription preparation of the EXPECTORANT agent GUAIPHENESIN. It can be used for the relief of chesty coughs and nasal congestion, and is available as an oral

liquid. It is not to be given to children under six years, except on medical advice.

Robitussin Chesty Cough with Congestion

(Whitehall) is a proprietary, non-prescription preparation of the EXPECTORANT agent GUAIPHENESIN and the SYMPATHOMIMETIC and DECONGESTANT pseudoephedrine hydrochloride. It can be used for the relief of chesty coughs and nasal congestion, and is available as an oral liquid. It is not to be given to children under six years, except on medical advice.

➕▲ Side-effects/warning: See PSEUDOEPHEDRINE HYDROCHLORIDE.

Robitussin Dry Cough

(Whitehall) is a proprietary, non-prescription preparation of the (OPIOID) NARCOTIC ANALGESIC and ANTITUSSIVE dextromethorphan hydrobromide. It can be used for the symptomatic relief of persistent dry, irritant cough, and is available as an oral liquid. It is not to be given to children under six years, except on medical advice.

➕▲ Side-effects/warning: See DEXTROMETHORPHAN HYDROBROMIDE.

Robitussin Junior Persistent Cough Medicine

(Whitehall) is a proprietary, non-prescription preparation of the (OPIOID) NARCOTIC ANALGESIC and ANTITUSSIVE dextromethorphan hydrobromide. It can be used for the symptomatic relief of persistent dry, irritant cough in children, and is available as an oral liquid. It is not to be given to children under one year, except on medical advice.

➕▲ Side-effects/warning: See DEXTROMETHORPHAN HYDROBROMIDE.

RoC Total Sunblock Cream

(RoC) is a proprietary, non-prescription SUNSCREEN which contains constituents that protect the skin from ultraviolet radiation. It contains several agents, including avobenzone and ethylhexyl-

R

methoxycinnamate. A patient whose skin condition requires this sort of protection may be prescribed it at the discretion of his or her doctor.

Rocaltrol

(Roche) is a proprietary, prescription-only preparation of calcitriol, which is a VITAMIN D analogue. It can be used to treat a deficiency of vitamin D, and is available as capsules.

+▲ Side-effects/warning: See CALCITRIOL.

Roccal

(Sanofi Winthrop) is a proprietary, non-prescription preparation of the ANTISEPTIC benzalkonium chloride. It can be used to cleanse wounds and the skin before operations, and is available as a solution.

+▲ Side-effects/warning: See BENZALKONIUM CHLORIDE.

Roccal Concentrate 10X

(Sanofi Winthrop) is a proprietary, non-prescription preparation of the ANTISEPTIC benzalkonium chloride. It can be used to cleanse wounds and the skin before operations, and is available as a solution.

+▲ Side-effects/warning: See BENZALKONIUM CHLORIDE.

Rocephin

(Roche) is a proprietary, prescription-only preparation of the ANTIBACTERIAL and (CEPHALOSPORIN) ANTIBIOTIC drug ceftriaxone. It can be used to treat bacterial infections and to prevent infection arising during and after surgery. It is available in a form for injection.

+▲ Side-effects/warning: See CEFTRIAXONE.

rocuronium bromide

is a *non-depolarizing* SKELETAL MUSCLE RELAXANT which is used to induce muscle paralysis during surgery. Administration is by injection.

+▲ Side-effects/warning: See TUBOCURARINE CHLORIDE; but with less cardiovascular side-effects. Administer with

care to patients with kidney and liver impairment.

○ Related entry: Esmeron.

Roferon-A

(Roche) is a proprietary, prescription-only preparation of interferon (in the form of alpha-2a, rbe). It can be used as an ANTICANCER drug in the treatment of hairy cell leukaemias, myelogenous leukaemia, certain renal cell carcinoma, cutaneous T-cell lymphoma, chronic active hepatitis B and AIDS-related Kaposi's sarcoma. It is available in a form for injection.

+▲ Side-effects/warning: See INTERFERON.

Rogitine

(Ciba) is a proprietary, prescription-only preparation of the ALPHA-ADRENOCEPTOR BLOCKER phentolamine mesylate. It can be used as an ANTIHYPERTENSIVE and in the diagnosis of phaeochromocytoma. It is available in a form for injection.

+▲ Side-effects/warning: See PHENTOLAMINE MESYLATE.

Rohypnol

(Roche) is a proprietary, prescription-only preparation of the BENZODIAZEPINE flunitrazepam. It can be used as a HYPNOTIC for the short-term treatment of insomnia, and is available as tablets.

+▲ Side-effects/warning: See FLUNITRAZEPAM.

Rommix

(Ashbourne) is a proprietary, prescription-only preparation of the ANTIBACTERIAL and (MACROLIDE) ANTIBIOTIC erythromycin. It can be used to treat and prevent many forms of infection, and is available as tablets and a liquid oral mixture.

+▲ Side-effects/warning: See ERYTHROMYCIN.

Ronicol

(Tillomed) is a proprietary, non-prescription preparation of the VASODILATOR nicotinyl alcohol. It can be used to help improve blood circulation to the hands and feet when this is impaired, for example, in peripheral vascular disease (Raynaud's phenomenon). It is available as a suspension and tablets, and as the stronger *Timespan* tablets.

✚▲ Side-effects/warning: See NICOTINYL ALCOHOL.

ropinirole

is a recently introduced ANTIPARKINSONISM drug (a *dopamine receptor agonist*) which is similar to BROMOCRIPTINE in that it is used to improve symptoms and signs of the disease, often in combination with LEVODOPA. Administration is oral.

✚ Side-effects: Nausea and vomiting; sleepiness; oedema of the legs; abdominal pain; sometimes severe hypotension and bradycardia; reports of hallucinations and confusion.

▲ Warning: It should not be administered to patients with severe kidney and liver disease; or to those who are pregnant or breast-feeding. Administer with caution where there is severe cardiovascular disease or major psychiatric disease. It may affect the performance of skilled tasks, such as driving. Avoid an abrupt withdrawal of treatment.

✪ Related entry: Requip.

rose bengal

is a dye which is used for ophthalmic diagnostic procedures in the eye. Administration is by topical application in the form of eye-drops.

✪ Related entry: Minims Rose Bengal.

Rowachol

(Monmouth) is a proprietary, prescription-only preparation of plant oils, including terpenes (borneol, camphene, cineole, mendone, menthol and pipene in olive oil). It can be administered to treat gallstones and bile and liver disorders in cases where surgery is not possible. It is available as capsules.

✚▲ Side-effects/warning: See TERPENES.

Rowatinex

(Monmouth) is a proprietary, prescription-only preparation of plant oils, including terpenes. It can be used to help expulsion of urinary tract calculi (stones), and is available as capsules.

✚▲ Side-effects/warning: See TERPENES.

Rub/Vac

is an abbreviation for RUBELLA VACCINE.

rubefacients ▨

are agents that are also known as COUNTER-IRRITANTS. The name derives from the fact that these agents cause a reddening of the skin by causing the blood vessels of the skin to dilate, which gives a soothing feeling of warmth. The term *counter-irritant* refers to the idea that irritation of the sensory nerve endings alters or offsets pain in the underlying muscle or joints that are served by the same nerves.

Rubella Immunoglobulin

(SNBTS) (Antirubella Immunoglobulin Injection) is a non-proprietary, prescription-only preparation of a SPECIFIC IMMUNOGLOBULIN. It can be used in IMMUNIZATION to give immediate immunity against infection by rubella (German Measles). It is available in a form for intramuscular injection.

✚▲ Side-effects/warning: See IMMUNIZATION.

rubella immunoglobulin, human

is a SPECIFIC IMMUNOGLOBULIN which is used in IMMUNIZATION to give immediate *passive immunity* against infection by rubella (German measles), for example, in pregnancy. It is generally not required since most people have established immunity through vaccination with RUBELLA VACCINE at an early age. Administration is by intramuscular injection.

✚▲ Side-effects/warning: See IMMUNIZATION.

✪ Related entry: Rubella Immunoglobulin.

R

rubella vaccine

(Rub/Vac) is a VACCINE used for
IMMUNIZATION against rubella (German
mealses). It is medically recommended for
pre-pubertal girls between 10 and 14 years,
for medical staff who, as potential carriers,
might put pregnant women at risk from
infection and also for women of child-
bearing age, because German measles
during pregnancy constitutes a serious risk
to the foetus. As a precaution, vaccination
should not take place if the patient is
pregnant or likely to become pregnant
within the following three months. The
vaccine is prepared as a freeze-dried
suspension of live, but attenuated, viruses
grown in cell cultures. Administration is by
injection. The substitution of a universal
vaccination programme in schools for boys
and girls by the combined MR vaccine
(against measles and rubella) and the MMR
programme for infants has meant that the
rubella vaccination treatment alone is likely
to become obsolete.
○ Related entry: Almevax.

Rusyde

(CP) is a proprietary, prescription-only
preparation of the (*loop*) DIURETIC
frusemide. It can be used to treat oedema,
particularly pulmonary (lung) oedema, in
patients with chronic heart failure and low
urine production due to kidney failure
(oliguria). It is available as tablets.
✚▲ Side-effects/warning: See FRUSEMIDE.

rutosides

also known as oxerutins, are derivatives
of rutin, which is a vegetable substance.
They are thought to work by reducing the
fragility and permeability of certain blood
vessels and may therefore be effective in
preventing small haemorrhages and
swellings (though there are some doubts as
to their efficacy). In mixtures, called
OXERUTINS, they are administered to treat
oedema associated with chronic venous
insufficiency.
✚ Side-effects: Flushing, rashes, headache

and gastrointestinal disturbances.
○ Related entry: Paroven.

Rynacrom

(Fisons) is a proprietary, non-prescription
preparation of the ANTI-ALLERGIC drug
sodium cromoglycate. It can be used in the
prevention of allergic rhinitis (inflamed
lining of the nose), and is available as a
nasal spray and nose-drops.
✚▲ Side-effects/warning: See SODIUM
CROMOGLYCATE.

Rynacrom Compound

(Fisons) is a proprietary, non-prescription
COMPOUND PREPARATION of the ANTI-ALLERGIC
drug sodium cromoglycate and the
SYMPATHOMIMETIC and DECONGESTANT
xylometazoline hydrochloride. It can be
used in the prevention of allergic rhinitis,
and is available as a nasal spray and nasal-
drops
✚▲ Side-effects/warning: See SODIUM
CROMOGLYCATE; XYLOMETAZOLINE
HYDROCHLORIDE.

Rythmodan

(Roussel) is a proprietary, prescription-
only preparation of the ANTI-ARRHYTHMIC
disopyramide (as disopyramide
phosphate), and is available as capsules
and in a form for injection.
✚▲ Side-effects/warning: See
DISOPYRAMIDE.

Rythmodan Retard

(Roussel) is a proprietary, prescription-
only preparation of the ANTI-ARRHYTHMIC
disopyramide (as disopyramide
phosphate), and is available as modified-
release tablets.
✚▲ Side-effects/warning: See
DISOPYRAMIDE.

S

Sabril

(Merrell) is a proprietary, prescription-only preparation of the ANTICONVULSANT and ANTI-EPILEPTIC drug vigabatrin. It can be used to assist in the control of seizures that have not responded to other anti-epileptic drugs. It is available as tablets and a powder for oral administration.

✚▲ Side-effects/warning: See VIGABATRIN.

Saizen

(Serono) is a proprietary, prescription-only preparation of somatropin, which is the biosynthetic form of the pituitary HORMONE human growth hormone. It can be used to treat hormonal deficiency and associated symptoms (in particular, short stature), and is available in a form for injection.

✚▲ Side-effects/warning: See SOMATROPIN.

Salactol

(Dermal) is a proprietary, non-prescription preparation of the KERATOLYTIC agent salicylic acid (with lactic acid). It can be used to remove warts and hard skin, and is available as a liquid paint.

✚▲ Side-effects/warning: See SALICYLIC ACID.

Salagen

(Chiron) is a proprietary, prescription-only preparation of the PARASYMPATHOMIMETIC pilocarpine. It can be used to alleviate the symptoms of salivary gland hypofunction in dry mouth following irradiation for head and neck cancer. It is available as tablets.

✚▲ Side-effects/warning: See PILOCARPINE.

Salamol

(Norton) is a proprietary, prescription-only preparation of the BETA-RECEPTOR STIMULANT salbutamol. It can be used as a BRONCHODILATOR in reversible obstructive airways disease, as an ANTI-ASTHMATIC treatment in severe acute asthma and for the alleviation of symptoms of chronic bronchitis and emphysema. It is available as a breath-actuated, metered aerosol inhalant.

✚▲ Side-effects/warning: See SALBUTAMOL.

Salatac

(Dermal) is a proprietary, non-prescription preparation of the KERATOLYTIC agent salicylic acid (with lactic acid). It can be used to remove warts and hard skin, and is available as a gel.

✚▲ Side-effects/warning: See SALICYLIC ACID.

Salazopyrin

(Pharmacia) is a proprietary, prescription-only preparation of the AMINOSALICYLATE sulphasalazine. It can be used to treat active rheumatoid arthritis, ulcerative colitis and Crohn's disease. It is available as tablets, enteric-coated tablets, an oral suspension, suppositories and a retention enema.

✚▲ Side-effects/warning: See SULPHASALAZINE.

Salazopyrin EN-Tabs

(Pharmacia) is a proprietary, prescription-only preparation of the AMINOSALICYLATE sulphasalazine. It can be used to treat active rheumatoid arthritis and ulcerative colitis, and is available as enteric-coated tablets.

✚▲ Side-effects/warning: See SULPHASALAZINE.

Salbulin

(3M) is a proprietary, prescription-only preparation of the BETA-RECEPTOR STIMULANT salbutamol (as salbutamol sulphate). It can be used as a BRONCHODILATOR in reversible obstructive airways disease, as an ANTI-ASTHMATIC treatment in severe acute asthma

S

and for the alleviation of symptoms of chronic bronchitis and emphysema. It is available as a metered aerosol inhalant.

✚▲ Side-effects/warning: See SALBUTAMOL.

salbutamol

is a SYMPATHOMIMETIC and BETA-RECEPTOR STIMULANT with good beta$_2$-receptor selectivity. It is mainly used as a BRONCHODILATOR in reversible obstructive airways disease and as an ANTI-ASTHMATIC treatment in severe acute asthma. It can also be used for the alleviation of symptoms of chronic bronchitis and emphysema, and in obstetrics to prevent or delay premature labour by relaxing the uterus.
Administration can be oral, by inhalation or by injection or infusion.

✚▲ Side-effects/warning: There may be a fine muscle tremor, particularly of the hands; headache and nervous tension, palpitations, dilation of blood vessels in the extremities, a speeding of the heart (normally minimal with aerosol administration) and very occasionally muscle cramps. Infusion or high doses can lead to a lowering of blood potassium levels. Some hypersensitivity reactions have been reported, including (paradoxical) bronchoconstriction, urticaria and angio-oedema. Administer with caution to patients with certain disorders of the thyroid gland and heart, with hypertension, diabetes (in intravenous use) and who are breast-feeding or pregnant (except when used to delay premature labour). Blood potassium levels should be monitored in severe asthma. There may be pain at the site of injection. For its use in labour, see RITODRINE HYDROCHLORIDE.

◎ Related entries: Aerocrom; Aerolin Autohaler; Airomir; Asmaven; Maxivent; Salamol; Salbulin; Steri-Neb Salamol; Ventide; Ventodisks; Ventolin; Volmax.

salcatonin

is a synthetic form of the THYROID HORMONE calcitonin (in the same form that is found in salmon). Its function is to lower the levels of calcium and phosphate in the blood and to regulate these levels with the correspondingly opposite action of a parathyroid hormone parathormone. Therapeutically, it has the same effect and is used to lower blood levels of calcium when they are abnormally high (hypercalcaemia) and to treat Paget's disease of the bone.

✚▲ Side-effects/warning: See CALCITONIN.

◎ Related entries: Calsynar; Miacalcic.

salicylates ⓐ

are a class of drugs that are chemically related to salicylic acid, which is a simple, single-ringed, organic molecule that occurs naturally as a component of salicin (a glycoside found in willow bark) and methyl salicylate (in oil of wintergreen). These natural products have been known for centuries to have antirheumatic actions, which derives from an inherent ANTI-INFLAMMATORY activity. Both the two natural medicines are irritant and poisonous if taken by mouth and the salt SODIUM SALICYLATE is rather irritant if administered orally. However, in 1899, the semi-synthetic drug the ester acetylsalicylic acid, was introduced under the name *Aspirin* as an ANALGESIC, ANTIPYRETIC and ANTIRHEUMATIC drug. Today, aspirin is still widely used as a generic drug and has been joined by a number of other salicylate drugs with similar actions and uses, for example, the aspirin-paracetamol ester BENORYLATE and the recently introduced DIFLUNISAL.

From the use of oil of wintergreen (containing methyl salicylate) as a topically applied treatment for muscle and joint aches and pains, several similar derivatives were developed with similar actions, for example, CHOLINE SALICYLATE, ETHYL SALICYLATE and GLYCOL SALICYLATE. Although it is not clear how these drugs act, it seems probable that they act as COUNTER-IRRITANTS, also known as RUBEFACIENTS.

Further uses of salicylates include the AMINOSALICYLATES (containing a 5-aminosalicylic acid component) which are used to treat active Crohn's disease and to induce and maintain remission of the symptoms of ulcerative colitis, and are also sometimes used to treat rheumatoid arthritis. Drugs in this group include MESALAZINE, OLSALAZINE SODIUM and SULPHASALAZINE, which combines within the one chemical both 5-aminosalicylic acid and the antibacterial SULPHONAMIDE.

In strong solution, salicylic acid is the standard, classic KERATOLYTIC agent, which can be used in the treatment of acne and to clear the skin of thickened, horny patches (hyperkeratoses) and scaly areas that occur in some forms of eczema, ichthyosis and psoriasis.

salicylic acid

is a KERATOLYTIC agent that also has some ANTIFUNGAL activity. It can be used to treat minor skin infections, such as athlete's foot, and psoriasis. It is also incorporated into some topical preparations that are rubbed into the skin as a COUNTER-IRRITANT, or RUBEFACIENT, treatment to relieve pain in soft tissues, including underlying muscle and joints. It is also used to remove warts and calluses. Administration is by topical application in a variety of forms.

✚ Side-effects: There may be excessive drying, sensitivity and local irritation. After prolonged use there may be systemic effects.

▲ Warning: Avoid broken or inflamed skin. Certain preparations of this drug should not be used by diabetics or those with impaired blood circulation.

✪ Related entries: Acnisal; Anthranol; Aserbine; Baltar; Benzoic Acid Ointment, Compound, BP; Capasal; Coal Tar and Salicylic Acid Ointment, BP; Cocois; Cuplex; Diprosalic; Dithrolan; Duofilm; Gelcosal; Ionil T; Monphytol; Movelat Cream; Occlusal; Phytex; Posalfilin; Pragmatar; Psorin; Pyralvex; Radian B Heat Spray; Radian B Muscle Lotion; Salactol; Salatac; Verrugon; Zinc and Salicylic Acid Paste, BP.

Saliva Orthana

(Nycomed) is a proprietary, non-prescription preparation of gastric mucin (porcine). It can be used as a form of ARTIFICIAL SALIVA for application to the membranes of the mouth and throat in conditions that make the mouth abnormally dry. It is available as an aerosol and lozenges.

Salivace

(Penn) is a proprietary, non-prescription COMPOUND PREPARATION of CARMELLOSE SODIUM and various other salts and constituents. It is used as a form of ARTIFICIAL SALIVA for application to the membranes of the mouth and throat in conditions that make the mouth abnormally dry (including after radiotherapy or in sicca syndrome). It is available as an aerosol.

Salivix

(Thames) is a proprietary, non-prescription COMPOUND PREPARATION of acacia, malic acid and various other constituents. It is used as a form of ARTIFICIAL SALIVA for application to the membranes of the mouth and throat in conditions that make the mouth abnormally dry (including after radiotherapy or in sicca syndrome). It is available as pastilles.

salmeterol

is a recently introduced SYMPATHOMIMETIC and BETA-RECEPTOR STIMULANT with β_2-receptor selectivity. It is mainly used as a BRONCHODILATOR in reversible obstructive airways disease and as an ANTI-ASTHMATIC treatment in severe acute asthma. It can also be used for the alleviation of symptoms of chronic bronchitis and emphysema. It is similar to salbutamol but has a much longer duration of action. Therefore it may be used to prevent asthma attacks throughout the night after inhalation before going to bed and also for long-duration prevention of exercise-induced bronchospasm. It is administered by inhalation as an aerosol or powder. It would normally be used in conjunction with long-term ANTI-INFLAMMATORY prophylactic (preventive) therapy (eg with CORTICOSTEROIDS or SODIUM CROMOGLYCATE).

S

Patients should be cautioned that this drug should not be used for the relief of acute attacks and that corticosteroid treatment must be continued. Patients should also be cautioned not to exceed the stated dose and if a previously effective dose fails to relieve symptoms they should consult their doctor.

+▲ Side-effects/warning: See SALBUTAMOL; but the effects are more prolonged. There is a significant incidence of (paradoxical) bronchospasm.

❍ Related entry: Serevent.

Salofalk

(Thames) is a proprietary, prescription-only preparation of the AMINOSALICYLATE mesalazine. It can be used to treat ulcerative colitis, and is available as tablets.

+▲ Side-effects/warning: See MESALAZINE.

Saluric

(Merck Sharp & Dohme) is a proprietary, prescription-only preparation of the (THIAZIDE) DIURETIC chlorothiazide. It can be used, either alone or in conjunction with other drugs, in the treatment of oedema and as an ANTIHYPERTENSIVE. It is available as tablets.

+▲ Side-effects/warning: See CHLOROTHIAZIDE.

Salzone

(Wallace) is a proprietary, non-prescription preparation of the NON-NARCOTIC ANALGESIC and ANTIPYRETIC paracetamol. It can be used to relieve mild to moderate pain and to reduce temperature in fever. It is available as a paediatric oral solution.

+▲ Side-effects/warning: See PARACETAMOL.

Sandimmun

(Sandoz) is a proprietary, prescription-only preparation of the IMMUNOSUPPRESSANT cyclosporin. It can be used to prevent tissue rejection in transplant patients, to treat severe, active rheumatoid arthritis and certain severe, resistant skin conditions (under specialist supervision). It is available as capsules, an oral solution and

in a form for injection.

+▲ Side-effects/warning: See CYCLOSPORIN.

Sando-K

(Sandoz) is a proprietary, non-prescription MINERAL SUPPLEMENT that contains POTASSIUM CHLORIDE (with potassium bicarbonate). It is used to make up deficient blood levels of potassium (hyperkalaemia), and is available as effervescent tablets.

Sandocal

(Sandoz) is a proprietary, non-prescription preparation of calcium carbonate, calcium lactate gluconate, calcium carbonate and citric acid. It can be used as a MINERAL SUPPLEMENT in cases of calcium deficiency. It is available as effervescent tablets in two strengths, *Sandocal-400* and *Sandocal-1000*.

+▲ Side-effects/warning: See CALCIUM CARBONATE.

Sandostatin

(Sandoz) is a proprietary, prescription-only preparation of octreotide. It can be used as an ANTICANCER drug to treat the symptoms following the release of hormones from certain carcinoid tumours. It is available in a form for injection.

+▲ Side-effects/warning: See OCTREOTIDE.

Sanomigran

(Sandoz) is a proprietary, prescription-only preparation of the ANTIMIGRAINE drug pizotifen. It can be used to treat headache, particularly migraine and cluster headache, and is available as tablets and an elixir.

+▲ Side-effects/warning: See PIZOTIFEN.

saquinavir

is a (*protease inhibitor*) ANTIVIRAL drug, which is often used together with other (*reverse transcriptase*) antivirals, and can be used in the treatment of progressive or advanced AIDS. Administration is oral.

+ Side-effects: Nausea, diarrhoea, abdominal pain; mouth ulceration; loss of appetite; headache, rash or skin eruptions;

dizziness, muscle weakness and loss of sensation in the extremities; changes in kidney function, blood changes and a number of other reported symptoms.

▲ Warning: It should not be given to patients who are breast-feeding. Administer with caution to those with certain kidney or liver disturbances, or haemophilia.

✪ Related entry: Invirase.

Saventrine

(Pharmax) is a proprietary, prescription-only preparation of the SYMPATHOMIMETIC isoprenaline (as isoprenaline hydrochloride). It can be used as a CARDIAC STIMULANT to treat a dangerously low heart rate or heart block. It is available as tablets and also in a form for infusion (as *Saventrine IV*).

✚▲ Side-effects/warning: See ISOPRENALINE.

Savlon Antiseptic Cream

(Zyma) is a proprietary, non-prescription preparation of the ANTISEPTICS chlorhexidine (as gluconate) and cetrimide. It can be used to clean lesions, ranging from minor skin disorders or blisters to minor burns and small wounds, and to prevent all types of infection from developing. It is available as a cream.

✚▲ Side-effects/warning: See CETRIMIDE; CHLORHEXIDINE.

Savlon Dry

(Zyma) is a proprietary, non-prescription preparation of the ANTISEPTIC povidone-iodine. It can be used for first aid treatment of cuts, grazes, minor burns and scalds, and is available as a spray.

✚▲ Side-effects/warning: See POVIDONE-IODINE.

scabicidals ⬛

are agents administered to kill the mites that cause scabies, which is an infestation by the itch-mite *Sarcoptes scabiei*. The female mite tunnels into the top surface of the skin in order to lay her eggs, causing severe irritation as she does so. Newly hatched mites, which also cause a considerable amount of irritation with their secretions, then pass easily from person to person on direct contact. Every member of an infected household must be treated and clothing and bedding should be disinfected thoroughly. Treatment is usually with local application of a cream containing LINDANE, MALATHION or PERMETHRIN, which kills the mites. BENZYL BENZOATE may also be used, but can be an irritant itself.

Schering PC4

(Schering) is a proprietary, prescription-only ORAL CONTRACEPTIVE (also known as the 'morning-after' pill) that contains an OESTROGEN and a PROGESTOGEN, in this case ethinyloestradiol and levonorgestrel. It can be used after sexual intercourse has taken place.

✚▲ Side-effects/warning: See ETHINYLOESTRADIOL; LEVONORGESTREL.

Scheriproct

(Schering) is a proprietary, prescription-only COMPOUND PREPARATION of the CORTICOSTEROID prednisolone (as hexanoate) and the LOCAL ANAESTHETIC cinchocaine (as dibucaine hydrochloride). It can be used by topical application to treat haemorrhoids, and is available as an ointment and suppositories.

✚▲ Side-effects/warning: See CINCHOCAINE; PREDNISOLONE.

Scholl Athlete's Foot Cream

(Scholl) is a proprietary, non-prescription preparation of the ANTIFUNGAL drug tolnaftate. It can be used to prevent and treat fungal infections responsible for athlete's foot, and is available as a cream.

✚▲ Side-effects/warning: See TOLNAFTATE.

Scholl Athlete's Foot Powder

(Scholl) is a proprietary, non-prescription preparation of the ANTIFUNGAL drug

S

tolnaftate. It can be used to prevent and treat fungal infections responsible for athlete's foot, and is available as a powder.

+▲ Side-effects/warning: See TOLNAFTATE.

Scholl Athlete's Foot Solution

(Scholl) is a proprietary, non-prescription preparation of the ANTIFUNGAL drug tolnaftate. It can be used to prevent and treat fungal infections responsible for athlete's foot, and is available as a solution.

+▲ Side-effects/warning: See TOLNAFTATE.

Scholl Athlete's Foot Spray Liquid

(Scholl) is a proprietary, non-prescription preparation of the ANTIFUNGAL drug tolnaftate. It can be used to prevent and treat athlete's foot, and is available as an aerosol spray.

+▲ Side-effects/warning: See TOLNAFTATE.

Scoline

(Evans) is a proprietary, prescription-only preparation of the (*depolarizing*) SKELETAL MUSCLE RELAXANT suxamethonium chloride. It can be used to induce muscle paralysis during surgery, and is available in a form for injection.

+▲ Side-effects/warning: See SUXAMETHONIUM CHLORIDE.

Scopoderm TTS

(Ciba) is a proprietary, prescription-only preparation of the ANTICHOLINERGIC drug hyoscine (as base). It can be used as an ANTINAUSEANT in the treatment of motion sickness. It is available as a self-adhesive patch that is placed on a hairless area of skin (usually behind an ear) and the drug is then released and absorbed through the skin.

+▲ Side-effects/warning: See HYOSCINE HYDROBROMIDE.

scopolamine hydrobromide

is another name, which is standard in the USA, for hyoscine hydrobromide.

Sea-Legs

(Seton) is a proprietary, non-prescription preparation of the ANTIHISTAMINE and ANTINAUSEANT drug meclozine hydrochloride. It can be used to treat motion sickness, and is available as tablets. It is not normally given to children under two years, except on medical advice.

+▲ Side-effects/warning: See MECLOZINE HYDROCHLORIDE.

Secaderm

(Fisons) is a proprietary, non-prescription COMPOUND PREPARATION of the ANTISEPTIC agent phenol, TURPENTINE OIL and terebene (with melaleuca oil). It can be used to improve underlying blood circulation and is therefore used to treat such disorders as chilblains or varicose veins. It is available as an ointment (salve) for topical application.

+▲ Side-effects/warning: See PHENOL.

Secadrex

(Rhône-Poulenc Rorer) is a proprietary, prescription-only COMPOUND PREPARATION of the BETA-BLOCKER acebutolol and the (THIAZIDE) DIURETIC hydrochlorothiazide. It can be used as an ANTIHYPERTENSIVE for raised blood pressure, and is available as tablets.

+▲ Side-effects/warning: See ACEBUTOLOL; HYDROCHLOROTHIAZIDE.

Seconal Sodium

(Lilly) is a proprietary, prescription-only preparation of the BARBITURATE quinalbarbitone sodium, and is on the Controlled Drugs List. It can be used as a HYPNOTIC to treat persistent and intractable insomnia, and is available as capsules.

+▲ Side-effects/warning: See QUINALBARBITONE SODIUM.

Sectral

(Rhône-Poulenc Rorer) is a proprietary, prescription-only preparation of the BETA-BLOCKER acebutolol. It can be used as an ANTIHYPERTENSIVE for raised blood pressure, as an ANTI-ANGINA treatment to relieve symptoms and improve exercise tolerance and as an ANTI-ARRHYTHMIC to regularize heartbeat and to treat myocardial infarction. It is available as capsules and tablets.

✚▲ Side-effects/warning: See ACEBUTOLOL.

Securon

(Knoll) is a proprietary, prescription-only preparation of the CALCIUM-CHANNEL BLOCKER verapamil hydrochloride. It can be used as an ANTIHYPERTENSIVE, as an ANTI-ANGINA drug in the prevention of attacks and as an ANTI-ARRHYTHMIC to correct certain heart irregularities. It is available as tablets and in a form for injection.

✚▲ Side-effects/warning: See VERAPAMIL HYDROCHLORIDE.

Securon SR

(Knoll) is a proprietary, prescription-only preparation of the CALCIUM-CHANNEL BLOCKER verapamil hydrochloride. It can be used as an ANTIHYPERTENSIVE and as an ANTI-ANGINA drug in the prevention of attacks. It is available as modified-release tablets.

✚▲ Side-effects/warning: See VERAPAMIL HYDROCHLORIDE.

Securopen

(Bayer) is a proprietary, prescription-only preparation of the ANTIBACTERIAL and (PENICILLIN) ANTIBIOTIC azlocillin. It is mainly used to treat pseudomonal infections of the urinary tract, upper respiratory tract and septicaemia. It is available in a form for infusion or injection.

✚▲ Side-effects/warning: See AZLOCILLIN.

sedatives ▨

are drugs that calm and soothe, relieving anxiety and nervous tension and disposing a patient towards drowsiness. They are used particularly as a premedication prior to surgery. Many sedatives are HYPNOTICS (such as the BARBITURATES), but are administered in doses lower than those used to induce sleep. The terms *minor tranquillizer* or

ANXIOLYTIC are commonly used to describe benzodiazepine sedatives that relieve anxiety without causing excessive sleepiness.

Seldane

(Hoechst Marrion Roussel) is a proprietary, non-prescription preparation of the ANTIHISTAMINE terfenadine. It can be used to treat the symptoms of allergic disorders, such as hay fever, and allergic skin conditions. It is available as tablets and is not normally given to children, except on medical advice.

✚▲ Side-effects/warning: See TERFENADINE. Just prior to publication the Department of Health announced that it would be reviewing whether terfenadine should become available only on prescription rather than OTC without a prescription. If you have any doubts about using this drug, consult your doctor.

Select-A-Jet Dopamine

(IMS) is a proprietary, prescription-only preparation of the SYMPATHOMIMETIC and CARDIAC STIMULANT dopamine (as dopamine hydrochloride). It can be used to treat cardiogenic shock following a heart attack or during heart surgery. It is available as a liquid in vials for dilution and infusion.

✚▲ Side-effects/warning: See DOPAMINE.

selegiline

is an ENZYME INHIBITOR which is administered in ANTIPARKINSONISM treatment because it inhibits the enzyme that breaks down the neurotransmitter DOPAMINE in the brain. It is thought that dopamine deficiency in the brain causes Parkinson's disease. It is frequently given in combination with LEVODOPA (which is converted to dopamine in the brain) to treat the symptoms of parkinsonism. Its enzyme-inhibiting property, in effect, supplements and extends the action of levodopa and (in many but not all patients) it also minimizes some side-effects. Administration is oral.

✚ Side-effects: Hypotension, nausea and vomiting, confusion and agitation.
▲ Warning: In some patients, side-effects are aggravated by the combination of selegiline and levodopa, and the dose of levodopa may have to be adjusted accordingly.
✪ Related entry: Eldepryl.

selenium sulphide

is a substance that is used as an anti-dandruff agent in some shampoos.
✪ Related entries: Lenium; Selsun.

Selsun

(Abbott) is a proprietary, non-prescription shampoo which contains SELENIUM SULPHIDE, and is used as an anti-dandruff agent.

Semi-Daonil

(Hoechst) is a proprietary, prescription-only preparation of the SULPHONYLUREA glibenclamide. It is used in DIABETIC TREATMENT for Type II diabetes (non-insulin-dependent diabetes mellitus; NIDDM; maturity-onset diabetes), and is available as tablets (at half the strength of *Daonil*).
✚▲ Side-effects/warning: See GLIBENCLAMIDE.

Semitard MC

(Novo Nordisk) is a proprietary, non-prescription preparation of highly purified porcine INSULIN ZINC SUSPENSION (AMORPHOUS). It is used in DIABETIC TREATMENT to treat and maintain diabetic patients, and is available in vials for injection and has an intermediate duration of action.
✚▲ Side-effects/warning: See INSULIN.

Semprex

(Wellcome) is a proprietary, prescription-only preparation of the ANTIHISTAMINE acrivastine. It can be used to treat the symptoms of allergic disorders, such as hay fever and urticaria, and is available as capsules.
✚▲ Side-effects/warning: See ACRIVASTINE.

Senlax

(Intercare) is a proprietary, non-prescription preparation of the (*stimulant*) LAXATIVE senna. It can be used to relieve constipation, and is available as a chocolate bar. It is not normally given to children under six years, except on medical advice.
✚▲ Side-effects/warning: See SENNA.

senna

is a traditional, powerful (*stimulant*) LAXATIVE which is still in fairly widespread use. It works by increasing the muscular activity of the intestinal walls and may take from 8 to 12 hours to have any relieving effect on constipation. Senna preparations can also be administered to evacuate the bowels before an abdominal X-ray or prior to endoscopy or surgery.
✚ Side-effects: It may cause griping, abdominal cramp and discoloured urine.
▲ Warning: It should not be administered to patients who suffer from intestinal blockage.
✪ Related entries: Calfig California Syrup of Figs; Manevac; Nylax Tablets; Pripsen Powder; Rhuaka Herbal Syrup; Senlax; Senokot Granules; Senokot Syrup; Senokot Tablets.

Senokot Granules

(Reckitt & Coleman) is a proprietary, non-prescription preparation of the (*stimulant*) LAXATIVE senna. It can be used to relieve constipation, and is available as granules. It is not normally given to children under six years, except on medical advice.
✚▲ Side-effects/warning: See SENNA.

Senokot Syrup

(Reckitt & Coleman) is a proprietary, non-prescription preparation of the (*stimulant*) LAXATIVE senna. It can be used to relieve constipation, and is available as a syrup. It is not normally given to children under six years, except on medical advice.
✚▲ Side-effects/warning: See SENNA.

Senokot Tablets

(Reckitt & Coleman) is a proprietary, non-prescription preparation of the (*stimulant*) LAXATIVE senna. It can be used to relieve constipation, and is available as tablets. It is not normally given to children, except on medical advice.

+▲ Side-effects/warning: See SENNA.

Septrin

(Wellcome) is a proprietary, prescription-only COMPOUND PREPARATION of the (SULPHONAMIDE) ANTIBACTERIAL sulphamethoxazole and the antibacterial trimethoprim, which is a combination called co-trimoxazole. It can be used to treat bacterial infections, especially infections of the urinary tract, prostatitis and bronchitis. It is available as tablets, soluble tablets, a suspension (in adult and paediatric strengths) and in a form for intravenous infusion.

+▲ Side-effects/warning: See CO-TRIMOXAZOLE.

Serc

(Duphar) is a proprietary, prescription-only preparation of betahistine hydrochloride, which has ANTINAUSEANT properties. It can be used to treat nausea associated with vertigo, tinnitus and hearing loss in Ménière's disease, and is available as tablets.

+▲ Side-effects/warning: See BETAHISTINE HYDROCHLORIDE.

Serdolect

(Lundbeck) is a proprietary, prescription-only preparation of the recently introduced ANTIPSYCHOTIC drug sertindole. It can be used to tranquillize patients suffering from schizophrenia, and is available as tablets.

+▲ Side-effects/warning: See SERTINDOLE.

Serenace

(Baker Norton) is a proprietary, prescription-only preparation of the ANTIPSYCHOTIC drug haloperidol. It can be used to treat psychotic disorders, especially schizophrenia and the hyperactive, euphoric condition mania, and to tranquillize patients undergoing behavioural disturbance. It can also be used in the short-term treatment of severe anxiety, for some involuntary motor disturbances and for intractable hiccup. It is available as a liquid, tablets, capsules and in a form for injection.

+▲ Side-effects/warning: See HALOPERIDOL.

Serevent

(Allen & Hanburys) is a proprietary, prescription-only preparation of the BETA-RECEPTOR STIMULANT salmeterol (as xinafoate; hydroxynaphthoate). It can be used as a BRONCHODILATOR in reversible obstructive airways disease and as an ANTI-ASTHMATIC treatment. It is a recently introduced drug with unusual properties, in that it has a very prolonged duration of action. Therefore it is not to be used for the relief of acute attacks, but instead is largely used to give overnight protection (though it should be taken in conjunction with corticosteroids or similar drugs). It is available as an aerosol and as a powder for inhalation using the *Diskhaler* or *Accuhaler* devices. (Patients should be cautioned that this drug should not be used for the relief of acute attacks and that corticosteroid treatment must be continued. Patients should also be cautioned not to exceed the stated dose and if a previously effective dose fails to relieve symptoms they should consult their doctor.)

+▲ Side-effects/warning: See SALMETEROL.

sermorelin

is an analogue of growth hormone releasing-hormone (somatorelin; GHRH). It is used therapeutically in a newly introduced test primarily to assess secretion of growth hormone. Administration is by injection.

+ Side-effects: It may cause flushing of the face and pain at the injection site.

▲ Warning: Administer with care to patients with epilepsy, hypothyroidism or

S

who are being treated with antithyroid drugs. Do not use in pregnancy or breast-feeding. Caution must be taken when prescribing to those who are obese, hyperglycaemic or have increased fatty acids in their blood.

✪ Related entry: Geref 50.

Serophene

(Serono) is a proprietary, prescription-only preparation of the HORMONE ANTAGONIST and ANTI-OESTROGEN clomiphene citrate. It can be used as an infertility treatment, and is available as tablets.

✛▲ Side-effects/warning: See CLOMIPHENE CITRATE.

serotonin

(5-HT; 5-hydroxytryptamine) is a natural mediator in the body with NEUROTRANSMITTER and LOCAL HORMONE roles. As a neurotransmitter in the brain, it mediates chemical messages on its release to excite or inhibit other nerves. It also interacts with a wide range of RECEPTORS (specific types of recognition sites on cells). A number of important drug classes have been developed that work by mimicking, modifying or antagonizing serotonin's actions, including drugs that selectively modify its effect at receptors. Serotonin levels in the brain are thought to be an important determinant of mood and ANTIDEPRESSANTS modify levels of serotonin (and other monoamines, such as NORADRENALINE). The most recently developed class of antidepressant, the SSRI class (eg FLUOXETIEN), is named after the drugs' mechanisms of action – selective serotonin re-uptake inhibitors. The recently introduced ANXIOLYTIC, BUSPIRONE HYDROCHLORIDE is thought to work by stimulating a certain type of serotonin receptor in the brain and can be used for the short-term relief of anxiety. Serotonin is also involved in the process of perception and its function is thought to be disrupted in psychotic illness (eg schizophrenia); part of the evidence for this is that drugs such as

LSD both induce mental states with psychotic features and are able to interact with some types of serontin receptors.

Serotonin and its receptors also have other important roles. For example, a newly developed class of ANTINAUSEANTS and ANTI-EMETICS are $5-HT_3$-receptor antagonists (eg GRANISETRON, ONDANSETRON and TROPISETRON) and are of particular value in treating vomiting caused by radiotherapy and chemotherapy by, in part, blocking the local hormone actions of serotonin in the intestine. SUMATRIPTAN, another recently developed drug, can be injected to treat acute migraine attacks. It works by producing a rapid constriction of blood vessels surrounding the brain through stimulating serotonin ($5-HT_1$) receptors.

Seroxat

(SmithKline Beecham) is a proprietary, prescription-only preparation of the (SSRI) ANTIDEPRESSANT paroxetine, which has less SEDATIVE effects than some other antidepressants. It is available as tablets.

✛▲ Side-effects/warning: See PAROXETINE.

sertindole

is a recently introduced ANTIPSYCHOTIC drug which can be used to tranquillize patients suffering from schizophrenia. Administration is oral.

✛▲ Side-effects/warning: See CHLORPROMAZINE HYDROCHLORIDE; but less sedation and extrapyramidal symptoms; some effects on heart rhythm; postural hypotension; oedema; dizziness and some other side-effects.

✪ Related entry: Serdolect.

sertraline

is an ANTIDEPRESSANT drug of the recently developed SSRI group. It is used to treat depressive illness and unlike some other antidepressant drugs it has relatively less SEDATIVE and ANTICHOLINERGIC side-effects. Administration is oral.

✛▲ Side-effects/warning: See FLUOXETINE.

✪ Related entry: Lustral.

Setlers Tablets Peppermint Flavour

(Stafford Miller) is a proprietary, non-prescription preparation of the ANTACID calcium carbonate. It can be used for the relief of heartburn, indigestion, dyspepsia, nausea and flatulence. It is available as tablets and is not normally given to children under 12 years, except on medical advice.
+▲ Side-effects/warning: See CALCIUM CARBONATE.

sevoflurane

is a recently introduced GENERAL ANAESTHETIC which is a rapid acting volatile liquid anaesthetic. Administration is by inhalation.
+▲ Side-effects/warning: See DESFLURANE. Also, agitation is common in children.
✪ Related entry: Sevoflurane.

Sevoflurane

(Abbott) is a proprietary, prescription-only preparation of the GENERAL ANAESTHETIC sevoflurane. It can be used for the induction and maintenance of anaesthesia, and is available in a form for inhalation.
+▲ Side-effects/warning: See SEVOFLURANE.

Sevredol

(Napp) is a proprietary, prescription-only preparation of the (OPIOID) NARCOTIC ANALGESIC morphine sulphate, and is on the Controlled Drugs List. It can be used primarily to relieve pain following surgery, or the pain experienced during the final stages of terminal malignant disease. It is available as tablets.
+▲ Side-effects/warning: See MORPHINE SULPHATE.

sex hormones 🔋

are endocrine (blood-borne) HORMONES that largely determine the development of the internal and external genitalia and secondary sexual characteristics (growth of hair, breasts and depth of voice). For convenience they are divided into male and female hormones, but both groups are produced to some extent by both sexes.

They are all STEROIDS and chemically very similar. The main *male sex hormones* are called ANDROGENS, of which TESTOSTERONE is the principal member. In men, androgens are produced primarily by the testes; in both men and women, they are also produced by the adrenal glands; and in women, small quantities are secreted by the ovaries. In medicine, there are a number of synthetic androgens that are administered to make up hormonal deficiency and which can also be used in ANTICANCER treatment.

Female sex hormones are called OESTROGENS and PROGESTERONE. They are produced and secreted mainly by the ovary and the placenta during pregnancy; and, though to a lesser extent, in men and women, by the adrenal cortex; and, in men, by the testes.

Natural and synthetic oestrogens are used therapeutically, sometimes in combination with PROGESTOGENS, to treat menstrual, menopausal or other gynaecological problems, as ORAL CONTRACEPTIVES (and as parenteral contraceptives by injection or implantation) and for HRT (hormone replacement therapy). See also ANTI-ANDROGENS; ANTI-OESTROGENS; CONTRACEPTIVES.

silver sulphadiazine

is a compound ANTIBACTERIAL preparation of silver and the SULPHONAMIDE sulphadiazine. It has a broad spectrum of antibacterial activity, as well as the astringent and antiseptic properties of the silver. It is used primarily to inhibit infection of burns and bedsores. Administration is by topical application.
+ Side-effects: These are rare, but there may be sensitivity reactions, for instance, rashes.
▲ Warning: It should not be administered to patients who are allergic to sulphonamides; it should be administered with caution to those with impaired function of the liver or kidneys.
✪ Related entry: Flamazine.

S

simethicone
is a name for activated DIMETHICONE.

simple eye ointment
is a non-proprietary, bland, sterile preparation of liquid paraffin and wool fat in yellow soft paraffin. It is used as an eye treatment both as a night-time eye lubricant (in conditions that cause dry eyes) and to soften the crusts caused by infections of the eyelids (blepharitis).
+▲ Side-effects/warning: See WOOL FAT.

Simplene
(Smith & Nephew) is a proprietary, prescription-only preparation of the SYMPATHOMIMETIC hormone adrenaline. It can be used in the treatment of glaucoma, but not closed-angle glaucoma, and is available as eye-drops.
+▲ Side-effects/warning: See ADRENALINE.

simvastatin
is used as a LIPID-LOWERING DRUG in hyperlipidaemia to reduce the levels, or change the proportions, of various lipids in the bloodstream. It is usually administered only to patients in whom a strict and regular dietary regime, alone, is not having the desired effect. Administration is oral.
+ Side-effects: Constipation or diarrhoea; nausea and headache; flatulence with abdominal discomfort, rash; insomnia; rarely, liver and other complaints.
▲ Warning: It should not be administered to patients who are pregnant or breast-feeding (and avoid pregnancy for at least one month after stopping treatment). Patients should be checked for normal liver function before and during treatment; avoid high alcohol consumption and report any muscle pain.
✪ Related entry: Zocor.

Sinemet
(Du Pont) is a proprietary, prescription-only COMPOUND PREPARATION of levodopa and carbidopa, which is a combination called co-careldopa. It can be used to treat parkinsonism, but not the parkinsonian symptoms induced by drugs (see ANTIPARKINSONISM), and is available as tablets with a carbidopa/levodopa ratio of 10:100 (mg).
+▲ Side-effects/warning: See LEVODOPA.

Sinemet CR
(Du Pont) is a proprietary, prescription-only COMPOUND PREPARATION of levodopa and carbidopa, which is a combination called co-careldopa. It can be used to treat parkinsonism, but not the parkinsonian symptoms induced by drugs (see ANTIPARKINSONISM), and is available as modified-release tablets with a levodopa/carbidopa ratio of 50:200 (mg).
+▲ Side-effects/warning: See LEVODOPA.

Sinemet LS
(Du Pont) is a proprietary, prescription-only COMPOUND PREPARATION of levodopa and carbidopa, which is a combination called co-careldopa. It can be used to treat parkinsonism, but not the parkinsonian symptoms induced by drugs (see ANTIPARKINSONISM), and is available as tablets with a levodopa/carbidopa ratio of 12.5:50 (mg).
+▲ Side-effects/warning: See LEVODOPA.

Sinemet-Plus
(Du Pont) is a proprietary, prescription-only COMPOUND PREPARATION of levodopa and carbidopa, which is a combination called co-careldopa. It can be used to treat parkinsonism, but not the parkinsonian symptoms induced by drugs (see ANTIPARKINSONISM), and is available as tablets with a carbidopa/levodopa ratio of 25:100 (mg).
+▲ Side-effects/warning: See LEVODOPA.

Sinequan
(Pfizer) is a proprietary, prescription-only preparation of the (TRICYCLIC) ANTIDEPRESSANT doxepin. It can be used to treat depressive illness, especially in cases where sedation is required, and is available

as capsules.

+▲ Side-effects/warning: See DOXEPIN.

Sinthrome

(Geigy) is a proprietary, prescription-only preparation of the synthetic ANTICOAGULANT nicoumalone. It can be used to prevent the formation of clots in heart disease, after heart surgery (especially following implantation of prosthetic heart valves) and to prevent venous thrombosis and pulmonary embolism. It is available as tablets.

+▲ Side-effects/warning: See NICOUMALONE.

Sinutab Tablets

(Warner Wellcome) is a proprietary, non-prescription, COMPOUND PREPARATION of the NON-NARCOTIC ANALGESIC paracetamol and the SYMPATHOMIMETIC and DECONGESTANT phenylpropanolamine hydrochloride. It can be used for the symptomatic relief of sinus pain, nasal congestion, hay fever, colds and flu. It is available as tablets and is not normally given to children, except on medical advice.

+▲ Side-effects/warning: See PARACETAMOL; PHENYLPROPANOLAMINE HYDROCHLORIDE.

Siopel

(Zeneca) is a proprietary, non-prescription preparation of the ANTISEPTIC cetrimide and the ANTIFOAMING AGENT dimethicone. It can be used as a BARRIER CREAM to treat and dress itching or infected skin, nappy rash and bedsores, and also to protect and sanitize a stoma (an outlet on the skin surface following the surgical curtailment of the intestines). It is available as a cream.

+▲ Side-effects/warning: See CETRIMIDE; DIMETHICONE.

skeletal muscle relaxants ⊡

act to reduce tone or spasm in the voluntary (skeletal) muscles of the body. They include those drugs – called *neuromuscular blocking drugs* – that are used in surgical operations to paralyse skeletal muscles that are normally under voluntary nerve control (but because the muscles involved in respiration are also paralysed, the patient usually needs to be artificially ventilated). The use of these drugs means that lighter levels of anaesthesia are required. Drugs of this sort work by acting at *nicotinic* RECEPTORS on the muscle that recognize ACETYLCHOLINE, the NEUROTRANSMITTER released from nerves to contract the muscle. There are two sorts of drug that achieve this effect, the *non-depolarizing* skeletal muscle relaxants (eg GALLAMINE TRIETHIODIDE, TUBOCURARINE CHLORIDE and VECURONIUM BROMIDE) and the *depolarizing* skeletal muscle relaxants (eg SUXAMETHONIUM CHLORIDE). The action of the non-depolarizing blocking agents may be reversed at the end of the operation, so that normal respiration may return, by administering an ANTICHOLINESTERASE drug (eg NEOSTIGMINE). DANTROLENE SODIUM acts directly on skeletal muscle and can be used to relieve muscle spasm.

There are some quite different drugs (eg BACLOFEN and DIAZEPAM) that effect muscle tone but do not work in the same way as the skeletal muscle relaxants discussed above, instead they act at some site in the central nervous system to reduce nervous activity and indirectly lower muscle tone. These drugs are used when some defect or disease causes spasm in muscle. All the drugs discussed in this entry are quite distinct from SMOOTH MUSCLE RELAXANTS.

Skelid

(Sanofi Winthrop) is a proprietary, prescription-only preparation of the CALCIUM METABOLISM MODIFIER tiludronic acid (as tiludronate sodium). It can be used to treat Paget's disease of the bone, and is available as tablets.

+▲ Side-effects/warning: See TILUDRONIC ACID.

Skinoren

(Schering) is a proprietary, prescription-

S

only preparation of azelaic acid, which has mild ANTIBACTERIAL and KERATOLYTIC properties. It can be used to treat skin conditions, such as acne, and is available as a cream.

✚▲ Side-effects/warning: See AZELAIC ACID.

Slo-Indo

(Generics) is a proprietary, prescription-only preparation of the (NSAID) NON-NARCOTIC ANALGESIC and ANTIRHEUMATIC indomethacin. It can be used to relieve the pain and inflammation of rheumatic disease, acute gout and other inflammatory musculoskeletal disorders and also period pain. It is available as modified-release capsules.

✚▲ Side-effects/warning: See INDOMETHACIN.

Slo-Phyllin

(Lipha) is a proprietary, non-prescription preparation of the BRONCHODILATOR theophylline. It can be used as an ANTI-ASTHMATIC and chronic bronchitis treatment, and is available as modified-release capsules for prolonged effect.

✚▲ Side-effects/warning: See THEOPHYLLINE.

Sloprolol

(CP) is a proprietary, prescription-only preparation of the BETA-BLOCKER propranolol hydrochloride. It can be used as an ANTIHYPERTENSIVE for raised blood pressure, as an ANTI-ANGINA treatment to relieve symptoms and improve exercise tolerance and as an ANTI-ARRHYTHMIC to regularize heartbeat and to treat myocardial infarction. It can also be used as an ANTITHYROID drug for the short-term treatment of thyrotoxicosis, as an ANTIMIGRAINE treatment to prevent attacks, as an ANXIOLYTIC, particularly for symptomatic relief of tremor and palpitations, and, with an ALPHA-ADRENOCEPTOR BLOCKER, in the acute treatment of phaeochromocytoma. It is available as modified-release capsules.

✚▲ Side-effects/warning: See PROPRANOLOL HYDROCHLORIDE.

Slow-Fe

(Ciba) is a proprietary, non-prescription preparation of ferrous sulphate. It can be used as an IRON supplement in iron deficiency ANAEMIA TREATMENT, and is available as modified-release tablets.

✚▲ Side-effects/warning: See FERROUS SULPHATE.

Slow-Fe Folic

(Ciba) is a proprietary, non-prescription COMPOUND PREPARATION of ferrous fumarate and folic acid. It can be used as an IRON and folic acid supplement during pregnancy, and is available as tablets.

✚▲ Side-effects/warning: See FERROUS SULPHATE; FOLIC ACID.

Slow-K

(Ciba) is a proprietary, non-prescription preparation of POTASSIUM CHLORIDE. It can be used as a potassium supplement to make up a blood deficiency of potassium (hypokalaemia), and is available as modified-release tablets.

Slow-Trasicor

(Ciba) is a proprietary, prescription-only preparation of the BETA-BLOCKER oxprenolol hydrochloride. It can be used as an ANTIHYPERTENSIVE for raised blood pressure, as an ANTI-ANGINA treatment to relieve symptoms and improve exercise tolerance and as an ANTI-ARRHYTHMIC to regularize heartbeat and to treat myocardial infarction. It can also be used as an ANXIOLYTIC, particularly for symptomatic relief of tremor and palpitations. It is available as modified-release tablets.

✚▲ Side-effects/warning: See OXPRENOLOL HYDROCHLORIDE.

Slozem

(Lipha) is a proprietary, prescription-only preparation of the CALCIUM-CHANNEL BLOCKER diltiazem hydrochloride. It can be used as an ANTIHYPERTENSIVE and ANTI-ANGINA treatment, and is available as modified-release capsules.

+▲ Side-effects/warning: See DILTIAZEM HYDROCHLORIDE.

smallpox vaccine

(Var/Vac) consists of a suspension of live (but attenuated) viruses and was used in IMMUNIZATION to prevent infection with smallpox. It is no longer required for public innoculation anywhere in the world because global eradication of smallpox has now been achieved. However, smallpox vaccine also works against other poxes (such as *vaccinia*) and is still used for specialist centres where researchers work with dangerous viruses. Technically, therefore, smallpox vaccine is still available on prescription.

+▲ Side-effects/warning: See VACCINES.

smooth muscle relaxants ⊘

act on smooth (involuntary) muscles (such as the intestines and blood vessels) throughout the body to reduce spasm (ANTISPASMODICS), cause relaxation and to decrease motility. They can work by a variety of mechanisms, though the term is often reserved for those drugs that act directly on smooth muscle, rather than those that work indirectly through blocking or modifying the action of vasoconstrictor HORMONES or NEUROTRANSMITTERS (eg ACE INHIBITORS, ALPHA-ADRENOCEPTOR BLOCKERS and BETA-BLOCKERS). Smooth muscle relaxants may be used for a number of purposes: drugs that dilate blood vessels may be used as ANTIHYPERTENSIVES to lower blood pressure (eg CALCIUM-CHANNEL BLOCKERS and HYDRALAZINE HYDROCHLORIDE for long-term treatment and SODIUM NITROPRUSSIDE for a hypertensive crisis); in ANTI-ANGINA treatment to treat angina pectoris (eg calcium-channel blockers for long-term prevention and GLYCERYL TRINITRATE for acute attacks); to improve circulation in the extremities in the treatment of peripheral vascular disease

(eg INOSITOL NICOTINATE and OXPENTIFYLLINE); in ANTI-ASTHMATIC treatment as BRONCHODILATORS (eg BETA-RECEPTOR STIMULANTS and THEOPHYLLINE); to reduce spasm or colic of the intestine (eg MEBEVERINE HYDROCHLORIDE); and to relax the uterus in premature labour (beta-receptor stimulants). Drugs of the smooth muscle relaxant class are quite distinct from SKELETAL MUSCLE RELAXANTS.

Sno Phenicol

(Smith & Nephew) is a proprietary, prescription-only preparation of the ANTIBACTERIAL and ANTIBIOTIC chloramphenicol. It can be used to treat bacterial infections in the eye, and is available as eye-drops.

+▲ Side-effects/warning: See CHLORAMPHENICOL.

Sno Pilo

(Smith & Nephew) is a proprietary, prescription-only preparation of the PARASYMPATHOMIMETIC pilocarpine. It can be used in GLAUCOMA TREATMENT and to facilitate inspection of the eye. It is available as eye-drops.

+▲ Side-effects/warning: See PILOCARPINE.

Sno Tears

(Smith & Nephew) is a proprietary, non-prescription preparation of POLYVINYL ALCOHOL. It can be used as artificial tears where there is dryness of the eye due to disease, and is available as eye-drops.

sodium acid phosphate

is a mineral salt which is mainly administered in combination either with other phosphorus salts as a phosphorus supplement or a proprietary enema to treat various infections of the urinary tract. It is available in proprietary LAXATIVE preparations as an enema, suppositories and as tablets.

✪ Related entries: Carbalax; Fleet Phospho-soda; Fleet Ready-to-use Enema; Fletchers' Phosphate Enema; Phosphate-Sandoz.

S

Sodium Amytal

(Lilly) is a proprietary, prescription-only preparation of the BARBITURATE amylobarbitone (as the sodium salt), and is on the Controlled Drugs List. It can be used as a HYPNOTIC to treat persistent and intractable insomnia, and is available as capsules and in a form for injection.

+▲ Side-effects/warning: See AMYLOBARBITONE.

sodium aurothiomalate

is a form in which gold can be used as an ANTI-INFLAMMATORY and ANTIRHEUMATIC drug in the treatment of severe conditions of active rheumatoid arthritis and juvenile arthritis. It works extremely slowly and takes several months to have any beneficial effect. Administration is by injection.

+ Side-effects: Severe reactions in a few patients and blood disorders; skin reactions, mouth ulcers; rarely, peripheral nerve disorders, fibrosis, liver toxicity and jaundice, hair loss and colitis.

▲ Warning: It should not be administered to patients with blood disorders or bone marrow disease, severe kidney or liver disease; certain skin disorders, lupus erythematosus, fibrosis; or who are pregnant or breast-feeding. Regular blood counts and monitoring of a wide range of body functions during treatment is necessary.

✪ Related entry: Myocrisin.

sodium bicarbonate

is an ANTACID and is used for the rapid relief of indigestion. It is a constituent of many proprietary preparations that are used to relieve hyperacidity, dyspepsia and for the symptomatic relief of heartburn and a peptic ulcer. It is also sometimes used in infusion media to replace lost electrolytes or to relieve conditions of severe metabolic acidosis – when the acidity of body fluids is badly out of balance with the alkalinity – which may occur in kidney failure or diabetic coma. Administration is oral.

+ Side-effects: Belching, when used as an antacid.

▲ Warning: It should not be taken by patients with impaired kidney function or who are on a low-sodium diet.

✪ Related entries: Actron; Alka-Seltzer Original; Bismag Tablets; Bisodol Antacid Powder; Bisodol Antacid Tablets; Bisodol Extra Tablets; Bisodol Heartburn; Caved-S; Eno; Gastrocote; Gaviscon 250; Gaviscon 500; Gaviscon Liquid; Japps Health Salts; Min-I-Jet Sodium Bicarbonate; Phosphate-Sandoz; Pyrogastrone; Sodium Bicarbonate, BP.

Sodium Bicarbonate, BP

is an a non-proprietary, non-prescription liquid formulation of sodium bicarbonate and can be used as an ANTACID. It is rapidly acting and, as with other antacids containing carbonate, causes belching and alkalosis if taken in excessive doses. It is available as a solution.

+▲ Side-effects/warning: See SODIUM BICARBONATE.

sodium calciumedetate

is a CHELATING AGENT which is used as an ANTIDOTE to poisoning by heavy metals, especially lead. It works by forming a chemical complex that is inactive and is excreted safely from the body. Administration is by injection.

+ Side-effects: Nausea, cramp and kidney damage in overdosage.

▲ Warning: Administer with caution to patients with impaired kidney function.

✪ Related entry: Ledclair.

sodium carboxymethyl cellulose

see CARMELLOSE SODIUM

sodium cellulose phosphate

is used to reduce high calcium levels in the bloodstream (hypercalcaemia) by inhibiting calcium absorption from food. Administration is oral.

+ Side-effects: It may cause diarrhoea and occasionally produces magnesium deficiency.

▲ Warning: Do not use in patients with congestive heart failure or certain other heart conditions, or where dietary sodium is restricted. Administer with care to patients who are breast-feeding, pregnant, who have certain kidney disorders and in growing children.
✪ Related entry: Calcisorb.

sodium chlodronate
is a (a BIPHOSPHONATE) CALCIUM METABOLISM MODIFIER that affects calcium metabolism and is used to treat high calcium levels associated with malignant tumours and bone lesions. Administration can be either oral or by slow intravenous infusion. Dietary counselling of patients is advised, particularly with regard to avoiding food containing calcium during oral treatment.
✚ Side-effects: There may be nausea and diarrhoea and skin reactions. There may be lowered calcium levels (hypocalcaemia).
▲ Warning: It should not be administered to patients with certain kidney disorders or who are pregnant or breast-feeding. Kidney and liver function and white cell count should be monitored; an adequate fluid intake should be maintained.
✪ Related entries: Bonefos; Loron.

sodium chloride
is an essential constituent of the human body for both blood and tissues. It is the major form in which the mineral element sodium appears. Sodium is involved in the balance of body fluids, in the nervous system and is essential for the functioning of the muscles. Sodium chloride, or salt, is contained in many foods, but too much salt can lead to oedema, dehydration and/or hypertension. Therapeutically, sodium chloride is widely used as saline solution (0.9%) or dextrose saline (to treat dehydration and shock), as a medium with which to effect bladder irrigation, as a sodium supplement in patients with low sodium levels, as an eye-wash, nose-drops, a mouthwash and by topical application in solution as a cleansing lotion.

✚ Side-effects: Overdosage can lead to hypertension, dehydration or oedema.
▲ Warning: It should be administered with caution to patients with heart failure, hypertension, fluid retention or impaired kidney function.
✪ Related entries: Balanced Salt Solution; Diocalm Replenisher; Dioralyte; Glandosane; Minims Sodium Chloride.

sodium citrate
is an alkaline compound which is used to treat mild infections of the urinary tract (especially cystitis) in which the urine is acid. It is available in several proprietary compound LAXATIVE preparations. Administration is oral.
✚ Side-effects: There may be dry mouth and mild diuresis.
▲ Warning: It should be administered with caution to patients with impaired kidney function, heart disease or who are pregnant.
✪ Related entries: Balanced Salt Solution; Diocalm Replenisher; Fleet Micro-enema; KLN Suspension; Lemsip; Micolette Micro-enema; Micralax Micro-enema; Relaxit Micro-enema; Vicks Original Cough Syrup (Chesty).

sodium cromoglicate
see SODIUM CROMOGLYCATE

sodium cromoglycate
(sodium cromoglicate) is an ANTI-ALLERGIC drug. It is used to prevent recurrent asthma attacks (but not to treat acute attacks) and allergic symptoms in the eye (eg allergic conjunctivitis), intestine (eg food allergy) and elsewhere. It is not clear how it works, but its ANTI-INFLAMMATORY activity appears to involve a reduction in the release of inflammatory mediators. Administration can be by inhalation, from an applicator that squirts dry powder, eye-drops, eye ointment, nose-drops or a nasal spray.
✚ Side-effects: Depending on the route of administration, there may be coughing or transient bronchospasm. Inhalation of the dry powder preparation may cause irritation

S

of the throat. Local irritation in the nose. Nausea, vomiting or joint pain.

○ Related entries: Aerochrom; Brol-eze Eye Drops; Hay-Crom; Intal; Nalcrom; Opticrom; Opticrom Allergy Eye Drops; Optrex Hayfever Allergy Eye Drops; Resiston One; Rynacrom; Rynacrom Compound; Vividrin.

sodium fusidate

see FUSIDIC ACID

Sodium Fusidate Gauze Dressing, BP

see FUCIDIN INTERTULLE

sodium hyaluronate

is a visco-elastic polymer that is normally present in the aqueous and vitreous humour of the eye. It can be used during surgical procedures on the eye. Administration is by injection.

✚ Side-effects: Occasional hypersensitivity reactions and short-lived rise in intraocular pressure (pressure in the eyeball).

○ Related entries: Healonid; Ophthalin.

sodium hypochlorite

is a powerful oxidizing agent which can be used in solution as an ANTISEPTIC for cleansing abrasions, burns and ulcers. It is not commonly used today because it can be an irritant to some people, but there are a number of non-proprietary solutions available in various concentrations.

✚▲ Side-effects/warning: It can have an irritant effect and can bleach fabrics.

○ Related entry: Chlorasol.

sodium nitrite

is a compound that is used in the emergency treatment of cyanide poisoning and often in combination with sodium thiosulphate. Administration is by injection. See ANTIDOTE.

✚ Side-effects: Flushing and headache.

Sodium Nitroprusside

(David Bull) is a proprietary, prescription-only, preparation of the VASODILATOR sodium nitroprusside. It can be used as an acute ANTIHYPERTENSIVE, as a HEART FAILURE TREATMENT and as a HYPOTENSIVE for controlling blood pressure in surgery. It is available in the form of a powder for reconstitution as a medium for infusion.

✚▲ Side-effects/warning: See SODIUM NITROPUSSIDE.

sodium nitroprusside

is a VASODILATOR drug which can be used acutely as an ANTIHYPERTENSIVE treatment to control severe hypertensive crises, as a HEART FAILURE TREATMENT and as a HYPOTENSIVE for controlled low blood pressure in surgery. Administration is by infusion.

✚ Side-effects: Headache, dizziness, sweating, nausea and retching, and palpitations. There may also be abdominal pain, anxiety and blood disorders.

▲ Warning: It should not be administered to patients with severe impaired liver function or vitamin B_{12} deficiency; it should be administered with caution to those with impaired kidney function, impaired brain blood circulation, hypothyroidism, who are elderly, pregnant or breast-feeding; or have ischaemic heart disease.

sodium perborate

is an ANTISEPTIC which is used in solution as a mouthwash.

▲ Warning: It should not be used continuously or borate poisoning may occur; use with care in those with renal impairment.

○ Related entry: Bocasan.

sodium picosulfate

see SODIUM PICOSULPHATE

sodium picosulphate

(sodium picosulfate) is a (*stimulant*) LAXATIVE which works by stimulating motility of the intestine and can be used to relieve constipation and to prepare patients for X-ray, endoscopy or surgery. Administration is oral.

S

+ Side-effects: Abdominal cramps.
▲ Warning: It should not be administered to patients who suffer from intestinal blockage.
○ Related entries: Laxoberal; Picolax.

sodium salicylate

is a soluble (NSAID) NON-NARCOTIC ANALGESIC and ANTIRHEUMATIC drug. It can be used to treat rheumatic disease and other musculoskeletal disorders. Administration is oral. See also SALICYLATES and SALICYLIC ACID.
+▲ Side-effects/warning: See NSAID.
○ Related entries: Doan's Backache Pills; Jackson's Febrifuge.

sodium stibogluconate

is an ANTIPROTOZOAL drug which can be used to treat various forms of the tropical disease leishmaniasis, or kala-azar, which is caused by parasitic protozoa transmitted in sandfly bites and leaves extensive, unsightly lesions on the skin. Administration is by slow intravenous or intramuscular injection.
+ Side-effects: There may be vomiting, coughing and chest pain or anorexia. The injection may be painful.
▲ Warning: It should not be administered to patients with pneumonia, certain heart, liver or kidney disorders.
○ Related entry: Pentostam.

sodium tetradecyl sulphate

is a drug used in sclerotherapy, which is a technique to treat varicose veins by the injection of an irritant solution. Administration is by injection.
+▲ Side-effects/warning: See ETHANOLAMINE OLEATE.
○ Related entry: STD.

sodium thiosulphate

is a compound that is administered in the emergency treatment of cyanide poisoning and often in combination with sodium nitrite. Administration is by injection. See ANTIDOTE.

sodium valproate

is an ANTICONVULSANT and ANTI-EPILEPTIC drug. It is a valuable drug for treating nearly all forms of epilepsy, particularly tonic-clonic seizures (grand mal) in primary generalized epilepsy. Administration can be either oral or by injection.
+ Side-effects: Nausea and gastric irritation, unsteady gait and muscle tremor, increased appetite and weight gain, temporary hair loss, oedema, blood changes, impaired liver function, effects on blood and liver, menstrual disorders, rashes, growth of breasts in men.
▲ Warning: It should not be administered to patients who have liver disease or a family history of liver dysfunction. Administer with caution to patients who are pregnant or breast-feeding, or who have porphyria or lupus erythematosus.
○ Related entries: Convulex; Epilim; Epilim Chrono; Epilim Intravenous; Orlept.

Sofradex

(Roussel) is a proprietary, prescription-only COMPOUND PREPARATION of the broad-spectrum ANTIBACTERIAL and (AMINOGLYCOSIDE) ANTIBIOTIC drug framycetin sulphate and the ANTI-INFLAMMATORY and CORTICOSTEROID dexamethasone. It can be used to treat inflammation and infection in the eye or outer ear, and is available as drops and an ointment.
+▲ Side-effects/warning: See DEXAMETHASONE; FRAMYCETIN SULPHATE.

Soframycin

(Roussel) is a proprietary, prescription-only preparation of the broad-spectrum, ANTIBACTERIAL and (AMINOGLYCOSIDE) ANTIBIOTIC drug framycetin sulphate. It can be used to treat various infections of the skin, an open wound or of the eye, and is available as eye-drops and an eye ointment.
+▲ Side-effects/warning: See FRAMYCETIN SULPHATE.

S

Solarcaine
(Schering-Plough) is a proprietary, non-prescription COMPOUND PREPARATION of the LOCAL ANAESTHETIC benzocaine and the ANTISEPTIC triclosan. It can be used to treat local pain and skin irritation, and is available as a cream, a lotion and a spray.

+▲ Side-effects/warning: See BENZOCAINE; TRICLOSAN.

Solpadeine Capsules
(Sterling) is a proprietary, non-prescription COMPOUND PREPARATION of the NON-NARCOTIC ANALGESIC paracetamol, the (OPIOID) NARCOTIC ANALGESIC codeine phosphate (a combination known as co-codamol) and the STIMULANT caffeine. It can be used to relieve headache, period pain and rheumatic and musculoskeletal pain. It is available as capsules and is not to be given to children under 12 years, except on medical advice.

+▲ Side-effects/warning: See CAFFEINE; CODEINE PHOSPHATE; PARACETAMOL.

Solpadeine Soluble Tablets
(Sterling) is a proprietary, non-prescription COMPOUND PREPARATION of the NON-NARCOTIC ANALGESIC paracetamol, the (OPIOID) NARCOTIC ANALGESIC codeine phosphate (a combination known as co-codamol) and the STIMULANT caffeine. It can be used to relieve headache, period pain and rheumatic and musculoskeletal pain. It is available as soluble tablets and is not to be given to children under seven years, except on medical advice.

+▲ Side-effects/warning: See CAFFEINE; CODEINE PHOSPHATE; PARACETAMOL.

Solpadeine Tablets
(Sterling) is a proprietary, non-prescription COMPOUND PREPARATION of the NON-NARCOTIC ANALGESIC paracetamol, the (OPIOID) NARCOTIC ANALGESIC codeine phosphate (a combination known as co-codamol) and the STIMULANT caffeine. It can be used to relieve headache, period pain and rheumatic and musculoskeletal pain. It is

available as tablets and is not to be given to children under 12 years, except on medical advice.

+▲ Side-effects/warning: See CAFFEINE; CODEINE PHOSPHATE; PARACETAMOL.

Solpadol
(Sterling-Winthrop) is a proprietary, prescription-only COMPOUND ANALGESIC preparation of the (OPIOID) NARCOTIC ANALGESIC and ANTITUSSIVE codeine phosphate and the NON-NARCOTIC ANALGESIC paracetamol (a combination known as co-codamol). It can be used as a painkiller, and is available as tablets (*Caplets*).

+▲ Side-effects/warning: See CODEINE PHOSPHATE; PARACETAMOL.

Solu-Cortef
(Upjohn) is a proprietary, prescription-only preparation of the CORTICOSTEROID and ANTI-INFLAMMATORY hydrocortisone (as sodium succinate). It can be used to treat inflammation, allergic symptoms and shock, and is available in a form for injection.

+▲ Side-effects/warning: See HYDROCORTISONE.

Solu-Medrone
(Upjohn) is a proprietary, prescription-only preparation of the CORTICOSTEROID and ANTI-INFLAMMATORY methylprednisolone (as acetate). It can be used in the treatment of allergic disorders, shock and cerebral oedema, and is available in a form for injection.

+▲ Side-effects/warning: See METHYLPREDNISOLONE.

soluble insulin
(neutral insulin; insulin injection) is a form of animal (porcine or bovine) or human insulin prepared as a sterile solution and used in DIABETIC TREATMENT to treat and maintain diabetic patients. It is available in vials for injection and has a short duration of action. It is the form of insulin that is used in diabetic emergencies.

+▲ Side-effects/warning: See INSULIN.

⚙ Related entries: Human Actrapid; Human Velosulin; Humulin S; Hypurin Neutral; Pur-In Neutral; Velosulin.

somatotropin

is a name for the pituitary HORMONE human growth hormone (HGH). It was isolated from the pituitary glands of cadavers, which when used to treat short stature (dwarfism) brought with it the risk of acquiring Creutzfeldt-Jakob disease due to contamination. It has now been replaced in the UK by SOMATROPIN, which is a biosynthetic form of human growth hormone and so has no risk of contamination.

somatropin

(biosynthetic human growth hormone) is the name given to the synthetic form of the pituitary HORMONE human growth hormone. The name is used to distinguish it from the natural human product somatotropin (HGH) that it replaced in the UK. Somatotropin was isolated from the pituitary glands of cadavers and consequently brought with it the risk of acquiring Creutzfeldt-Jakob disease due to contamination. Somatropin is used to treat short stature (dwarfism) when the condition is due to growth hormone deficiency (eg in Turner syndrome). It is only used when the bones are still forming and is administered by injection.

+ Side-effects: There may be reactions at injection sites and swelling due to accumulation of lymph in tissues (in Turner syndrome).

▲ Warning: It should not be used by pregnant women and given with caution to those with diabetes, other pituitary hormone deficiencies, or open bone epiphyses.

⚙ Related entries: Genotropin; Humatrope; Norditropin; Saizen; Zomacton.

Sominex

(SmithKline Beecham) is a proprietary, non-prescription preparation of the ANTIHISTAMINE promethazine hydrochloride, which is a PHENOTHIAZINE with marked SEDATIVE properties. It can be used to help induce sleep in the treatment of temporary sleep disturbances, and is available as tablets. It is not normally given to children under 16 years, except on medical advice.

+▲ Side-effects/warning: See PROMETHAZINE HYDROCHLORIDE.

Somnite

(Norgine) is a proprietary, prescription-only preparation of the BENZODIAZEPINE nitrazepam. It can be used as a relatively long-acting HYPNOTIC for the short-term treatment of insomnia, where a degree of sedation during the daytime is acceptable. It is available as an oral suspension.

+▲ Side-effects/warning: See NITRAZEPAM.

Soneryl

(Rhône-Poulenc Rorer) is a proprietary, prescription-only preparation of the BARBITURATE butobarbitone, and is on the Controlled Drugs List. It can be used as a HYPNOTIC to treat persistent and intractable insomnia, and is available as tablets.

+▲ Side-effects/warning: See BUTOBARBITONE.

Sootheye

(Rhône-Poulenc Rorer) is a proprietary, non-prescription preparation of the ASTRINGENT zinc sulphate. It can be used for the symptomatic relief of minor eye irritation, and is available as eye-drops for topical application.

+▲ Side-effects/warning: See ZINC SULPHATE.

Sorbichew

(Stuart) is a proprietary, non-prescription preparation of the VASODILATOR and ANTI-ANGINA drug isosorbide dinitrate. It can be used in HEART FAILURE TREATMENT and to treat and, in particular, prevent angina pectoris. It is available as chewable tablets.

+▲ Side-effects/warning: See ISOSORBIDE DINITRATE.

S

Sorbid SA

(Stuart) is a proprietary, non-prescription preparation of the VASODILATOR and ANTI-ANGINA drug isosorbide dinitrate. It can be used to treat and, in particular, prevent angina pectoris. It is available as modified-release sublingual tablets in two strengths, *Sorbid-20 SA* and *Sorbid-20 SA*.

✚▲ Side-effects/warning: See ISOSORBIDE DINITRATE.

sorbitol

is a sweet-tasting carbohydrate which is used as a sugar-substitute (particularly by diabetics) and as the carbohydrate component in some nutritional supplements that are administered by injection or infusion. It is also used as a constituent of ARTIFICIAL SALIVA.

✪ Related entries: Glandosane; Luborant.

Sorbitrate

(Stuart) is a proprietary, non-prescription preparation of the VASODILATOR and ANTI-ANGINA drug isosorbide dinitrate. It can be used in HEART FAILURE TREATMENT and to treat and, in particular, prevent angina pectoris. It is available as tablets.

✚▲ Side-effects/warning: See ISOSORBIDE DINITRATE.

Sotacor

(Bristol-Myers) is a proprietary, prescription-only preparation of the BETA-BLOCKER sotalol hydrochloride. It is used as an ANTI-ARRHYTHMIC to regularize heartbeat and to treat myocardial infarction, and is available as tablets and in a form for injection.

✚▲ Side-effects/warning: See SOTALOL HYDROCHLORIDE.

sotalol hydrochloride

is a BETA-BLOCKER which can be used as an ANTI-ARRHYTHMIC treatment to regularize heartbeat in life-threatening situations. Administration can be either oral or by injection.

✚▲ Side-effects/warning: See PROPRANOLOL

HYDROCHLORIDE. It may cause abnormal heart rhythms, and care must be taken to avoid low blood potassium when used with diuretics.

✪ Related entries: Beta-Cardone; Sotacor.

Sparine

(Wyeth) is a proprietary, prescription-only preparation of the ANTIPSYCHOTIC drug promazine hydrochloride. It can be used to soothe agitated and restless patients, particularly elderly patients, and is available as tablets, a suspension and in a form for injection

✚▲ Side-effects/warning: See PROMAZINE HYDROCHLORIDE.

spasmolytic

see ANTISPASMODIC

Spasmonal

(Norgine) is a proprietary, non-prescription preparation of the ANTISPASMODIC alverine citrate. It can be used to treat muscle spasm of the gastrointestinal tract, and is available as capsules.

✚▲ Side-effects/warning: See ALVERINE CITRATE.

specific immunoglobulin

is used to give immediate *passive immunity*. Protection is achieved by administering a blood component prepared in much the same way as NORMAL IMMUNOGLOBULIN (HNIG), except that the blood plasma pooled is from donors with high levels of the particular antibody that is required (eg for hepatitis B, rabies, rubella, tetanus or varicella-zoster). Administration is by injection.

✚▲ Side-effects/warning: See IMMUNIZATION.

✪ Related entries: anti-D (Rh$_0$) immunoglobulin; hepatitis B immunoglobulin (HBIG); rabies immunoglobulin; rubella immunoglobulin; tetanus immunoglobulin; varicella-zoster immunoglobulin (VZIG).

spectinomycin

is an ANTIBACTERIAL and ANTIBIOTIC drug, which is administered almost exclusively to treat gonorrhoea caused by Gram-negative organisms resistant to penicillin, or in patients who are allergic to penicillin. It is an AMINOGLYCOSIDE-like antibiotic, because it is related both in structure and by the method of its action to that group of drugs. Administration is by deep intramuscular injection.

✚ Side-effects: There may be nausea and vomiting; high temperature and dizziness; urticaria; fever.

▲ Warning: It is essential that both sexual partners undergo treatment, even if only one of them shows any symptoms. Spectinomycin must be administered with caution to patients who are pregnant or breast-feeding.

✪ Related entry: Trobicin.

Spectraban Lotion

(Stiefel) is a proprietary, non-prescription SUNSCREEN lotion. It contains constituents that protect the skin from ultraviolet radiation, including padimate-O and aminobezoic acid, with UVB protection (SPF25). A patient whose skin condition requires this sort of protection may be prescribed it at the discretion of his or her doctor.

✚▲ Side-effects/warning: See AMINOBENZOIC ACID.

Spectraban Ultra

(Stiefel) is a proprietary, non-prescription SUNSCREEN lotion. It conatins constituents that protect the skin from ultraviolet radiation, including padimate-O, aminobenzoic acid, oxybenzone and butylmethoxydibenzoyl, with both UVB (SPF28) and UVA protection (SPF 6). A patient whose suffers from a skin condition that requires this sort of protection may be prescribed the preparation at the discretion of his or her doctor.

✚▲ Side-effects/warning: See AMINOBENZOIC ACID.

spermicidal contraceptives 🔢

are drugs that kill sperm and are intended to be used as an adjunct to barrier methods of contraception, such as the condom (sheath) or diaphragm (Dutch cap), but should never be regarded as a sole means of contraception. Most spermicidal preparations consist of a spermicide, which is usually chemically an alcohol ester (eg NONOXINOL), within a jelly liquid or cream base. Administration is topical.

✪ Related entries: C-Film; Delfen; Double Check; Duracreme; Duragel; Gynol II; Ortho-Creme; Orthoforms.

Spiro-Co

(Baker Norton) is a proprietary, prescription-only COMPOUND PREPARATION of the (*aldosterone-antagonist* and *potassium-sparing*) DIURETIC spironolactone and the (*potassium-depleting* and THIAZIDE) diuretic hydroflumethiazide (a combination called co-flumactone 25/25). It can be used in congestive HEART FAILURE TREATMENT, and is available as tablets.

✚▲ Side-effects/warning: See HYDROFLUMETHIAZIDE; SPIRONOLACTONE.

Spiro-Co 50

(Baker Norton) is a proprietary, prescription-only COMPOUND PREPARATION of the (*aldosterone-antagonist* and *potassium-sparing*) DIURETIC spironolactone and the (*potassium-depleting* and THIAZIDE) diuretic hydroflumethiazide (a combination called co-flumactone 50/50). It can be used in congestive HEART FAILURE TREATMENT, and is available as tablets.

✚▲ Side-effects/warning: See HYDROFLUMETHIAZIDE; SPIRONOLACTONE.

Spiroctan

(Boehringer Mannheim) is a proprietary, prescription-only preparation of the (*potassium-sparing* and *aldosterone-antagonist*) DIURETIC spironolactone, which

S

is often used in conjunction with other types of diuretics, such as the THIAZIDES. It can be used to treat oedema associated with aldosteronism, in congestive heart failure, kidney disease and fluid retention and ascites caused by cirrhosis of the liver. It is available as tablets and capsules.

✚▲ Side-effects/warning: See SPIRONOLACTONE.

Spiroctan-M

(Boehringer Mannheim) is a proprietary, prescription-only preparation of the (*aldosterone-antagonist*) DIURETIC potassium canrenoate. It can be used to treat oedema associated with aldosteronism, heart disease and liver failure, and is available in a form for injection.

✚▲ Side-effects/warning: See POTASSIUM CANRENOATE.

Spirolone

(Berk) is a proprietary, prescription-only preparation of the (*aldosterone-antagonist* and *potassium-sparing*) DIURETIC spironolactone, which is often used in conjunction with other types of diuretics, such as the THIAZIDES. It can be used to treat oedema associated with aldosteronism, congestive heart failure, kidney disease and fluid retention and ascites caused by cirrhosis of the liver. It is available as tablets.

✚▲ Side-effects/warning: See SPIRONOLACTONE.

spironolactone

is a DIURETIC of the *aldosterone-antagonist* type. It is also *potassium-sparing* and so can be used in conjunction with other types of diuretic, such as the THIAZIDES, which cause loss of potassium, to obtain a more beneficial action. It can be used to treat oedema associated with aldosteronism (abnormal production of aldosterone by the adrenal gland), in congestive HEART FAILURE TREATMENT, kidney disease and fluid retention and ascites caused by cirrhosis of the liver. Administration is oral.

✚ Side-effects: Gastrointestinal disturbances, impotence and gynaecomastia (enlargements of breasts) in men; irregular periods in women; skin rashes, lethargy, raised blood potassium and lowered blood sodium levels; disturbances of liver, blood and bone function.

▲ Warning: It should not be used in patients with severe kidney failure; raised potassium or lowered sodium levels in the blood; who are pregnant or breast-feeding; or have Addison's disease. Administer with caution in certain liver or kidney disorders (blood electrolytes should be monitored).

✪ Related entries: Aldactide 25; Aldactide 50; Aldactone; Laractone; Lasilactone; Spiro-Co; Spiro-Co 50; Spiroctan; Spirolone; Spirospare.

Spirospare

(Ashbourne) is a proprietary, prescription-only preparation of the (*aldosterone-antagonist* and *potassium-sparing*) DIURETIC spironolactone, which is often used in conjunction with other types of diuretic, such as the THIAZIDES, that cause loss of potassium. It can be used in congestive HEART FAILURE TREATMENT, to treat oedema associated with aldosteronism, kidney disease and fluid retention and ascites caused by cirrhosis of the liver. It is available as tablets.

✚▲ Side-effects/warning: See SPIRONOLACTONE.

Sporanox

(Janssen) is a proprietary, prescription-only preparation of the ANTIFUNGAL drug itraconazole. It can be used for candidiasis infections of the vagina, vulva and oropharynx, and ringworm infections of the skin. It is available as a liquid and as capsules.

✚▲ Side-effects/warning: See ITRACONAZOLE.

Sprilon

(Perstorp) is a proprietary, non-prescription COMPOUND PREPARATION of zinc oxide, the ANTIFOAMING AGENT dimethicone, wool fat, wool alcohol and paraffins. It can be used as a BARRIER CREAM to treat leg ulcers, bedsores or applied to areas of the skin that require protection from urine or faeces (as in nappy rash or around a stoma – an outlet on the skin surface following the surgical curtailment of the intestines). It is available as an aerosol.

✚▲ Side-effects/warning: See DIMETHICONE; WOOL FAT.

SSRI ⚠

drugs are ANTIDEPRESSANTS which are used to relieve the symptoms of depressive illness (eg FLUOXETINE and PAROXETINE). Like the MONOAMINE-OXIDASE INHIBITORS (MAOIs) and TRICYCLICS, the SSRI antidepressants are thought to work by modifying the actions of a mood-modifying amine NEUROTRANSMITTERS in the brain. The abbreviation SSRI stands for *Selective Serotonin Re-uptake Inhibitor*, because the mechanism of action is thought to be principally through inhibiting the amine-pump responsible for the re-uptake of the neurotransmitter 5-hydroxytryptamine (5-HT, SEROTONIN) into nerve endings within the brain. This recently developed class of drug seems to be effective in many patients and has the advantage of being less SEDATIVE than the tricyclics and with less ANTICHOLINERGIC side-effects, such as effects on the heart. Treatment normally takes some weeks before any benefit is achieved. Treatment should not begin immediately before or after other types of antidepressant have been taken. Withdrawal of treatment must be gradual. See FLUOXETINE for principal actions and side-effects, though VENLAFAXINE also inhibits re-uptake of both serotonin and NORADRENALINE. See also CITALOPRAM, FLUVOXAMINE MALEATE and SERTRALINE.

Stafoxil

(Yamanouchi) is a proprietary, prescription-only preparation of the ANTIBACTERIAL and (PENICILLIN) ANTIBIOTIC flucloxacillin. It can be used to treat bacterial infections, especially staphylococcal infections resistant to penicillin, and is available as capsules.

✚▲ Side-effects/warning: See FLUCLOXACILLIN.

stanozolol

is an *anabolic* STEROID which can be used to assist the metabolic synthesis of protein in the body and to treat hereditary angio-oedema. Administration is oral.

✚▲ Side-effects/warning: See NANDROLONE; with headache, euphoria, dyspepsia, depression and cramp; there have been reports of hair loss and jaundice.

✪ Related entry: Stromba.

Staril

(Squibb) is a proprietary, prescription-only preparation of the ACE INHIBITOR fosinopril. It can be used as an ANTIHYPERTENSIVE, and is available as tablets.

✚▲ Side-effects/warning: See FOSINOPRIL.

stavudine

(d4T) is a recently introduced (*reverse transcriptase*) ANTIVIRAL drug which can be used in the treatment of AIDS (normally in cases where ZIDOVUDINE is not appropriate). Administration is oral.

✚ Side-effects: There may be peripheral neuropathy; pancreatitis; nausea and vomiting, diarrhoea, constipation and abdominal discomfort; chest pain and shortness of breath, muscle weakness; headache, insomnia, mood changes; muscular pain, flu symptoms; rash and other allergic syptoms; rarely, blood disturbances, neoplasms.

▲ Warning: It should not be administered to patients who are breast-feeding. Administer with caution to those with a history of neuropathy or pancreatitis, kidney impairment or who are pregnant.

✪ Related entry: Zerit.

STD

(STD Pharmaceutical) is a proprietary, prescription-only preparation of sodium

S

tetradecyl sulphate. It is used in scleropathy, which is a technique to treat varicose veins by the injection of an irritant solution, and is available in a form for injection.

✚▲ Side-effects/warning: See SODIUM TETRADECYL SULPHATE.

Stelazine

(SmithKline Beecham) is a proprietary, prescription-only preparation of the (PHENOTHIAZINE derivative) ANTIPSYCHOTIC drug trifluoperazine. It can be used to treat and tranquillize psychotic patients (such as schizophrenics), particularly those experiencing behavioural disturbances. The drug can also be used in the short-term treatment of severe anxiety and as an ANTI-EMETIC and ANTINAUSEANT for nausea and vomiting caused by an underlying disease or by drug therapies. It is available as tablets, a syrup and capsules (*Spansules*).

✚▲ Side-effects/warning: See TRIFLUOPERAZINE.

Stemetil

(Rhône-Poulenc Rorer) is a proprietary, prescription-only preparation of the PHENOTHIAZINE derivative prochlorperazine (as maleate or mesylate), which has a range of applications. In this preparation it is used as an ANTINAUSEANT to relieve the symptoms of nausea caused by cytotoxic drugs in the treatment of cancer and by the vertigo and loss of balance experienced due to infections of the inner and middle ear. It can also be used as an ANTIPSYCHOTIC for schizophrenia and other psychoses and for the short-term treatment of severe anxiety. It is available as tablets, effervescent granules, a syrup, suppositories and in a form for injection.

✚▲ Side-effects/warning: See PROCHLORPERAZINE.

Ster-Zac Bath Concentrate

(Hough) is a proprietary, non-prescription preparation of the ANTISEPTIC triclosan. It can be used for staphylococcal skin infections, and is available as concentrates for adding to a bath.

✚▲ Side-effects/warning: See TRICLOSAN.

sterculia

is a vegetable gum that can absorb large amounts of water and is used as a (*bulking-agent*) LAXATIVE. It works by increasing the overall mass of faeces and so stimulating bowel movement, though the full effect may not be achieved for several hours. It is a useful alternative for patients who cannot tolerate bran in treating a range of bowel conditions, including diverticular disease and irritable bowel syndrome. More controversially, sterculia is also used to treat serious obesity with the intention that small amounts of food ingested may be bulked up internally, so making the patient feel full. Administration is oral.

✚▲ Side-effects/warning: See ISPAGHULA HUSK.

✪ Related entries: Alvercol; Normacol; Normacol Plus; Prefil.

Steri-Neb Ipratropium

(Baker Norton) is a proprietary, prescription-only preparation of the ANTICHOLINERGIC and BRONCHODILATOR ipratropium bromide. It can be used to alleviate the symptoms of chronic bronchitis, and is available as a nebulizer solution unit.

✚▲ Side-effects/warning: See IPRATROPIUM BROMIDE.

Steri-Neb Salamol

(Baker Norton) is a proprietary, prescription-only preparation of the BETA-RECEPTOR STIMULANT salbutamol (as salbutamol sulphate). It can be used as a BRONCHODILATOR in reversible obstructive airways disease, as an ANTI-ASTHMATIC treatment in severe acute asthma and for the alleviation of symptoms caused by chronic bronchitis and emphysema. It is available as a nebulizer solution unit.

✚▲ Side-effects/warning: See SALBUTAMOL.

Steripod Chlorhexidine

(Seton) is a proprietary, non-prescription preparation of the ANTISEPTIC chlorhexidine (as gluconate). It can be used for swabbing and cleaning wounds and burns, and is available as a solution.

+▲ Side-effects/warning: See CHLORHEXIDINE.

steroids ?

are a class of naturally occurring and synthetic agents whose structure is based chemically on a steroid nucleus (a rather complex structure that consists of three six-member rings and one five-member ring). There are a number of important groups of chemicals in the body that are steroids, including all the CORTICOSTEROID hormones of the adrenal cortex (*glucocorticoids* or *mineralocorticoids*), all the SEX HORMONES (ANDROGENS, PROGESTOGENS and anabolic steroids), all VITAMINS of the VITAMIN D group (CALCIFEROL and analogues) and the bile acids (ie CHENODEOXYCHOLIC ACID and analogues). Synthetic chemical analogues of the majority of these have an important part in medicine.

Stesolid

(Dumex) is a proprietary, prescription-only preparation of the BENZODIAZEPINE diazepam. It can be used as an ANXIOLYTIC for the short-term treatment of anxiety, as a HYPNOTIC to relieve insomnia, as an ANTICONVULSANT and ANTI-EPILEPTIC for status epilepticus, as a SEDATIVE in preoperative medication, as a SKELETAL MUSCLE RELAXANT and to assist in the treatment of alcohol withdrawal symptoms. It is available as a rectal solution.

+▲ Side-effects/warning: See DIAZEPAM.

Stiedex

(Stiefel) is a proprietary, prescription-only preparation of the CORTICOSTEROID and ANTI-INFLAMMATORY desoxymethasone. It can be used to treat severe, acute inflammation and chronic skin disorders, including psoriasis, and is available as a lotion.

+▲ Side-effects/warning: See DESOXYMETHASONE.

Stiemycin

(Stiefel) is a proprietary, prescription-only preparation of the ANTIBACTERIAL and (MACROLIDE) ANTIBIOTIC erythromycin. It can be used to treat acne, and is available as a solution for topical application.

+▲ Side-effects/warning: See ERYTHROMYCIN.

stilboestrol

(diethylstilbestrol) is a synthetic SEX HORMONE with OESTROGEN activity. It is useful in HRT (hormone replacement therapy) in women following the menopause. It is sometimes administered in low dosage as an ANTICANCER treatment for cancer of the prostate gland in men and in postmenopausal women for breast cancer and vaginal atrophy. Administration can be either oral or as pessaries.

+ Side-effects: Nausea, thrombosis, fluid retention. In men, breast growth and impotence; in women, bleeding on withdrawal. There may be high blood calcium levels and bone pain when used for breast cancer.

▲ Warning: It should not be administered to patients with certain cardiovascular or liver disorders.

○ Related entries: Apstil; Tampovagan.

Stilnoct

(Lorex) is a proprietary, prescription-only preparation of the recently introduced HYPNOTIC drug zolpidem tartrate. It can be administered for the short-term treatment only of insomnia, and is available as tablets.

+▲ Side-effects/warning: See ZOLPIDEM TARTRATE.

stimulants ?

are drugs that activate body systems or functions. In general, the term is used to describe drugs that stimulate the central nervous system. Therapeutically, they can

S

be administered to treat patients suffering from narcolepsy (which is an extreme tendency to fall asleep when engaged in monotonous activities or when in quiet surroundings). There is a marked tendency for those who use stimulant drugs on a regular basis to become drug dependant and to experience a withdrawal syndrome when they stop taking the drug.

Preparations of DEXAMPHETAMINE SULPHATE, one of the most powerful and best-known stimulants, are on the Controlled Drugs List. CAFFEINE and related compounds are mild stimulants and for medical purposes caffeine is incorporated into several proprietary COMPOUND ANALGESIC preparations that are used as cold remedies.

Streptase

(Hoechst) is a proprietary, prescription-only preparation of the FIBRINOLYTIC drug streptokinase. It can be used to treat thrombosis and embolism, and is available in a form for injection.

✚▲ Side-effects/warning: See STREPTOKINASE.

streptokinase

is an ENZYME which is used therapeutically as a FIBRINOLYTIC drug, because it has the property of breaking up blood clots. It is administered rapidly in such serious conditions as venous thrombi, pulmonary embolism and myocardial infarction. Administration is by injection or infusion.

✚ Side-effects: Nausea, vomiting and bleeding. There may be allergic reaction such as a rash and a high temperature and also back pain.

▲ Warning: It should not be administered to patients with disorders of coagulation; who are liable to bleed (vaginal bleeding, peptic ulceration, recent trauma or surgery); acute pancreatitis or oesophageal varices. Administer with care to those who are pregnant.

✪ Related entries: Kabikinase; Streptase; Varidase Topical.

streptomycin

is an ANTIBACTERIAL and ANTIBIOTIC drug which is an original member of the AMINOGLYCOSIDE family. In the UK today, it is used almost exclusively for the treatment of tuberculosis, in combination with other antibiotics. Treatment takes between 6 and 18 months. Administration is normally by injection.

✚▲ Side-effects/warning: See GENTAMICIN; there may also be hypersensitivity reactions and loss of sensation in the mouth.

Stromba

(Sanofi Winthrop) is a proprietary, prescription-only preparation of the *anabolic* STEROID stanozolol. It can be used to treat angio-oedema and, is available as tablets.

✚▲ Side-effects/warning: See STANOZOLOL.

Stugeron

(Janssen) is a proprietary, non-prescription preparation of the ANTIHISTAMINE cinnarizine. It can be used as an ANTINAUSEANT to treat nausea and vomiting caused by the vertigo and loss of balance that is experienced in vestibular disease. It can also be used as a VASODILATOR to treat peripheral vascular disease (Raynaud's phenomenon). It is available as tablets.

✚▲ Side-effects/warning: See CINNARIZINE.

Sublimaze

(Janssen) is a proprietary, prescription-only preparation of the (OPIOID) NARCOTIC ANALGESIC fentanyl (as hydrochloride), and is on the Controlled Drugs List. It can be used to treat moderate to severe pain, mainly during operations and to enhance the effect of a BARBITURATE general anaesthetic. It is available in a form for injection.

✚▲ Side-effects/warning: See FENTANYL.

sucralfate

is a complex of aluminium hydroxide and sulphated sucrose, which can be used as a long-term treatment of gastric and duodenal ulcers. It has very little ANTACID action, but is thought to work as a CYTOPROTECTANT by forming a barrier over an ulcer, so protecting it from acid and the enzyme pepsin and allowing it to heal. Administration is oral.

✚ Side-effects: Constipation, diarrhoea, nausea, indigestion, gastric discomfort, dry mouth, skin rash and itching, insomnia, dizziness, vertigo and drowsiness.

▲ Warning: It should be administered with caution to patients with kidney disease or who are pregnant or breast-feeding.

◑ Related entry: Antepsin.

Sudafed Elixir

(Warner Wellcome) is a proprietary, non-prescription preparation of the SYMPATHOMIMETIC and DECONGESTANT pseudoephedrine hydrochloride. It can be used for the symptomatic relief of allergic and vasomotor rhinitis and colds and flu. It is available as a liquid and is not normally given to children under two years, except on medical advice.

✚▲ Side-effects/warning: See PSEUDOEPHEDRINE HYDROCHLORIDE.

Sudafed Expectorant

(Warner Wellcome) is a proprietary non-prescription COMPOUND PREPARATION of the SYMPATHOMIMETIC and DECONGESTANT pseudoephedrine hydrochloride and the EXPECTORANT agent GUAIPHENESIN. It can be used for the symptomatic relief of upper respiratory tract disorders accompanied by productive cough. It is available as a liquid and is not normally given to children under two years, except on medical advice.

✚▲ Side-effects/warning: See PSEUDOEPHEDRINE HYDROCHLORIDE.

Sudafed Linctus

(Warner Wellcome) is a proprietary, non-prescription COMPOUND PREPARATION of the SYMPATHOMIMETIC and DECONGESTANT pseudoephedrine hydrochloride and the (OPIOID) ANTITUSSIVE and NARCOTIC ANALGESIC dextromethorphan hydrobromide. It can be used for the symptomatic relief of dry coughs accompanied by congestion of the upper airways. It is available as a liquid and is not normally given to children under two years, except on medical advice.

✚▲ Side-effects/warning: See DEXTROMETHORPHAN HYDROBROMIDE; PSEUDOEPHEDRINE HYDROCHLORIDE.

Sudafed Nasal Spray

(Warner Wellcome) is a proprietary, non-prescription preparation of the SYMPATHOMIMETIC and VASOCONSTRICTOR oxymetazoline hydrochloride. It can be used as a NASAL DECONGESTANT for symptomatic relief of nasal congestion associated with a wide variety of upper respiratory tract disorders. It is available as a nasal spray and is not normally given to children under six years, except on medical advice.

✚▲ Side-effects/warning: See OXYMETAZOLINE HYDROCHLORIDE.

Sudafed Tablets

(Warner Wellcome) is a proprietary, non-prescription preparation of the SYMPATHOMIMETIC and DECONGESTANT pseudoephedrine hydrochloride. It can be used for the symptomatic relief of allergic rhinitis, colds and flu. It is available as tablets and is not normally given to children under 12 years, except on medical advice.

✚▲ Side-effects/warning: See PSEUDOEPHEDRINE HYDROCHLORIDE.

Sudafed-Co Tablets

(Warner Wellcome) is a proprietary, non-prescription COMPOUND PREPARATION of the SYMPATHOMIMETIC and DECONGESTANT pseudoephedrine hydrochloride and the NON-NARCOTIC ANALGESIC paracetamol. It can be used for the symptomatic relief of conditions where upper respiratory congestion is associated with raised body temperature or pain, including colds and flu. It is available as tablets and is not normally given to children under six years, except on medical advice.

S

+▲ Side-effects/warning: See PARACETAMOL; PSEUDOEPHEDRINE HYDROCHLORIDE.

Sudocrem Antiseptic Cream

(Pharmax) is a proprietary, non-prescription COMPOUND PREPARATION of ZINC OXIDE, benzyl alcohol, benzyl benzoate, hypoallergenic lanolin and various other minor constituents. It can be used as an EMOLLIENT and a BARRIER CREAM for nappy rash and incontinence dermatitis.

+▲ Side-effects/warning: See BENZYL BENZOATE; LANOLIN.

sulconazole nitrate

is an (AZOLE) ANTIFUNGAL drug which is administered in order to treat skin infections, particularly those caused by tinea. Administration is by topical application.

+▲ Side-effects/warning: See CLOTRIMAZOLE. Avoid contact with the eyes.
○ Related entry: Exelderm.

Suleo-C

(Napp) is a proprietary, non-prescription preparation of the PEDICULICIDAL drug carbaryl. It can be used to treat infestations of the scalp and pubic hair by lice (pediculosis). It is available as a lotion and a shampoo and is not normally used for children under six months, except on medical advice.

+▲ Side-effects/warning: See CARBARYL.

Suleo-M

(Napp) is a proprietary, non-prescription preparation of the SCABICIDAL and PEDICULICIDAL drug malathion. It can be used to treat infestations of the scalp and pubic hair by lice (pediculosis) and of the skin by itch-mites (scabies). It is available as a lotion and is not normally used for children under six months, except on medical advice.

+▲ Side-effects/warning: See MALATHION.

sulfadiazine

see SULPHADIAZINE

sulfadoxine

is a long-acting (SULPONAMIDE) ANTIBACTERIAL drug, which is used solely in combination with the ANTIMALARIAL drug PYRIMETHAMINE to prevent or treat malaria.

+▲ Side-effects/warning: There may be serious side-effects; administer with caution to patients who are pregnant or breast-feeding.
○ Related entry: Fansidar.

sulfametopyrazine

is a long-acting (SULPHONAMIDE) ANTIBACTERIAL drug which is used primarily in the treatment of chronic bronchitis and infections of the urinary tract. Administration is oral.

+▲ Side-effects/warning: See CO-TRIMOXAZOLE.
○ Related entry: Kelfizine W.

sulfasalazine

see SULPHASALAZINE

sulfinpyrazone

see SULPHINPYRAZONE

sulindac

is a (NSAID) NON-NARCOTIC ANALGESIC and ANTIRHEUMATIC drug. It is used to treat pain and inflammation in rheumatic disease and other musculoskeletal disorders. Administration is oral.

+▲ Side-effects/warning: see NSAID. Administer with care to patients who have had kidney stones. An adequate fluid intake must be maintained.
○ Related entry: Clinoril.

sulpha drugs

see SULPHONAMIDES

sulphabenzamide

is a (SULPHONAMIDE) ANTIBACTERIAL drug which is combined with two similar drugs, sulphacetamide and sulphathiazole, in a proprietary preparation that can be administered to treat various bacterial infections of the vagina and the cervix, and to prevent infection following gynaecological surgery. Administration is by topical application.

✚ Side-effects: There may be sensitivity reactions.

▲ Warning: It should not be administered to patients with severe kidney damage or who are pregnant.

۞ Related entry: Sultrin.

sulphacetamide

is a (SULPHONAMIDE) ANTIBACTERIAL drug which is combined with two similar drugs, sulphabenzamide and sulphathiazole, in a proprietary preparation that can be administered to treat various bacterial infections of the vagina and the cervix, and to prevent infection following gynaecological surgery. Administration is by topical application.

✚ Side-effects: There may be sensitivity reactions.

▲ Warning: It should not be used by patients with severe kidney damage or who are pregnant.

۞ Related entry: Sultrin.

sulphadiazine

(sulfadiazine) is a (SULPHONAMIDE) ANTIBACTERIAL drug which can be administered to treat serious bacterial infections, particularly meningococcal meningitis, and to prevent recurrence of rheumatic fever. Administration is either oral or by injection or infusion. It is available as two non-proprietary, prescription-only preparations, *Sulphadiazine* (CP) as tablets and *Sulphadiazine* (Rhône-Poulenc Rorer) in a form for injection.

✚▲ Side-effects/warning: See CO-TRIMOXAZOLE.

sulphadimethoxine

is a (SULPHONAMIDE) ANTIBACTERIAL drug which can be administered to treat the eye disorder trachoma, which is common in underdeveloped countries. Administration is oral. (It is not available in the UK.)

sulphadimidine

is a (SULPHONAMIDE) ANTIBACTERIAL drug which can be used to treat serious bacterial infections, particularly infections of the urinary tract. Administration is oral. It is available as a non-proprietary, prescription-only preparation, *Sulphadimidine* (CP).

✚▲ Side-effects/warning: See CO-TRIMOXAZOLE.

sulphamethoxazole

is a (SULPHONAMIDE) ANTIBACTERIAL drug which can be used, in combination with another antibacterial drug trimethoprim (a combination called co-trimoxazole), to treat a wide range of serious infections, especially of the urinary tract, the upper respiratory tract and prostate.

✚▲ Side-effects/warning: See CO-TRIMOXAZOLE.

۞ Related entries: Bactrim; Chemotrim; Comixco; Comox; Fectrim; Laratrim; Septrin.

sulphasalazine

(sulfasalazine) is an AMINOSALICYLATE which combines within the one chemical a SULPHONAMIDE constituent (with ANTIBACTERIAL properties) and an aminosalicylate (5-aminosalicylic acid) component. It can be used to treat active Crohn's disease and to induce and maintain remission of the symptoms of ulcerative colitis. It is also sometimes used to treat rheumatoid arthritis. Administration can be either oral or topical as suppositories or a retention enema.

✚ Side-effects: Nausea, vomiting and discomfort in the upper abdomen; rash, headache; rarely, fever, blood disorders and a number of other complaints.

▲ Warning: It should not be administered to patients known to be sensitive to salicylates (aspirin-type drugs) or to sulphonamides; it should be administered with caution to those with liver or kidney disease, G6PD deficieny or who are pregnant or breast-feeding.

۞ Related entries: Salazopyrin; Salazopyrin EN-Tabs.

S

sulphathiazole

is a (SULPHONAMIDE) ANTIBACTERIAL drug which is combined with two similar drugs, sulphacetamide and sulphabenzamide, in a proprietary preparation that can be used to treat bacterial infections of the vagina and the cervix, and to prevent infection following gynaecological surgery. Administration is by topical.

✚ Side-effects: There may be sensitivity reactions.

▲ Warning: It should not be used by patients with severe kidney damage, or who are pregnant.

❍ Related entry: Sultrin.

sulphinpyrazone

(sulfinpyrazone) is a drug that is used to treat and prevent gout and renal hyperurea. It works by promoting the excretion of uric acid in the urine. Administration is oral.

✚ Side-effects: Gastrointestinal disturbances, allergic skin reactions, salt and water retention, rarely blood disorders, ulceration and bleeding in the gastrointestinal tract, kidney failure and changes in liver function.

▲ Warning: See PROBENECID. Regular blood counts are advisable and avoid using in patients with NSAID hypersensitivity or heart disease.

❍ Related entry: Anturan.

sulphonamides ▢

(sulpha or sulfa drugs) are derivatives of a red dye called prontosil, which is metabolized to sulphanilamide, that has the property of preventing the growth of bacteria. They were the first group of drugs suitable for ANTIMICROBIAL use as relatively safe ANTIBACTERIAL agents. Today, they, along with other similar synthetic classes of chemotherapeutic drugs, are commonly referred to as ANTIBIOTICS, although, strictly speaking, they are not *antibiotics* (in the literal sense of agents produced by, or obtained from, micro-organisms that inhibit the growth of, or destroy, other micro-organisms). Their antibacterial action

stems from their chemical similarity to a compound required by bacteria to generate the essential growth factor, folic acid. This similarity inhibits the production of folic acid by bacteria (and therefore growth), while the human host is able to utilize folic acid in the diet. Most sulponamides are administered orally and are rapidly absorbed into the blood. They are short-acting and may have to be taken several times a day. Their quick progress through the body and excretion in the urine makes them particularly suited for the treatment of urinary tract infections. One or two sulphonamides are long-acting (and may be used to treat diseases such as malaria or leprosy) and another one or two are poorly absorbed (consequently, they were, until recently, used to treat intestinal infections). The best-known and most-used sulphonamides include SULPHADIAZINE, SULPHADIMIDINE and SULFAMETOPYRAZINE. Sulphonamides tend to cause side-effects, particularly nausea, vomiting, diarrhoea and headache, some of which (especially sensitivity reactions) may become serious. For instance, bone-marrow damage may result from prolonged treatment. Such serious hypersensitivity reactions are more of a risk with the longer-acting sulphonamides, which can accumulate in the body. As a general rule, patients being treated with sulphonamides should try to avoid sunlight. The sulphonamides are largely being replaced by newer antibacterials with greater activity, fewer problems with bacterial resistance and less risk of side-effects. See CO-TRIMOXAZOLE; SILVER SULPHADIAZINE; SULFADOXINE; SULPHADIMETHOXINE; SULPHAMETHOXAZOLE; SULPHONE.

sulphones ▢

are drugs closely related to the SULPHONAMIDES. They have similar therapeutic action and are therefore used for similar purposes. They are particularly successful in preventing the growth of the bacteria responsible for leprosy, malaria and tuberculosis. The only member of this group that is still commonly used is the valuable drug DAPSONE.

sulphonylureas ⁊

are drugs that were derived from a SULPHONAMIDE and have the effect of reducing blood levels of glucose, so they can be used orally in DIABETIC TREATMENT. They work by promoting the secretion of INSULIN from the pancreas and are thus useful in treating the form of hyperglycaemia that occurs in Type II diabetes (non-insulin-dependent diabetes mellitus; NIDDM; maturity-onset diabetes) where there is still some insulin production. They should be used in conjunction with a modified diet. See CHLORPROPAMIDE; GLIBENCLAMIDE; GLICLAZIDE; GLIPIZIDE; GLIQUIDONE; TOLAZAMIDE; TOLBUTAMIDE.

sulphur

is a non-metallic element which was thought to be active against external parasites and fungal infections of the skin, but this would now appear to have little scientific basis. Consequently, sulphur now has a less common use in creams, ointments and lotions for treating skin disorders, such as acne, dermatitis and psoriasis.
✪ Related entries: Cocois; Eskamel; Pragmatar.

sulpiride

is an ANTIPSYCHOTIC drug which is used to treat the symptoms of schizophrenia (to increase an apathetic and withdrawn patient's awareness) and, quite separately from its antipsychotic uses, disorders that may cause tremor, tics, involuntary movements or involuntary utterances (such as Gilles de la Tourette syndrome). Administration is oral.
✚▲ Side-effects/warning: See CHLORPROMAZINE HYDROCHLORIDE; but is less sedating and does not cause jaundice or skin reactions. Administer with care to

patients with porphyria and avoid its use in those who are breast-feeding.
✪ Related entries: Dolmatil; Sulpitil.

Sulpitil

(Pharmacia) is a proprietary, prescription-only preparation of the ANTIPSYCHOTIC drug sulpiride. It can be used, at a low dose, to treat the symptoms of schizophrenia (to increase an apathetic and withdrawn patient's awareness) and at a higher dose, and quite separately from its antipsychotic uses, to treat other conditions that may cause tremor, tics, involuntary movements or involuntary utterances (such as Gilles de la Tourette syndrome). It is available as tablets.
✚▲ Side-effects/warning: See SULPIRIDE.

Sultrin

(Cilag) is a proprietary, prescription-only COMPOUND PREPARATION of the (SULPHONAMIDE) ANTIBACTERIAL drugs sulphacetamide, sulphabenzamide and sulphathiazole. It can be used to treat bacterial infections of the vagina and cervix, and to prevent infection following gynaecological surgery. It is available as a cream.
✚▲ Side-effects/warning: See SULPHACETAMIDE; SULPHABENZAMIDE; SULPHATHIAZOLE.

sumatriptan

is a recently introduced ANTIMIGRAINE drug which is used to treat acute migraine attacks (but not to prevent attacks) and cluster headache. It works by producing a rapid constriction of blood vessels surrounding the brain (by stimulating SEROTONIN receptors). Administration can be either oral or by self-injection.
✚ Side-effects: Chest pain and tightness in the chest (sometimes intense, angina-like pain), sensation of tingling, heaviness, pressure, heat, flushing, dizziness, a feeling of weakness, loss of sensation in the extremities, drowsiness and fatigue, changes in liver function, reports of nausea and

S

vomiting, also transient pain at the injection site.

▲ Warning: It should not be given to the elderly or children, or to patients with ischaemic heart disease or a history of heart attack, coronary vasospasm, certain types of angina or uncontrolled hypertension. Administer with care to patients with conditions predisposing to coronary heart disease, liver or kidney impairment, or who are pregnant or breast-feeding. Drowsiness may impair the performance of skilled tasks, such as driving.

✚ Related entry: Imigran.

Sun E45

(Crookes) is the name of a range of proprietary, non-prescription SUNSCREEN lotions. They contain TITANIUM DIOXIDE, aminobenzoic acid, padimate-O, oxybenzone and butylmethoxydibenzoyl, which provide protection from ultraviolet radiation (factors 15-25; but with both UVA and UVB protection). *Sun E45* is available as *Sunblock Cream (SPF25)* and *Ultra Protection Lotion (SPF15)* and both are water resistant. A patient whose skin condition requires this sort of preparation may be prescribed it at the discretion of his or her doctor.

✚▲ Side-effects/warning: See AMINOBENZOIC ACID.

sunscreens ⚑

are creams and lotions that contain chemical agents which partly block the passage of ultraviolet radiation from the sun and in certain radiation therapies to the skin. Ultraviolet radiation harms the skin and exacerbates many skin conditions. It can be divided into two wavelength bands: UVB causes sunburn and contributes to skin cancer and ageing; UVA causes problems by sensitizing the skin to certain drugs and, in the long term, may contribute to skin cancers. A number of substances offer protection against UVB, but are less effective against UVA. Some preparations also contain substances, such as TITANIUM

DIOXIDE, which are reflective and provide some protection against UVA. The sun-protection factor, or SPF, of a preparation indicates the degree of protection against burning by UVB. For example, an SPF of 4 allows a person to stay in the sun four-times longer than an unprotected person without burning. A star-rating system is used by some sunscreens to indicate the degree of protection against UVA relative to UVB. For example, a rating of 4 stars means equal protection against UVA and UVB; lower ratings mean greater protection against UVB than UVA. Sunscreens with an SPF greater than 15 may be prescribed for patients whose skin condition require this sort of preparation (eg those abnormally sensitive to UV radiation due to genetic disorders, or to radiotherapy, or those with recurrent or chronic herpes simplex labialis).

✚ Related entries: Coppertone Ultrashade 23; Piz Buin SPF 20 Sun Block Lotion; RoC Total Sunblock Cream; Spectraban Lotion; Spectraban Ultra; Sun E45; Uvistat.

Suprane

(Pharmacia) is a proprietary, prescription-only preparation of the inhalant GENERAL ANAESTHETIC desflurane. It can be used for the induction and maintenance of anaesthesia, and is available in a form for inhalation.

✚▲ Side-effects/warning: See DESFLURANE.

Suprax

(Lederle) is a proprietary, prescription-only preparation of the ANTIBACTERIAL and (CEPHALOSPORIN) ANTIBIOTIC cefixime. It can be used to treat acute bacterial infections by Gram-positive and Gram-negative organisms, particularly infections of the urinary tract. It is available as capsules, tablets and a paediatric oral suspension.

✚▲ Side-effects/warning: See CEFIXIME.

Suprecur

(Hoechst) is a proprietary, prescription-only preparation of the HORMONE buserelin, which is a form of gonadotrophin-releasing hormone. It can be used in women to treat endometriosis and in men as an ANTICANCER treatment for cancer of the prostate gland. It is available as a nasal spray (it is absorbed into the systemic circulation from the nasal mucosa).

+▲ Side-effects/warning: See BUSERELIN.

Suprefact

(Hoechst) is a proprietary, prescription-only preparation of the HORMONE buserelin, which is a form of gonadotrophin-releasing hormone. It can be used in men as an ANTICANCER treatment for cancer of the prostate gland and in women for endometriosis. It is available as a nasal spray (it is adsorbed into the systemic circulation through the nasal mucosa) and in a form for injection.

+▲ Side-effects/warning: See BUSERELIN.

Surgam

(Roussel) is a proprietary, prescription-only preparation of the (NSAID) NON-NARCOTIC ANALGESIC and ANTIRHEUMATIC tiaprofenic acid. It can be used to treat the pain of rheumatic disease and other musculoskeletal disorders. It is available as tablets and modified-release capsules (*Surgam SA*).

+▲ Side-effects/warning: See TIAPROFENIC ACID.

Surmontil

(Rhône-Poulenc Rorer) is a proprietary, prescription-only preparation of the (TRICYCLIC) ANTIDEPRESSANT trimipramine. It can be used to treat depressive illness, especially in cases where there is a need for sedation. It is available as tablets and as capsules (in the form of trimipramine maleate).

+▲ Side-effects/warning: See TRIMIPRAMINE.

Suscard

(Pharmax) is a proprietary, non-prescription preparation of the VASODILATOR and ANTI-ANGINA drug glyceryl trinitrate. It

can be used in HEART FAILURE TREATMENT and to treat and prevent angina pectoris. It is available as modified-release buccal tablets (which dissolve between the upper lip and gums).

+▲ Side-effects/warning: See GLYCERYL TRINITRATE.

Sustac

(Pharmax) is a proprietary, non-prescription preparation of the VASODILATOR and ANTI-ANGINA drug glyceryl trinitrate. It can be used to treat and prevent angina pectoris, and is available as modified-release tablets.

+▲ Side-effects/warning: See GLYCERYL TRINITRATE.

Sustamycin

(Boehringer Mannheim) is a proprietary, prescription-only preparation of the ANTIBACTERIAL and (TETRACYCLINE) ANTIBIOTIC tetracycline. It can be used to treat infections of many kinds, and is available as modified-release capsules.

+▲ Side-effects/warning: See TETRACYCLINE.

Sustenon 100

(Organon) is a proprietary, prescription-only preparation of the ANDROGEN (male SEX HORMONE) testosterone (as propionate, isocaproate and phenylpropionate). It can be used to treat testosterone deficiency in men, and is available in a form for depot (long-lasting) injection.

+▲ Side-effects/warning: See TESTOSTERONE.

Sustenon 250

(Organon) is a proprietary, prescription-only preparation of the ANDROGEN (male SEX HORMONE) testosterone (as propionate and phenylpropionate). It can be used to treat testosterone deficiency in men, and is available in a form for depot (long-lasting) injection.

+▲ Side-effects/warning: See TESTOSTERONE.

S

suxamethonium chloride

(succinylcholine chloride) is a
(*depolarizing*) SKELETAL MUSCLE RELAXANT
which is used to induce muscle paralysis
during surgery. Administration is by
injection.

✚ Side-effects: There may be muscle pain
afterwards and repeated doses may cause
prolonged muscle paralysis.

▲ Warning: It should not be administered
to patients with severe liver disease or severe
burns. Prolonged paralysis occurs
infrequently where there is abnormal
plasma cholinesterases and under certain
other circumstances.

✪ Related entries: Anectine; Scoline.

Symmetrel

(Geigy) is a proprietary, prescription-only
preparation of the ANTIPARKINSONISM drug
amantadine hydrochloride, which also has
some ANTIVIRAL activity. It is used to treat
parkinsonism, but not the parkinsonian
symptoms induced by drugs. It can also be
used to prevent certain types of influenza
and to treat herpes zoster (shingles). It is
available as capsules and as a syrup.

✚▲ Side-effects/warning: See AMANTADINE
HYDROCHLORIDE.

sympathomimetics ▣

are drugs that have effects that mimic those
of the sympathetic nervous system. There
are two main types (though several
sympathomimetics belong to both types):
the alpha-adrenoceptor stimulants (eg
PHENYLEPHRINE HYDROCHLORIDE and
OXYMETAZOLINE HYDROCHLORIDE) are
VASOCONSTRICTORS and are used particularly
in NASAL DECONGESTANTS and preparations for
relieving cold symtpoms; the other type is
the BETA-RECEPTOR STIMULANTS (eg
SALBUTAMOL, ORCIPRENALINE SULPHATE,
TERBUTALINE SULPHATE) which are widely
used as BRONCHODILATORS, particularly in
ANTI-ASTHMATIC treatment and also as
CARDIAC STIMULANTS (eg ISOPRENALINE). A
distinction may be made between the *direct
sympathomimetics* such as those examples

given above, which achieve selectivity of
action within the body by only acting at one
receptor type (recognition site for
HORMONES or NEUROTRANSMITTERS), as
compared to the *indirect
sympathomimetics* (eg EPHEDRINE
HYDROCHLORIDE and PSEUDOEPHEDRINE
HYDROCHLORIDE) that work by releasing
NORADRENALINE and ADRENALINE from nerves
of the sympathetic nervous system and
adrenal medulla and consequently show no
selectivity of action, which therapeutically is
a disadvantage. See DOBUTAMINE
HYDROCHLORIDE; DOPAMINE; FENOTEROL
HYDROBROMIDE; METARAMINOL; METHOXAMINE
HYDROCHLORIDE; PIRBUTEROL; REPROTEROL
HYDROCHLORIDE; RIMITEROL HYDROCHLORIDE.

Synacthen

(Ciba) is a proprietary, prescription-only
preparation of tracosactrin, which is an
analogue of the pituitary HORMONE
CORTICOTROPHIN (ACTH) that stimulates the
adrenal gland to produce corticosteroid
hormones. It may be therapeutically useful
to stimulate the adrenal gland when it is
suppressed by chronic corticosteroid
administration, however, the primary use
of this drug is to test adrenal gland
function. It is available in a form for
injection.

✚▲ Side-effects/warning: See
TRACOSACTRIN.

Synacthen Depot

(Ciba) is a proprietary, prescription-only
preparation of tracosactrin (and a zinc
complex), which is an analogue of the
pituitary HORMONE CORTICOTROPHIN (ACTH)
that stimulates the adrenal gland to produce
corticosteroid hormones. It may be
therapeutically useful to stimulate the
adrenal gland when it is suppressed by
chronic corticosteroid administration,
however, the primary use of this drug
is to test adrenal gland function. It is
available in a form for injection.

✚▲ Side-effects/warning: See
TRACOSACTRIN.

Synalar

(Zeneca) is a proprietary, prescription-only preparation of the CORTICOSTEROID and ANTI-INFLAMMATORY drug fluocinolone acetonide. It can be used to treat severe, acute inflammatory skin disorders, such as eczema and psoriasis. It is available as a cream, gel or ointment in three different strengths under the names *Synalar*, *Synalar 1 in 4 Dilution* and *Synalar 1 in 10 Dilution*.

+▲ Side-effects/warning: See FLUOCINOLONE ACETONIDE.

Synalar C

(Zeneca) is a proprietary, prescription-only COMPOUND PREPARATION of the CORTICOSTEROID and ANTI-INFLAMMATORY drug fluocinolone acetonide and the ANTIMICROBIAL clioquinol. It can be used to treat skin infections with inflammation, and is available as an ointment and a cream for topical application.

+▲ Side-effects/warning: See CLIOQUINOL; FLUOCINOLONE ACETONIDE.

Synalar N

(Zeneca) is a proprietary, prescription-only COMPOUND PREPARATION of the CORTICOSTEROID and ANTI-INFLAMMATORY drug fluocinolone acetonide and the ANTIBACTERIAL and (AMINOGLYCOSIDE) ANTIBIOTIC neomycin sulphate. It can be used to treat skin infections with inflammation, and is available as an ointment and a cream for topical application.

+▲ Side-effects/warning: See FLUOCINOLONE ACETONIDE; NEOMYCIN SULPHATE.

Synarel

(Syntex) is a proprietary, prescription-only preparation of nafarelin, which is an analogue of the hypothalamic HORMONE GONADORELIN (gonadothrophin-releasing hormone; GnRH). It can be used to treat endometriosis, and is available as a nasal spray.

+▲ Side-effects/warning: See NAFARELIN.

Syndol

(Hoechst Marion Roussel) is a proprietary, non-prescription COMPOUND PREPARATION of the NON-NARCOTIC ANALGESIC paracetamol, the (OPIOID) NARCOTIC ANALGESIC codeine phosphate, the ANTIHISTAMINE doxylamine succinate and the STIMULANT caffeine. It can be used to treat mild to moderate pain, including tension headache, toothache, period pain, muscle pain, neuralgia and pain following surgery. It is available as tablets and is not normally given to children, except on medical advice.

+▲ Side-effects/warning: See CAFFEINE; CODEINE PHOSPHATE; DOXYLAMINE SUCCINATE; PARACETAMOL.

Synflex

(Syntex) is a proprietary, prescription-only preparation of the (NSAID) NON-NARCOTIC ANALGESIC and ANTIRHEUMATIC naproxen (as the sodium salt). It can be used to relieve pain and inflammation, particularly rheumatic and arthritic pain and also of acute gout, other musculoskeletal disorders and period pain. It is available as tablets.

+▲ Side-effects/warning: See NAPROXEN.

Synkavit

(Cambridge) is a proprietary, non-prescription preparation of menadiol sodium phosphate (vitamin K_3). It can be used to treat certain types of vitamin K deficiency, and is available as tablets.

+▲ Side-effects/warning: See MENADIOL SODIUM PHOSPHATE.

Synphase

(Syntex) is a proprietary, prescription-only COMPOUND PREPARATION which can be used as a (*triphasic*) ORAL CONTRACEPTIVE (and also for certain menstrual problems) of the type that combines an OESTROGEN and a PROGESTOGEN, in this instance ethinyloestradiol and norethisterone. It is available as tablets contained in a calendar pack.

+▲ Side-effects/warning: See ETHINYLOESTRADIOL; NORETHISTERONE.

S

S

Syntaris

(Syntex) is a proprietary, prescription-only preparation of the CORTICOSTEROID flunisolide. It can be used to treat nasal allergy (such as hay fever), and is available as a nasal spray.

✚▲ Side-effects/warning: See FLUNISOLIDE.

Syntex Menophase

(Syntex) is a proprietary, prescription-only COMPOUND PREPARATION of the female SEX HORMONES mestranol (an OESTROGEN) and norethisterone (a PROGESTOGEN). It can be used in HRT, and is available in the form of tablets in a calendar pack.

✚▲ Side-effects/warning: See MESTRANOL; NORETHISTERONE.

Syntocinon

(Sandoz) is a proprietary, prescription-only preparation of the natural pituitary HORMONE oxytocin, which causes increased contraction of the uterus during labour and stimulates lactation. It can be administered therapeutically to induce or assist labour and, in conjunction with ergometrine maleate (*Syntometrine*), to control bleeding following incomplete abortion and to aid delivery of the placenta under medical supervision. It is available in a form for injection or infusion.

✚▲ Side-effects/warning: See OXYTOCIN.

Syntometrine

(Sandoz) is a proprietary, prescription-only COMPOUND PREPARATION of the ALKALOID ergometrine maleate and the natural HORMONE oxytocin. It can be usd to assist the third and final stage of labour (delivery of the placenta) and to control postnatal bleeding following incomplete abortion. It is available in a form for injection.

✚▲ Side-effects/warning: See ERGOMETRINE MALEATE; OXYTOCIN.

Syntopressin

(Sandoz) is a proprietary, prescription-only preparation of lypressin, which is an analogue of the pituitary HORMONE vasopressin (antidiuretic hormone, ADH). It may be used as a pituitary-originated DIABETES INSIPIDUS TREATMENT, and is available as a nasal spray (it is absorbed into the systemic circulation from the nasal mucosa).

✚▲ Side-effects/warning: See LYPRESSIN.

Syscor MR

(Bayer) is a proprietary, prescription-only preparation of the CALCIUM-CHANNEL BLOCKER nisoldipine. It can be used as an ANTI-ANGINA treatment in the prevention of attacks and as an ANTIHYPERTENSIVE. It is available as tablets.

✚▲ Side-effects/warning: See NISOLDIPINE.

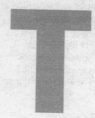

T/Gel

(Neutrogena) is a proprietary, non-prescription preparation of coal tar. It can be used to treat such skin conditions as dandruff and psoriasis of the scalp, and is available as a shampoo.a

✚▲ Side-effects/warning: See COAL TAR.

tacalcitol

is an analogue of vitamin D which is used as a skin treatment for plaque psoriasis. Administration is topical.

✚ Side-effects: There may be local irritation including itching, burning, erythema and loss of sensation.

▲ Warning: It should not be used in patients with disorders of calcium metabolism. Administer with care to those who are pregnamt. Avoid the scalp or contact with eyes and other body areas.
○ Related entry: Curatoderm.

tacrolimus

is an IMMUNOSUPPRESSANT drug (a MACROLIDE ANTIBIOTIC) that is used particularly to limit tissue rejection during and following organ transplant surgery (particularly of liver or kidney). Administration is either oral or by intravenous infusion.

✚▲ Side-effects/warning: See CYCLOSPORIN. Do not administer to patients who are sensitive to macrolide antibiotics, pregnant or breast-feeding. Monitor body function.
○ Related entry: Prograf.

Tagamet

(SmithKline Beecham) is a proprietary preparation of the H₂-ANTAGONIST and ULCER-HEALING DRUG cimetidine. It is available on prescription or without a prescription in a limited amount for short-term uses only. It can be used to treat benign peptic ulcers (in the stomach or duodenum), gastro-oesophageal reflux, dyspepsia and associated conditions. It is available as tablets, effervescent tablets, a syrup and in a form for injection or infusion.

✚▲ Side-effects/warning: See CIMETIDINE.

Tagamet Dual Action Liquid

(SmithKline Beecham) is a proprietary COMPOUND PREPARATION of the H₂-ANTAGONIST and ULCER-HEALING DRUG cimetidine and ALGINIC ACID (as sodium alginate). It can be used for the short-term treatment of dyspepsia, regurgitation and heartburn, and is available as a liquid.

✚▲ Side-effects/warning: See CIMETIDINE.

Tambocor

(3M) is a proprietary, prescription-only preparation of the ANTI-ARRHYTHMIC flecainide acetate. It can be used to treat heartbeat irregularities, and is available as tablets and in a form for injection.

✚▲ Side-effects/warning: See FLECAINIDE ACETATE.

Tamofen

(Pharmacia) is a proprietary, prescription-only preparation of the sex HORMONE ANTAGONIST tamoxifen. It inhibits the effect of OESTROGENS and because of this is used primarily as an ANTICANCER drug for cancers that depend on the presence of oestrogen in women, particularly breast cancer. It may also be used to treat certain conditions of infertility. It is available as tablets.

✚▲ Side-effects/warning: See TAMOXIFEN.

tamoxifen

is a sex HORMONE ANTAGONIST, an ANTI-OESTROGEN, which antagonizes the natural oestrogens present in the body by blocking the RECEPTORS and can be useful in treating infertility in women whose condition is

T

linked to the persistent presence of oestrogens and a consequent failure to ovulate. A second, and major use, is as an ANTICANCER drug in the treatment of existing oestrogen-dependent breast cancer (both in pre- and postmenopausal women). A related, but still experimental, use is as a prophylactic (preventive) treatment in women considered to be at risk of breast cancer. Administration is oral.

✚ Side-effects: Hot flushes, vaginal bleeding or discharge, suppression of menstruation, itching vulva, gastrointestinal upsets, oedema, hair loss, blood disturbances (fall in platelet count and porphyria), visual disturbances and liver dysfunction. Some patients with breast cancer may have pain.

▲ Warning: It should not be administered to patients who are pregnant or breast-feeding. There may be swelling within the ovaries, raised blood calcium (associated with bone cancer) or adverse changes in the endometrial lining of the uterus.

✪ Related entries: Emblon; Noltam; Nolvadex; Oestrifen; Tamofen.

Tampovagan

(Norgine) is a proprietary, prescription-only preparation of a form of stilboestrol, which is a SEX HORMONE analogue with OESTROGEN activity. It can be used to treat conditions of the vagina caused by hormonal deficiency (generally atrophic vaginitis in the menopause). It is available as vaginal inserts (pessaries).

✚▲ Side-effects/warning: See STILBOESTROL.

tamsulosin hydrochloride

is a selective ALPHA-ADRENOCEPTOR BLOCKER which can be used to treat urinary retention in benign prostatic hypertrophy. Administration is oral.

✚▲ Side-effects/warning: See PRAZOSIN HYDROCHLORIDE.

✪ Related entry: Flomax MR.

Tancolin

(Roche) is a proprietary, non-prescription

preparation of the (OPIOID) ANTITUSSIVE and NARCOTIC ANALGESIC dextromethorphan hydrobromide and vitamin C. It can be used for the symptomatic relief of coughs, particularly those associated with infection in the upper respiratory tract. It is available as a liquid and is not to be given to children under six months.

✚▲ Side-effects/warning: See DEXTROMETHORPHAN HYDROBROMIDE.

Tarcortin

(Stafford-Miller) is a proprietary, prescription-only COMPOUND PREPARATION of the CORTICOSTEROID hydrocortisone and coal tar. It can be used to treat eczema and psoriasis, and is available as a cream for topical application.

✚▲ Side-effects/warning: See COAL TAR; HYDROCORTISONE.

Targocid

(Merrell) is a proprietary, prescription-only preparation of the ANTIBACTERIAL and ANTIBIOTIC drug teicoplanin. It can be used for serious infections, such as endocarditis, dialysis-associated peritonitis and infections due to *Staphylococcus aureus*. It is available in a form for injection.

✚▲ Side-effects/warning: See TEICOPLANIN.

Tarivid

(Hoechst, Roussel) is a proprietary, prescription-only preparation of the ANTIBACTERIAL and (QUINOLONE) ANTIBIOTIC ofloxacin. It can be used to treat infections, particularly complicated infections of the urinary tract, cervical infections, septicaemia and gonorrhoea. It is available as tablets and in a form for intravenous infusion.

✚▲ Side-effects/warning: See OFLOXACIN.

Tavegil

(Sandoz) is a proprietary, non-prescription preparation of the ANTIHISTAMINE drug clemastine (as hydrogen fumarate). It can be administered to relieve the symptoms of allergic disorders, such as hay fever and urticaria, and is available as tablets and a liquid.

+▲ Side-effects/warning: See CLEMASTINE.

Taxol

(Bristol-Myers; Squibb) is a proprietary, prescription-only preparation of the (CYTOTOXIC) ANTICANCER drug paclitaxel. It can be used to treat ovarian and breast cancer, and is available in a form for intravenous infusion.

+▲ Side-effects/warning: See PACLITAXEL.

Taxotere

(Rhône-Poulenc Rorer) is a proprietary, prescription-only preparation of the *taxane* (CYTOTOXIC) ANTICANCER drug docetaxel. It can be used to treat breast cancer, and is available in a form for intravenous infusion.

+▲ Side-effects/warning: See DOCETAXEL.

Tazocin

(Lederle) is a proprietary, prescription-only COMPOUND PREPARATION of the broad-spectrum ANTIBACTERIAL and (PENICILLIN) ANTIBIOTIC piperacillin and the PENICILLLINASE INHIBITOR tazobactam, which, by preventing degradation by bacterium-derived beta-lactamase enzyme, confers *penicillinase-resistance* to the antibiotic. It can be used to treat many serious or compound forms of bacterial infection, including skin infections, septicaemia and of the respiratory and urinary tracts, particularly infections caused by *Pseudomonas aeruginosa*. It is available in a form for injection or infusion.

+▲ Side-effects/warning: See PIPERACILLIN.

TCP Antiseptic Throat Pastilles (Blackcurrant Flavour)

(Charwell) is a proprietary, non-prescription preparation of TCP liquid antiseptic, which contains the ANTISEPTIC agent phenol (with halogenated phenols). It can be used for the relief of minor sore throats.

+▲ Side-effects/warning: See PHENOL.

TCP Liquid Antiseptic

(Charwell) is a proprietary, non-prescription preparation of the ANTISEPTIC agent phenol (with halogenated phenols). It can be used for the symptomatic relief of sore throat, including those associated with colds and flu, and is available as a solution for use as a gargle.

+▲ Side-effects/warning: See PHENOL.

Tears Naturale

(Alcon) is a proprietary, non-prescription preparation of HYPROMELLOSE (with dextran '70'). It can be used as artificial tears for tear deficiency, and is available as eye-drops.

Teejel Gel

(Seton) is a proprietary, non-prescription COMPOUND PREPARATION of the ANTISEPTIC cetalkonium chloride and choline salicylate, which is a COUNTER-IRRITANT, or RUBEFACIENT. It can be applied to the mouth for the symptomatic relief of pain from mouth ulcers, cold sores, denture irritation, inflammation of the tongue and teething in infants. It is not normally given to children under four months, except on medical advice.

+▲ Side-effects/warning: See CHOLINE SALICYLATE.

Tegretol

(Geigy) is a proprietary, prescription-only preparation of the ANTICONVULSANT and ANTI-EPILEPTIC drug carbamazepine. It can be used in the preventive treatment of most forms of epilepsy (except absence seizures), for trigeminal neuralgia, in the treatment of diabetes insipidus and in the management of manic-depressive illness. It is available as tablets, chewable tablets, a liquid, suppositories and as modified-release tablets called *Tegretol Retard*.

+▲ Side-effects/warning: See CARBAMAZEPINE.

teicoplanin

is an ANTIBACTERIAL and ANTIBIOTIC drug of

T

the glycopeptide family. It is similar to VANCOMYCIN, but with a longer duration of action so it can be taken only once a day. It has activity primarily against Gram-positive bacteria and works by inhibiting the synthesis of components of the bacterial cell wall. It can be used in the treatment of serious infections, including endocarditis, dialysis-associated peritonitis, severe burns and for infections caused by *Staphylococcus aureus*. Administration is by injection or infusion.

✚ Side-effects: There may be diarrhoea, nausea and vomiting, headache; severe allergic reactions, bronchospasm, fever and rash; blood disorders; ringing in the ears and mild loss of hearing; local reactions at the injection site; loss of balance has been reported.

▲ Warning: Tests on liver and kidney function are required, also blood counts and hearing tests. Administer with caution to patients who are elderly, pregnant or breast-feeding. Its use may have deleterious effects on the organs of the ear, on the kidney and liver; blood concentrations of the drug in the blood, along with liver and kidney function, should be monitored during treatment.

✪ Related entry: Targocid.

Telfast

(Hoechst Marion Roussel) is a proprietary, prescription-only preparation of the ANTIHISTAMINE fexofenadine. It can be used to treat allergic symptoms, such as the rhinitis of hay fever, and is available as tablets.

✚▲ Side-effects/warning: See FEXOFENADINE.

temazepam

is a BENZODIAZEPINE which is used as a relatively short-acting HYPNOTIC for the short-term treatment of insomnia and as a preoperative medication. Administration is oral.

✚▲ Side-effects/warning: See BENZODIAZEPINES.

Temgesic

(Reckitt & Colman) is a proprietary, prescription-only preparation of the (OPIOID) NARCOTIC ANALGESIC buprenorphine (as hydrochloride), and is on the Controlled Drugs List. It can be used to treat all forms of pain, and is available as sublingual tablets (to be retained under the tongue) and in a form for injection.

✚▲ Side-effects/warning: See BUPRENORPHINE.

temocillin

is a new ANTIBACTERIAL (PENICILLIN) ANTIBIOTIC which is used primarily to treat forms of infection that other penicillins are incapable of countering, due to the production of the enzyme penicillinase by the bacteria concerned. Temocillin is not inactivated by the penicillinase enzymes produced, for example, by certain Gram-negative bacteria (but not *Pseudomonas aeruginosa*), however, it is not active against Gram-positive bacteria, such as in infections of the urinary tract. It is therefore classed as a *penicillinase-resistant* penicillin. Administration can be either oral or by injection.

✚▲ Side-effects/warning: See BENZYLPENICILLIN.

✪ Related entry: Temopen.

Temopen

(Bencard) is a proprietary, prescription-only preparation of the ANTIBACTERIAL and (PENICILLIN) ANTIBIOTIC temocillin. It can be used to treat bacterial infections, especially certain Gram-negative bacterial infections that prove to be resistant to penicillin, but is not active against Gram-positive bacteria. It is available in a form for injection.

✚▲ Side-effects/warning: See TEMOCILLIN.

Tenben

(Galen) is a proprietary, prescription-only COMPOUND PREPARATION of the BETA-BLOCKER atenolol and the DIURETIC bendrofluazide. It can be used as an ANTIHYPERTENSIVE, and is available as capsules.

+▲ Side-effects/warning: See ATENOLOL; BENDROFLUAZIDE.

Tenchlor

(Berk) is a proprietary, prescription-only COMPOUND PREPARATION of the BETA-BLOCKER atenolol and the DIURETIC chlorthalidone (a combination called co-tenidone). It can be used as an ANTIHYPERTENSIVE for raised blood pressure, and is available as tablets.
+▲ Side-effects/warning: See ATENOLOL; CHLORTHALIDONE.

Tenif

(Stuart) is a proprietary, prescription-only COMPOUND PREPARATION of the BETA-BLOCKER atenolol and the CALCIUM-CHANNEL BLOCKER nifedipine. It can be used as an ANTIHYPERTENSIVE for raised blood pressure, and is available as capsules.
+▲ Side-effects/warning: See ATENOLOL; NIFEDIPINE.

Tenoret 50

(Stuart) is a proprietary, prescription-only COMPOUND PREPARATION of the BETA-BLOCKER atenolol and the DIURETIC chlorthalidone. It can be used as an ANTIHYPERTENSIVE, and is available as tablets.
+▲ Side-effects/warning: See ATENOLOL; CHLORTHALIDONE.

Tenoretic

(Stuart) is a proprietary, prescription-only COMPOUND PREPARATION of the BETA-BLOCKER atenolol and the DIURETIC chlorthalidone. It can be used as an ANTIHYPERTENSIVE, and is available as tablets.
+▲ Side-effects/warning: See ATENOLOL; CHLORTHALIDONE.

Tenormin

(Stuart) is a proprietary, prescription-only preparation of the BETA-BLOCKER atenolol. It can be used as an ANTIHYPERTENSIVE for raised blood pressure, as an ANTI-ANGINA treatment to relieve symptoms and improve exercise tolerance and as an ANTI-ARRHYTHMIC to regularize heartbeat and to treat myocardial infarction. It is available as tablets, a syrup and in a form for injection.
+▲ Side-effects/warning: See ATENOLOL.

tenoxicam

is a (NSAID) NON-NARCOTIC ANALGESIC and ANTIRHEUMATIC drug. It has a long duration of action and is used to treat pain and inflammation in rheumatic disease and other musculoskeletal disorders. Administration can be either oral or by injection.
+▲ Side-effects/warning: See NSAID.
✪ Related entry: Mobiflex.

Tensium

(DDSA Pharmaceuticals) is a proprietary, prescription-only preparation of the BENZODIAZEPINE diazepam. It can be used as an ANXIOLYTIC for the short-term treatment of anxiety, as a HYPNOTIC to relieve insomnia, as an ANTICONVULSANT and ANTI-EPILEPTIC for status epilepticus, as a SEDATIVE in preoperative medication, as a SKELETAL MUSCLE RELAXANT and to assist in the treatment of alcohol withdrawal symptoms. It is available as tablets.
+▲ Side-effects/warning: See DIAZEPAM.

Teoptic

(CIBA Vision) is a proprietary, prescription-only preparation of the BETA-BLOCKER carteolol hydrochloride. It can be used for GLAUCOMA TREATMENT, and is available as eye-drops.
+▲ Side-effects/warning: See CARTEOLOL HYDROCHLORIDE.

terazosin

is a selective ALPHA-ADRENOCEPTOR BLOCKER drug which is administered as an ANTIHYPERTENSIVE and also, because of its SMOOTH MUSCLE RELAXANT properties, in the treatment of urinary retention (eg in benign prostatic hyperplasia). Administration is oral.
+▲ Side-effects/warning: See PRAZOSIN HYDROCHLORIDE.
✪ Related entries: Hytrin; Hytrin BPH.

T

terbinafine

is an ANTIFUNGAL drug which is used to treat ringworm infections of the skin and fungal infections of the nails. Unlike most other antifungals it can be taken by mouth and so is available as tablets as well as a cream.

✚ Side-effects: There may be loss of appetite, abdominal discomfort, nausea and diarrhoea, headache, muscle and joint ache and urticaria, unusual skin disturbances, light sensitivity, taste disturbances and liver disorders.

▲ Warning: It should be administered with care to patients with abnormal liver or kidney function, who are pregnant or breast-feeding. Avoid contact of the cream with the eyes.

✿ Related entry: Lamisil.

terbutaline sulphate

is a SYMPATHOMIMETIC and a BETA-RECEPTOR STIMULANT with good beta₂-receptor selectivity. It is mainly used as a BRONCHODILATOR in reversible obstructive airways disease, as an ANTI-ASTHMATIC treatment in severe acute asthma and for the alleviation of symptoms of chronic bronchitis and emphysema. It can also be used in obstetrics to prevent or delay premature labour by relaxing the uterus. Administration is oral, by injection or inhalation.

✚▲ Side-effects/warning: See SALBUTAMOL (and RITODRINE HYDROCHLORIDE for use in labour).

✿ Related entries: Bricanyl; Monovent.

terfenadine

is a recently developed ANTIHISTAMINE which has less sedative side-effects than some of the older members of its class. It can be administered for the symptomatic relief of allergic symptoms, such as hay fever and urticaria. Administration is oral in the form of tablets or as a suspension. Just prior to publication of this book the Committee on Safety of Medicines announced that it would be reviewing whether this drug and its proprietary preparations should become available only on prescription rather than OTC without a prescription.

✚▲ Side-effects/warning: See ANTIHISTAMINES. Although the incidence of sedative and anticholinergic effects is low, there may still be some drowsiness which may impair the performance of skilled tasks, such as driving and operating machinery. Certain serious disturbances of heart rhythm have been observed after excessive dose and when used in combination with certain other drugs (including a number of antibiotics, antidepressants, antipsychotics, anti-arrhythmics and astemizoles). Hair loss has been reported. If you have any doubts about using this drug, consult your doctor.

✿ Related entries: Aller-eze Clear; Seldane; Terfenor; Triludan.

Terfenor

(Norton) is a proprietary, non-prescription preparation of the ANTIHISTAMINE terfenadine. It can be used to treat the symptoms of allergic disorders, such as hay fever and urticaria, and is available as tablets in three strengths (the weakest is called *Terfenor 30* and the strongest *Terfenor Forte*).

✚▲ Side-effects/warning: See TERFENADINE. Just prior to publication the Department of Health announced that it would be reviewing whether terfenadine should become available only on prescription rather than OTC without a prescription. If you have any doubts about using this drug, consult your doctor.

terlipressin

is a form of the pituitary HORMONE antidiuretic hormone (ADH) or vasopressin. It can be used as a VASOCONSTRICTOR type of HAEMOSTATIC drug to treat bleeding from varices (varicose veins) in the oesophagus. Administration is by injection.

✚▲ Side-effects/warning: See VASOPRESSIN; but side-effects are usually milder.

✿ Related entry: Glypressin.

terpenes ☆

are chemically unsaturated hydrocarbons that are found in terpene plant oils and resins. Examples include CINEOLE, MENTHOL, pinene and squalene. Examples that are chemically larger include the caratenoids and VITAMIN A. Mixtures of some terpenes are used to treat gallstone disorders. Menthol, which is the most widely used of all the terpenes, is included in inhalant preparations intended to clear nasal or catarrhal congestion in conditions such as colds, rhinitis or sinusitis. It is also included in some COUNTER-IRRITANT, or RUBEFACIENT, preparations that are rubbed into the skin to relieve muscle or joint pain.
➕▲ Side-effects/warning: There seem to be only a few adverse reactions with topical application, even though their action would appear to involve irritation of sensory nerve endings. Some interact with contraceptives or coagulants that are administered orally.

Terra-Cortril

(Pfizer) is a proprietary, prescription-only COMPOUND PREPARATION of the ANTI-INFLAMMATORY and CORTICOSTEROID hydrocortisone (as acetate) and the ANTIBACTERIAL and (TETRACYCLINE) ANTIBIOTIC oxytetracycline. It can be used for local or topical application to treat skin disorders in which bacterial or other infection is also implicated. It is available as a topical ointment.
➕▲ Side-effects/warning: See HYDROCORTISONE; OXYTETRACYCLINE.

Terra-Cortril Nystatin

(Pfizer) is a proprietary, prescription-only COMPOUND PREPARATION of the ANTI-INFLAMMATORY and CORTICOSTEROID hydrocortisone (as acetate), the ANTIFUNGAL and ANTIBIOTIC nystatin and the ANTIBACTERIAL and (TETRACYCLINE) antibiotic oxytetracycline. It can be used to treat skin disorders caused by fungal or bacterial infection, and is available as a cream.
➕▲ Side-effects/warning: See HYDROCORTISONE; NYSTATIN; OXYTETRACYCLINE.

Terramycin

(Pfizer) is a proprietary, prescription-only preparation of the ANTIBACTERIAL and (TETRACYCLINE) ANTIBIOTIC oxytetracycline. It can be used to treat a wide range of infections, and is available as tablets and capsules.
➕▲ Side-effects/warning: See OXYTETRACYCLINE.

Tertroxin

(Link) is a proprietary, prescription-only preparation of liothyronine sodium, which is a form of the THYROID HORMONE triiodothyronine. It can be used to make up hormonal deficiency (hypothyroidism) and therefore to treat the associated symptoms. It is available as tablets.
➕▲ Side-effects/warning: See LIOTHYRONINE SODIUM.

Testosterone

(Organon) is a proprietary, prescription-only preparation of the ANDROGEN (male SEX HORMONE) testosterone (as propionate and phenylpropionate). It can be used to treat testosterone deficiency in men and women (as part of HRT), and is available as an implant.
➕▲ Side-effects/warning: See TESTOSTERONE.

testosterone

is an ANDROGEN and the principal male SEX HORMONE. It is produced (in men) mainly in the testes with other androgens that promote the development and maintenance of the male sex organs and in the development of the secondary male sexual characteristics. It is also made in small amounts in women. Therapeutically, it can be administered to treat hormonal deficiency, for instance for delayed puberty, certain cancers (eg breast cancer in women) and in HRT (hormone replacement therapy) in menopausal women. Administration can be either oral or by injection.
➕▲ Side-effects/warning: See ANDROGENS.

⭕ Related entries: Primoteston Depot;
Restandol; Sustenon 100; Sustenon 250;
Testosterone; Virormone.

Tet/Vac/Ads

is an abbreviation for ADSORBED TETANUS
VACCINE.

Tet/Vac/FT

is an abbreviation for TETANUS VACCINE, which
is prepared from tetanus formol toxoid, the
plain vaccine and is not adsorbed onto a
carrier.

Tetabulin

(Immuno) (Tetanus Immunoglobulin
Injection) is a proprietary, prescription-
only preparation of tetanus immunoglobulin, human (HTIG), which is a
SPECIFIC IMMUNOGLOBULIN. It can be used in
IMMUNIZATION to give immediate *passive
immunity* against infection by the tetanus
organism. Administration is by
intramuscular injection.
➕▲ Side-effects/warning: See
IMMUNIZATION.

Tetanus Immunoglobulin

(BLS; SNBTS) (Antitetanus Immunoglobulin
Injection) is a non-proprietary,
prescription-only preparation of tetanus
immunoglobulin, human (HTIG), which is a
SPECIFIC IMMUNOGLOBULIN that can be used in
immunization to give immediate *passive
immunity* against infection by the tetanus
organism. Administration is by
intramuscular injection.
➕▲ Side-effects/warning: See
IMMUNIZATION.

Tetanus Immunoglobulin for Intravenous Use

(SNBTS) is a non-proprietary, prescription-
only preparation of TETANUS
IMMUNOGLOBULIN, HUMAN (HTIG), which is a
SPECIFIC IMMUNOGLOBULIN that can be
administered in IMMUNIZATION to give
immediate passive immunity against
infection by the tetanus organism.

Administration is by intravenous injection.
➕▲ Side-effects/warning: See
IMMUNIZATION.

tetanus immunoglobulin, human

(HTIG) is a SPECIFIC IMMUNOGLOBULIN, which
is a form of immunoglobulin used for
IMMUNIZATION to give immediate *passive
immunity* against infection by tetanus. It is
mostly used as an added precaution in
treating patients with contaminated wounds.
It can be considered just a precautionary
measure because today almost everybody
has established immunity through a VACCINE
administered at an early age and
vaccination is in any case readily available
for those at risk. Administration is by
intramuscular injection.
➕▲ Side-effects/warning: See
IMMUNIZATION.
⭕ Related entries: Tetabulin; Tetanus
Immunoglobulin; Tetanus Immunoglobulin
for Intravenous Use.

Tetanus Immunoglobulin Injection

see TETABULIN

tetanus toxoid

see TETANUS VACCINE

tetanus vaccine

(tetanus toxoid) is used in IMMUNIZATION to
provide protection against infection by the
tetanus organism. It is a *toxoid-type*
VACCINE, which is a vaccine made from a
toxin produced by a microbe, in this case
tetanus bacteria, that is modified to make it
non-infective and which then stimulates the
body to form the appropriate antitoxin
(antibody). In tetanus vaccine, the bacterial
toxoid is adsorbed onto a mineral carrier
and is usually given as one constituent of
the *triple vaccine* ADSORBED DIPTHERIA,
TETANUS AND PERTUSSIS VACCINE
(DTPer/Vac/Ads) or the *double vaccine*
ADSORBED DIPTHERIA AND TETANUS VACCINE
(DT/Vac/Ads), which are administered

during early life. However, tetanus vaccine can be administered by itself at any age for those who are at special risk from being infected. Administration is by injection, and a 'booster' injection is given after ten years.
○ Related entries: Adsorbed Diphtheria and Tetanus Vaccine; Adsorbed Diphtheria and Tetanus Vaccine for Adults and Adolescents; Adsorbed Tetanus Vaccine; Clostet; Tetanus Vaccine; Trivax-AD.

Tetanus Vaccine

(Evans) (Tet/Vac/FT) is a non-proprietary, prescription-only VACCINE preparation of the *toxoid-type* tetanus vaccine. It can be used to provide active immunization against tetanus, and is available in a form for injection.
✚▲ Side-effects/warning: See TETANUS VACCINE.

tetrabenazine

is a drug that is used to assist a patient to regain voluntary control of movement, or at least to lessen the extent of involuntary movements, in Huntingdon's chorea and related disorders. It is thought to work by reducing the amount of DOPAMINE in the nerves in the brain. Administration is oral.
✚ Side-effects: Drowsiness, gastrointestinal disturbance, depression, hypotension, extrapyramidal symptoms (muscle tremor and rigidity).
▲ Warning: Administer with caution to patients who are pregnant and avoid its use in those who are breast-feeding. Because of its drowsiness effect, the performance of skilled tasks, such as driving, may be impaired.
○ Related entry: Nitoman.

Tetrachel

(Berk) is a proprietary, prescription-only preparation of the ANTIBACTERIAL and (TETRACYCLINE) ANTIBIOTIC tetracycline. It can be used to treat various infections, and is available as capsules and tablets.
✚▲ Side-effects/warning: See TETRACYCLINE.

tetracosactide

see TRACOSACTRIN

tetracycline

is a broad-spectrum ANTIBACTERIAL and ANTIBIOTIC of the TETRACYCLINE family, and gave its name to this family of similar antibiotics. It can be used to treat many forms of infection, for example, infections of the urinary and respiratory tracts, of the genital organs, ears, eyes, mouth ulcers and skin (acne). Administration can be either oral or by infusion.
✚ Side-effects: There may be nausea and vomiting with diarrhoea; headache and visual disturbances. Occasionally, there is sensitivity to light or other sensitivity reactions, such as rashes (if so, discontinue treatment). Rarely, pancreatitis and colitis.
▲ Warning: It should not be administered to patients who are aged under 12 years, because of tooth colouration, or who are pregnant or breast-feeding. Administer with caution to those with impaired liver or kidney function.
○ Related entries: Achromycin; Deteclo; Sustamycin; Tetrachel; Topicycline.

tetracyclines ⊟

are a group of very broad-spectrum ANTIBACTERIAL and ANTIBIOTIC drugs. Apart from being effective against bacteria, they also inhibit the growth of chlamydia (a virus-like bacterium that causes genitourinary tract infections, eye infections and psittacosis *Chlamydia psittaci*), rickettsia (a virus-like bacterium that causes, for example, Q fever and typhus *Rickettsia typhi*) and mycoplasma (a minute nonmotile organism that causes, for example, mycoplasmal pneumonia *Mycoplasma pneumoniae*). The tetracyclines act by inhibiting protein biosynthesis in sensitive micro-organisms and penetrate human macrophages and are therefore useful in combating micro-organisms, such as mycoplasma, that can survive and multiply within macrophages. Although they have been used to treat a very

T

wide range of infections, the development of bacterial resistance has meant that their uses have become more specific. Treatment of atypical pneumonia due to chlamydia, rickettsia or mycoplasma is a notable indication for tetracyclines, while treatment of chlamydial urethritis and pelvic inflammatory disease is another. They are also used to treat brucellosis and Lyme disease, and are effective in treating exacerbations of chronic bronchitis and acne. Most tetracyclines are more difficult to absorb in a stomach that contains milk, antacids (calcium salts or magnesium salts) or IRON salts (eg in ANAEMIA TREATMENT); and most (except doxycycline and minicycline) may exacerbate kidney failure and so should be avoided when treating patients with kidney disease. They may be deposited in growing bone and teeth (causing staining and potential deformity), and should therefore not be administered to children under 12 years or to pregnant women. The best-known and most-used tetracyclines include TETRACYCLINE (which they were all named after), DOXYCYCLINE and OXYTETRACYCLINE. The members of the tetracycline family have generic names ending -*cycline*. Administration is oral. See CHLORTETRACYCLINE; DEMECLOCYCLINE HYDROCHLORIDE; LYMECYCLINE; MINOCYCLINE.

Tetralysal 300

(Pharmacia) is a proprietary, prescription-only preparation of the ANTIBACTERIAL and (TETRACYCLINE) ANTIBIOTIC lymecycline. It can be used to treat infections of many kinds, and is available as capsules.
✚▲ Side-effects/warning: See LYMECYCLINE.

Theo-Dur

(Astra) is a proprietary, non-prescription preparation of the BRONCHODILATOR theophylline. It can be used as an ANTI-ASTHMATIC and for the treatment of chronic bronchitis, and is available as modified-release tablets.
✚▲ Side-effects/warning: See THEOPHYLLINE.

theophylline

is a BRONCHODILATOR drug which is mainly used as an ANTI-ASTHMATIC and for the treatment of bronchitis. Chemically, it is classed as a xanthine. Administration is oral as tablets and capsules (mainly modified-release forms capable of maintaining actions for up to 12 hours), as a liquid and in a form for injection. It is also available in the form of chemical derivatives, eg AMINOPHYLLINE.
✚ Side-effects: There may be nausea and gastrointestinal disturbances, headache, an increase or irregularity in the heartbeat and/or insomnia; convulsions may occur when given intravenously.
▲ Warning: Safety depends very much on the concentration in the blood, but this depends on many factors, including whether the patient smokes or drinks, his or her age and concurrent drug therapy. For this reason treatment should initially be gradual and progressively increased until control of bronchospasm is achieved. Administer with caution to patients who suffer from certain heart or liver disorders, who are pregnant or breast-feeding, and where there is a risk of low blood potassium (hypokalaemia). It should not be used in patients with porphyria.
✪ Related entries: Anestan Bronchial Tablets; Do-Do Chesteze; Franol; Franol Plus; Franolyn For Chesty Coughs; Lasma; Nuelin; Nuelin SA; Slo-Phyllin; Theo-Dur; Uniphyllin Continus.

Thephorin

(Sinclair) is a proprietary, non-prescription preparation of the ANTIHISTAMINE phenindamine tartrate. It can be used to treat the symptoms of allergic disorders, such as hay fever and urticaria, and is available as tablets.
✚▲ Side-effects/warning: See PHENINDAMINE TARTRATE.

thiabendazole

(tiabendazole) is an (AZOLE) ANTHELMINTIC drug. It is used in the treatment of infestations by worm parasites, particularly those of the *Strongyloides* species that reside in the intestines but may migrate into the tissues. It is also used to treat other worm infestations resistant to common drugs. The usual course of treatment is intensive.

✚ Side-effects: There may be nausea, vomiting, diarrhoea and anorexia; dizziness and drowsiness; and headache and itching. Possible hypersensitivity reactions include fever with chills, rashes and other skin disorders and occasionally tinnitus or liver damage.

▲ Warning: It should be administered with caution to patients with impaired kidney or liver function. Treatment should be stopped if hypersensitivity reactions occur. It is not to be administered to pregnant women. It may impair the performance of skilled tasks, such as driving.

✪ Related entry: Mintezol.

thiazides ⊡

have a DIURETIC action: they inhibit sodium reabsorption at the beginning of the distal convoluted tubule of the kidney and may be used for prolonged periods. Their uses include as ANTIHYPERTENSIVES (either alone or in conjunction with other types of diuretic or other drugs) and the treatment of oedema associated with congestive heart failure. There may be a certain amount of depletion of potassium, but this can be treated with potassium supplements or the co-administering of *potassium-sparing* diuretics. Administration is oral. See BENDROFLUAZIDE; BENZTHIAZIDE; CHLOROTHIAZIDE; CHLORTHALIDONE; CLOPAMIDE; CYCLOPENTHIAZIDE; HYDROCHLOROTHIAZIDE; HYDROFLUMETHIAZIDE; INDAPAMIDE; MEFRUSIDE; METOLAZONE; POLYTHIAZIDE; XIPAMIDE.

thioguanine

is a CYTOTOXIC drug and is used as an ANTICANCER treatment of acute leukaemias. Administration is oral.

✚▲ Side-effects/warning: See CYTOTOXICS.
✪ Related entry: Lanvis.

thiopental sodium
see THIOPENTONE SODIUM

thiopentone sodium

(thiopental sodium) is a BARBITURATE which can be used as a GENERAL ANAESTHETIC for induction and maintenance of anaesthesia during very short operations. Administration is by injection.

✚▲ Side-effects/warning: See BARBITURATES. It is not to be given to patients with porphyria.

✪ Related entries: Intraval Sodium; Thiopentone Sodium.

Thiopentone Sodium

(IMS) is a proprietary, prescription-only preparation of the GENERAL ANAESTHETIC thiopentone sodium. It can be used for the induction of anaesthesia, and is available in a form for injection.

✚▲ Side-effects/warning: See THIOPENTONE SODIUM.

thioridazine

is a recently introduced ANTIPSYCHOTIC drug, which is used to treat and tranquillize psychotic patients (such as schizophrenics), particularly those experiencing behavioural disturbances. The drug may also be used for the short-term treatment of anxiety and to calm agitated, elderly patients. Administration is oral.

✚▲ Side-effects/warning: See CHLORPROMAZINE HYDROCHLORIDE; but has less sedative, hypothermia and extrapyramidal (muscle tremor and rigidity) symptoms; but is more likely to cause hypotension and there may be eye disorders and sexual dysfunction. Avoid its use in patients with porphyria.

✪ Related entries: Melleril; Rideril.

thiotepa

is a CYTOTOXIC drug which is used as an ANTICANCER drug in the treatment of tumours in the bladder and sometimes for breast cancer. It works by interfering with the DNA of new-forming cells, so preventing cell

T

replication. Administration is by instillation in the body cavity.

+▲ Side-effects/warning: See CYTOTOXICS.

○ Related entry: Thiotepa.

Thiotepa

(Lederle) is a proprietary, prescription-only preparation of the (CYTOTOXIC) ANTICANCER drug thiotepa. It can be used in the treatment of tumours in the bladder or other body cavities. It is available in a form for instillation into the body cavity.

+▲ Side-effects/warning: See THIOTEPA.

thrombolytic drugs

break up or dissolve thrombi (blood clots). See FIBRINOLYTICS.

thymol

is obtained from the essential oil of the plant thyme. It can be used as a weak ANTISEPTIC, particularly in mouthwash preparations for oral or dental hygiene, and also in DECONGESTANT preparations for inhalation. It is sometimes used in combination with the essential oils of other plants.

○ Related entries: Compound Thymol Glycerin, BP; Karvol Decongestant Capsules.

thymoxamine

(moxisylyte) is an ALPHA-ADRENOCEPTOR BLOCKER which can be used, because of its VASODILATOR properties, in the treatment of peripheral vascular disease (Raynaud's phenomenon). Administration is oral.

+ Side-effects: See PRAZOSIN HYDROCHLORIDE. There may also be diarrhoea, liver toxicity and flushing.

▲ Warning: It should not be administered to patients with certain liver disorders. Administer with caution to patients with diabetes.

○ Related entry: Opilon.

thyroid hormones ☒

are secreted by the thyroid gland at the base of the neck. There are two major forms, both containing iodine: THYROXINE

(l-thyroxine; T_4 (80%) and TRIIODOTHYRONINE (L-tri-iodothronine; T_3(20%). They are transported in the bloodstream to control functions throughout the body. Both these hormones, in the form of their sodium salts, are used therapeutically to make up a hormonal deficiency on a regular maintenance basis and to treat associated symptoms. They may also be used in the treatment of goitre, thyroid cancer, myxoedema and cretinism. A third hormone, CALCITONIN, is secreted by a different cell type in the thyroid gland and has a different physiological role. It is concerned with lowering calcium levels in the blood (an action which is used therapeutically).

thyroid-stimulating hormone

see THYROTROPHIN

thyrotrophin

(thyroid-stimulating hormone; TSH) is an anterior pituitary HORMONE. It controls the release of THYROID HORMONES from the thyroid gland and is itself controlled by the hypothalamic hormone TRH (thyrotrophin-releasing hormone) and by high levels of thyroid hormone in the blood. In the case of clinical defects at some stage in this system of control, diagnostic tests are necessarily a matter for specialist clinics. Nowadays, it is considered less helpful to make direct diagnosis using thyrotrophin itself in stimulation tests, because it is easier to chemically measure the concentration of thyrotrophin and thyroid hormones (T_3 and T_4) in the blood.

thyrotrophin-releasing hormone

see PROTIRELIN

thyroxine

is one of the natural blood-borne (endocrine) HORMONES released by the thyroid gland. The other major THYROID HORMONE is TRIIODOTHYRONINE. In turn, the release of these hormones is regulated by the endocrine hormone THYROTROPHIN (thyroid-stimulating hormone; TSH), which is secreted by the pituitary gland. Therapeutically, thyroxine is used in the form of THYROXINE SODIUM (sodium l-throxine; T_4).

thyroxine sodium

(sodium l-thyroxine; T_4) is a preparation of THYROXINE, which is one of the two main natural THYROID HORMONES. It is used therapeutically to make up a hormonal deficiency on a regular maintenance basis and to treat associated symptoms. It may also be used in the treatment of goitre and thyroid cancer. Administration is oral.
✚ Side-effects: There may be heartbeat irregularities and increased heart rate, angina pain; headache, muscle cramp, flushing and sweating, diarrhoea, restlessness and weight loss.
▲ Warning: Administer with caution to patients with certain cardiovascular disorders, impaired adrenal glands or prolonged myxoedema.
✪ Related entry: Eltroxin.

tiabendazole

see THIABENDAZOLE

tiaprofenic acid

is a (NSAID) NON-NARCOTIC ANALGESIC and ANTIRHEUMATIC drug, which is used to treat pain and inflammation in rheumatic disease and other musculoskeletal disorders. Administration is oral.
✚▲ Side-effects/warning: See NSAID. It may cause cystitis and bladder irritation and so should not be used where there is a history of urinary tract disorders and treatment must be stopped if adverse effects occur (such as increased frequency of urination, pain or blood in the urine).
✪ Related entry: Surgam.

tibolone

(Organon) is a drug that has both OESTROGEN and PROGESTOGEN activity. It can

be used to treat menopausal problems in HRT (hormone replacement therapy). Administration is oral.
✚▲ Side-effects/warning: See OESTROGENS; PROGESTOGEN.
✪ Related entry: Livial.

Ticar

(Link) is a proprietary, prescription-only preparation of the ANTIBACTERIAL and (PENICILLIN) ANTIBIOTIC ticarcillin. It can be used to treat serious infections, such as septicaemia and peritonitis, and also infections of the respiratory and urinary tracts. It is available in a form for injection or infusion.
✚▲ Side-effects/warning: See TICARCILLIN.

ticarcillin

is an ANTIBACTERIAL and (PENICILLIN) ANTIBIOTIC drug. It has improved activity against a number of important Gram-negative bacteria, including *Pseudomonas aeruginosa*. It can be used to treat serious infections, such as septicaemia and peritonitis, and also infections of the respiratory and urinary tracts. One of its proprietary forms also contains CLAVULANIC ACID. Administration is by injection or infusion.
✚▲ Side-effects/warning: See BENZYLPENICILLIN.
✪ Related entries: Ticar; Timentin.

Tilade

(Fisons) is a proprietary, prescription-only preparation of the ANTI-ASTHMATIC drug nedocromil sodium. It can be used to prevent recurrent attacks of asthma, and is available in a form for inhalation.
✚▲ Side-effects/warning: See NEDOCROMIL SODIUM.

Tilarin

(Fisons) is a proprietary, prescription-only preparation of the ANTI-ALLERGIC drug nedocromil sodium. It can be used to prevent seasonal allergic rhinitis, and is available in the form of a nasal spray

T

+▲ Side-effects/warning: See NEDOCROMIL SODIUM.

Tildiem

(Lorex) is a proprietary, prescription-only preparation of the CALCIUM-CHANNEL BLOCKER drug diltiazem hydrochloride. It can be used as as an ANTIHYPERTENSIVE treatment and as an ANTI-ANGINA drug. It is available as tablets.
+▲ Side-effects/warning: See DILTIAZEM HYDROCHLORIDE.

Tildiem LA

(Lorex) is a proprietary, prescription-only preparation of the CALCIUM-CHANNEL BLOCKER drug diltiazem hydrochloride. It can be used as as an ANTIHYPERTENSIVE treatment and as an ANTI-ANGINA drug. It is available as modified-release capsules.
+▲ Side-effects/warning: See DILTIAZEM HYDROCHLORIDE.

Tildiem Retard

(Lorex) is a proprietary, prescription-only preparation of the CALCIUM-CHANNEL BLOCKER drug diltiazem hydrochloride. It can be used as as an ANTIHYPERTENSIVE treatment and as an ANTI-ANGINA drug. It is available as modified-release tablets.
+▲ Side-effects/warning: See DILTIAZEM HYDROCHLORIDE.

tiludronate disodium

see tiludronic acid

tiludronic acid

is a CALCIUM METABOLISM MODIFIER (a biphosphonate) used (as tiludronate disodium) for the HORMONE disorder Paget's disease of the bone. Administration is oral.
+ Side-effects: Stomach pain and nausea, diarrhoea; rarely dizziness, headache and skin reactions.
▲ Warning: Administer with caution to patients with certain kidney disorders. It should not be given to those who are pregnant or breast-feeding.
540 ○ Related entry: Skelid.

Timecef

(Roussel) is a proprietary, prescription-only preparation of the ANTIBACTERIAL and (CEPHALOSPORIN) ANTIBIOTIC cefodizime. It can be used to treat infections of the lower respiratory tract, such as pneumonia and bronchopneumonia, and of the urinary tract, including cystitis and pyelonephritis. It is available in a form for injection.
+▲ Side-effects/warning: See CEFODIZIME.

Timentin

(Beecham) is a proprietary, prescription-only COMPOUND PREPARATION of the ANTIBACTERIAL and (PENICILLIN) ANTIBIOTIC ticarcillin and the PENICILLINASE INHIBITOR clavulanic acid, which inhibits enzymes produced by some bacteria and thereby imparting *penicillinase-resistance* on ticarcillin. This combination can be used to treat serious infections that occur in patients whose immune systems are undermined by disease or drugs, and where the responsible micro-organism is resistant to ticarcillin alone. (Patients with such conditions are generally in hospital.) It is available in a form for injection or infusion.
+▲ Side-effects/warning: See TICARCILLIN.

Timodine

(Reckitt & Colman) is a proprietary, prescription-only COMPOUND PREPARATION of the CORTICOSTEROID hydrocortisone, the ANTIFUNGAL and ANTIBIOTIC nystatin and the ANTISEPTIC benzalkonium chloride. It can be used to treat fungal infections and mild skin inflammation, and is available as a cream for topical application.
+▲ Side-effects/warning: See BENZALKONIUM CHLORIDE; HYDROCORTISONE; NYSTATIN.

timolol maleate

is a BETA-BLOCKER which can be administered as an ANTIHYPERTENSIVE for raised blood pressure, as an ANTI-ANGINA treatment to relieve symptoms and improve exercise tolerance and as an ANTI-ARRHYTHMIC to regularize heartbeat and to treat and prevent myocardial infarction. It can also be used as an ANTIMIGRAINE treatment to prevent attacks. Administration is oral. Additionally, it can be administered as a GLAUCOMA TREATMENT and is administered as eye-drops. It is also available, as an antihypertensive, in the form of a COMPOUND PREPARATION with a DIURETIC.

✚▲ Side-effects/warning: See PROPRANOLOL HYDROCHLORIDE.

○ Related entries: Betim; Blocadren; Glaucol; Moducren; Prestim; Prestim Forte; Timoptol.

Timoptol

(Merck Sharp & Dohme) is a proprietary, prescription-only preparation of the BETA-BLOCKER timolol maleate. It can be used for GLAUCOMA TREATMENT, and is available as eye-drops (in *Ocumeter* units). Another eye-drop preparation, *Timoptol-LA*, is also available.

✚▲ Side-effects/warning: See TIMOLOL MALEATE.

Timpron

(Berk) is a proprietary, prescription-only preparation of the (NSAID) NON-NARCOTIC ANALGESIC and ANTIRHEUMATIC drug naproxen. It can be used to relieve the pain of various musculoskeletal disorders, particularly rheumatic and arthritic pain and acute gout. It is available as tablets.

✚▲ Side-effects/warning: See NAPROXEN.

Tinaderm Cream

(Schering-Plough) is a proprietary, non-prescription preparation of the ANTIFUNGAL drug tolnaftate. It can be used to treat athlete's foot, and is available as a cream.

✚▲ Side-effects/warning: See TOLNAFTATE.

Tinaderm Plus Powder

(Schering-Plough) is a proprietary, non-prescription preparation of the ANTIFUNGAL drug tolnaftate. It can be used to treat athlete's foot, and is available as a powder.

✚▲ Side-effects/warning: See TOLNAFTATE.

Tinaderm Plus Powder Aerosol

(Schering-Plough) is a proprietary, non-prescription preparation of the ANTIFUNGAL drug tolnaftate. It can be used to treat athlete's foot, and is available as a powder spray.

✚▲ Side-effects/warning: See TOLNAFTATE.

Tinaderm-M

(Schering-Plough) is a proprietary, prescription-only COMPOUND PREPARATION of the ANTIFUNGAL and ANTIBIOTIC nystatin and the antifungal tolnaftate. It can be used to treat *Candida* fungal infections of the skin and nails, and is available as a cream.

✚▲ Side-effects/warning: See NYSTATIN; TOLNAFTATE.

tinidazole

is an (AZOLE) ANTIMICROBIAL drug with ANTIBACTERIAL and ANTIPROTOZOAL properties. It can be used to treat anaerobic infections, such as bacterial vaginitis, and protozoal infections, such as giardiasis, trichomoniasis and amoebiasis. It can also be used to treat acute ulcerative gingivitis and to prevent infection following abdominal surgery. Administration is oral.

✚▲ Side-effects/warning: See METRONIDAZOLE.

○ Related entry: Fasigyn.

tinzaparin

is a LOW MOLECULAR WEIGHT HEPARIN. It has some advantages as an ANTICOAGULANT when used for long-term prevention of venous thrombo-embolism, particularly in orthopaedic use. Administration is by injection.

✚▲ Side-effects/warning: See HEPARIN.

○ Related entry: Innohep.

tioconazole

is an (AZOLE) ANTIFUNGAL drug which is administered in order to treat fungal infections of the nails. It is available as a lotion and a cream, which are applied to the nails and surrounding area.

T + Side-effects: There may be local irritation.
○ Related entry: Trosyl.

Tisept

(Seton) is a proprietary, non-prescription COMPOUND PREPARATION of the ANTISEPTICS chlorhexidine (as gluconate) and cetrimide. It can be used as a general skin disinfectant and as an antiseptic for cleaning wounds. It is available as a solution.
+▲ Side-effects/warning: See CETRIMIDE; CHLORHEXIDINE.

titanium dioxide

is a white pigment incorporated into several SUNSCREEN preparations. It provides some degree of protection from ultraviolet UVA and UVB radiation.
○ Related entries: Piz Buin SPF 20 Sun Block Lotion; Sun E45.

Tixylix Catarrh Syrup

(Intercare) is a proprietary, non-prescription preparation of the ANTIHISTAMINE diphenhydramine hydrochloride (with menthol). It can be used for the relief of catarrh and congestion. It is available as a syrup and is not normally given to children under one year, except on medical advice.
+▲ Side-effects/warning: See DIPHENHYDRAMINE HYDROCHLORIDE.

Tixylix Chesty Cough

(Intercare) is a proprietary, non-prescription preparation of the EXPECTORANT agent GUAIPHENESIN. It can be used for the relief of chesty coughs, sore throats and hoarseness. It is available as a linctus. It is not normally given to children under one year, except on medical advice.

Tixylix Cough and Cold

(Intercare) is a proprietary, non-prescription COMPOUND PREPARATION of the (OPIOID) ANTITUSSIVE pholcodine, the ANTIHISTAMINE chlorpheniramine maleate

and the SYMPATHOMIMETIC and DECONGESTANT pseudoephedrine hydrochloride. It can be used for the relief of dry, tickly coughs, runny nose and congestion. It is available as a syrup and is not normally given to children under one year, except on medical advice.
+▲ Side-effects/warning: See CHLORPHENIRAMINE MALEATE; PHOLCODINE; PSEUDOEPHEDRINE HYDROCHLORIDE.

Tixylix Daytime

(Intercare) is a proprietary, non-prescription preparation of the (OPIOID) ANTITUSSIVE pholcodine. It can be used for the symptomatic relief of tickly coughs without drowsiness. It is available as a linctus and is not normally given to children under one year, except on medical advice.
+▲ Side-effects/warning: See PHOLCODINE.

Tixylix Inhalant

(Intercare) is a proprietary, non-prescription COMPOUND PREPARATION of aromatic oils (TURPENTINE OILS, eucalyptus oil, CAMPHOR and MENTHOL). It can be used for the symptomatic relief of colds, catarrh, flu and hay fever. It is available as capsules that are sprinkled over bed linen or nightwear, or inhaled after being mixed with hot water. It is not normally given to children under three months, except on medical advice.

Tixylix Night-Time

(Intercare) is a proprietary, non-prescription COMPOUND PREPARATION of the (OPIOID) ANTITUSSIVE pholcodine and the ANTIHISTAMINE promethazine hydrochloride. It can be used for the sympomatic relief tickly coughs. It is available as a linctus and is not normally given to children under one year or over ten years, except on medical advice.
+▲ Side-effects/warning: See PHOLCODINE; PROMETHAZINE HYDROCHLORIDE.

Tobralex

(Alcon) is a proprietary, prescription-only

preparation of the ANTIBACTERIAL and (AMINOGLYCOSIDE) ANTIBIOTIC tobramycin. It can be used to treat bacterial infections of the eye, and is available as eye-drops.

✚▲ Side-effects/warning: See TOBRAMYCIN.

tobramycin

is an ANTIBACTERIAL and ANTIBIOTIC drug of the AMINOGLYCOSIDE group. It is effective against some Gram-positive and Gram-negative bacteria and is used primarily for the treatment of serious Gram-negative infections caused by *Pseudomonas aeruginosa*, because it is significantly more active against this organism than gentamicin (the most commonly used of this class of antibiotic). Like other aminoglycosides, it is not absorbed from the intestine (except in the case of local infection or liver failure) and so is administered by injection when treating systemic disease. It is also available as eye-drops to treat bacterial infections of the eye.

✚▲ Side-effects/warning: See GENTAMICIN.
⊘ Related entries: Nebcin; Tobralex.

tocainide hydrochloride

is an ANTI-ARRHYTHMIC drug that is an analogue of the LOCAL ANAESTHETIC drug LIGNOCAINE HYDROCHLORIDE. It can be used to treat heartbeat irregularities, but, because of its high incidence of blood toxicity, generally only when more common drugs have been found to be ineffective. Administration is oral.

✚ Side-effects: There may be nausea, vomiting and gastrointestinal disturbance; a number of blood disturbances, tremor and liver impairment; visual hallucinations and confusion; dizziness and loss of sensation can occur and may lead to convulsions.

▲ Warning: It should not be used in patients with heart block; and given with extreme caution to those with severely impaired liver or kidney function, heart failure or who are elderly or pregnant. Regular and frequent blood counts are essential.

⊘ Related entry: Tonocard.

tocopherol

(vitamin E) is a general name that is used to describe a group of substances known collectively as vitamin E. Good food sources include eggs, vegetable oils, wheat germ and green vegetables. Although deficiency is rare, it can be caused by malabsorption in conditions such as cystic fibrosis, abetalipoproteinaemia and chronic cholestasis. The form of tocopherol most used in therapy to make up vitamin deficiency is ALPHA TOCOPHERYL ACETATE. Administration is oral.

✚▲ Side-effects/warning: See ALPHA TOCOPHERYL ACETATE.
⊘ Related entry: Vitamin E Suspension.

tocopheryl acetate

see ALPHA TOCOPHERYL ACETATE

Tofranil

(Geigy) is a proprietary, prescription-only preparation of the (TRICYCLIC) ANTIDEPRESSANT imipramine hydrochloride. It can be used to treat depressive illness, particularly in patients who are withdrawn and apathetic, and may also be used to treat bed-wetting at night by children. It is available as tablets and a syrup.

✚▲ Side-effects/warning: See IMIPRAMINE HYDROCHLORIDE.

Tolanase

(Upjohn) is a proprietary, prescription-only preparation of the SULPHONYLUREA tolazamide. It is used in DIABETIC TREATMENT for Type II diabetes (non-insulin-dependent diabetes mellitus; NIDDM; maturity-onset diabetes), and is available as tablets.

✚▲ Side-effects/warning: See TOLAZAMIDE.

tolazamide

is a SULPHONYLUREA used in DIABETIC TREATMENT for Type II diabetes (non-insulin-dependent diabetes mellitus; NIDDM; maturity-onset diabetes). Administration is oral.

✚▲ Side-effects/warning: See GLIBENCLAMIDE.
⊘ Related entry: Tolanase.

T

tolbutamide

is a SULPHONYLUREA which is used in DIABETIC TREATMENT for Type II diabetes (non-insulin-dependent diabetes mellitus; NIDDM; maturity-onset diabetes). Administration is oral.

+▲ Side-effects/warning: See GLIBENCLAMIDE; but it may be used in renal impairment and the elderly.
✿ Related entry: Rastinon.

Tolectin

(Cilag) is a proprietary, prescription-only preparation of the (NSAID) NON-NARCOTIC ANALGESIC and ANTIRHEUMATIC tolmetin. It can be used to treat the pain and inflammation of rheumatic disease and other musculoskeletal disorders. It is available as capsules.

+▲ Side-effects/warning: See TOLMETIN.

tolmetin

is a (NSAID) NON-NARCOTIC ANALGESIC and ANTIRHEUMATIC drug. It is used to treat the pain of rheumatic disease and other musculoskeletal disorders in juvenile arthritis. Administration is oral.

+▲ Side-effects/warning: See NSAID.
✿ Related entry: Tolectin.

tolnaftate

is a mild ANTIFUNGAL drug which is used primarily in the topical treatment of infections caused by the tinea species (eg athlete's foot). Administration is by topical application

+▲ Side-effects/warning: Rarely, sensitivity reactions.

✿ Related entries: Mycil Athlete's Foot Ointment; Mycil Athlete's Foot Spray; Mycil Powder; Scholl Athlete's Foot Cream; Scholl Athlete's Foot Powder; Scholl Athlete's Foot Solution; Scholl Athlete's Foot Spray Liquid; Tinaderm Cream; Tinaderm Plus Powder; Tinaderm Plus Powder Aerosol; Tinaderm-M.

Tomudex

(Zeneca) is a proprietary, prescription-only preparation of the CYTOTOXIC drug raltitrexed. It is used as an ANTICANCER treatment for cancer of the colon, and is available in a form for injection.

+▲ Side-effects/warning: See RALTITREXED.

Tonocard

(Astra) is a proprietary, prescription-only preparation of the ANTI-ARRHYTHMIC drug tocainide hydrochloride. It can be used to correct heart irregularities, and is available as tablets.

+▲ Side-effects/warning: See TOCAINIDE HYDROCHLORIDE.

Topal

(Novex) is a proprietary, non-prescription COMPOUND PREPARATION of the ANTACIDS aluminium hydroxide and magnesium carbonate and the DEMULCENT agent ALGINIC ACID. It can be used to treat heartburn, severe indigestion and the symptoms of hiatus hernia. It is available as chewable tablets.

+▲ Side-effects/warning: See ALUMINIUM HYDROXIDE; MAGNESIUM CARBONATE.

Topamax

(Janssen-Cilag) is a proprietary, prescription-only preparation of the recently introduced ANTI-EPILEPTIC drug topiramate. It can be used in the treatment of partial seizures that are not satisfactorily controlled with other anti-epileptics. It is available as tablets.

+▲ Side-effects/warning: See TOPIRAMATE.

Topicycline

(Monmouth) is a proprietary, prescription-only preparation of the ANTIBACTERIAL and (TETRACYCLINE) ANTIBIOTIC tetracycline (as hydrochloride). It can be used to treat acne, and is available as a solution for topical application.

+▲ Side-effects/warning: See TETRACYCLINE.

topiramate

is a recently introduced ANTI-EPILEPTIC drug which is used in the treatment of partial seizures that are not satisfactorily controlled with other anti-epileptics. Administration is oral.

✚▲ Side-effects: Impaired gait, confusion, poor concentration and abnormal thinking; dizziness, fatigue and sleepiness; agitation, emotional instability, depression; loss of sensation in the extremities, effects on kidneys; also amnesia, anorexia, double vision and other eye disorders, nausea, speech disorders, taste alteration and loss of weight.

▲ Warning: It should not be administered to patients who are breast-feeding. Use with care in those who are pregnant or have kidney impairment. Withdrawal of treatment should be gradual.

◑ Related entry: Topamax.

Toradol

(Syntex) is a proprietary, prescription-only preparation of the (NSAID) NON-NARCOTIC ANALGESIC ketorolac trometamol. It can be used in the short-term management of moderate to severe acute postoperative pain, and is available as tablets and in a form for injection.

✚▲ Side-effects/warning: See KETOROLAC TROMETAMOL.

torasemide

is a powerful (*loop*) DIURETIC which can be used to treat oedema, particularly pulmonary (lung) oedema in patients with chronic heart failure, low urine production due to kidney failure (oliguria) and as an ANTIHYPERTENSIVE. Administration can be either oral or by injection or infusion.

✚▲ Side-effects/warning: See FRUSEMIDE. It should not be used by patients who are pregnant or breast-feeding.

◑ Related entry: Torem.

Torem

(Boehringer Mannheim) is a proprietary, prescription-only preparation of the (*loop*) DIURETIC torasemide. It can be used to treat oedema, particularly pulmonary (lung) oedema in patients with chronic heart

failure and low urine production due to kidney failure (oliguria). It is available as tablets and in a form for injection or infusion.

✚▲ Side-effects/warning: See TORASEMIDE.

toremifene

is a sex HORMONE ANTAGONIST, an ANTI-OESTROGEN. It antagonizes the natural oestrogen present in the body and is used in treating hormone-dependent metastatic breast cancer in postmenopausal women. Administration is oral.

✚▲ Side-effects/warning: See TAMOXIFEN. It is not to be administered to patients with severe liver impairment, endometrial hyperplasia or a history of thrombo-embolic disease.

◑ Related entry: Fareston.

Totamol

(CP) is a proprietary, prescription-only preparation of the BETA-BLOCKER atenolol. It can be used as an ANTIHYPERTENSIVE for raised blood pressure, as an ANTI-ANGINA treatment to relieve symptoms and improve exercise tolerance and as an ANTI-ARRHYTHMIC to regularize heartbeat and to treat myocardial infarction. It is available as tablets.

✚▲ Side-effects/warning: See ATENOLOL.

tracosactrin

(tetracosactide) is a synthetic HORMONE, an analogue of the pituitary hormone corticotrophin (ACTH), which acts on the adrenal glands to release corticosteroids, especially HYDROCORTISONE. It is used to test adrenal function. Administration is oral.

✚▲ Side-effects/warning: See CORTICOSTEROIDS. There is a risk of anaphylaxis.

◑ Related entries: Synacthen; Synacthen Depot.

Tracrium

(Wellcome) is a proprietary, prescription-only preparation of the (*non-depolarizing*) SKELETAL MUSCLE RELAXANT

T

atracurium besylate. It can be used to induce muscle paralysis during surgery, and is available in a form for injection.

+▲ Side-effects/warning: See ATRACURIUM BESYLATE.

Tramadol

(ASTA Medica) is a proprietary, prescription-only preparation of the (OPIOID) NARCOTIC ANALGESIC tramadol hydrochloride. It can be used to relieve pain, but seems to differ from typical opioids in its mode of action. It is available as capsules.

+▲ Side-effects/warning: See TRAMADOL HYDROCHLORIDE.

tramadol hydrochloride

is a recently introduced NARCOTIC ANALGESIC which is similar to morphine in relieving pain, but probably with fewer side-effects. However, there seem to be some differences in the mechanism by which it produces analgesia and it may not represent a typical OPIOID. Administration can be either oral or by injection.

+▲ Side-effects/warning: See OPIOIDS. Hypotension, hypertension and anaphylactic reactions have been reported. Administer with care to epileptics since convulsions have been reported. It should not be given to those who are pregnant or breast-feeding.

۞ Related entries: Tramadol; Tramake; Zydol.

Tramake

(Galen) is a proprietary, prescription-only preparation of the (OPIOID) NARCOTIC ANALGESIC tramadol hydrochloride. It can be used to relieve pain, but seems to differ from typical opioids in its mode of action, and is available as capsules.

+▲ Side-effects/warning: See TRAMADOL HYDROCHLORIDE.

tramazoline hydrochloride

is a SYMPATHOMIMETIC and VASOCONSTRICTOR drug which can be used as a NASAL DECONGESTANT to treat allergic rhinitis.

Administration is topical as an aerosol.

+▲ Side-effects/warning: See EPHEDRINE HYDROCHLORIDE.

۞ Related entry: Dexa-Rhinaspray.

Tramil 500 Analgesic Capsules

(Whitehall) is a proprietary, non-prescription preparation of the NON-NARCOTIC ANALGESIC and ANTIPYRETIC paracetamol. It can be used to treat many forms of pain, including headache, migraine, muscular pain and period pain, and also to relieve the symptoms of feverish colds and flu. It is available as tablets and is not normally given to children under 12 years, except on medical advice.

+▲ Side-effects/warning: See PARACETAMOL.

Trandate

(DF) is a proprietary, prescription-only preparation of the mixed BETA-BLOCKER and ALPHA-ADRENOCEPTOR BLOCKER labetalol hydrochloride. It can be used as an ANTIHYPERTENSIVE to reduce blood pressure, including in pregnancy, after myocardial infarction, in angina and during surgery. It is available as tablets and in a form for injection.

+▲ Side-effects/warning: See LABETALOL HYDROCHLORIDE.

trandolapril

is an ACE INHIBITOR and acts as a VASODILATOR. It can be used as an ANTIHYPERTENSIVE and often in conjunction with other classes of drug, particularly (THIAZIDE) DIURETICS. Administration is oral.

+▲ Side-effects/warning: See CAPTOPRIL.

۞ Related entries: Gopten; Odrik.

tranexamic acid

is an antifibrinolytic and HAEMOSTATIC drug which is used to stem bleeding in circumstances such as dental extraction in a haemophiliac patient or menorrhagia (excessive period bleeding). It works by inhibiting plasminogen, which is one of the blood's natural anticoagulant factors.

Administration can be either oral or by injection.

✚ Side-effects: There may be nausea and vomiting with diarrhoea; an injection may cause temporary giddiness.

▲ Warning: It should be administered with caution to those with impaired kidney function. Prolonged treatment requires regular eye checks and liver function tests.

○ Related entry: Cyklokapron.

tranquillizers ⊡

are drugs that calm, soothe and relieve anxiety, and many also cause some degree of sedation. Although it is somewhat misleading, they are often classified in two groups *major tranquillizers* and *minor tranquillizers*. The major tranquillizers, which are also called NEUROLEPTICS or ANTIPSYCHOTICS, are used primarily to treat severe mental disorders, such as psychoses (including schizophrenia and mania). They are extremely effective in restoring a patient to a calmer, less-disturbed state of mind. The hallucinations, both auditory and visual, the gross disturbance of logical thinking and to some extent the delusions typical of psychotic states are generally well controlled by these drugs. Violent, aggressive behaviour that presents a danger to the patients themselves and to those that look after them, is also effectively treated by major tranquillizers. For this reason they are often used in the *management* of difficult, aggressive, antisocial individuals. Major tranquillizers that are commonly administered include the PHENOTHIAZINE derivatives (eg CHLORPROMAZINE HYDROCHLORIDE, PROCHLORPERAZINE and THIORIDAZINE) and such drugs as FLUPENTHIXOL, FLUSPIRILENE and HALOPERIDOL. Minor tranquillizers are also *calming drugs*, but they are ineffective in the treatment of psychotic states. Their principal applications are as ANXIOLYTICS, HYPNOTICS and SEDATIVES. The best-known and most-used minor tranquillizers are undoubtedly the BENZODIAZEPINES (eg DIAZEPAM and CHLORDIAZEPOXIDE). However, prolonged treatment with minor tranquillizers can lead to dependence (addiction).

Transiderm-Nitro

(Geigy) is a proprietary, non-prescription preparation of the VASODILATOR and ANTI-ANGINA drug glyceryl trinitrate. It can be used to treat and prevent angina pectoris and to prevent phlebitis (inflammation in the veins). It is available as a self-adhesive dressing (patch), which, when placed on the chest, allows the drug to be absorbed through the skin (transdermally) to give lasting relief.

✚▲ Side-effects/warning: See GLYCERYL TRINITRATE.

Transvasin Heat Rub

(Seton) is a proprietary, non-prescription COMPOUND PREPARATION of the COUNTER-IRRITANT, or RUBEFACIENT, ethyl salicylate (with terahydrofurfuryl salicylate and hexyl nicotinate). It can be used for the symptomatic relief of muscular aches and pains, and is available as a cream for topical application to the skin.

✚▲ Side-effects/warning: See ETHYL SALICYLATE.

Transvasin Heat Spray

(Seton) is a proprietary, non-prescription COMPOUND PREPARATION of the COUNTER-IRRITANT, or RUBEFACIENT, methyl nicotinate (with terahydrofurfuryl salicylate and hexyl nicotinate). It can be used for the symptomatic relief of muscular aches and pains, and is available as a cream for topical application to the skin. It is not to be used on children under five years.

✚▲ Side-effects/warning: See METHYL NICOTINATE.

Tranxene

(Boehringer Ingelheim) is a proprietary, prescription-only preparation of the ANXIOLYTIC clorazepate dipotassium. It can be used principally for short-term treatment of anxiety, and is available as capsules.

T

+▲ Side-effects/warning: See CLORAZEPATE DIPOTASSIUM.

tranylcypromine

is an ANTIDEPRESSANT of the MONOAMINE-OXIDASE INHIBITOR (MAOI) class. It has, however, some STIMULANT effect and so is not as frequently used as other antidepressants. Administration is oral.
+▲ Side-effects/warning: See PHENELZINE; but do not use in patients with overactive thyroid secretion. It can cause hypertensive crisis, throbbing headache and insomnia (if taken in the evenings), but is less likely to cause liver damage.
✪ Related entries: Parnate; Parstelin.

Trasicor

(Ciba) is a proprietary, prescription-only preparation of the BETA-BLOCKER oxprenolol hydrochloride. It can be used as an ANTIHYPERTENSIVE for raised blood pressure, as an ANTI-ANGINA treatment to relieve symptoms and improve exercise tolerance and as an ANTI-ARRHYTHMIC to regularize heartbeat and to treat myocardial infarction. It can also be used as an ANXIOLYTIC, particularly for symptomatic relief of tremor and palpitations. It is available as tablets.
+▲ Side-effects/warning: See OXPRENOLOL HYDROCHLORIDE.

Trasidrex

(Ciba) is a proprietary, prescription-only COMPOUND PREPARATION of the BETA-BLOCKER oxprenolol hydrochloride and the (THIAZIDE) DIURETIC cyclopenthiazide. It can be used as an ANTIHYPERTENSIVE for raised blood pressure, and is available as tablets.
+▲ Side-effects/warning: See CYCLOPENTHIAZIDE; OXPRENOLOL HYDROCHLORIDE.

Trasylol

(Bayer) is a proprietary, prescription-only preparation of aprotinin, which is an antifibrinolytic drug used to prevent life-threatening bleeding, for instance, in open-heart surgery, removal of tumours and in surgical procedures in patients with certain blood disorders (hyperplasminaemias). It is available in a from for injection.
+▲ Side-effects/warning: See APROTININ.

Travasept 100

(Baxter) is a proprietary, non-prescription COMPOUND PREPARATION of the ANTISEPTICS cetrimide and chlorhexidine (as acetate). It can be used for cleaning wounds and burns, and is available as a solution.
+▲ Side-effects/warning: See CETRIMIDE; CHLORHEXIDINE.

Travogyn

(Schering) is a proprietary, prescription-only preparation of the ANTIFUNGAL drug isoconazole (as nitrate). It can be used in the treatment of fungal infections of the vagina, and is available as vaginal tablets (pessaries).
+▲ Side-effects/warning: See ISOCONAZOLE.

Traxam

(Lederle) is a proprietary, prescription-only preparation of felbinac (an active metabolite of fenbufen), which has (NSAID) NON-NARCOTIC ANALGESIC and COUNTER-IRRITANT, or RUBEFACIENT, actions. It can be used for the symptomatic relief of underlying muscle or joint pain, and is available as a foam or gel for topical application to the skin. A non-prescription version, *Traxam Pain Relief*, is now available. It is not normally used for children, except on medical advice.
+▲ Side-effects/warning: See FENBUFEN; but adverse effects on topical application are limited.

trazodone hydrochloride

is a TRICYCLIC-related ANTIDEPRESSANT which is used to treat depressive illness, particularly in cases where some degree of SEDATION is required. Administration is oral.
+▲ Side-effects/warning: See AMITRIPTYLINE HYDROCHLORIDE; but it has less ANTICHOLINERGIC actions. Occasionally, it

may cause prolonged penile erection (priapism).

○ Related entry: Molipaxin.

Trental

(Hoechst) is a proprietary, prescription-only preparation of the VASODILATOR oxpentifylline. It can be used to help improve blood circulation to the hands and feet when this is impaired, for example, in peripheral vascular disease (Raynaud's phenomenon). It is available as tablets.

✚▲ Side-effects/warning: See OXPENTIFYLLINE.

treosulfan

is a CYTOTOXIC drug which is used as an ANTICANCER treatment specifically of ovarian cancer. It works by interfering with the DNA of new-forming cells and so preventing cell replication. Administration can be either oral or by injection.

✚▲ Side-effects/warning: See CYTOTOXICS.

○ Related entry: Treosulfan.

Treosulfan

(Medac) is a proprietary, prescription-only preparation of the (CYTOTOXIC) ANTICANCER drug treosulfan. It can be used in the treatment of ovarian cancer, and is available as capsules and in a form for injection.

✚▲ Side-effects/warning: See TREOSULFAN.

tretinoin

is chemically a retinoid (a derivative of RETINOL, or vitamin A) and can be used to treat acne. Administration is by topical application.

✚ Side-effects: There may be irritation or skin peeling, redness, changes in skin pigmentation and sensitivity to light.

▲ Warning: It should not be applied to broken skin. It should be kept away from the eyes, mouth and mucous membranes. It is not to be used in combination with other keratolytics, or with sun-ray lamps. Do not use if pregnant, or where there is eczema or sunburned skin.

○ Related entry: Retin-A.

TRH

see PROTIRELIN

TRH-Cambridge

(Roche) is a proprietary, prescription-only preparation of the natural pituitary HORMONE thyrotrophin-releasing hormone (TRH or protirelin). It can be used primarily in diagnosing thryoid function in patients who suffer from over-activity of the thyroid gland (hyperthyroidism), or under-activity of the pituitary gland (hypopituitarism). It is available in a form for injection.

✚▲ Side-effects/warning: See PROTIRELIN.

Tri-Adcortyl

(Squibb) is a proprietary, prescription-only COMPOUND PREPARATION of the ANTI-INFLAMMATORY and CORTICOSTEROID triamcinolone acetonide, the ANTIBACTERIAL and ANTIBIOTIC drugs gramicidin and neomycin sulphate and the ANTIFUNGAL and antibiotic nystatin. It can be used for the treatment of various severe infective skin inflammation, such as eczema and psoriasis, especially in patients whose condition has not responded to less-powerful therapies. It is available as a cream and an ointment for topical application.

✚▲ Side-effects/warning: See GRAMICIDIN; NEOMYCIN SULPHATE; NYSTATIN; TRIAMCINOLONE ACETONIDE.

Tri-Adcortyl Otic

(Squibb) is a proprietary, prescription-only COMPOUND PREPARATION of the ANTI-INFLAMMATORY and CORTICOSTEROID triamcinolone acetonide, the ANTIBACTERIAL and ANTIBIOTIC drugs gramicidin and neomycin sulphate and the ANTIFUNGAL and antibiotic nystatin. It can be used for the treatment of severe infective inflammation of the outer ear, and is available as an ear ointment.

✚▲ Side-effects/warning: See GRAMICIDIN; NEOMYCIN SULPHATE; NYSTATIN; TRIAMCINOLONE ACETONIDE.

T

Tri-Minulet

(Wyeth) is a proprietary, prescription-only COMPOUND PREPARATION which can be used as a (*triphasic*) ORAL CONTRACEPTIVE (and for also certain menstrual problems) of the type that combines an OESTROGEN and a PROGESTOGEN, in this case ethinyloestradiol and gestodene. It is available as tablets in a calendar pack.

✚▲ Side-effects/warning: See ETHINYLOESTRADIOL; GESTODENE.

Triadene

(Schering) is a proprietary, prescription-only COMPOUND PREPARATION which can be used as a (*triphasic*) ORAL CONTRACEPTIVE (and also for certain menstrual problems) of the type that combines an OESTROGEN and a PROGESTOGEN, in this case ethinyloestradiol and gestodene. It is available as tablets in a calendar pack.

✚▲ Side-effects/warning: See ETHINYLOESTRADIOL; GESTODENE.

Triam-Co

(Baker Norton) is a proprietary, prescription-only COMPOUND PREPARATION of the (THIAZIDE) DIURETIC hydrochlorothiazide and the (*potassium-sparing*) diuretic triamterine (a combination called co-triamterzide 50/25). It can be used in the treatment of oedema and as an ANTIHYPERTENSIVE. It is available as tablets.

✚▲ Side-effects/warning: See HYDROCHLOROTHIAZIDE; TRIAMTERINE.

triamcinolone

is a synthetic CORTICOSTEROID with ANTI-INFLAMMATORY and ANTI-ALLERGIC properties. It is used to suppress the symptoms of inflammation, especially when it is caused by allergic disorders. Administration can be either oral or by injection.

✚▲ Side-effects/warning: See CORTICOSTEROIDS.

✪ Related entries: Ledercort; Pevaryl TC.

triamcinolone acetonide

is a synthetic CORTICOSTEROID with ANTI-INFLAMMATORY and ANTI-ALLERGIC properties. It is used to suppress the symptoms of inflammation, especially when it is caused by allergic disorders. It is sometimes administered as a systemic medication (in the form of an injection) to relieve conditions such as hay fever and asthma, but it is usually given by local injection to treat skin inflammation due to rheumatoid arthritis and bursitis. There are several proprietary cream preparations available that are mainly used to treat severe, non-infective skin inflammation, such as eczema, but one or two are used for treating inflammation in the mouth.

✚▲ Side-effects/warning: See CORTICOSTEROIDS. The type and severity of any side-effects depends on the route of administration.

✪ Related entries: Adcortyl; Adcortyl in Orabase;Adcortyl Intra-articular/Intradermal; Adcortyl with Graneodin; Audicort; Aureocort; Kenalog; Kenalog Intra-articular/Intramuscular; Nystadermal; Tri-Adcortyl; Tri-Adcortyl Otic.

triamcinolone hexacetonide

is a CORTICOSTEROID with ANTI-INFLAMMATORY and ANTI-ALLERGIC properties. It is used to suppress the symptoms of inflammation in soft tissues. Administration is by injection.

✚▲ Side-effects/warning: See CORTICOSTEROIDS.

✪ Related entry: Lederspan.

triamterene

is a mild DIURETIC of the *potassium-sparing* type and so causes the retention of potassium. It is therefore used as an alternative to or, more commonly, in combination with other diuretics that normally cause a loss of potassium from the body (such as the THIAZIDE and *loop* diuretics). It can be used to treat oedema, as an ANTIHYPERTENSIVE (in combination with other drugs) and in congestive HEART FAILURE TREATMENT.

✚ Side-effects: Gastrointestinal upsets, skin rashes, dry mouth, fall in blood pressure on standing and raised blood potassium. There are also reports of blood disorders and light-sensitivity.

▲ Warning: See AMILORIDE HYDROCHLORIDE. Blood tests for potassium and urea are required, particularly in the elderly or in patients with impaired kidney function. The urine may be coloured blue.

✪ Related entries: Dyazide; Dytac; Dytide; Frusene; Kalspare; Triam-Co.

triazoles 🛈

are members of a chemical family, a type of AZOLE, that includes the ANTIFUNGAL drugs FLUCYTOSINE and ITRACONAZOLE. They work by damaging the fungal cell membrane by inhibiting an enzyme called demethylase.

tribavirin

(ribavirin) is an ANTIVIRAL drug which inhibits a wide range of DNA and RNA viruses. It can be used to treat severe bronchiolitis caused by the syncytial virus in infants and certain other serious diseases (including lassa fever). It is administered by either nebulization or aerosol inhalation.

✚ Side-effects: Reticulocytosis and effects on the respiratory system.

▲ Warning: It should not be used during pregnancy.

✪ Related entry: Virazid.

Tribiotic

(3M) is a proprietary, prescription-only COMPOUND PREPARATION of the ANTIBACTERIAL and ANTIBIOTIC drugs neomycin sulphate, polymyxin B sulphate and bacitracin zinc. It can be used to treat infections of the skin, and is available as a spray.

✚▲ Side-effects/warning: See BACITRACIN ZINC; NEOMYCIN SULPHATE; POLYMYXIN B SULPHATE.

triclofos elixir

see TRICLOFOS ORAL SOLUTION, BP

Triclofos Oral Solution, BP

(triclofos elixir) is a non-proprietary, prescription-only preparation of the HYPNOTIC triclofos sodium. It is used to treat insomnia in children and the elderly, and is available as an elixir.

✚▲ Side-effects/warning: See TRICLOFOS SODIUM.

triclofos sodium

is used as a HYPNOTIC to treat insomnia. Administration is oral.

✚▲ Side-effects/warning: See CHLORAL HYDRATE; but with less stomach irritation.

triclosan

is an ANTISEPTIC agent which is used to prevent the spread of an infection on the skin. It is available as a hand rub and a powder to be added to a bath.

✚▲ Side-effects/warning: Avoid contact with the eyes.

✪ Related entries: Solarcaine; Ster-Zac Bath Concentrate.

tricyclics 🛈

are one of the three main, original classes of ANTIDEPRESSANT drugs that are used to relieve the symptoms of depressive illness. They are well established class of drugs, having been used for many years, but they do have SEDATIVE actions and many other side-effects. Since depression is commonly associated with loss of appetite and sleep disorders, an early benefit of tricyclic treatment may be an improvement of these symptoms. Some are also useful in the management of panic attacks and bed-wetting in children. Chemically, they are mainly dibenzazepine or dibenzcycloheptene derivatives and notable examples include AMITRIPTYLINE HYDROCHLORIDE, DOTHIEPIN HYDROCHLORIDE, DOXEPIN and IMIPRAMINE HYDROCHLORIDE. Some examples are chemically not tricyclics because they do not have the characteristic three-ringed structure, but are pharmacologically similar and so are often classed under this heading (eg MIANSERIN HYDROCHLORIDE). Treatment often takes some weeks to show maximal beneficial effects. Anxious or agitated patients respond

T

better to those tricyclics which have more pronounced sedative properties (eg amitriptyline and doxepin), whereas withdrawn patients are prescribed less-sedative tricyclics (eg imipramine). See AMITRIPTYLINE HYDROCHLORIDE for principal uses and side-effects.

Tridestra

(Sanofi Winthrop) is a proprietary, prescription-only COMPOUND PREPARATION of the female SEX HORMONES oestradiol (as valerate; an OESTROGEN) and medroxyprogesterone acetate (a PROGESTOGEN). It can be used to treat menopausal problems in HRT, and is available as tablets.
+▲ Side-effects/warning: See MEDROXYPROGESTERONE ACETATE; OESTRADIOL.

trientine dihydrochloride

is a CHELATING AGENT which is used to reduce the abnormally high levels of copper in the body that occur in Wilson's disease. It is given to patients who cannot tolerate the more commonly used PENICILLAMINE. Administration is oral.
+ Side-effects: Nausea.
▲ Warning: Administer with care to patients who are pregnant.
۞ Related entry: Trientine Dihydrochloride Capsules.

Trientine Dihydrochloride Capsules

(K & K-Greeff) is a proprietary, prescription-only preparation of the CHELATING AGENT trientine dihydrochloride. It can be used to reduce the abnormally high levels of copper in the body that occur in Wilson's disease. It is given to patients who cannot tolerate the more commonly used PENICILLAMINE, and is available as capsules.
+▲ Side-effects/warning: See TRIENTINE DIHYDROCHLORIDE.

trifluoperazine

is chemically a PHENOTHIAZINE derivative. It is used as a powerful ANTIPSYCHOTIC drug to treat and tranquillize psychotic patients (such as schizophrenics), particularly those experiencing some form of behavioural disturbance. It can also be used for the short-term treatment of severe anxiety and as an ANTI-EMETIC and ANTINAUSEANT for severe nausea and vomiting caused by underlying disease or drug therapies. Administration can be either oral or by injection.
+▲ Side-effects/warning: See CHLORPROMAZINE HYDROCHLORIDE; but with less sedation, hypotension, hypothermia and anticholinergic effects; though there is a greater frequency of various movement disturbances, including extrapyramidal symptoms (muscle tremor and rigidity).
۞ Related entries: Parstelin; Stelazine.

trifluperidol

is a powerful ANTIPSYCHOTIC drug which is used to treat and tranquillize psychotic patients (such as schizophrenics), particularly those experiencing manic, behavioural disturbances. Administration is oral.
+▲ Side-effects/warning: See HALOPERIDOL.
۞ Related entry: Triperidol.

Trifyba

(Sanofi Winthrop) is a proprietary, non-prescription preparation of the natural (*bulking-agent*) LAXATIVE bran (wheat fibre), and is available as a powder.
+▲ Side-effects/warning: See BRAN.

trihexyphenidyl hydrochloride

see BENZHEXOL HYDROCHLORIDE

triiodothyronine

(L-tri-iodothyronine; T_3) is the natural form of one of the two main THYROID HORMONES. Therapeutically, as liothyronine sodium, it is used to make up hormonal deficiency (hypothyroidism) and to treat associated symptoms (myxoedema). It may also be used in the treatment of goitre and thyroid cancer.

+▲ Side-effects/warning: See THYROXINE SODIUM.

Triiodothyronine

(Link) is a proprietary, prescription-only preparation of liothyronine sodium, which is a form of the THYROID HORMONE triiodothyronine. It can be used to make up hormonal deficiency (hypothyroidism) and to treat the associated symptoms. It is available in a form for injection.
+▲ Side-effects/warning: See LIOTHYRONINE SODIUM.

trilostane

is an ENZYME INHIBITOR which inhibits the production of both *glucocorticoid* and *mineralocorticoid* CORTICOSTEROIDS by the adrenal glands. It can therefore be used to treat conditions that result from the excessive secretion of corticosteroids into the bloodstream (such as Cushing's syndrome). It can also be used to treat postmenopausal breast cancer. Administration is oral.
+ Side-effects: Flushing, swelling and tingling of the mouth, congested nose, nausea, vomiting, diarrhoea; rarely, rashes and blood changes.
▲ Warning: It is not to be given to patients who are pregnant, breast-feeding or children; administer with caution to those with breast cancer (concurrent corticosteroids are required) or impaired liver or kidney function.
○ Related entry: Modrenal.

Triludan

(Hoechst Marion Rousell) is a proprietary, non-prescription preparation of the ANTIHISTAMINE terfenadine. It can be used to treat the symptoms of allergic disorders, such as hay fever and urticaria. It is available as tablets in two strengths (the stronger preparation is called *Triludan Forte*) and as a suspension for dilution.
+▲ Side-effects/warning: See TERFENADINE. Just prior to publication the Department of Health announced that it would be

reviewing whether terfenadine should become available only on prescription rather than OTC without a prescription. If you have any doubts about using this drug, consult your doctor.

TrimaxCo

(Ashbourne) is a proprietary prescription-only COMPOUND PREPARATION of the (*potassium-sparing*) DIURETIC triamterine and the (THIAZIDE) diuretic hydrochlorothiazide (a combination also called co-triamterzide 50/25). It can be used in the treatment of oedema and as an ANTIHYPERTENSIVE. It is available as tablets.
+▲ Side-effects/warning: See HYDROCHLOROTHIAZIDE; TRIAMTERINE.

trimeprazine tartrate

(alimemazine tartrate) is an ANTIHISTAMINE which is chemically a PHENOTHIAZINE derivative. It can be used to treat the symptoms of allergic disorders, particularly urticaria and pruritis. It also has SEDATIVE and ANTINAUSEANT properties and is used as a premedication prior to surgery. Administration is oral.
+▲ Side-effects/warning: See ANTIHISTAMINES. Because of its sedative property, the performance of skilled tasks, such as driving, may be impaired.
○ Related entry: Vallergan.

trimetaphan camsilate

see TRIMETAPHAN CAMSYLATE

trimetaphan camsylate

(trimetaphan camsilate) is a GANGLION-BLOCKER drug which lowers blood pressure by reducing vascular tone normally induced by the sympathetic nervous system. It is short-acting and can be used as a HYPOTENSIVE for controlled blood pressure during surgery. Administration is by injection or intravenous infusion.
+ Side-effects: There may be an increase in the heart rate and depression of respiration, increased intraocular pressure, dilated pupils and constipation.

T

▲ Warning: It should be administered with caution to patients with certain heart or kidney disorders, diabetes, Addison's disease, degenerative disease of the brain and in the elderly. It is not to be given to patients who are pregnant or with severe arteriosclerosis.
○ Related entry: Arfonad.

trimethoprim

is an ANTIBACTERIAL drug which is similar to the SULPHONAMIDES. It is used to treat and prevent the spread of many forms of bacterial infection, but particularly infections of the urinary and respiratory tracts. It has been used in combination with the sulphonamide SULPHAMETHOXAZOLE, because the combined effect is considered to be greater than twice the individual effect of either drug. This is the basis of the medicinal compound CO-TRIMOXAZOLE. More recently there has been a move away from the compound preparation to the use of trimethoprim alone. It is effective in many situations and lacks the side-effects of sulphamethoxazole. Administration can be either oral or by injection.
✚ Side-effects: There may be nausea, vomiting and gastrointestinal disturbances; rashes may break out with pruritus (itching) and there may be effects on blood constituents.
▲ Warning: It should not be administered to newborn babies; to patients who are pregnant; who have severely impaired kidney function or porphyria. Dosage should be reduced for patients with poor kidney function or who are breast-feeding. Prolonged treatment requires frequent blood counts.
○ Related entries: Bactrim; Chemotrim; Comixco; Comox; Fectrim; Ipral; Laratrim; Monotrim; Polytrim; Septrin; Trimogal; Trimopan; Triprimix.

trimetrexate

is a recently introduced ANTIPROTOZOAL drug. It is used to treat pneumonia caused by the protozoan micro-organism *Pneumocystis carinii* in patients whose immune system has been suppressed as in AIDS (normally where standard treatment is not appropriate). Administration is by injection.
✚ Side-effects: Diarrhoea, vomiting, mouth and gastrointestinal ulceration; changes in blood counts and salts including low haemoglobin; fever; confusion, rarely seizures, disturbed liver enzymes and blood electrolytes, rash and very rarely anaphylactic shock.
▲ Warning: It should not be administered to patients who are pregnant or breast-feeding, and (for men and women) avoid conception for at least six months after treatment. Administration requires concurrent use of calcium folinate and specialist monitoring.
○ Related entry: Neutrexin.

trimipramine

is an ANTIDEPRESSANT of the TRICYCLIC class. It is used to treat depressive illness, especially in cases where SEDATION is required. Administration is oral.
✚▲ Side-effects/warning: See AMITRIPTYLINE HYDROCHLORIDE.
○ Related entry: Surmontil.

Trimogal

(Lagap) is a proprietary, prescription-only preparation of the ANTIBACTERIAL drug trimethoprim. It can be used to treat infections of the upper respiratory tract (particularly bronchitis) and the urinary tract. It is available as tablets.
✚▲ Side-effects/warning: See TRIMETHOPRIM.

Trimopan

(Berk) is a proprietary, prescription-only preparation of the ANTIBACTERIAL drug trimethoprim. It can be used to treat infections of the upper respiratory tract (particularly bronchitis) and the urinary tract. It is available as a sugar-free suspension.
✚▲ Side-effects/warning: See TRIMETHOPRIM.

Trimovate

(Glaxo) is a proprietary, prescription-only COMPOUND PREPARATION of the CORTICOSTEROID clobetasone butyrate, the ANTIBACTERIAL and (TETRACYCLINE) ANTIBIOTIC drug oxytetracycline and the ANTIFUNGAL and antibiotic drug nystatin. It can be administered to treat various skin infections, and is available as a cream for topical application.
+▲ Side-effects/warning: See CLOBETASONE BUTYRATE; NYSTATIN; OXYTETRACYCLINE.

Trinordiol

(Wyeth) is a proprietary, prescription-only COMPOUND PREPARATION which can be used as a (*triphasic*) ORAL CONTRACEPTIVE (and also for certain menstrual problems) of the type that combines an OESTROGEN and a PROGESTOGEN, in this case it is a combination of ethinyloestradiol and levonorgestrel. It is available as tablets contained in a calendar pack.
+▲ Side-effects/warning: See ETHINYLOESTRADIOL; LEVONORGESTREL.

TriNovum

(Ortho) is a proprietary, prescription-only COMPOUND PREPARATION which can be used as a (*triphasic*) ORAL CONTRACEPTIVE (and also for certain menstrual problems) of the type that combines an OESTROGEN and a PROGESTOGEN, in this case ethinyloestradiol and norethisterone. It is available as tablets in a calendar pack.
+▲ Side-effects/warning: See ETHINYLOESTRADIOL; NORETHISTERONE.

TriNovum ED

(Ortho) is a proprietary, prescription-only COMPOUND PREPARATION which can be used as a (*triphasic*) ORAL CONTRACEPTIVE (and also for certain menstrual problems) of the type that combines an OESTROGEN and a PROGESTOGEN, in this case ethinyloestradiol and norethisterone. It is available as tablets in a calendar pack.
+▲ Side-effects/warning: See ETHINYLOESTRADIOL; NORETHISTERONE.

Triogesic Tablets

(Intercare) is a proprietary, non-prescription COMPOUND PREPARATION of the NON-NARCOTIC ANALGESIC paracetamol and the SYMPATHOMIMETIC and DECONGESTANT phenylpropanolamine hydrochloride. It can be used to treat nasal and sinus congestion and associated pain, and, unlike many decongestants, is available as tablets. It is not normally given to children under six years, except on medical advice.
+▲ Side-effects/warning: See PARACETAMOL; PHENYLPROPANOLAMINE HYDROCHLORIDE.

Triominic Tablets

(Intercare) is a proprietary, non-prescription COMPOUND PREPARATION of the SYMPATHOMIMETIC and VASOCONSTRICTOR phenylpropanolamine hydrochloride and the ANTIHISTAMINE pheniramine maleate. It can be used as a NASAL DECONGESTANT for the relief of nasal congestion and allergic rhinitis. It is available as tablets and is not normally given to children under six years, except on medical advice.
+▲ Side-effects/warning: See PHENIRAMINE MALEATE; PHENYLPROPANOLAMINE HYDROCHLORIDE.

Triperidol

(Lagap) is a proprietary, prescription-only preparation of the ANTIPSYCHOTIC drug trifluperidol. It can be used to treat psychotic patients (including schizophrenics), particularly those experiencing manic, behavioural disturbances, and is available as tablets.
+▲ Side-effects/warning: See TRIFLUPERIDOL.

tripotassium dicitratobismuthate

(bismuth chelate) is a CYTOPROTECTANT drug. It coats the mucosa of the stomach and can be used as an ULCER-HEALING DRUG for benign peptic ulcers in the stomach and duodenum. It may have a specific action on the bacterial organism *Helicobacter pylori*, which is associated with peptic ulcers.

Administration is oral.

✚ Side-effects: The compound may darken the tongue and the faeces and cause nausea and vomiting.

▲ Warning: It should not be given to patients with kidney impairment or who are pregnant.

✪ Related entries: De-Nol; De-Noltab.

Triprimix

(Ashbourne) is a proprietary, prescription-only preparation of the ANTIBACTERIAL trimethoprim. It can be used to treat infections of the upper respiratory tract (particularly bronchitis) and the urinary tract. It is available as tablets.

✚▲ Side-effects/warning: See TRIMETHOPRIM.

triprolidine hydrochloride

is an ANTIHISTAMINE which can be administered for the symptomatic relief of allergic symptoms, such as hay fever and urticaria. It is also used in some cough and decongestant preparations. Administration is oral.

✚▲ Side-effects/warning: See ANTIHISTAMINES. Because of its sedative property, the performance of skilled tasks, such as driving and operating machinery, may be impaired.

✪ Related entries: Actifed Compound Linctus; Actifed Expectorant; Actifed Junior Cough Relief; Actifed Syrup; Actifed Tablets.

Triptafen

(Forley) is a proprietary, prescription-only COMPOUND PREPARATION of the ANTIDEPRESSANT amitriptyline hydrochloride and the ANTIPSYCHOTIC perphenazine, in the ratio of 12.5:1. It can be used to treat depressive illness, particularly in association with anxiety, and is available as tablets. *Triptafen-M* is a similar preparation but with a lower proportion of amitriptyline hydrochloride (5:1).

✚▲ Side-effects/warning: See AMITRIPTYLINE HYDROCHLORIDE; PERPHENAZINE.

triptorelin

is an analogue of GONADORELIN (gonadothrophin-releasing hormone; GnRH), which is a hypothalamic HORMONE. On prolonged administration it acts as an indirect HORMONE ANTAGONIST in that it reduces the pituitary gland's secretion of gonadotrophin (after an initial surge), which results in reduced secretion of SEX HORMONES by the ovaries or testes. It can be used to treat endometriosis (a growth of the lining of the uterus at inappropriate sites) and is also used as an ANTICANCER drug for cancer of the prostate gland. Administration is by injection.

✚▲ Side-effects/warning: See BUSERELIN. There may also be transient hypertension, fatigue, phlebitis, peripheral oedema, fever, sweating, insomnia and effects on salivation. There may be irritation at the injection site.

✪ Related entry: De-capeptyl sr.

Trisequens

(Novo Nordisk) is a proprietary, prescription-only COMPOUND PREPARATION of the female SEX HORMONES oestradiol and oestriol (both OESTROGENS) and norethisterone (as acetate; a PROGESTOGEN). It can be used to treat menopausal problems, including in HRT. It is available as tabletsin a calendar pack and also in a higher strength form, *Trisequens Forte*.

✚▲ Side-effects/warning: See NORETHISTERONE; OESTRADIOL; OESTRIOL.

trisodium edetate

is a CHELATING AGENT that binds to calcium and forms an inactive complex. It can therefore be used as an ANTIDOTE to treat conditions in which there is excessive calcium in the bloodstream (hypercalcaemia), and can also be used in the form of a solution to treat calcification of the cornea, or lime burns, of the eye. Administration for treating hypercalcaemia is by intravenous infusion and for the eye it is by topical application as a solution.

✚ Side-effects: Nausea, diarrhoea and

cramps; pain in the limb where it is injected. An overdose may lead to kidney damage.

▲ Warning: Do not give to patients with impaired kidney function.

○ Related entry: Limclair.

Tritace

(Hoechst) is a proprietary, prescription-only preparation of the ACE INHIBITOR ramipril. It can be used as an ANTIHYPERTENSIVE and in HEART FAILURE TREATMENT, often in conjunction with other classes of drug, and is available as capsules.

✚▲ Side-effects/warning: See RAMIPRIL.

Trivax-AD

(Evans) is a proprietary, prescription-only version of the VACCINE preparation known as ADSORBED DIPHTHERIA, TETANUS AND PERTUSSIS VACCINE (DTPer/Vac/Ads), when supplied direct by District Health Authorities and which is commonly referred to as *triple vaccine*, because it combines the (*toxoid*) vaccines for diphtheria and pertussis (whooping cough) with the TETANUS VACCINE adsorbed onto a mineral carrier. It is available in a form for injection.

✚▲ Side-effects/warning: See DIPHTHERIA VACCINES; PERTUSSIS VACCINE; TETANUS VACCINE.

Trobicin

(Upjohn) is a proprietary, prescription-only preparation of the ANTIBACTERIAL and (AMINOGLYCOSIDE) ANTIBIOTIC spectinomycin. It is used specifically in the treatment of gonorrhoea in patients who are allergic to penicillins, or in cases resistant to penicillins. It is available in a form for injection.

✚▲ Side-effects/warning: See SPECTINOMYCIN.

tropicamide

is a short-acting ANTICHOLINERGIC drug, which can be used to dilate the pupil and paralyse the focusing of the eye for ophthalmic examination. Administration is topical as eye-drops.

✚▲ Side-effects/warning: See ATROPINE SULPHATE; but there should be few side-effects because of topical administration, apart from blurred vision. It should not be used in patients with raised intraocular pressure (pressure in the eyeball) .

○ Related entries: Minims Tropicamide; Mydriacyl; NODS Tropicamide.

tropisetron

is a recently introduced ANTI-EMETIC and ANTINAUSEANT drug. It gives relief from nausea and vomiting, especially in patients receiving radiotherapy or chemotherapy and where other drugs have been ineffective. It acts by blocking the action of the naturally occurring mediator SEROTONIN. Administration can be either oral or by injection

✚ Side-effects: Constipation, diarrhoea, abdominal pain, headache, fatigue and dizziness (which may impair the performance of skilled tasks, such as driving).

▲ Warning: Administer with care to patients with hypertension or who are pregnant or breast-feeding.

○ Related entry: Navoban.

Tropium

(DDSA) is a proprietary, prescription-only preparation of the BENZODIAZEPINE chlordiazepoxide. It can be used as an ANXIOLYTIC for the short-term treatment of anxiety and to alleviate acute alcohol withdrawal symptoms. It is available as capsules.

✚▲ Side-effects/warning: See CHLORDIAZEPOXIDE.

Trosyl

(Pfizer) is a proprietary, prescription-only preparation of the ANTIFUNGAL drug tioconazole. It can be used to treat fungal infections of the nails, and is available as a cream and a nail solution.

✚▲ Side-effects/warning: See TIOCONAZOLE.

Trusopt

(Merck Sharp & Dohme) is a proprietary, prescription-only preparation of the CARBONIC ANHYDRASE INHIBITOR dorzolamide. It is used in GLAUCOMA TREATMENT, and is available as eye-drops.

✚▲ Side-effects/warning: See DORZOLAMIDE.

Tryptizol

(Morson) is a proprietary, prescription-only preparation of the (TRICYCLIC) ANTIDEPRESSANT amitriptyline hydrochloride. It can be used in the treatment of depressive illness, especially in cases where a degree of sedation is required and appropriate, and also to prevent bed-wetting at night by children. It is available as tablets, as a sugar-free liquid for dilution and in a form for injection.

✚▲ Side-effects/warning: See AMITRIPTYLINE HYDROCHLORIDE.

tryptophan

is an amino acid present in an ordinary, well-balanced diet and from which the natural body substance serotonin (5-hydroxytryptamine; 5-HT) is derived. Dysfunction of serotonin, in its NEUROTRANSMITTER role in nerve-tracts in the brain, is thought to contribute to depression. Therapeutic administration of tryptophan has been used in ANTIDEPRESSANT treatment, but was withdrawn from use because of an association with a dangerous side-effect called eosinophilia-myalgia syndrome. It has been reintroduced for administration to patients only where no alternative treatment is suitable and with registration and constant blood-monitoring. Administration is oral.

✚ Side-effects: Light-headedness, drowsiness, headache, nausea, eosinophilia-myalgia syndrome.

▲ Warning: It should not be administered to patients known to have defective metabolism of tryptophan in the diet, or who have a history of eosinophilia-myalgia syndrome. Administer with caution to those

who are pregnant or breast-feeding.

⊙ Related entry: Optimax.

TSH

see THYROTROPHIN

Tub/Vac/BCG (Dried)

is an abbreviation for the freeze-dried version of BCG VACCINE (against tuberculosis), which is administered by intradermal injection. See also TUB/VAC/BCG (PERC).

Tub/Vac/BCG (Perc)

is an abbreviation for a VACCINE, the live version of BCG VACCINE (against tuberculosis) for *percutaneous* administration by multiple puncture of the skin. See TUB/VAC/BCG (DRIED).

tubocurarine chloride

is a *non-depolarizing* SKELETAL MUSCLE RELAXANT which is used to induce muscle paralysis during surgery. Administration is by injection.

✚ Side-effects: Histamine may be released, causing a rash on the chest and neck; there may be a fall in blood pressure.

Tuinal

(Lilly) is a proprietary, prescription-only COMPOUND PREPARATION of the BARBITURATES amylobarbitone (as sodium) and quinalbarbitone sodium, and is on the Controlled Drugs List. It can be used as a HYPNOTIC to treat persistent and intractable insomnia, and is available as tablets.

✚▲ Side-effects/warning: See AMYLOBARBITONE; QUINALBARBITONE SODIUM.

tulobuterol hydrochloride

is a SYMPATHOMIMETIC and BETA-RECEPTOR STIMULANT. It is mainly used as a BRONCHODILATOR in reversible obstructive airways disease and as an ANTI-ASTHMATIC treatment in severe acute asthma. It can also be used for the alleviation of symptoms of chronic bronchitis and emphysema. Administration is oral.

+▲ Side-effects/warning: See SALBUTAMOL. Avoid in pregnancy and certain kidney or liver disorders.
۞ Related entry: Respacal.

turpentine oil

is a COUNTER-IRRITANT, or RUBEFACIENT, agent. It is included in certain COMPOUND PREPARATIONS that are used for the symptomatic relief of pain associated with rheumatism, neuralgia, fibrosis and sprains and stiffness of the joints. It is also used, along with other constituents, as an inhalant in DECONGESTANT preparations for the relief of cold symptoms.
۞ Related entries: BN Liniment; Ellimans Universal Embrocation; Goddard's Embrocation; Mentholatum Deep Heat Rub; Secaderm; Tixylix Inhalant.

Tylex

(Cilag) is a proprietary, prescription-only COMPOUND ANALGESIC preparation of the (OPIOID) NARCOTIC ANALGESIC and ANTITUSSIVE codeine phosphate and the NON-NARCOTIC ANALGESIC paracetamol (a combination known as co-codamol 30/500). It can be used as a painkiller, and is available as capsules.
+▲ Side-effects/warning: See CODEINE PHOSPHATE; PARACETAMOL.

Typhim VI

(Merieux) is a proprietary, prescription-only VACCINE preparation of the typhoid vaccine, and is available in a form for injection.
+▲ Side-effects/warning: See TYPHOID VACCINE.

typhoid vaccine

is a suspension of dead typhoid bacteria. However, full protection is not guaranteed and travellers at risk are advised not to eat uncooked food or to drink untreated water. Administration can be either oral or by deep subcutaneous or intramuscular injection.
۞ Related entry: Typhim VI; Typhoid Vaccine.

Typhoid Vaccine

(Department of Health) is a non-proprietary, prescription-only VACCINE preparation of the typhoid vaccine, and is available in a form for injection.
+▲ Side-effects/warning: See TYPHOID VACCINE.

Tyrocane Junior Antiseptic Lozenges

(Seton) is a proprietary, non-prescription preparation of the ANTISEPTIC agent CETYLPYRIDINIUM CHLORIDE. It can be used for the relief of minor throat infections and is not normally given to children under six years, except on medical advice.
▲ Warning: See CETYLPYRIDINIUM CHLORIDE.

tyrothricin

is a weak ANTISEPTIC agent which is incorporated in some lozenges for sore throats.
۞ Related entry: Tyrozets.

Tyrozets

(Johnson & Johnson) is a proprietary, non-prescription COMPOUND PREPARATION of the ANTISEPTIC agent TYROTHRICIN and the LOCAL ANAESTHETIC benzocaine. It can be used to relieve minor mouth and throat irritations, and is available as lozenges. It is not normally given to children under three years, except on medical advice.
+▲ Side-effects/warning: See BENZOCAINE.

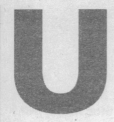

Ubretid

(Rhône-Poulenc Rorer) is a proprietary, prescription-only preparation of the ANTICHOLINESTERASE and PARASYMPATHOMIMETIC distigmine bromide. It can be used to stimulate bladder and intestinal activity and to treat myasthenia gravis. It is available as tablets.

✚▲ Side-effects/warning: See DISTIGMINE BROMIDE.

Ucerax

(UCB Pharma) is a proprietary, prescription-only preparation of the ANTIHISTAMINE hydroxyzine hydrochloride, which has some additional ANXIOLYTIC properties. It can be administered for the relief of allergic symptoms, such as itching and mild rashes, and also for short-term treatment of anxiety. It is available as tablets and a syrup.

✚▲ Side-effects/warning: See HYDROXYZINE HYDROCHLORIDE.

Ukidan

(Serono) is a proprietary, prescription-only preparation of the FIBRINOLYTIC urokinase. It can be used to treat such serious conditions as venous thrombi, pulmonary embolism, peripheral vascular occlusion, clots in the eye and myocardial infarction. It is available in a form for injection.

✚▲ Side-effects/warning: See UROKINASE.

Ulc-Aid Gel

(Seton) is a proprietary, non-prescription COMPOUND PREPARATION of the LOCAL ANAESTHETIC lignocaine hydrochloride and the ANTISEPTIC agent CETYLPYRIDINIUM CHLORIDE. It can be used for the temporary relief of the pain and discomfort caused by teething, denture irritation and mouth ulcers, and is available as a gel for topical application. It is not to be used for babies under three months.

✚▲ Side-effects/warning: See LIGNOCAINE HYDROCHLORIDE.

ulcer-healing drugs 🗗

are administered to promote healing of ulceration of the gastric (stomach) and duodenal (first part of small intestine) linings and so are used in the treatment of peptic ulcers. A number of classes of drugs may be used, including H_2-ANTAGONISTS (eg CIMETIDINE and RANITIDINE), PROTON-PUMP INHIBITORS (eg OMEPRAZOLE), selective ANTICHOLINERGIC drugs (eg PIRENZEPINE), PROSTAGLANDIN analogues (eg MISOPROSTOL), BISMUTH CHELATE compounds (eg TRIPOTASSIUM DICITRATOBISMUTHATE) and certain other drugs with poorly understood modes of action, including LIQUORICE derivatives (eg CARBENOXOLONE SODIUM). The first three classes act principally by reducing the secretion of peptic acid by the stomach's mucosal lining. The other drugs have complex actions that include a beneficial increase in blood flow to the mucosa, alterations in natural protective secretions, or antimicrobial actions against an infection by the bacterial organism *Helicobacter pylori*, which is associated with peptic ulcers. These classes may be combined in treatment, and RANITIDINE BISMUTH CITRATE combines two actions in one chemical compound. Other types of drug may reduce the discomfort of peptic ulcers without necessarily being ulcer-healing drugs (eg ANTACIDS and non-specific anticholinergics).

Ultec

(Berk) is a proprietary preparation of the H_2-ANTAGONIST and ULCER-HEALING DRUG cimetidine. It is available on prescription or without a prescription in a limited amount and for short-term uses only. It can be used to treat benign peptic ulcers (in the stomach or duodenum), gastro-oesophageal reflux, dyspepsia and associated conditions. It is available as tablets.

✚▲ Side-effects/warning: See CIMETIDINE.

Ultiva

(GlaxoWellcome) is a proprietary, prescription-only preparation of the (OPIOID) NARCOTIC ANALGESIC remifentanil (as hydrochloride). It can be used for the induction of anaesthesia and during surgery to supplement the effect of GENERAL ANAESTHETICS. It is available in a form for intravenous infusion.

✚▲ Side-effects/warning: See REMIFENTANIL.

Ultra Clearasil Maximum Strength

(Procter & Gamble) is a proprietary, non-prescription preparation of the KERATOLYTIC and ANTIMICROBIAL benzoyl peroxide (10%). It can be used to treat acne, spots and pimples, and is available as a cream for topical application.

✚▲ Side-effects/warning: See BENZOYL PEROXIDE.

Ultra Clearasil Regular Strength

(Procter & Gamble) is a proprietary, non-prescription preparation of the KERATOLYTIC and ANTIMICROBIAL benzoyl peroxide (5%). It can be used to treat acne, spots and pimples, and is available as a cream for topical application.

✚▲ Side-effects/warning: See BENZOYL PEROXIDE.

Ultralanum Plain

(Schering) is a proprietary, prescription-only preparation of the CORTICOSTEROID and ANTI-INFLAMMATORY fluocortolone (as fluocortolone hexanoate and fluocortolone pivalate). It can be used to treat various

severe, inflammatory skin disorders, such as eczema and psoriasis, and is available as a cream and an ointment for topical application.

✚▲ Side-effects/warning: See FLUOCORTOLONE.

Ultraproct

(Schering) is a proprietary, prescription-only COMPOUND PREPARATION of the CORTICOSTEROID and ANTI-INFLAMMATORY fluocortolone (as hexanoate) and the LOCAL ANAESTHETIC cinchocaine (as dibucaine hydrochloride). It can be used to treat haemorrhoids, and is available as an ointment and suppositories for topical application.

✚▲ Side-effects/warning: See CINCHOCAINE; FLUOCORTOLONE.

undecenoate

see UNDECENOIC ACID

undecenoic acid

and its salts (eg zinc undecenoate) have ANTIFUNGAL activity and are incorporated into a number of topical preparations for the treatment of fungal infections of the skin, particularly athlete's foot. Administration is by topical application.

○ Related entries: Ceanel Concentrate; Mycota Cream; Mycota Powder; Mycota Spray.

Unguentum Merck

(Merck) is a proprietary, non-prescription COMPOUND PREPARATION of LIQUID PARAFFIN, WHITE SOFT PARAFFIN and several other constituents. It can be used as an EMOLLIENT for dry skin and related disorders, and is available as a cream.

Unihep

(Leo) is a proprietary, prescription-only preparation of the ANTICOAGULANT heparin (as heparin sodium). It can be used to treat various forms of thrombosis, and is available in a form for injection.

✚▲ Side-effects/warning: See HEPARIN.

U

Uniparin
(CP) is a proprietary, prescription-only preparation of the ANTICOAGULANT heparin (as heparin sodium). It can be used to treat various forms of thrombosis, and is available in a form for injection.
✚▲ Side-effects/warning: See HEPARIN.

Uniparin Calcium
(CP) is a proprietary, prescription-only preparation of the ANTICOAGULANT heparin (as heparin calcium). It can be used to treat various forms of thrombosis, and is available in a form for injection.
✚▲ Side-effects/warning: See HEPARIN.

Uniphyllin Continus
(Napp) is a proprietary, non-prescription preparation of the BRONCHODILATOR theophylline. It can be used as an ANTI-ASTHMATIC and to treat bronchitis. It is available as modified-release tablets for prolonged effect and lower dose tablets for children.
✚▲ Side-effects/warning: See THEOPHYLLINE.

Uniroid-HC
(Unigreg) is a proprietary, prescription-only COMPOUND PREPARATION of the CORTICOSTEROID hydrocortisone and the LOCAL ANAESTHETIC cinchocaine. It can be used by topical application to treat haemorrhoids, and is available as an ointment and as suppositories.
✚▲ Side-effects/warning: See CINCHOCAINE; HYDROCORTISONE.

Unisept
(Seton) is a proprietary, non-prescription preparation of the ANTISEPTIC chlorhexidine (as gluconate). It can be used to clean wounds, and is available in sachets for making up into a solution.
✚▲ Side-effects/warning: See CHLORHEXIDINE.

Unisomnia
(Unigreg) is a proprietary, prescription-only preparation of the BENZODIAZEPINE nitrazepam. It can be used as a relatively long-acting HYPNOTIC for the short-term treatment of insomnia, where a degree of sedation during the daytime is acceptable. It is available as tablets.
✚▲ Side-effects/warning: See NITRAZEPAM.

Univer
(Rhône-Poulenc Rorer) is a proprietary, prescription-only preparation of the CALCIUM-CHANNEL BLOCKER verapamil hydrochloride. It can be used as as an ANTIHYPERTENSIVE and an ANTI-ANGINA drug in the prevention of attacks. It is available as modified-release capsules.
✚▲ Side-effects/warning: See VERAPAMIL HYDROCHLORIDE.

urea
is a chemical incorporated as a HYDRATING AGENT into a number of skin preparations; for example, creams that are used to treat eczema and psoriasis. It is also included in ear-drop preparations used for dissolving and washing out earwax.
✪ **Related entries: Alphaderm; Aquadrate; Calmurid; Calmurid HC; Exterol; Nutraplus; Otex Ear Drops.**

Uriben
(RP) is a proprietary, prescription-only preparation of the ANTIBACTERIAL and (QUINOLONE) ANTIBIOTIC nalidixic acid. It can be used to treat infections, particularly those of the urinary tract, and is available as an oral suspension.
✚▲ Side-effects/warning: See NALIDIXIC ACID.

Urispas
(Syntex) is a proprietary, prescription-only preparation of the ANTICHOLINERGIC drug flavoxate hydrochloride. It can be used as an ANTISPASMODIC in the treatment of urinary frequency and incontinence, and is available as tablets.
✚▲ Side-effects/warning: See FLAVOXATE HYDROCHLORIDE.

urofollitrophin

is a form of the pituitary HORMONE, FOLLICLE-STIMULATING HORMONE (FSH), which is also found in and can be prepared from urine from menopausal women. Urofollitrophin is used as an infertility treatment in women whose infertility is due to abnormal pituitary gland function, or who do not respond to the commonly used fertility drug CLOMIPHENE CITRATE. It is also used in superovulation treatment for assisted conception, such as in *in vitro* fertilization (IVF).

✚▲ Side-effects/warning: See HUMAN MENOPAUSAL GONADOTROPHINS.

✪ Related entries: Metrodin High Purity; Orgafol.

Urokinase

(Leo) is a proprietary, prescription-only preparation of the FIBRINOLYTIC drug urokinase. It can be used to treat such serious conditions as venous thrombi, pulmonary embolism, peripheral vascular occlusion, clots in the eye and myocardial infarction. It is available in a form for injection.

✚▲ Side-effects/warning: See UROKINASE.

urokinase

is an ENZYME which is used therapeutically as a FIBRINOLYTIC drug, because it has the property of breaking up blood clots by activating plasmin formation, which then digests the fibrin that forms the clot. It can be used rapidly in the treatment of such serious conditions as venous thrombi, pulmonary embolism, peripheral vascular occlusion and clots in the eye. Administration is by injection.

✚ Side-effects: Nausea, vomiting and bleeding.

▲ Warning: It should not be administered to patients with disorders of coagulation; who are liable to bleed (vaginal bleeding, peptic ulceration, recent trauma or surgery); acute pancreatitis, oesophageal varices or who are pregnant.

✪ Related entries: Ukidan; Urokinase.

Uromitexan

(ASTA Medica) is a proprietary, prescription-only preparation of the synthetic drug mesna. It is administered to combat haemorrhagic cystitis, which is a serious complication caused by certain CYTOTOXIC drugs. It is available as tablets and in a form for injection.

✚▲ Side-effects/warning: See MESNA.

ursodeoxycholic acid

is a drug which can dissolve some gallstones *in situ*. Administration is oral.

✚▲ Side-effects/warning: See CHENODEOXYCHOLIC ACID; though liver changes have not been reported and diarrhoea is rare.

✪ Related entries: Combidol; Destolit; Lithofalk; Ursofalk.

Ursofalk

(Thames) is a proprietary, prescription-only preparation of ursodeoxycholic acid. It can be used to dissolve gallstones, and is available as capsules.

✚▲ Side-effects/warning: See URSODEOXYCHOLIC ACID.

Utinor

(Merck Sharp & Dohme) is a proprietary, prescription-only preparation of the ANTIBACTERIAL and (QUINOLONE) ANTIBIOTIC drug norfloxacin. It can be administered to treat various infections, particularly of the urinary tract, and is available as tablets.

✚▲ Side-effects/warning: See NORFLOXACIN.

Utovlan

(Syntex) is a proprietary, prescription-only preparation of the PROGESTOGEN norethisterone. It can be administered to treat uterine bleeding, abnormally heavy menstruation, endometriosis, premenstrual tension syndrome and several other menstrual problems. It is available as tablets.

✚▲ Side-effects/warning: See NORETHISTERONE.

V

Uvistat

(Windsor) is the name of a range of proprietary, non-prescription SUNSCREEN preparations. The preparations contain TITANIUM DIOXIDE, ethylhexyl-methoxycinnaminate and avobenzone, which protect the skin from UVA and UVB ultraviolet radiation. They are available as skin creams (SPF30), a water-resistant cream (SPF20), babysun cream (SPF22) and as a lipscreen (SPF15). A patient whose skin condition requires one of these preparations may be prescribed it at the discretion of his or her doctor.

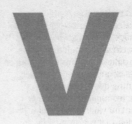

vaccines ▨

are preparations that are used for IMMUNIZATION, to confer what is known as *active immunity* against specific infections: that is, they cause a patient's own body to create a defence, in the form of antibodies, against the microbe or its toxic products. Vaccines can be one of three types. The first type of vaccines are those administered in the form of a suspension of *dead* viruses (eg INFLUENZA VACCINE) or bacteria (eg TYPHOID VACCINE). The second type may be *live* but weakened, or 'attenuated', viruses (eg RUBELLA VACCINE) or bacteria (eg BCG VACCINE). The third and final type of vaccines are *toxoids*, which are suspensions containing extracts of the toxins released by the invading organism, which then stimulate the formation of antibodies against the toxin of the disease, rather than the organism itself. Vaccines that incorporate dead micro-organisms or toxoids generally require a series of administrations (usually three) to build up a sufficient supply of antibodies in the body. 'Booster' shots may thereafter be necessary at regular intervals to reinforce immunity, for example, after ten years in the case of the tetanus vaccine. Vaccines that incorporate live micro-organisms may confer immunity with a single dose, because the organisms multiply within the body, although some live vaccines still require three administrations, for example, oral *poliomyelitis vaccine*.

✚ Side-effects: These range from little or no reactions to severe discomfort, high temperature and pain; a mild form of the disease (eg measles) and, rarely, anaphylactic shock.

▲ Warning: Vaccination should not be administered to patients who have a febrile (feverish) illness or any form of infection. Vaccines containing live material should not be administered routinely to patients who are pregnant, or who are known to have an immunodeficiency disorder.
○ Related entries: adsorbed diphtheria and tetanus vaccine; adsorbed diphtheria, anthrax vaccine; cholera vaccine; diphtheria vaccines; hepatitis B vaccine; measles vaccine; meningococcal polysaccharide vaccine; MMR vaccine; MR vaccine; pertussis vaccine; pneumococcal vaccine; poliomyelitis vaccine; rabies vaccine; smallpox vaccine; tetanus and pertussis vaccine; tetanus vaccine; yellow fever vaccine.

Vagifem
(Novo Nordisk) is a proprietary, prescription-only preparation of the female SEX HORMONE oestradiol (an OESTROGEN). It can be administered to treat conditions of the vagina caused by hormonal deficiency (generally, atrophic vaginitis in the menopause). It is available as vaginal tablets (pessaries) that come with disposable applicators.
✚▲ Side-effects/warning: See OESTRADIOL.

Vaginyl
(DDSA Pharmaceuticals) is a proprietary, prescription-only preparation of the ANTIMICROBIAL metronidazole, which has both ANTIPROTOZOAL and ANTIBACTERIAL properties. It can be used to treat a range of infections, including those that may occur following surgery, vaginosis and dental infections and ulcers. The antiprotozoal activity is effective against the organisms that cause amoebic dysentery, giardiasis and trichomoniasis. It is available as tablets.
✚▲ Side-effects/warning: See METRONIDAZOLE.

valaciclovir
is a pro-drug of aciclovir, an ANTIVIRAL drug. It can be used to treat herpes zoster and herpes simplex infections of the skin and mucous membranes (including initial and recurrent genital herpes). Administration is oral.
✚▲ Side-effects/warning: See ACICLOVIR; nausea and headache have been reported.
○ Related entry: Valtrex.

Valclair
(Sinclair) is a proprietary, prescription-only preparation of the BENZODIAZEPINE diazepam. It can be administered as an ANXIOLYTIC for the short-term treatment of anxiety, as a HYPNOTIC to relieve insomnia, as an ANTICONVULSANT and ANTI-EPILEPTIC for status epilepticus, as a SEDATIVE in preoperative medication, as a SKELETAL MUSCLE RELAXANT and to help alleviate alcohol withdrawal symptoms. It is available as suppositories.
✚▲ Side-effects/warning: See DIAZEPAM.

Valenac
(Shire) is a prescription-only, non-proprietary version of the (NSAID) NON-NARCOTIC ANALGESIC and ANTIRHEUMATIC diclofenac sodium. It can be used to treat arthritic and rheumatic pain and other musculoskeletal disorders. It is available as tablets.
✚▲ Side-effects/warning: See DICLOFENAC SODIUM.

Valium
(Roche) is a proprietary, prescription-only preparation of the BENZODIAZEPINE diazepam. It can be used as an ANXIOLYTIC for the short-term treatment of anxiety, as a HYPNOTIC to relieve insomnia, as an ANTICONVULSANT and ANTI-EPILEPTIC for status epilepticus, as a SEDATIVE in preoperative medication, as a SKELETAL MUSCLE RELAXANT and to help alleviate alcohol withdrawal symptoms. It is available as tablets, an oral solution and a form for injection.
✚▲ Side-effects/warning: See DIAZEPAM.

V

Vallergan
(Rhône-Poulenc Rorer) is a proprietary, prescription-only preparation of the ANTIHISTAMINE trimeprazine tartrate. It can be used to treat the symptoms of allergic disorders, particularly urticaria and pruritis. It also has SEDATIVE and ANTINAUSEANT properties and can be used for premedication prior to surgery. It is available as tablets and a syrup.
✚▲ Side-effects/warning: See TRIMEPRAZINE TARTRATE.

Valoid
(Wellcome) is a proprietary preparation of the ANTIHISTAMINE and ANTINAUSEANT drug cyclizine (as lactate). It can be administered to treat nausea, vomiting, vertigo, motion sickness and disorders of the balance function of the inner ear. It is available in two forms: without prescription as tablets; and in a form for injection only on prescription.
✚▲ Side-effects/warning: See CYCLIZINE.

valproic acid
see SODIUM VALPROATE

Valrox
(Shire) is a proprietary, prescription-only preparation of the (NSAID) NON-NARCOTIC ANALGESIC and ANTIRHEUMATIC naproxen. It can be used to relieve the pain of musculoskeletal disorders, particularly rheumatic and arthritic pain, and acute gout. It is available as tablets.
✚▲ Side-effects/warning: See NAPROXEN.

valsartan
is an ANGIOTENSIN-RECEPTOR BLOCKER, which is a fairly recently introduced class of drugs that work by blocking angiotensin receptors in the body. Angiotensin II is a circulating HORMONE that has powerful VASOCONSTRICTOR properties and so blocking its effects leads to a fall in blood pressure. Valsartan can therefore be administered as an ANTIHYPERTENSIVE treatment. Administration is oral.

✚▲ Side-effects/warning: See LOSARTAN POTASSIUM.
◉ Related entry: Diovan.

Valtrex
(Wellcome) is a proprietary, prescription-only preparation of the ANTIVIRAL drug valaciclovir, which is a pro-drug of acyclovir. It can be used to treat herpes zoster and herpes simplex infections of skin and mucous membranes (including initial and recurrent genital herpes).
Administration is oral.
✚▲ Side-effects/warning: See VALACICLOVIR.

Vancocin
(Lilly) is a proprietary, prescription-only preparation of the ANTIBACTERIAL and ANTIBIOTIC vancomycin (as hydrochloride). It can be used to treat certain infections, such as pseudomembranous colitis and certain types of endocarditis. It is available as capsules (*Matrigel*) and in a form for injection.
✚▲ Side-effects/warning: See VANCOMYCIN.

vancomycin
is an ANTIBACTERIAL and ANTIBIOTIC drug which is primarily active against Gram-positive bacteria and works by inhibiting the synthesis of components of the bacterial cell wall. It is only used in special situations, for example, in the treatment of pseudomembranous colitis (a superinfection of the gastrointestinal tract), which can occur after treatment with broad-spectrum antibiotics. Another use is in the treatment of multiple-drug-resistant staphylococcal infections, particularly endocarditis. Administration is oral to treat colitis and by infusion for systemic infections.
✚ Side-effects: These include kidney damage and tinnitus. There may be blood disorders, chills, fever, rashes and other complications.
▲ Warning: It should not be administered to patients with impaired kidney function, or who are deaf. Administer with caution to

patients who are pregnant or breast-feeding. Blood counts, kidney function tests and hearing tests are required.
○ Related entry: Vancocin.

Var/Vac

is an abbreviation for variola vaccine (in fact made from *vaccinia* virus). See SMALLPOX VACCINE.

varicella-zoster immunoglobulin (VZIG)

is a SPECIFIC IMMUNOGLOBULIN, which is a form of immunoglobulin that is used in IMMUNIZATION to give immediate *passive immunity* against infection by the varicella-zoster virus (chickenpox), but is used only in immunosuppressed patients at risk, including infants and pregnant women. (Varicella VACCINE is also available, but only on a 'named-patient' basis). Administration is by intramuscular injection.
✚▲ Side-effects/warning: See IMMUNIZATION.
○ Related entry: Varicella-Zoster Immunoglobulin (VZIG).

Varicella-Zoster Immunoglobulin (VZIG)

(Public Health Laboratory Service) (Antivaricella-Zoster Immunoglobulin) is a non-proprietary, prescription-only preparation of a SPECIFIC IMMUNOGLOBULIN and is used to give immediate immunity against infection by varicella-zoster (chickenpox) virus. Administration is by intramuscular injection.
✚▲ Side-effects/warning: See IMMUNIZATION.

Varidase Topical

(Lederle) is a proprietary, prescription-only preparation of the powdered ENZYMES streptokinase and streptodornase. It can be used, with a desloughing agent, to cleanse and soothe skin ulcers. It can also be administered through a catheter to dissolve clots in the urinary bladder. It is available as a powder.

✚▲ Side-effects/warning: See STREPTOKINASE.

Vascace

(Roche) is a proprietary, prescription-only preparation of the ACE INHIBITOR cilazapril. It can be used as an ANTIHYPERTENSIVE in conjunction with other classes of drug, particularly (THIAZIDE) DIURETICS, and is available as tablets.
✚▲ Side-effects/warning: See CILAZAPRIL.

Vaseline Dermacare

(Elida Gibbs) is a proprietary, non-prescription COMPOUND PREPARATION of WHITE SOFT PARAFFIN and dimethicone. It can be used as an EMOLLIENT for dry skin, eczema, scaly or itchy skin and related disorders. It is available as a cream and a lotion.
✚▲ Side-effects/warning: DIMETHICONE.

vasoconstrictors ?

are drugs that cause a narrowing (constricting) of the blood vessels and therefore a reduction in blood flow and an increase in blood pressure. They are used to increase blood pressure in circulatory disorders, in cases of shock or in cases where pressure has fallen during lengthy or complex surgery. Different vasoconstrictors work in different ways, but many are SYMPATHOMIMETICS with alpha-adrenoceptor stimulant properties. Most vasoconstrictors have an effect on mucous membranes and therefore may be used to relieve nasal congestion (eg OXYMETAZOLINE HYDROCHLORIDE and XYLOMETAZOLINE HYDROCHLORIDE). Some are used to prolong the effects of local anaesthetics (eg ADRENALINE). Vasoconstrictors used in circulatory shock include METHOXAMINE HYDROCHLORIDE, NORADRENALINE and PHENYLEPHRINE HYDROCHLORIDE.

vasodilators ?

are drugs that dilate blood vessels and thereby increase blood flow. Theoretically, they would be expected to be HYPOTENSIVE

V

and therefore could be used to lower blood pressure. However, in practice, there may be compensatory mechanisms that maintain blood pressure by redistributing blood within the body, or by changing heart function. Drugs of this class work in a number of different ways: some are SMOOTH MUSCLE RELAXANTS that act directly on the blood vessels (eg nitrite and nitrate compounds and CALCIUM-CHANNEL BLOCKERS); whereas others act indirectly by blocking or modifying the action of HORMONES or NEUROTRANSMITTERS (eg ALPHA-ADRENOCEPTOR BLOCKERS and ACE INHIBITORS). Vasodilator drugs are used for a number of purposes, including as ANTI-ANGINA drugs (eg GLYCERYL TRINITRATE), in acute hypertensive crisis (eg SODIUM NITROPRUSSIDE), as ANTIHYPERTENSIVES to treat chronic raised blood pressure (eg HYDRALAZINE HYDROCHLORIDE and NIFEDIPINE) and to treat poor circulation in the extremities (peripheral vascular disease, or Raynaud's Phenomenon: eg INOSITOL NICOTINATE).

Vasogen Cream

(Pharmax) is a proprietary, non-prescription COMPOUND PREPARATION of ZINC OXIDE, dimethicone and CALAMINE. It can be used for nappy rash, bedsores and the skin around a stoma (an outlet on the skin surface following surgical curtailment of the intestines). It is available as a cream.
✚▲ Side-effects/warning: See DIMETHICONE.

vasopressin

is one of the pituitary HORMONES secreted by the posterior lobe of the pituitary gland. It is also known as *antidiuretic hormone*, or ADH. Therapeutically, it is used mainly in pituitary-originated DIABETES INSIPIDUS TREATMENT, but it is a powerful VASOCONSTRICTOR and can also be used to treat bleeding from varices (varicose veins) of the oesophagus. There are several forms of vasopressin (DESMOPRESSIN, LYPRESSIN and TERLIPRESSIN), which all differ in their duration of action and uses. Administration can be either topical (for example, as a

nasal spray) or by injection.
✚ Side-effects: Peripheral vasoconstriction with pallor of skin; nausea, belching, abdominal cramps and an urge to defecate; hypersensitivity reactions, constriction of coronary arteries (possibly leading to angina and heart pain).
▲ Warning: Dosage should be adjusted to individual response in order to balance water levels in the body. Administer with great care to those patients patients with asthma, epilepsy, certain kidney disorders, migraine, heart failure, who are pregnant or have certain vascular disorders. Treatment must not be prolonged and should be carefully and regularly monitored; intermittent treatment is needed to avoid water overloading.
⊘ Related entry: Pitressin.

Vasoxine

(Wellcome) is a proprietary, prescription-only preparation of the SYMPATHOMIMETIC and VASOCONSTRICTOR methoxamine hydrochloride. It can be used to treat cases of acute hypotension, particularly where blood pressure has dropped because of induction of general anaesthesia, and is available in a form for injection or infusion.
✚▲ Side-effects/warning: See METHOXAMINE HYDROCHLORIDE.

Vectavir

(SmithKline Beecham) is a proprietary, prescription-only preparation of the ANTIVIRAL drug penciclovir. It can be used to treat herpes labialis, and is available in a cream for topical application.
✚▲ Side-effects/warning: See PENCICLOVIR.

vecuronium bromide

is a (*non-depolarizing*) SKELETAL MUSCLE RELAXANT which is used to induce muscle paralysis during surgery. Administration is by injection.
✚▲ Side-effects/warning: See TUBOCURARINE CHLORIDE; but it does not generally cause the release of histamine.
⊘ Related entry: Norcuron.

Veganin Tablets

(Warner Wellcome) is a proprietary, non-prescription COMPOUND ANALGESIC preparation of the NON-NARCOTIC ANALGESIC and ANTIRHEUMATIC drug aspirin, the non-narcotic analgesic and ANTIPYRETIC paracetamol and the (OPIOID) NARCOTIC ANALGESIC and ANTITUSSIVE codeine phosphate. It can be administered to treat the symptoms of flu, headache, rheumatism, toothache and period pain. It is available as tablets and is not to be given to children under 12 years, except on medical advice.

+▲ Side-effects/warning: See ASPIRIN; CODEINE PHOSPHATE; PARACETAMOL.

Veil

(Blake) is a proprietary, non-prescription preparation which is used to mask scars and other skin disfigurements. It is available as a cream and a powder and may be obtained on prescription under certain circumstances.

Velbe

(Lilly) is a proprietary, prescription-only preparation of the (CYTOTOXIC) ANTICANCER drug vinblastine sulphate. It can be used in the treatment of cancers, particularly lymphomas, acute leukaemias and some solid tumours. It is available in a form for injection.

+▲ Side-effects/warning: See VINBLASTINE SULPHATE.

Velosef

(Squibb) is a proprietary, prescription-only preparation of the ANTIBACTERIAL and (CEPHALOSPORIN) ANTIBIOTIC cephradine. It can be used to treat a wide range of bacterial infections, particularly streptococcal infections of the skin and soft tissues, the urinary and upper respiratory tracts and middle ear; and also to prevent infection during surgery. It is available as capsules, a syrup and in a form for injection.

+▲ Side-effects/warning: See CEPHRADINE.

Velosulin

(Novo Nordisk, Wellcome) is a proprietary form of highly purified porcine SOLUBLE INSULIN. It is used in DIABETIC TREATMENT for treating and maintaining diabetic patients, and is available in the form of vials for injection; it has a short duration of action.

+▲ Side-effects/warning: See INSULIN.

venlafaxine

is an ANTIDEPRESSANT of the SSRI group. It can be used to treat depressive illness and has the advantage over some other antidepressants in that it works by inhibiting uptake of the NEUROTRANSMITTERS SEROTONIN and NORADRENALINE and so has less sedative and ANTICHOLINERGIC side-effects. Administration is oral.

+▲ Side-effects/warning: See FLUOXETINE. There may also be changes in liver enzymes.

○ Related entry: Efexor.

Veno's Cough Mixture

(SmithKline Beecham) is a proprietary, non-prescription preparation of a syrup containing glucose and treacle. It is not normally given to children under three years, except on medical advice.

Veno's Expectorant

(SmithKline Beecham) is a proprietary, non-prescription preparation of the EXPECTORANT agent GUAIPHENESIN with glucose and treacle. It is not normally given to children under three years, except on medical advice.

Veno's Honey and Lemon

(SmithKline Beecham) is a proprietary, non-prescription preparation of a syrup containing lemon juice, honey and glucose. It is not normally given to children under one year, except on medical advice.

Ventide

(Allen & Hanburys) is a proprietary, prescription-only COMPOUND PREPARATION of the CORTICOSTEROID beclomethasone dipropionate and the SYMPATHOMIMETIC,

V

V

BRONCHODILATOR and BETA-RECEPTOR STIMULANT salbutamol. It can be used as a treatment for the symptomatic relief of obstructive airways disease, as an ANTI-ASTHMATIC and to treat chronic bronchitis. It is available as an aerosol inhalant.

✚▲ Side-effects/warning: See BECLOMETHASONE DIPROPIONATE; SALBUTAMOL.

Ventodisks

(Allen & Hanburys) is a proprietary, prescription-only preparation of the BETA-RECEPTOR STIMULANT salbutamol (as salbutamol sulphate). It can be used as a BRONCHODILATOR in reversible obstructive airways disease, as an ANTI-ASTHMATIC treatment in severe acute asthma and for the alleviation of the symptoms of chronic bronchitis and emphysema. It is available in the form of disks for use with the *Diskhaler* device.

✚▲ Side-effects/warning: See SALBUTAMOL.

Ventolin

(Allen & Hanburys) is a proprietary, prescription-only preparation of the BETA-RECEPTOR STIMULANT salbutamol (as salbutamol sulphate). It can be used as a BRONCHODILATOR in reversible obstructive airways disease, as an ANTI-ASTHMATIC treatment in severe acute asthma and for the alleviation of the symptoms of chronic bronchitis and emphysema. It is available in many forms: as tablets, a sugar-free syrup, ampoules for injection, an infusion fluid, an aerosol-metered inhalant, as ampoules for nebulization spray (under the name *Nebules*), as a respirator solution and as a powder for inhalation (under the name *Rotacaps*).

✚▲ Side-effects/warning: See SALBUTAMOL.

Vepesid

(Bristol-Myers) is a proprietary, prescription-only preparation of the (CYTOTOXIC) ANTICANCER drug etoposide. It can be used in the treatment of cancers, particularly lymphoma or small cell carcinoma of the bronchus or testicle. It is available as capsules and in a form for injection.

✚▲ Side-effects/warning: See ETOPOSIDE.

Veracur

(Typharm) is a proprietary, non-prescription preparation of the KERATOLYTIC agent formaldehyde. It can be used to treat warts, especially verrucas (plantar warts), and is available as a gel.

✚▲ Side-effects/warning: See FORMALDEHYDE.

verapamil hydrochloride

is a CALCIUM-CHANNEL BLOCKER which is used as an ANTI-ANGINA drug in the prevention and treatment of attacks, as an ANTI-ARRHYTHMIC to correct heart irregularities and as an ANTIHYPERTENSIVE. Administration can be either oral or by injection or infusion.

✚ Side-effects: There may be constipation, nausea and vomiting; headache, dizziness, flushing, fatigue; swollen ankles; rarely, there may be impairment of liver function; allergic skin reactions; gynaecomastia (enlargement of breasts in males); abnormal growth of the gums on prolonged treatment. After intravenous injection there may be a fall in blood pressure, a slowing of the heart, heart block or heart irregularities.

▲ Warning: It should not be taken by patients with certain heart disorders or porphyria. Administer with caution in patients with certain liver disorders or who are pregnant or breast-feeding.

✪ Related entries: Berkatens; Cordilox; Geangin; Half Securon SR; Securon; Securon SR; Univer.

Veripaque

(Sanofi Winthrop) is a proprietary, non-prescription preparation of the (*stimulant*) LAXATIVE oxyphenisatin. It can be used to promote bowel movement (for instance, before colonic surgery or a barium enema), and is available as an enema.

✚▲ Side-effects/warning: See OXYPHENISATIN.

Vermox

(Janssen) is a proprietary, prescription-only preparation of the ANTHELMINTIC drug mebendazole. It can be used to treat infections by roundworm, threadworm, whipworm and hookworm and similar intestinal parasites. It is available as chewable tablets and a liquid oral suspension.

✚▲ Side-effects/warning: See MEBENDAZOLE.

Verrugon

(Pickles) is a proprietary, non-prescription preparation of the KERATOLYTIC agent salicylic acid. It can be used to used to remove warts and hard skin, and is available as an ointment for topical application.

✚▲ Side-effects/warning: See SALICYLIC ACID.

Verucasep

(Galen) is a proprietary, non-prescription preparation of the KERATOLYTIC agent glutaraldehyde. It can be used to treat warts and to remove hard, dead skin. It is available as a gel for topical application to the skin.

✚▲ Side-effects/warning: See GLUTARALDEHYDE.

Vibramycin

(Invicta) is a proprietary, prescription-only preparation of the ANTIBACTERIAL and (TETRACYCLINE) ANTIBIOTIC drug doxycycline. It can be administered to treat an extensive range of infections, and is available as capsules.

✚▲ Side-effects/warning: See DOXYCYCLINE.

Vibramycin D

(Invicta) is a proprietary, prescription-only preparation of the ANTIBACTERIAL and (TETRACYCLINE) ANTIBIOTIC drug doxycycline. It can be administered to treat a wide range of infections, and is available as soluble tablets.

✚▲ Side-effects/warning: See DOXYCYCLINE.

Vicks Medinite

(Procter & Gamble) is a proprietary, non-prescription COMPOUND PREPARATION of the NON-NARCOTIC ANALGESIC and ANTIPYRETIC paracetamol, the ANTITUSSIVE and (OPIOID) NARCOTIC ANALGESIC dextromethorphan hydrobromide and the SYMPATHOMIMETIC and DECONGESTANT pseudoephedrine hydrochloride (with doxylamine succinate). It can be used for the symptomatic relief of colds and flu, and is available as a syrup. It is not normally given to children under ten years, except on medical advice.

✚▲ Side-effects/warning: See DEXTROMETHORPHAN HYDROBROMIDE; PARACETAMOL; PSEUDOEPHEDRINE HYDROCHLORIDE.

Vicks Original Cough Syrup (Chesty)

(Procter & Gamble) is a proprietary, non-prescription COMPOUND PREPARATION of the EXPECTORANT agent GUAIPHENESIN, the ANTISEPTIC agent CETYLPYRIDINIUM CHLORIDE (and sodium citrate). It can be used for relieving a productive cough and is available as a syrup. It is not normally given to children under six years, except on medical advice.

✚▲ Side-effects/warning: See SODIUM CITRATE.

Vicks Sinex Decongestant Nasal Spray

(Procter & Gamble) is a proprietary, non-prescription preparation of the SYMPATHOMIMETIC and VASOCONSTRICTOR oxymetazoline hydrochloride, along with MENTHOL and CINEOLE. It can be used as a NASAL DECONGESTANT for the symptomatic relief of nasal congestion associated with a wide variety of upper respiratory tract disorders, such as hay fever and colds. It is available as a nasal spray and is not normally given to children under six years, except on medical advice.

✚▲ Side-effects/warning: See OXYMETAZOLINE HYDROCHLORIDE.

V | Vicks Ultra Chloraseptic

(Procter & Gamble) is a proprietary, non-prescription preparation of the LOCAL ANAESTHETIC drug benzocaine, and can be administered for the short-term, symptomatic relief of a sore throat. It is available as a spray, and is not normally given to children under six years, except on medical advice.

✚▲ Side-effects/warning: See BENZOCAINE.

Vicks Vaposyrup for Chesty Coughs

(Procter & Gamble) is a proprietary, non-prescription preparation of the EXPECTORANT agent GUAIPHENESIN. It can be used for relieving coughs and to loosen the throat and is available as a syrup. It is not normally given to children under two years, except on medical advice.

Vicks Vaposyrup for Chesty Coughs and Nasal Congestion

(Procter & Gamble) is a proprietary, non-prescription COMPOUND PREPARATION of the SYMPATHOMIMETIC and DECONGESTANT phenylpropanolamine hydrochloride and the EXPECTORANT agent GUAIPHENESIN. It can be used for the short-term, symptomatic relief of nasal congestion and upper airways infections. It is available as a syrup and is not normally given to children under six years, except on medical advice.

✚▲ Side-effects/warning: See PHENYLPROPANOLAMINE HYDROCHLORIDE.

Vicks Vaposyrup for Dry Coughs

(Procter & Gamble) is a proprietary, non-prescription preparation of the (OPIOID) ANTITUSSIVE and NARCOTIC ANALGESIC dextromethorphan hydrobromide. It can be used for relieving and calming coughs and is available as a syrup. It is not normally given to children under six years, except on medical advice.

✚▲ Side-effects/warning: See DEXTROMETHORPHAN HYDROBROMIDE.

Vicks Vaposyrup for Dry Coughs and Nasal Congestion

(Procter & Gamble) is a proprietary, non-prescription preparation of the (OPIOID) ANTITUSSIVE and NARCOTIC ANALGESIC dextromethorphan hydrobromide and the SYMPATHOMIMETIC and DECONGESTANT phenylpropanolamine hydrochloride. It can be used for the symptomatic relief of short-term upper airways infections. It is available as a syrup and is not normally given to children under six years, except on medical advice.

✚▲ Side-effects/warning: See DEXTROMETHORPHAN HYDROBROMIDE; PHENYLPROPANOLAMINE HYDROCHLORIDE.

Videne

(DePuy) is a proprietary, non-prescription preparation of the ANTISEPTIC povidone-iodine. It can be used on the skin, and is available as a dusting powder.

✚▲ Side-effects/warning: See POVIDONE-IODINE.

Videx

(Bristol-Myers) is a proprietary, prescription-only preparation of the ANTIVIRAL drug didanosine. It can be used in the treatment of AIDS, and is available as tablets.

✚▲ Side-effects/warning: See DIDANOSINE.

Vidopen

(Berk) is a proprietary, prescription-only preparation of the broad-spectrum ANTIBACTERIAL and (PENICILLIN) ANTIBIOTIC ampicillin. It can be used to treat systemic bacterial infections, infections of the upper respiratory tract, of the ear, nose and throat and the urinogenital tracts. It is available as capsules.

✚▲ Side-effects/warning: See AMPICILLIN.

vigabatrin

is an ANTI-EPILEPTIC drug which is used to treat chronic epilepsy, especially in cases where other anti-epileptic drugs have not been effective. Administration is oral.

✚ Side-effects: There may be fatigue, dizziness, drowsiness, depression, headache, nervousness and irritability, confusion, aggression, memory, visual and gastrointestinal disturbances; weight gain; psychotic episodes and excitation and agitation in children.

▲ Warning: Administer with caution to patients with kidney impairment, or where there is a history of psychosis or behavioural problems.

○ Related entry: Sabril.

viloxazine hydrochloride

is a TRICYCLIC-related ANTIDEPRESSANT which has less SEDATIVE effects than many other antidepressants, and dosage must be carefully monitored to maintain the optimum effect for each patient. Administration is oral.

✚▲ Side-effects/warning: See AMITRIPTYLINE HYDROCHLORIDE; but it has less sedative, anticholinergic and cardiovascular actions. Headache and nausea may occur.

○ Related entry: Vivalan.

vinblastine sulphate

is a CYTOTOXIC drug and one of the VINCA ALKALOIDS. It can be used as an ANTICANCER treatment of acute leukaemias, lymphomas and some solid tumours. Administration is by injection.

✚▲ Side-effects/warning: See CYTOTOXICS.

○ Related entry: Velbe.

Vinca alkaloids 🔁

are a type of CYTOTOXIC drug derived from the periwinkle *Vinca rosea*. They work by halting the process of cell replication and are therefore used as ANTICANCER drugs, particularly for acute leukaemias, lymphomas and some solid tumours. Their toxicity inevitably causes some serious side-effects, in particular, some loss of neural nerve function at the extremities, constipation and bloating, all of which may be severe. See VINBLASTINE SULPHATE; VINCRISTINE SULPHATE; VINDESINE SULPHATE.

vincristine sulphate

is a CYTOTOXIC drug and one of the VINCA ALKALOIDS. It is used as an ANTICANCER drug, particularly in the treatment of acute leukaemias, lymphomas and some solid tumours. Administration is by injection.

✚▲ Side-effects/warning: See CYTOTOXICS. It causes little myelosuppression.

○ Related entry: Oncovin.

vindesine sulphate

is a CYTOTOXIC drug and one of the VINCA ALKALOIDS. It is used as an ANTICANCER drug, particularly in the treatment of leukaemias, lymphomas and some solid tumours. Administration is by injection.

✚▲ Side-effects/warning: See CYTOTOXICS.

○ Related entry: Eldisine.

Vioform-Hydrocortisone

(Zyma) is a proprietary, prescription-only COMPOUND PREPARATION of the CORTICOSTEROID hydrocortisone and the ANTIMICROBIAL clioquinol. It can be used to treat inflammatory skin disorders, and is available as a water-based cream and an ointment.

✚▲ Side-effects/warning: See CLIOQUINOL; HYDROCORTISONE.

Viraferon

(Schering-Plough) is a proprietary, prescription-only preparation of the IMMUNOMODULATOR interferon (in the form alpha-2b, rbe). It can be used in the treatment of chronic active hepatitis B and chronic hepatitis, and is available in a form for injection.

✚▲ Side-effects/warning: See INTERFERON.

Virazid

(Britannia) is a proprietary, prescription-only preparation of the ANTIVIRAL drug tribavirin. It can be used to treat severe bronchiolitis caused by the syncytial virus in infants and some other serious diseases (including lassa fever). It is available in a form for inhalation.

✚▲ Side-effects/warning: See TRIBAVIRIN.

V

Viridal

(Schwarz) is a PROSTAGLANDIN, alprostadil
(PGE$_1$). It is a recently introduced,
prescription-only treatment for men to
manage penile erectile dysfunction. It is
administered by intracavernosal injection
into the penis, and is available in a form for
injection.

+▲ Side-effects/warning: See ALPROSTADIL.

Virormone

(Paines & Byrne) is a proprietary,
prescription-only preparation of the male
SEX HORMONE testosterone (as testosterone
propionate). In men, it can be used in
hormone replacement therapy and for
delayed puberty; in women, as an
ANTICANCER drug for breast cancer. It is
available in a form for injection.

+▲ Side-effects/warning: See
TESTOSTERONE.

Visclair

(Sinclair) is a proprietary, non-prescription
preparation of the MUCOLYTIC and
EXPECTORANT methyl cysteine hydrochloride.
It can be used to reduce the viscosity of
sputum and thus facilitate expectoration in
patients with chronic asthma or bronchitis.
It is available as tablets.

+▲ Side-effects/warning: See METHYL
CYSTEINE HYDROCHLORIDE.

Viscotears

(CIBA Vision) is a proprietary, non-
prescription preparation of CARBOMER. It
can be used as artificial tears where there is
dryness of the eye due to disease (eg
ketanoconjunctivitis). It is available as a
liquid gel for application to the eye.

Viskaldix

(Sandoz) is a proprietary, prescription-only
COMPOUND PREPARATION of the BETA-BLOCKER
pindolol and the DIURETIC clopamide. It can
be used as an ANTIHYPERTENSIVE for raised
blood pressure, and is available as tablets.

+▲ Side-effects/warning: See CLOPAMIDE;
PINDOLOL.

Visken

(Sandoz) is a proprietary, prescription-only
preparation of the BETA-BLOCKER pindolol. It
can be used as an ANTIHYPERTENSIVE for
raised blood pressure and as an ANTI-ANGINA
treatment to relieve symptoms and improve
exercise tolerance. It can also be used as an
ANTIMIGRAINE drug to prevent attacks. It is
available as modified-release tablets.

+▲ Side-effects/warning: SEE PINDOLOL.

Vista-Methasone

(Daniels) is a proprietary, prescription-only
preparation of the CORTICOSTEROID and
ANTI-INFLAMMATORY betamethasone (as
sodium phosphate). It can be used to treat
inflammation in the ear, eye or nose, and is
available as drops.

+▲ Side-effects/warning: See
BETAMETHASONE.

Vista-Methasone-N

(Daniel) is a proprietary, prescription-
only COMPOUND PREPARATION of the
ANTI-INFLAMMATORY and CORTICOSTEROID
betamethasone (as sodium phosphate) and
the ANTIBACTERIAL and (AMINOGLYCOSIDE)
ANTIBIOTIC neomycin sulphate. It can be
used to treat inflammation in the ear, eye,
or nose, and is available as drops.

+▲ Side-effects/warning: See
BETAMETHASONE; NEOMYCIN SULPHATE.

vitamin A

is another term for RETINOL.

vitamin B

is the collective term for a number of water-
soluble vitamins, which are found
particularly in dairy products, cereals and
liver. See CYANOCOBALAMIN; FOLIC ACID;
NICOTINAMIDE; NICOTINIC ACID.

vitamin C

see ASCORBIC ACID

vitamin D

occurs in four main forms, D$_1$, D$_2$, D$_3$ and
D$_4$, which are produced in plants or in

human skin by the action of sunlight. Vitamin D facilitates the absorption of calcium and, to a lesser extent, phosphorus from the intestine and so promotes good deposition into the bones. A deficiency of vitamin D therefore results in bone deficiency disorders, such as rickets in children. It is readily available in a normal, well-balanced diet and particularly good sources include eggs, milk, cheese and fish-liver oil, which can be used as a dietary supplement. Vitamin D deficiency is commonly found in communities eating unleavened bread, in the elderly and where certain diseases prevent proper absorption from food. The preferred therapeutic method (despite the cost) of replacing vitamin D in cases of severe deficiency is by using quantities of one of the synthetic vitamin D analogues, such as ALFACALCIDOL, CALCITRIOL, DIHYDROTACHYSTEROL and ERGOCALCIFEROL. However, as with most vitamins, prolonged administration of large doses can produce adverse effects (hypervitaminosis).

✚ Side-effects: There may be nausea, vomiting, anorexia, lassitude, diarrhoea, weight loss, sweating, headache, thirst, dizziness and vertigo.

▲ Warning: An overdose may cause kidney damage. Calcium levels should be monitored and use with care in those who are breast-feeding (high levels of calcium may reach the baby).

vitamin E
see TOCOPHEROL

Vitamin E Suspension
(Cambridge) is a proprietary, prescription-only preparation of alpha tocopheryl acetate (a form of vitamin E). It can be used to treat vitamin E deficiency, and is available in the form of an oral suspension.

✚▲ Side-effects/warning: See ALPHA TOCOPHERYL ACETATE.

vitamin K
is a fat-soluble vitamin that occurs naturally in two forms, vitamin K_1 (also called PHYTOMENADIONE) and vitamin K_2 and is an essential requirement for a healthy body. Vitamin K_1 is found in food and particularly good sources include fresh root vegetables, fruit, seeds, dairy products and meat. Vitamin K_2 is synthesized in the intestine by bacteria and this source supplements the dietary form. Vitamin K is necessary for blood-clotting factors and is also important for the proper calcification of bone.

Both forms of the vitamin require the secretion of bile salts by the liver and fat absorption from the intestine in order to be taken up into the body. For this reason, when treating vitamin K deficiency due to malabsorption disorders (eg due to obstruction of the bile ducts or in liver disease) a synthetic form, vitamin K_3 (usually called MENADIOL SODIUM PHOSPHATE) is administered, because it is water-soluble and therefore effective when taken orally in such disease states. However, in adults, deficiency of vitamin K is rare because it is so readily available in a normal, balanced diet, but medical administration may be required in fat malabsorption states where the intestinal flora is disturbed by ANTIBIOTICS or certain ANTICOAGULANTS (eg nicoumalone). Vitamin K is given routinely to newborn babies to prevent vitamin-K-deficiency bleeding. Chronic overdose due to vitamin supplements (hypervitaminosis) can be dangerous.

✚ Side-effects: There may be liver damage if high doses are taken for a long period.

▲ Warning: It should be administered with caution to patients who are pregnant or susceptible to red-blood-cell haemolysis due to G6PD enzyme deficiency or vitamin E deficiency.

vitamins ▨
are substances required in small quantities for growth, development and proper functioning of the metabolism. Because many of the vitamins cannot be synthesized by the body, they must be obtained from a normal, well-balanced diet. The lack of any

V one vitamin causes a specific deficiency disorder, which may be treated by the use of vitamin supplements.

Vivalan

(Zeneca) is a proprietary, prescription-only preparation of the (TRICYCLIC-related) ANTIDEPRESSANT viloxazine hydrochloride. It can be used to treat depressive illness, particularly where a less SEDATIVE effect is required, and is available as tablets.
+▲ Side-effects/warning: See VILOXAZINE HYDROCHLORIDE.

Vividrin

(Novex) is a proprietary, prescription-only preparation of the ANTI-ALLERGIC drug sodium cromoglycate. It can be used to treat allergic conjunctivitis and is available as eye-drops, an eye ointment and a nasal spray. (It is available without a prescription subject to certain conditions of quantity and use.)
+▲ Side-effects/warning: See SODIUM CROMOGLYCATE.

Vivotif

(Evans) is a proprietary, prescription-only VACCINE preparation of typhoid vaccine as a *live* (attenuated) oral vaccine. It is available as capsules.
+▲ Side-effects/warning: See TYPHOID VACCINE.

Volital

(LAB) is a proprietary, prescription-only preparation of the weak STIMULANT pemoline. It can be used to treat hyperkinesis (hyperactivity) in children, and is available as tablets.
+▲ Side-effects/warning: See PEMOLINE.

Volmax

(DF) is a proprietary, prescription-only preparation of the BETA-RECEPTOR STIMULANT salbutamol (as salbutamol sulphate). It can be used as a BRONCHODILATOR in reversible obstructive airways disease, as an ANTI-ASTHMATIC treatment in severe acute asthma and for the alleviation of symptoms of chronic bronchitis and emphysema. It is available as tablets.
+▲ Side-effects/warning: See SALBUTAMOL.

Volraman

(Eastern) is a prescription-only non-proprietary version of the (NSAID) NON-NARCOTIC ANALGESIC and ANTIRHEUMATIC diclofenac sodium. It can be used to treat arthritic and rheumatic pain, other musculoskeletal disorders and acute gout. It is available as tablets.
+▲ Side-effects/warning: See DICLOFENAC SODIUM.

Voltarol

(Geigy) is a proprietary, prescription-only preparation of the (NSAID) NON-NARCOTIC ANALGESIC and ANTIRHEUMATIC diclofenac sodium. It can be used to treat arthritic and rheumatic pain and other musculoskeletal disorders. It is available as tablets, modified-release tablets (*Voltarol 75 mg SR*, *Voltarol Retard*), suppositories, paediatric suppositories and in a form for injection.
+▲ Side-effects/warning: See DICLOFENAC SODIUM.

Voltarol Emulgel

(Geigy) is a proprietary, prescription-only preparation of the (NSAID) NON-NARCOTIC ANALGESIC diclofenac sodium (as diethylammonium), which also has COUNTER-IRRITANT, or RUBEFACIENT, actions. It can be used for the symptomatic relief of underlying muscle or joint pain and is available as a gel for topical application to the skin. It is not normally used on children, except on medical advice.
+▲ Side-effects/warning: See DICLOFENAC SODIUM; but adverse effects on topical application are limited.

Voltarol Optha

(CIBA Vision) is a proprietary, prescription-only preparation of the (NSAID) NON-NARCOTIC ANALGESIC diclofenac sodium. It

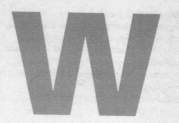

can be used by topical application to inhibit contraction of the pupil of the eye, and is available as eye-drops.

✚▲ Side-effects/warning: See DICLOFENAC SODIUM.

VZIG

see VARICELLA-ZOSTER IMMUNOGLOBULIN (VZIG)

warfarin sodium

is an ANTICOAGULANT which can be used to prevent clot formation in heart disease, after heart surgery (especially following implantation of prosthetic heart valves) and venous thrombosis and pulmonary embolism. Administration is oral.

✚ Side-effects: Haemorrhaging.

▲ Warning: It should be administered with care to patients with certain kidney or liver disorders and after recent operations. It should not be used by patients with severe hypertension, bacterial endocarditis, peptic ulcer or who are pregnant.

✪ Related entries: Marevan; Warfarin WBP.

Warfarin WBP

(Boehringer Ingelheim) is a proprietary, prescription-only preparation of the synthetic ANTICOAGULANT warfarin sodium. It can be used to prevent the formation of clots in heart disease, after heart surgery (especially following implantation of prosthetic heart valves) and venous thrombosis and pulmonary embolism. It is available as tablets.

✚▲ Side-effects/warning: See WARFARIN SODIUM.

Warticon

(Perstorp) is a proprietary, prescription-only preparation of the KERATOLYTIC agent podophyllotoxin. It can be used by topical application to treat and remove penile warts, and is available as a solution.

✚▲ Side-effects/warning: See PODOPHYLLUM.

W

Warticon Fem

(Perstorp) is a proprietary, prescription-only preparation of the KERATOLYTIC agent podophyllotoxin. It can be used to treat and remove warts on the external genitalia of women, and is available as a solution for topical application.

✚▲ Side-effects/warning: See PODOPHYLLUM.

Waxsol Ear Drops

(Norgine) is a proprietary, non-prescription preparation of docusate sodium. It can be used for the dissolution and removal of earwax, and is available as ear-drops.

✚▲ Side-effects/warning: See DOCUSATE SODIUM.

Welldorm

(Smith & Nephew) is a proprietary, prescription-only preparation of the HYPNOTIC drug chloral hydrate (in the form of chloral betaine). It can be used as a short-term treatment only of insomnia in children and the elderly, and is available as tablets and an elixir.

✚▲ Side-effects/warning: See CHLORAL HYDRATE.

Wellferon

(Wellcome) is a proprietary, prescription-only preparation of the IMMUNOMODULATOR interferon (in the form alpha-N1, lns). It can be used as ANTICANCER drug in the treatment of hairy cell leukaemia and chronic active hepatitis B. It is available in a form for injection.

✚▲ Side-effects/warning: See INTERFERON.

Wellvone

(Wellcome) is a proprietary, prescription-only preparation of the ANTIPROTOZOAL drug atovaquone. It can be used to treat pneumonia caused by the protozoan micro-organism *Pneumocystis carinii* in patients whose immune system has been suppressed. It is available as tablets.

✚▲ Side-effects/warning: See ATOVAQUONE.

white soft paraffin

is used as a base for ointments and is also incorporated into EMOLLIENT preparations.

✪ Related entries: E45 Cream; Lacri-Lube; Unguentum Merck; Vaseline Dermacare; Zinc and Salicylic Acid Paste, BP; zinc paste.

Whitfield's Ointment

see BENZOIC ACID OINTMENT, COMPOUND, BP

Windcheaters Capsules

(Seton) is a proprietary, non-prescription preparation of the ANTIFOAMING AGENT dimethicone (as simethicone). It can be used for the sympomatic relief of wind pains, flatulence and associated pain, and is available as capsules.

✚▲ Side-effects/warning: SeeDIMETHICONE.

wool alcohol

see WOOL FAT

wool fat

which contains lanolin, is a greasy preparation of hydrous wool fat in a yellow soft paraffin base. It is used as a protective BARRIER CREAM on cracked, dry or scaling skin and encourages hydration.

✚▲ Side-effects/warning: See LANOLIN. Local reactions may occur in sensitive people.

✪ Related entries: E45 Cream; Hewletts Cream; Massé Breast Cream; Panda Baby Cream & Castor Oil Cream with Lanolin; simple eye ointment; Sprilon.

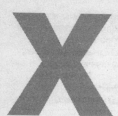

Xalatan

(Pharmacia; Upjohn) is proprietary prescription-only preparation of the PROSTAGLANDIN analogue latanoprost. It can be used as a GLAUCOMA TREATMENT in open-angle glaucoma and ocular hypertension, and is available as eye-drops.

+▲ Side-effects/warning: See LATANOPROST.

xamoterol

is a SYMPATHOMIMETIC and a weak BETA-RECEPTOR STIMULANT. It can be used as a CARDIAC STIMULANT in the treatment of heart conditions where moderate stimulation of the force of heartbeat is required, such as chronic moderate heart failure.
Administration is oral.

+ Side-effects: There may be headache, dizziness, hypotension and bronchospasm; there are some reports of palpitations and chest pains, rashes and cramps.

▲ Warning: It should not be given to patients with severe heart failure, who are breast-feeding or where certain other drugs are being used (especially cardiac glycosides and beta-receptor stimulant drugs for bronchoconstriction). Administer with caution in pregnancy, obstructive airways disease and certain heart and kidney disorders. Treatment will usually be initiated in hospital where full evaluation can be made.

✪ Related entry: Corwin.

Xanax

(Upjohn) is a proprietary, prescription-only preparation of the BENZODIAZEPINE alprazolam. It can be used as an ANXIOLYTIC for the short-term treatment of anxiety, and is available as tablets.

+▲ Side-effects/warning: See ALPRAZOLAM.

xanthine-oxidase inhibitors ▣

are ENZYME INHIBITORS which work by inhibiting the enzyme in the body that synthesizes uric acid and can therefore be administered in the treatment of gout (because gout is caused by the deposition of uric acid crystal in the tissues). The most commonly administered xanthine-oxidase inhibitor is ALLOPURINOL, which is administered for the long-term treatment of gout.

Xanthomax

(Ashbourne) is a proprietary, prescription-only preparation of the ENZYME INHIBITOR allopurinol, which is a XANTHINE-OXIDASE INHIBITOR. It can be used to treat excess uric acid in the blood and so prevent renal stones and attacks of gout. It is available as tablets.

+▲ Side-effects/warning: See ALLOPURINOL.

Xatral

(Lorex) is a proprietary, prescription-only preparation of the ALPHA-ADRENOCEPTOR BLOCKER drug alfuzosin. It can be used to treat urinary retention (eg in benign prostatic hyperplasia), and is available as tablets.

+▲ Side-effects/warning: See ALFUZOSIN.

xipamide

is a DIURETIC of the THIAZIDE-related class. It can be used as an ANTIHYPERTENSIVE (either alone or in conjunction with other drugs) and also in congestive HEART FAILURE TREATMENT and associated oedema.
Administration is oral.

+▲ Side-effects/warning: See BENDROFLUAZIDE. Also, there may be mild dizziness, gastrointestinal upsets and giddiness.

✪ Related entry: Diurexan.

Xylocaine

(Astra) is a series of proprietary, mainly prescription-only preparations of the LOCAL ANAESTHETIC lignocaine hydrochloride. They can be used for inducing anaesthesia or relieving pain by a variety of methods of application and at a number of sites. Some preparations include adrenaline as a SYMPATHOMIMETIC and VASOCONSTRICTOR. Solutions and forms for injection are available only on prescription (including dental cartridges); ointment, gel and spray preparations are available without prescription.

✚▲ Side-effects/warning: See LIGNOCAINE HYDROCHLORIDE.

Xylocard

(Astra) is a proprietary, prescription-only preparation of the LOCAL ANAESTHETIC lignocaine hydrochloride. It can be used as an ANTI-ARRHYTHMIC to treat irregularities in the heartbeat, especially after a heart attack, and is available in a form for injection.

✚▲ Side-effects/warning: See LIGNOCAINE HYDROCHLORIDE.

xylometazoline hydrochloride

is an alpha-adrenoceptor stimulant and SYMPATHOMIMETIC drug with VASOCONSTRICTOR properties, which is why it is mainly used as a NASAL DECONGESTANT. It is available as nose-drops and as a nasal spray, and is also a constituent of some eye-drop preparations that are used to treat allergic conjunctivitis.

✚▲ Side-effects/warning: See EPHEDRINE HYDROCHLORIDE.

✪ Related entries: Otrivine-Antistin; Otrivine Adult Formula Drops; Otrivine Adult Formula Spray; Otrivine Children's Formula Drops; Otrivine Menthol Nasal Spray; Otrivine Metered Dose Sinusitis Spray; Resiston One; Rynacrom Compound.

Xyloproct

(Astra) is a proprietary, prescription-only COMPOUND PREPARATION of the CORTICOSTEROID hydrocortisone and the LOCAL ANAESTHETIC lignocaine hydrochloride (with aluminium acetate). It can be used by topical application to treat haemorrhoids, and is available as an ointment and as suppositories.

✚▲ Side-effects/warning: See HYDROCORTISONE; LIGNOCAINE HYDROCHLORIDE.

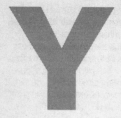

only preparation of the BETA-ADRENOCEPTOR STIMULANT drug ritodrine hydrochloride. It can be administered to prevent or delay premature labour, and is available either as tablets or in a form for intravenous infusion.

+▲ Side-effects/warning: See RITODRINE HYDROCHLORIDE.

Yel/Vac
is an abbreviation for YELLOW FEVER VACCINE.

yellow fever vaccine
(Yel/Vac) is a VACCINE administered for IMMUNIZATION that consists of a protein suspension which contains *live*, but weakened (attenuated), yellow fever viruses that have been cultured in chick embryos. Immunity lasts for at least ten years. The disease is still prevalent in parts of tropical Africa and northern South America. Administration is by subcutaneous injection.

+▲ Side-effects/warning: See VACCINES. It should not be administered to those who are pregnant.

◐ Related entry: Arilvax.

yellow soft paraffin
is used as a base for ointments and is also incorporated into many EMOLLIENT preparations, which are applied topically for the treatment of variety of skin conditions.

◐ Related entry: simple eye ointment.

Yomesan
(Bayer) is a proprietary, non-prescription preparation of the ANTHELMINTIC drug niclosamide. It can be used to treat infestation by tapeworms, and is available as chewable tablets.

+▲ Side-effects/warning: See NICLOSAMIDE.

Yutopar
(Duphar) is a proprietary, prescription-

581

Z

Zaditen

(Sandoz) is a proprietary, prescription-only preparation of ketotifen (as hydrogen fumarate). It can be used as an ANTI-ASTHMATIC treatment, and is available as capsules, tablets and an elixir.

+▲ Side-effects/warning: See KETOTIFEN.

Zadstat

(Lederle) is a proprietary, prescription-only preparation of the ANTIMICROBIAL drug metronidazole, which has ANTIPROTOZOAL and ANTIBACTERIAL properties. It can be used to treat anaerobic infections, including those that may occur following surgery, vaginitis, dental infections and mouth ulcers. The antiprotozoal activity is effective against the organisms that cause amoebic dysentery, giardiasis and trichomoniasis. It is available as tablets and suppositories.

+▲ Side-effects/warning: See METRONIDAZOLE.

Zagreb antivenom

is a prescription-only, non-proprietary ANTIVENOM preparation. It can be used as an ANTIDOTE to the poison from an adder's bite. However, the systemic effects of the venom are rarely serious enough to warrant the use of the antivenom. It is available in a form for injection.

+▲ Side-effects/warning: See ANTIVENOM.

zalcitabine

(ddC; DDC) is a (*reverse transcriptase inhibitor*) ANTIVIRAL drug which can be used as an AIDS treatment where

ZIDOVUDINE is not tolerated or has proven not to be beneficial. Administration is oral.

+ Side-effects: Peripheral neuropathy, nausea, vomiting, mouth ulcers, anorexia and weight loss; diarrhoea or constipation, abdominal pain; headache, dizziness and rash; mood changes and hearing and visual disorders, and other disorders.

▲ Warning: It should not be used in patients with peripheral neuropathy or who are breast-feeding. Administer with care where there is a history of pancreatitis, certain heart disorders or impaired liver or kidney function.

◐ Related entry: Hivid.

Zantac

(Glaxo), or Azantac, is a proprietary, prescription-only preparation of the H$_2$-ANTAGONIST and ULCER-HEALING DRUG ranitidine (as hydrochloride). It can be used to treat benign peptic ulcers (in the stomach or duodenum), gastro-oesophageal reflux, dyspepsia and associated conditions. It is available as tablets, effervescent tablets, a syrup and in a form for infusion or injection. (It is also available in limited amounts without prescription).

+▲ Side-effects/warning: See RANITIDINE.

Zantac 75

(Warner Wellcome) is a proprietary non-prescription preparation of the H$_2$-ANTAGONIST ranitidine (as hydrochloride). It can be used for the short-term relief of heartburn, dyspepsia and excess stomach acid. It is available as tablets.

+▲ Side-effects/warning: See RANITIDINE.

Zarontin

is a proprietary, prescription-only preparation of the ANTICONVULSANT and ANTI-EPILEPTIC drug ethosuximide. It can be used to treat absence (petit mal), myoclonic and some other types of seizure. It is available as capsules and a syrup.

+▲ Side-effects/warning: See ETHOSUXIMIDE.

Zavedos

(Pharmacia) is a proprietary, prescription-only preparation of the (CYTOTOXIC) ANTICANCER drug idarubicin hydrochloride. It can be used to treat various cancers, particularly leukaemias and breast cancer, and is available as capsules and in a form for injection.

✚▲ Side-effects/warning: See IDARUBICIN HYDROCHLORIDE.

Zerit

(Bristol-Myers) is a proprietary, prescription-only preparation of the ANTIVIRAL drug stavudine. It can be used in the treatment of AIDS, and is available as capsules.

✚▲ Side-effects/warning: See STAVUDINE.

Zestoretic

(Zeneca) is a proprietary, prescription-only COMPOUND PREPARATION of the ACE INHIBITOR lisinopril and the (THIAZIDE) DIURETIC hydrochlorothiazide. It can be used as an ANTIHYPERTENSIVE and is available as tablets in two strengths, *Zestoretic 10* and *Zestoretic 20*.

✚▲ Side-effects/warning: See HYDROCHLOROTHIAZIDE; LISINOPRIL.

Zestril

(Zeneca) is a proprietary, prescription-only preparation of the ACE INHIBITOR lisinopril. It can be used as an ANTIHYPERTENSIVE and in HEART FAILURE TREATMENT, and is available as tablets.

✚▲ Side-effects/warning: See LISINOPRIL.

zidovudine

(azidothymidine; AZT) is a (*reverse transcriptase inhibitor*) ANTIVIRAL drug which is used in the treatment of AIDS. Formerly, it was used for the treatment of advanced AIDS, but is now considered useful, by some, for the early forms of HIV virus infections before the full AIDS syndrome develops, including HIV-positive individuals who do not show symptoms of AIDS. It works by inhibiting the HIV virus replication and therefore delays progression of the disease, but does not cure it. Administration can be either oral or by intravenous infusion.

✚ Side-effects: There are many and may include disturbances in various blood cells, often to a degree requiring blood transfusions; nausea and vomiting, gastrointestinal disturbances, loss of appetite, headache, rashes, fever and sleep disturbances; abdominal pain, malaise, convulsions, pigmentation of the nails, skin and mouth.

▲ Warning: It should not be used where there is depression of neutrophils or haemoglobin, or when breast-feeding. Administer with care to those who are pregnant, have kidney or liver impairment, or are elderly. Avoid alcohol as its effects may be enhanced. Blood tests should be carried out.

○ Related entry: Retrovir.

Zimovane

(Rhône-Poulenc Rorer) is a proprietary, non-prescription preparation of the HYPNOTIC drug zopiclone. It can be used for the short-term treatment of insomnia, and is available as tablets.

✚▲ Side-effects/warning: See ZOPICLONE.

Zinacef

(Glaxo) is a proprietary, prescription-only preparation of the ANTIBACTERIAL and (CEPHALOSPORIN) ANTIBIOTIC cefuroxime. It can be used for bacterial infections and to prevent infection during and after surgery. It is available in a form for injection.

✚▲ Side-effects/warning: See CEFUROXIME.

Zinamide

(Merck Sharp & Dohme) is a proprietary, prescription-only preparation of the ANTIBACTERIAL pyrazinamide. It can be used as an ANTITUBERCULAR drug, usually in combination with other antitubercular drugs, and is available as tablets.

✚▲ Side-effects/warning: See PYRAZINAMIDE.

Z

Zinc and Salicylic Acid Paste, BP

(Lassar's paste) is a non-proprietary, non-prescription preparation of the ASTRINGENT agent ZINC OXIDE and the KERATOLYTIC salicylic acid, along with starch in WHITE SOFT PARAFFIN. It can be used in the treatment of psoriasis.

✚▲ Side-effects/warning: See SALICYLIC ACID.

zinc oxide

is a mild ASTRINGENT agent which is used primarily to treat skin disorders, such as nappy rash, urinary rash and eczema. It is available (without prescription) in any of a number of compound forms: as a cream with arachis oil, oleic acid and wool fat, or with ichthammol and wool fat; as an ointment and as an ointment with castor oil; as a dusting powder with starch and talc; as a paste with starch and white soft paraffin, or with starch and zinc and salicylic acid paste.

❂ Related entries: Anugesic-HC; Anusol; Anusol-HC; Caladryl Cream; Caladryl Lotion; Calamine Cream, Aqueous, BP; Germoline Ointment; Germoloids; Hemocane; Hewletts Cream; Morhulin Ointment; Panda Baby Cream & Caster Oil Cream with Lanolin; Sprilon; Ster-Zac Bath Concentrates; Sudocrem Antiseptic Cream; Vasogen Cream; Zinc and Salicylic Acid Paste, BP; zinc paste.

zinc paste

is a non-proprietary, ASTRINGENT compound made up of ZINC OXIDE and WHITE SOFT PARAFFIN (and starch). It is used as a base to which other active constituents can be added, especially within impregnated bandages. Of all such pastes that are compounded to treat and protect the lesions of skin diseases, such as eczema and psoriasis, zinc paste is the standard type. There are also pastes combining other active substances, including *zinc and ichthammol cream* and ZINC AND SALICYLIC ACID PASTE, BP.

zinc sulphate

is one form in which zinc supplements can be administered in order to make up a zinc deficiency in the body. There are several proprietary preparations that are all different in form, though all are adminsitered orally. In solution, zinc sulphate is also used as an ASTRINGENT and wound cleanser and also in eye-drops.

✚ Side-effects: There may be abdominal pain or mild gastrointestinal upsets.

❂ Related entries: Efalith; Sootheye.

zinc undecenoate

see UNDECENOIC ACID

Zineryt

(Yamanouchi) is a proprietary, prescription-only preparation of the ANTIBACTERIAL and (MACROLIDE) ANTIBIOTIC erythromycin. It can be used to treat acne, and is available as a solution for topical application.

✚▲ Side-effects/warning: See ERYTHROMYCIN.

Zinnat

(Glaxo) is a proprietary, prescription-only preparation of the ANTIBACTERIAL and (CEPHALOSPORIN) ANTIBIOTIC cefuroxime. It can be used to treat bacterial infections and to prevent infection during and following surgery. It is available as tablets, sachets and an oral suspension.

✚▲ Side-effects/warning: See CEFUROXIME.

Zirtek

(UCB Pharma) is a proprietary, prescription-only preparation of the ANTIHISTAMINE cetirizine. It can be used to treat the symptoms of allergic disorders, such as hay fever and urticaria, and is available as tablets and an oral solution.

✚▲ Side-effects/warning: See CETIRIZINE.

Zita

(Eastern) is a proprietary preparation of the H_2-ANTAGONIST and ULCER-HEALING DRUG cimetidine. It is available on prescription or without a prescription in a limited amount and for short-term uses only. It can be used to treat benign peptic ulcers (in the stomach or duodenum), gastro-oesophageal reflux, dyspepsia and associated conditions. It is available as tablets.

➕▲ Side-effects/warning: See CIMETIDINE.

Zithromax

(Richborough) is a proprietary, prescription-only preparation of the ANTIBACTERIAL and (MACROLIDE) ANTIBIOTIC azithromycin. It can be used to treat and prevent many forms of infection and is usually used as an alternative to penicillin-type antibiotics in patients who are allergic to penicillin, or whose infections are resistant to penicillin. It is available as capsules and an oral suspension.

➕▲ Side-effects/warning: See AZITHROMYCIN.

Zocor

(Merck Sharp & Dohme) is a proprietary, prescription-only preparation of the LIPID-LOWERING DRUG simvastatin. It can be used in hyperlipidaemia to reduce the levels, or change the proportions, of various lipids in the bloodstream. It is available as tablets.

➕▲ Side-effects/warning: See SIMVASTATIN.

Zofran

(Glaxo) is a proprietary, prescription-only preparation of the ANTI-EMETIC and ANTINAUSEANT ondansetron. It can be used to give relief from nausea and vomiting, especially in patients receiving radiotherapy or chemotherapy and where other drugs are ineffective. It is available as tablets or in a form for intravenous injection or infusion.

➕▲ Side-effects/warning: See ONDANSETRON.

Zoladex

(Zeneca) is a proprietary, prescription-only preparation of goserelin, which is an analogue of the pituitary HORMONE gonadortelin. It can be used as an

ANTICANCER drug for cancer of the prostate gland, breast and for uterine endometriosis. It is available in a form for implantation into the abdominal wall (with a syringe supplied).

➕▲ Side-effects/warning: See GOSERELIN.

zolpidem tartrate

is a newly introduced HYPNOTIC drug which works in the same way as the BENZODIAZEPINES. It can be used for the short-term treatment of insomnia. Administration is oral.

➕ Side-effects: Diarrhoea, nausea, vomiting, dizziness, vertigo, headache, drowsiness during the day, memory disturbances, nocturnal restlessness, nightmares, confusion, depression, double vision and other visual disturbances, tremor, unsteady gait and falls.

▲ Warning: It should not be administered to patients with pulmonary insufficiency, respiratory depression, severe liver impairment, myasthenia gravis or who are pregnant or breast-feedings. Administer with care to those with depression, a history of alcohol or drug abuse, or liver or kidney disorders. Drowsiness may impair the performance of skilled tasks, eg driving.

⊕ Related entry: Stilnoct.

Zomacton

(Ferring) is a proprietary, prescription-only preparation of somatropin, which is the biosynthetic form of the pituitary HORMONE human growth hormone. It can be used to treat hormonal deficiency and associated symptoms (in particular, short stature). It is available in a form for injection.

➕▲ Side-effects/warning: See SOMATROPIN.

Zonulysin

(Henleys) is a proprietary, prescription-only preparation of the ENZYME CHYMOTRYPSIN. It can be used to dissolve a suspensory ligament of the lens of the eye to aid surgical remove of the lens because of a cataract. It is available in a form for injection.

Z

Zopiclone
(Lagap) is a proprietary, non-prescription preparation of the HYPNOTIC drug zopiclone. It can be used for the short-term treatment of insomnia, and is available as tablets.
✚▲ Side-effects/warning: See ZOPICLONE.

zopiclone
is a newly introduced HYPNOTIC drug which works in the same way as the BENZODIAZEPINES. It can be used for the short-term treatment of insomnia. Administration is oral.
✚ Side-effects: Nausea, vomiting, gastrointestinal disturbances, a bitter or metallic taste in the mouth, drowsiness, light-headedness and affects coordination the next day, dizziness, depression, sensitivity reactions, including rashes; amnesia, hallucinations, irritability and behavioural disturbances, including aggression.
▲ Warning: Administer with care to patients with liver impairment, psychiatric disorders, who have a history of drug abuse or who are pregnant or breast-feeding. Avoid prolonged use. It may cause drowsiness and impair the performance of skilled tasks, such as driving.
✪ Related entries: Zimovane; Zopiclone.

Zoton
(Lederle) is a proprietary, prescription-only preparation of the PROTON-PUMP INHIBITOR lansoprazole. It can be used as an ULCER-HEALING DRUG and for associated conditions, such as gastro-oesophageal reflux, and is available as capsules.
✚▲ Side-effects/warning: See LANSOPRAZOLE.

Zovirax
(Wellcome) is a proprietary, prescription-only preparation of the ANTIVIRAL drug acyclovir. It can be used to treat various infections by the herpes simplex and herpes zoster viruses. It is available as tablets, an oral suspension, an eye ointment, a cream and in a form for intravenous infusion. (A

non-prescription ointment preparation for the treatment of cold sores is also available.)
✚▲ Side-effects/warning: See ACYCLOVIR.

Zovirax Cold Sore Cream
(Wellcome) is a proprietary, non-prescription preparation of the ANTIVIRAL drug acyclovir. It can be used to treat herpes simplex on the lip and face (cold sores), and is available as a cream for topical application.
✚▲ Side-effects/warning: See ACYCLOVIR.

zuclopenthixol acetate
is an ANTIPSYCHOTIC drug that is chemically one of the thioxanthenes, which have similar general actions to the PHENOTHIAZINE derivatives. It is administered for the short-term management of acute psychotic and mania disorders or for the exacerbation of chronic psychotic disorders. Administration is oral. See also ZUCLOPENTHIXOL DECANOATE.
✚▲ Side-effects/warning: See CHLORPROMAZINE HYDROCHLORIDE. Avoid its use in patients with porphyria.
✪ Related entry: Clopixol Acuphase.

zuclopenthixol decanoate
is an ANTIPSYCHOTIC drug that is chemically one of the thioxanthenes, which have similar general actions to the PHENOTHIAZINE derivatives. It is used for the long-term maintenance of schizophrenia and other psychotic disorders. Administration is by injection.
✚▲ Side-effects/warning: See CHLORPROMAZINE HYDROCHLORIDE; but is less sedating. Avoid its use in patients with porphyria.
✪ Related entries: Clopixol, Clopixol Conc.

zuclopenthixol dihydrochloride
is an ANTIPSYCHOTIC drug which is chemically one of the thioxanthenes, which have similar general actions to the PHENOTHIAZINE derivatives. It can be

administered to treat patients with psychotic disorders, such as schizophrenia, and is particularly effective for agitated and aggressive behaviour. Administration can be either oral or by injection.

✚▲ Side-effects/warning: See CHLORPROMAZINE HYDROCHLORIDE. However, do not administer to those patients with porphyria.

⊙ Related entry: Clopixol.

Zumenon

(Duphar) is a proprietary, prescription-only preparation of the OESTROGEN of oestradiol. It can be used in HRT, and is available as tablets contained in a calendar pack.

✚▲ Side-effects/warning: See OESTRADIOL.

Zydol

(Searle) is a proprietary, prescription-only preparation of the (OPIOID) NARCOTIC ANALGESIC tramadol hydrochloride. It can be used to relieve pain, but seems to differ from typical opioids in its mode of action. It is available as capsules and in a form for injection.

✚▲ Side-effects/warning: See TRAMADOL HYDROCHLORIDE.

Zyprexa

(Lilly) is a proprietary, prescription-only preparation of the recently introduced ANTIPSYCHOTIC drug olanzapine. It can be used to tranquillize patients suffering from schizophrenia, and is available as tablets.

✚▲ Side-effects/warning: See OLANZAPINE.

Z

GLOSSARY

*Terms **in bold** refer to related entries in the glossary*
Terms IN CAPITALS refer to the main Medicines A–Z section

abuse liability of drugs concerns their propensity to lead to drug-seeking behaviour. In the case of some drugs (especially OPIOIDS, such as heroin), there is a strong progression into drug **dependence** (addiction) with an associated **withdrawal syndrome**.

abuse of drugs denotes the non-medical use of drugs – without intent to treat or cure disease – ie recreational use. The term is commonly pejorative, reflecting the extent that drugs can seriously interfere with physical and mental health of the individual. See also **misuse of drugs**.

acute means short-term – in contrast to **chronic** (long-term) – and can be used to describe a disease or for how long a drug is taken.

addiction see **dependence**

adjuvants are drugs used in addition to other drugs to increase the latter's effectiveness.

adrenal means pertaining to the adrenal gland, which is an endocrine gland close to the kidney. It secretes hormones into the bloodstream from two main layers. Adrenocortical hormones – from the cortex, or outer layer – are usually called CORTICOSTEROIDS and are classified into two types, glucocorticoids and mineralocorticoids; eg CORTISONE, HYDROCORTISONE and ALDOSTERONE. Adrenomedullary hormones – from the medulla, or central core – include ADRENALINE and NORADRENALINE. See also **aldosteronism**.

adverse drug reactions are seriously unpleasant or harmful effects of drugs caused by doses used for normal therapeutic use. Relatively trivial side-effects, such as a dry mouth, are not normally referred to as adverse drug reactions. These reactions are divided into groups, including type A, dose-related and expected (often inevitable given the mode of action of the drug), and type B, rare and occurring only in some patients (sometimes called idiosyncratic reactions; often an allergic reaction).

aerosols are a means of administering drugs as fine droplets in a spray, often from a nebulizer (eg BETA-RECEPTOR STIMULANTS in asthma treatment).

aetiology is the cause of the disease, and the study of the factors involved in causing it.

aldosteronism is a disease caused by excessive production of aldosterone, a **hormone** produced by the cortex of the **adrenal** gland due to a **tumour** of the gland known as Conn's syndrome or sometimes as part of heart failure. Symptoms include **hypertension**, **oedema**, thirst and tiredness. Treatment includes the use of aldosterone antagonists (eg POTASSIUM CANRENOATE and SPIRONOLACTONE).

allergens are foreign proteins to which the body has become sensitive, and can cause an allergy in **hypersensitive** persons and thus an allergic reaction.

allergic reactions are caused by the reaction of **allergens** (often foreign proteins) with **antibodies** (formed by the body's protective immune system). These reactions may be local or generalized (as in **anaphylactic shock**). Treatment of allergic disease is with ANTI-ALLERGIC drugs, including CORTICOSTEROIDS and ANTIHISTAMINES. Also, there may be allergic reactions (type B **adverse drug reactions**) to some drugs, such as PENICILLINS and LOCAL ANAESTHETICS.

amenorrhoea is a stopping or absence of menstrual periods.

anaemia is a collection of conditions where there is a reduced capacity of the blood to carry oxygen, due to a reduction in haemoglobin levels. There may be many causes.

analogues are chemicals or drugs that are closely related in chemical structure.

anaphylactic shock see **anaphylaxis**

anaphylaxis is an extreme local reaction to drugs or **allergens** in **hypersensitive** people. An extreme generalized reaction (eg to bee stings), called anaphylactic shock, is treated as a medical emergency. Treatment is by injection of ANTI-ALLERGIC drugs, including CORTICOSTEROIDS, ANTIHISTAMINES and also ADRENALINE.

angina pectoris is a pain felt in the centre of the chest and sometimes spreading to the arm, shoulder or jaw. It often occurs with exercise, and is due to the demand for oxygen by the heart muscle exceeding the supply, for instance, when there is an obstruction of the cardiac arteries (**atheroma**). It may be treated with anti-angina drugs (eg BETA-BLOCKERS and VASODILATORS).

angioedema (angioneurotic oedema) is caused by **allergy** resulting in the rapid development of swellings similar to **urticaria** of the skin, but also other sites in the body (including the larynx). The most common causes are food allergy, insect stings, infections and drug allergy (eg PENICILLINS). Treatment is with CORTICOSTEROIDS and ANTIHISTAMINES.

anorexia is loss of appetite, and can be induced by APPETITE SUPPRESSANTS or anorectic agents. The psychological state anorexia nervosa is characterized by an unwillingness to eat, extreme weight loss and fear of becoming fat.

anoxia is a state where the tissues receive inadequate oxygen. This may result from many causes, including **anaemia**, inadequate oxygen in the atmosphere (eg with high altitude), in respiratory diseases (eg **asthma** and **bronchitis**), inadequate perfusion of the tissues (eg in **angina pectoris** where there is **atheroma** of the cardiac arteries). Treatment depends on the specific cause.

antibodies are special blood proteins (immunoglobulins) formed by lymphatic tissues in response to **antigens**, and circulating in the blood plasma they react with these foreign proteins to make them harmless. The production of antibodies with antigens underlies both **allergic reactions** and **immunity**.

antigens are proteins that are treated by the body as foreign; **antibodies** in the blood react with them, making them harmless.

aplasia means failure of development of an organ or tissue (eg aplastic **anaemia**).

arrhythmias (dysrrhythmias) are abnormalities of heart rhythm or rate of heartbeat. They are usually caused by disturbances of the electrical impulses and their conduction within the heart. There are a number of types of disturbance: ectopic beats are isolated irregular beats; tachycardias are where the heartbeat is too fast; and bradycardias where it is too slow. atrial flutter is a rapid beat originating within the atrium, and ventricular fibrillation is a form of cardiac arrest where the ventricles of the heart twitch in a disorganized manner. Treatment of each type of disorder is usually under specialist supervision and includes the use of classes of drugs such as ANTI-ARRHYTHMICS, BETA-BLOCKERS, CALCIUM-CHANNEL BLOCKERS and CARDIAC GLYCOSIDES.

asthma is an obstructive airways disease characterized by acute attacks of shortness of breath (caused by difficulty in exhalation), often with increased secretions in the airways. Bronchial asthma may be precipitated by **allergens**, noxious gases, cold, exercise and certain drugs (eg aspirin). It is treated with ANTI-ALLERGIC, ANTI-INFLAMMATORY and ANTI-ASTHMATIC drugs.

ataxia is clumsiness and a lack of coordination, with an unsteady gait, impaired eye and limb movements, and speech problems. There can be many causes, but mostly involving neurological damage. Several drugs may cause ataxia as a side-effect (eg BARBITURATES, HYPNOTICS and some ANTI-EPILEPTICS). Alcohol also has similar actions.

atheroma is a degeneration of the walls of blood vessels, causing atherosclerosis, characteristically by fatty deposits and scar tissue, and predisposes to tissue **anoxia** (eg in **angina pectoris**) and **thrombosis** (causing stroke, heart attacks, gangrene). Causal factors are thought to include smoking and a diet high in animal fats. Therapy includes a low-fat diet, bypass surgery, LIPID-LOWERING DRUGS and VASODILATORS.

atherosclerosis see atheroma

attention-deficit hyperactivity disorder is a condition in children characterized by hyperkinesis (hyperactivity). As part of a comprehensive treatment programme certain drugs, such as METHYLPHENIDATE HYDROCHLORIDE (Ritalin), may be administered.

autoimmune diseases are where there is an immune (see **immunity**) reaction of the subject's **antibodies** with certain of the subject's own cells, which act as **antigens**. An increasing number of diseases are now thought to involve such auto-antibodies, including **rheumatoid arthritis**, rheumatic fever, certain types of **anaemia** (pernicious anaemia, haemolytic anaemia), **lupus erythematosus** and Hashimoto's disease of the thyroid gland.

autonomic nervous system control of bodily function involves involuntary functions such as blood pressure, heart rate and the activity of muscles of internal organs (eg blood vessels, intestines and secretions). The sympathetic nervous system (utilizing the neurotransmitter NORADRENALINE and the hormone ADRENALINE) is primarily involved in excitation of these functions, often described as 'fight, fright and flight'. The parasympathetic nervous system (utilizing the neurotransmitter ACETYLCHOLINE) is more involved in functions such as digestive processes. See also ANTICHOLINERGIC; ANTISYMPATHETIC.

benign means, in general, harmless conditions within the body. In relation to tumours, it is used where the growth does not invade and destroy other cells or tissue, ie it is not **malignant** (cancerous).

bilirubin is the main pigment found in bile. It is formed from the breakdown of the blood pigment **haemoglobin** in the liver. It is yellow in colour and gives the characteristic colour of jaundice when it accumulates in the bloodstream in **hepatitis**, when liver function is impaired.

bioavailability of a pharmaceutical formulation is the amount that is biologically available, after administration and subsequent absorption etc., pharmacologically to act. See **formulation**.

biotechnology is a term that denotes application of biological techniques to chemical manufacture and is used in a variety of ways, eg **recombinant DNA technology (genetic engineering)**.

block/blocker refers to the process where an ANTAGONIST prevents an agonist drug exerting its effect, usually by preventing the action of the latter at a RECEPTOR (eg BETA-BLOCKERS, ALPHA-ADRENOCEPTOR BLOCKERS, ANGIOTENSIN-RECEPTOR BLOCKERS).

blood dyscrazias see dyscrazia

blood-brain barrier is the means by which the nerves within the brain are normally kept separate from the blood cells and large molecules within the blood. In some instances this barrier may be a disadvantage (eg certain antibiotics may not reach central nervous system cells when treating infections). However, sometimes unwanted side-effects of drugs caused by their effects on the brain can be avoided by deliberately designing new drugs that do not cross the blood-brain barrier; eg second-generation ANTIHISTAMINES do not cause drowsiness whereas earlier ones did.

BNF is the abbreviation for British National Formulary, which is an impartial and critical compendium of drug types and names sponsored by the British Medical Association and Pharmaceutical Society of Great Britain. It is issued every six months to prescribing doctors.

BP is the abbreviation for **British Pharmacopoeia**.

bradycardia is a decrease in the rate of heartbeat. See **arrhythmias**.

bradykinesia is slow and poor movement, as seen in Parkinson's disease and **extrapyramidal disorders** caused by several groups of drugs as a side-effect (eg PHENOTHIAZINES). See also **tardive dyskinesia**.

British Pharmacopoeia (BP) is a formulary of official preparation as used in the UK. It may differ in the drugs included, their names and further details from equivalent formulary of other countries or areas (eg **European Pharmacopoeia**).

bronchitis is an obstructive airways disease characterized by a chronic shortness of breath (caused by difficulty in exhalation) and coughing, with inflammation and increased secretions and blockage of the airways (often associated with infection by micro-organisms). It is associated with a history of smoking and air pollution. It is treated with ANTIBIOTIC, ANTI-INFLAMMATORY and ANTI-ASTHMATIC drugs.

bronchoconstriction (or bronchospasm) is a narrowing of the bronchioles of the lungs, caused by a contraction of the **smooth muscle** surrounding the airways and often exacerbated by excessive secretions within the airways. It is very characteristic of obstructive airways diseases, such as asthma, and in **allergic reaction** to **antigens** (of which an extreme example is **anaphylactic shock**). It may also be caused by drugs acting directly on the airways (eg PARASYMPATHOMIMETICS or ANTICHOLINESTERASES), in drug allergy (eg PENICILLINS) or other types of hypersensitivity (eg to NSAIDS). Treatment is with BRONCHODILATORS and, where allergy is involved, with CORTICOSTEROIDS and ANTIHISTAMINES.

brucellosis is a rare bacterial infection, normally caught from dairy products and farm animals. It is treated with ANTIBIOTICS.

cancer is where disease is due to unrestrained cancerous cell growth and tumours. They are described as **malignant**, as such cells or growths invade and destroys other cells or tissues. There are various types of cancers, such as **carcinoma**, **sarcoma**, **lymphoma** and **leukaemia**. If untreated, cancerous growths may be life-threatening.

capsules are gelatine or similar containers for

liquid or solid forms of drugs that are to be taken by mouth. They allow complex formulation of the constituent drug(s), including modified-release (especially sustained-release) versions where release is over a period of time and so reducing the frequency of dosing.

carcinoid tumours are cancerous growths of neuroendocrine glandular tissue leading to large and often dramatic release of potent autacoids. Argentochromaffin tumours of the gut, which release 5-hydroxytryptamine and other mediators causing asthma-like attacks, flushing and diarrhoea, where recognized early; but **phaeochromocytomas**, VIPomas and other neuroendocrine tumours are similar. Treatment is usually surgical.

carcinoma is a **malignant** type of **neoplasm**, a cancerous growth, which arises in the epithelium which lines the internal organs and skin (cf. **sarcoma**).

cardiac muscle is the type of striated muscle that makes up the contractile muscle of the heart (but not of the smooth muscle of the blood vessels within the heart). The muscle is controlled by the **autonomic nervous system**, through opposing excitatory actions of NORADRENALINE from the sympathetic nervous system versus the inhibitory actions of ACETYLCHOLINE from the parasympathomimetic nervous system.

central nervous system (CNS) is the division of the nervous system comprising the brain within the skull and spinal cord within the vertebrae. The remainder of the nervous system is the peripheral nervous system.

chemical drug names are not normally used outside technical circles, because although they are precise and unambiguous, they can be very large and unwieldy. In its place is substituted an official trivial or shortened name, a **generic drug name**, though this may unfortunately vary between countries. For instance, N-(4-hydroxyphenyl)acetamide is a chemical name for the analgesic drug given the generic name PARACETAMOL (UK) or acetaminophen (USA).

chemotherapy is the treatment or prevention of disease by means of chemical substances. The term is often restricted to the treatment of disease by drugs (eg antibiotics) or to the treatment of cancer (ie anticancer drugs) in contrast to radiotherapy.

chlamydial infection is caused by a group of small micro-organisms called clamydia (clamylidiae) which physically are larger than viruses but smaller than bacteria (though, like bacteria, their infection can be treated with ANTIBIOTICS). They cause a wide range of infections in humans and animals, and may spread between the two (eg psittacosis from birds). The commonest infection is by strains of Chlamydia trachomatis, causing various eye, lymph node and (sexually transmitted) genital infections.

cholestasis is a failure of the normal bile flow to the intestine causing jaundice. Causes include a physical obstructive jaundice due to a stone (extrahepatic biliary obstruction), liver disease (eg viral hepatitis) or drug-induced toxic reaction (intrahepatic cholestasis), for instance, in individuals abnormally sensitivity to chlorpromazine. The symptoms are jaundice with dark urine, pale faeces and skin itching. Treatment depends on the cause, and when due to **adverse drug reaction** normally reverses on discontinuing drug administration.

chronic describes a disease of long duration, usually of slow onset and slowly reversing (if at all). It does not mean severe. See **acute**.

cirrhosis of the liver is caused by chronic damage to its cells, leading to scarring and loss of function. One result is a loss of ability to metabolize toxic substances and drugs, and it may cause **hypertension**. The causes include **hepatitis** (an inflammation of the liver commonly caused by microbial infection) or heavy consumption of alcohol.

clinical pharmacology encompasses all aspects of the scientific study of drugs in humans.

clinical trial is a systematic study of medically active agents in humans. Such trials advance through early phases in normal volunteers (to determine duration of action and metabolism), to eventual studies in patients with disease. Commonly, new active agents are compared to existing standard treatments and to dummy treatments (placebos). To avoid bias, assessment of the efficacy of treatment may be single-blind (where either the patient or the doctor does not know the identity of treatments) or double-blind (where neither knows until the trial is finished).

colitis is inflammation of the colon of the gut. | **593**

Symptoms include pain, diarrhoea, and sometimes blood or mucous, and fever. It may be due to parasitic or bacterial infections or to ulcerative colitis and Crohn's disease. Treatment of ulcerative colitis is with AMINOSALICYLATES.

Committee on Safety of Medicines (CSM) is an independent group set up to give advice via the Medicines Control Agency (MCA), which administers the Medicines Act, to the licensing authorities under the Ministry of Health.

complementary medicine is a general term sometimes applied to traditional or alternative systems of medicine and healing, including herbal remedies, homeopathy, faith healing, hypnosis, acupuncture and aromatherapy. These alternative treatments are not normally administered by registered practitioners, and are not normally subject to objective proof of efficacy through **clinical trials**.

compliance is the extent to which patient behaviour accords with medical advice, and in relation to drugs relates to the accuracy and frequency of taking prescribed medicines (which can be surprisingly low).

constriction is a narrowing or obstruction of a hollow organ, commonly applied to blood vessels (vasoconstriction). See VASOCONSTRICTORS.

Crohn's disease see **colitis**

Cushing's syndrome is caused by raised levels of the hormones called CORTICOSTEROIDS in the bloodstream. It can be due to excess production by the adrenal gland due to a tumour of that gland, tumours in the lungs and elsewhere in the periphery, to a tumour of the pituitary gland leading to excess stimulation of the adrenal gland, or to prolonged medical administration of corticosteroid drugs (eg in advanced asthma in children). Characteristics of the syndrome include a moon-faced, rounded and red-faced appearance, obesity and humped shoulders, wasted limbs, thin and easily bruised skin, **osteoporosis**, hairiness in females, and a variety of other adverse effects including **diabetes**. The course of chosen treatment requires expert evaluation by an endocrinologist.

cycloplegic agents cause cycloplegia, which is paralysis of the smooth muscle of the eye that accommodate the lens (allowing the eye to focus on near objects), so leaving the eye focused for distant objects. ANTICHOLINERGIC drugs may be used for this purpose in the diagnosis and treatment of disease states, or alternatively cycloplegia may be an unavoidable side-effect of these drugs when used for other reasons. Often cycloplegia is accompanied by mydriaisis.

dependence on a drug (addiction) is a state where regular, repeated and probably excessive taking of an agent causes the individual to become accustomed to it, resulting in detrimental effects. Stopping dosing precipitates a **withdrawal syndrome** which may have marked psychological and/or physical symptoms. See **habituation**.

dialysis is separation of substances in liquid by virtue of differences in their capacities to pass through membranes. Haemodialysis is used in medicine to separate low molecular weight compounds (eg toxins or drugs and their metabolites in overdose) from blood. Peritoneal dialysis is a simpler procedure which can sometimes be used in drug overdose, in which saline solution is perfused continuously through the peritoneal cavity.

dilatation is a widening of a hollow organ, commonly applied to blood vessels (vasodilatation). See VASODILATORS.

diverticular disease is the presence of small pouches or sacs protruding into the intestine, commonly the colon. Diverticulosis is when inflammation is present, and if this becomes severe it can lead to perforation of the bowel wall. Treatment is surgical and with ANTIBIOTIC, ANTISPASMODIC and ANTI-INFLAMMATORY drugs.

dose is the amount of a drug administered, and is critical in order to achieve the desired therapeutic effect without unnecessary adverse effects or side-effects. An initial (loading) dose may be administered, followed by a smaller maintenance dose given at regular intervals appropriate to that particular drug and the metabolism and excretion (pharmacokinetics) in a particular patient.

drug interactions occur when one drug changes the magnitude of effect, or duration of action, of the other.

drug screening is the process of testing chemical agents for given types of pharmacological activity.

dys- as a prefix means abnormal or disturbed body function.

dyscrazia is a term that formerly referred to any disease state, but now is used only in relation to blood diseases for abnormalities of blood cells or their numbers (eg agranulocytosis, thrombocytopenia). A number of drugs cause blood dyscrazias as **adverse drug reactions**.

dysfunctional means abnormal or disturbed body function. See **dys-**.

dyskinesia is abnormal muscle movements, such as jerking and twitching; eg **tardive dyskinesia**.

dysmenorrhoea is the term used for the pain or discomfort just before or during menstrual periods, probably due to hormonal effects. In general, there are few effective drugs to treat it, though analgesics may be used to ease the discomfort. Sometimes, in older women, it can be caused by pelvic inflammatory disease and other disorders, which are treated with appropriate drugs. See also **amenorrhoea**.

dysphoria is a feeling or discomfort or lack of wellbeing (as opposed to **euphoria**).

dysrhythmia see **arrhythmia**

dystonia is a disorder of skeletal muscle tone (either increased or decreased), causing abnormal positions and movements. It is sometimes caused by disorders of the basal ganglia of the brain due to adverse drug reaction (eg PHENOTHIAZINES, ANTIPSYCHOTICS). See **extrapyramidal disorders**; **tardive dyskinesia**.

EC (European Community) has been replaced by the European Union (EU) for most regulatory purposes.

eclampsia is a condition of late pregnancy, or during or directly after delivery, characterized by convulsions (and preceded in pre-eclampsia by **hypertension**, **oedema** and **proteinurea**). It is treated by ANTICONVULSANTS and in pre-eclampsia by a low-sodium diet and ANTIHYPERTENSIVES.

ectopic means not in its right or normal position.

efficacy in therapeutics, is the capacity of a drug to produce the desired effect or result.

elixir is a medicated liquid preparation for taking by mouth, which is intended to disguise a potentially unpleasant taste by including a sweetening substance, such as glycerol or alcohol, and often with aromatic agents.

embolism is a condition where a blood clot (thrombus) lodges in an artery to obstruct blood flow. There are various types according to the area obstructed (eg pulmonary embolism in the case of the lung). Treatment can be by surgery, the use of drugs that can dissolve blood clots (FIBRINOLYTICS or thrombolytics) or by drugs that prevent formation of further clots (ANTICOAGULANTS). See also **thrombosis**.

emphysema is a lung disease where there is damage to the alveoli of the lungs (which are tiny air sacs in which oxygen exchange with the blood takes place), resulting in shortness of breath. It is often accompanied by chronic **bronchitis**, and can in turn lead to heart failure and respiratory failure. It is generally due to smoking, but exacerbated by air pollution (and a genetic predisposition in some individuals). The damage to the alveoli cannot be repaired, but symptomatic relief maybe given by BRONCHODILATORS, CORTICOSTEROIDS and DIURETICS.

encephalopathy is any of a group of disorders that affect the functioning of the brain.

endocarditis is inflammation of the endocardium (the lining of the heart), and occurs usually where there has been damage due to congenital heart disease or rheumatic fever, and where the immune system is damaged (as in AIDS). Endocarditis may be caused by a number or micro-organisms, including bacteria and fungi, particularly after dental extractions and heart surgery. ANTIBIOTICS may be used both prophylactically and in treatment.

endogenous means produced within the body; in contrast to exogenous agents that are administered to the body. Some agents (eg hormones, local hormones and neurotransmitters), though released endogenously, may be administered exogenously, as drugs, in medicine.

endometriosis is the abnormal presence of tissue similar to the endometrial lining of the uterus in various sites within the pelvis. The abnormal tissue may undergo similar responses to hormones as the endometrium, causing pain and **dysmenorrhoea**. Treatment is with HORMONE ANTAGONISTS or by surgery.

595

endometrium is the mucous membrane layer lining the uterus within the muscle layer (myometrium).

endothelium is the tissue that lines the blood vessels, heart and lymphatic ducts. See **epithelium**.

enema is an infusion of liquid into the rectum, via the anus, as a method of administering laxatives, diagnostic agents (eg radio-opaque agents) or therapeutic drugs to act locally (eg steroids in **colitis**) or sometimes agents for absorption for systemic effects (eg paraldehyde as an ANTI-EPILEPTIC).

enteral is pertaining to the intestinal tract.

enteric-coated tablets are covered with a layer (originally shellac varnish) that dissolves slowly. They are intended to prevent release until the tablet has left the stomach, where the active drug is gastro-irritant (eg aspirin) or is broken down by gastric juices.

epilepsy is a group of central nervous system diseases characterized by a tendency to recurrent seizures (fits), usually of sudden onset. There are various schemes of classification: Grand Mal is a generalized seizure in which the patient falls down unconscious; Petit Mal (absence seizure) is a generalized seizure characterized by momentary loss of consciousness without abnormal movements; Simple Partial Seizure is where consciousness is maintained during a partial physical seizure, including Jacksonian epilepsy where twitching occurs and spreads across the body in a pattern; Complex Partial Seizure (temporal lobe epilepsy) is where conscious contact with surroundings are lost and there may be stereotyped abnormal behaviour. Status epilepticus is an extension of one of these conditions to prolonged or repeated epileptic seizures without periods for recovery, and is a medical emergency. Treatment of some of these is with ANTI-EPILEPTIC drugs (ANTICONVULSANTS) appropriate to each type.

epithelium is the tissue that covers the entire external surface of the body and lines the hollow organs of the body (except blood vessels). See **endothelium**.

erythrocytes are red blood cells.

EU (European Union) has replaced the European Community (EC) for most purposes. Its official regulatory body, EMEA, has an important role in recommending various European drug regulatory matters.

euphoria is a feeling of confident wellbeing, the opposite of **dysphoria**. It can be induced by some OPIOIDS, such as morphine, and prolonged use of CORTICOSTEROIDS.

European Pharmacopoeia (Eur. P), like the British Pharmacopoeia (BP), lists official preparations of drugs. The BP and EP are likely to converge in their coverage.

exocrine glands secrete substances through a duct (eg the salivary glands), usually under the control of HORMONES or NEUROTRANSMITTERS.

extrapyramidal disorders of movement are caused by several groups of drugs as an adverse reaction that is commonly a foreseeable side-effect (that may be difficult to avoid with higher dose schedules). The syndrome is due to effects of drugs on the basal ganglia and associated structures within the brain (corpus striatum and substantia nigra), and is most commonly incurred with antipsychotic drugs, such as PHENOTHIAZINES working as dopamine-receptor antagonists. See also **tardive dyskinesia**.

extrapyramidal symptoms see **extrapyramidal disorders**

familial diseases are those found in some families, but not others, and are largely genetically determined.

favism is a disorder in some individuals characterized by a food intolerance to broad beans (Vicia fava), which contain a chemical that in the affected person causes rapid destruction of red blood cells (haemolytic anaemia). It is a genetically inherited condition and is relatively common in African, Indian and some Mediterranean peoples (in some areas it may affect up to 10% of the population). It is caused by an enzyme deficiency disorder (**G6PD deficiency**; glucose 6-phosphate dehydrogenase deficiency) which also predisposes to serious adverse drug reactions (eg to the antimalarial drug primaquine).

FDA (Food and Drug Authority) is the USA authority that is concerned in evaluating evidence of a drug's safety and efficacy, clinical trials and the general process of drug registration. Its regulations have an international impact.

formulary is a book (or increasingly a computer database) that details formulations or doses of drugs. See **British Pharmacopoeia**; **European Pharmacopoeia**.

formulation is the pharmaceutical term for the mode of presentation of a medicine: ie capsule, tablet, pill, cream, lotion, emulsion, solution, pessary, suppository, form for injection, etc. Modern medicines are often quite complex and sophisticated products that are stable, have reliable **bioavailability**, and acceptability (taste, etc.).

G6PD deficiency (glucose 6-phosphate dehydrogenase enzyme deficiency) is a genetically inherited condition and is relatively common among African, Indian and some Mediterranean peoples. Serious adverse reactions occur in affected people when they take quite a few drugs; for instance, the antimalarial drug primaquine causes red blood cell haemolysis in 5–10% of black men, leading to severe anaemia. Adverse reactions also occur to certain foodstuffs; see **favism**.

gastro-oesophageal reflux (acid reflux) is regurgitation of acid and enzymes into the oesophagus from the stomach, of which heartburn is a symptom, and is associated with oesophagitis (inflammation of the oesophagus). It is caused by a weakness in the sphincter muscle at the bottom of the oesophagus, by hiatus hernia and is common in pregnancy. Treatment is by ANTACIDS and by ULCER-HEALING DRUGS which reduce acid secretion.

gels are a colloidal formulation of a medicine as a jelly-like mass, and is convenient for **topical** application.

generations of drugs are 'created' when, in the development of a class of drugs, a significant advance occurs (in potency, duration of action, absorption, spectrum of action, etc.). Thus in a number of ANTIBIOTIC families there are first, second and third generations (eg the CEPHALOSPORINS).

generic drug name is the official or standard names for the active chemical(s) in a medicine, in contrast to the proprietary name (trade name), for a medicine. In the UK, doctors in general and hospital practice are encouraged to refer to, and prescribe, drugs by the generic name (correctly written without an initial capital letters). Under NHS recommendations for generic substitution, a prescription written for a proprietary drug (always written with initial capital letters) can be supplied in the form of a (cheaper) equivalent generic drug. However, during the period of the patent that is granted to the inventor (commonly 16–20 years for a new chemical entity or formulation, but depending on the country concerned), only a proprietary form of the drug may be available. In this case a generic prescription will be filled with a proprietary drug (complete with packaging, etc., in the latter name). Although the generic form has the same molecular structure as the proprietary form of the drug, concern has been expressed about the bioequivalence of preparations, and regulatory authorities normally require proof that, at a given dose, the generic drugs substituted for their parent proprietary drug have a **bioavailability** that ensures equivalent pharmacological effect. See also **names of drugs**.

genes that determine the genetic make-up of living organisms are contained in 23 pairs of chromosomes in humans. The Human Genome Project is concerned with identifying the entire gene sequence (c. 100,000 genes made up of a total of about 3000 million DNA base pairs). See **genotype**; **genome**.

genetic engineering is a modern term meaning the use of techniques (**recombinant DNA technology**) to modify the structure of genes, or to create or delete genes. Potentially, these techniques may be used to correct diseases in humans due to genetic defects (eg cystic fibrosis). Use in animal husbandry is now quite advanced.

genitourinary tract (also called the urogenital tract) comprises the sexual organs and bladder, and related structures. As a medical speciality, genitourinary medicine is often taken narrowly to mean the study and treatment of sexually transmitted diseases.

genome is the total genetic material of an organism, which in humans is the **genes** that are contained in 23 pairs of chromosomes.

genotype is the total genetic complement of a set of genes that an individual possesses (containing contributions from both parents). Not all this information is expressed. See also **phenotype**.

glaucoma is an eye condition characterized by a raised intraocular pressure in the eye, which if left untreated can damage the optic nerve. There are various forms, but the two common ones are: simple (open-angle) glaucoma, which is chronic, seen more commonly in middle-age and is often **familial**; and acute (closed-angle) glaucoma. The former is treated with BETA-BLOCKERS and certain other drugs or surgery. See also GLAUCOMA TREATMENT.

goitre is a collection of disease states characterized by an enlarged thyroid gland. Goitre has a number of causes: a shortage of iodine in the diet – endemic goitre; hyperplasia (tumour) of the gland – sporadic goitre; swelling due to overactivity in Grave's disease – exothalmic goitre; or autoimmune thyroiditis (Hashimoto's disease). Additionally, some chemicals and drugs may cause goitre as a side-effect.

grandfather drug is the original or archetype in a series, from which generations of successor drugs have been developed. See **generations of drugs**.

granulocytopenia see **neutropenia**

gynaecomastia is enlargement of breasts in the male. It can be caused by elevated levels of female sex hormones (OESTROGEN) in the blood. Some drugs may cause it as a side-effect (eg CIMETIDINE, DIGOXIN, SPIRONOLACTONE).

habituation to a drug is a state where regular (possibly excessive) taking of an agent causes the individual to become accustomed to it, but not to the extreme psychological or physical stage of **dependence** (addiction).

haemodialysis see **dialysis**

haemoglobin is the oxygen-carrying pigment of the red blood cells (erythrocytes) of the blood. Some familial abnormal forms cause anaemia (eg **sickle-cell disease**). Other abnormal forms that carry oxygen poorly and cause **anoxia** are caused by acute reaction with chemicals, for instance **methaemoglobin** by nitrates and a number of other drugs and chemicals, and carboxyhaemoglobin by carbon monoxide.

haemolysis is the destruction of red blood cells (erythrocytes). It may occur within the body through infection, poisoning, the action of antibodies or as an **adverse drug reaction**. Individuals with (normally **familial**) low levels of the enzyme glucose 6-phosphate (**G6PD-deficiency**) are particularly at risk from many drugs, including SULPHONAMIDES, SULPHONES and PRIMAQUINE.

haemorrhoids (piles) are an enlargement of the wall of the anus, sometimes caused as a consequence of prolonged constipation, and often following childbirth. There may be pain and bleeding. Treatment of first-degree haemorrhoids is normally through adjustment of diet, but second- and third-degree severity may require surgical or similar intervention.

hepatitis is inflammation of the liver, with accompanying damage or death of liver cells. It may be due to infection (eg viral hepatitis), toxic substances or immunological abnormalities. Infectious hepatitis is of several types: hepatitis A (infectious hepatitis) is mainly transmitted by faecal-contaminated food; hepatitis B (serum hepatitis) is transmitted by infected blood, needles and sexually. Further forms are hepatitis C (non-A, non-B hepatitis), hepatitis D and hepatitis E. Prevention by vaccination or immunization is recommended for those at risk, and treatments include avoidance of alcohol and occasionally use of INTERFERONS.

herpes is an inflammation with blistering of the skin or mucous membranes, caused by the herpesvirus. Herpes simplex virus (HSV) is of two sorts: type I causes the common cold sore around the lips (which is contagious by contact); and type II is associated with genital herpes (which is sexually transmitted). Herpes zoster (shingles), which is caused by the varicella-zoster virus, remains in a dormant form in sensory nerves following chickenpox, and can later be activated to affect the eye (ophthalmic zoster) or skin (dermosomes). Treatment of all forms of herpes is mainly with ACYCLOVIR.

herpesvirus see **herpes**

Hodgkin's disease is a **lymphoma**, a **malignant** disease, a **cancer** arising in lymphoid tissue, including lymph nodes and the spleen.

homeostasis is the physiological system that maintains the internal state of the body.

hyper- as a prefix in medical terms denotes above normal.

hyperaemia is excess blood in vessels supplying any part of the body. It may occur through drugs affecting blood supply or drainage from an organ; for example, the SYMPATHOMIMETIC drug APRACLONIDINE when used in the eye to control intraocular pressure.

hyperhidrosis is excessive sweating and may be localized to the armpits, feet, palms or face. It may be due to hormone imbalance, anxiety, nervous system disorders or as a side-effect of some drugs (eg PARASYMPATHOMIMETICS, ANTICHOLINESTERASES, LEVODOPA, BUSERELIN, AMITRIPTYLINE, THYROXINE). It is treated with **topical** application of ALUMINIUM CHLORIDE.

hyperlipidaemia is a clinical condition where the blood plasma contains very high levels of the lipids (fats) cholesterol and/or triglycerides (natural fats of the body). Deposition of lipids onto the lining of blood vessels leads to diseases such as coronary atherosclerosis (see **atheroma**) where plaques of lipid material narrow blood vessels, which contributes to angina pectoris attacks, and the formation of abnormal clots that go on to cause heart attacks (**myocardial infarction**) and strokes. Lipid in the blood may be lowered by appropriate modifications of diet, but LIPID-LOWERING DRUGS may be used (generally where there is a family history of hyperlipidaemia or clinical signs indicating the need for intervention).

hyperplasia is an increase in the production and growth of normal cells in a tissue, where the organ becomes bigger but retains its form (eg the breasts in pregnancy). See also **hypertrophy**; **neoplasm**.

hyperreactivity see **hypersensitivity**

hypersensitivity is when a pharmacological response occurs at lower than normal doses. The term is often used to denote an allergic component to the hypersensitivity.

hypertension is a higher than normal blood pressure for a person of that age. The World Health Organization defines hypertension as a blood pressure consistently exceeding 160/95 mm Hg (systolic/diastolic). However, because there is a considerable range of blood pressures for a population group, high blood pressure in itself may not denote hypertension, but a rising pressure with secondary pathology usually is an indication for treatment. Clinically hypertension is divided into a number of disease states each with different **aetiology**. Essential hypertension is the most common, and here the determinants of the disease are not well understood. Renal hypertension has its origins in kidney disease (eg a narrowing of the renal arteries). **Phaeochromocytoma** is characterized by episodes of extreme hypertension due to release of adrenaline and noradrenaline from a tumour of adrenal gland

tissue. Other specific causes of hypertension include Cushing's disease and pre-eclampsia. Treatment depends on cause and may involve ANTIHYPERTENSIVES.

hyperthyroidism is over-activity of the thyroid gland, with elevated levels of thyroid hormones (thyroxine) in the bloodstream. See **goitre**.

hypertrophy is an increase in the size of an organ or tissue brought about by an increase in the size of its cells (rather than of number) as in muscles with exercise) or due to tumours. See also **hyperplasia**; **neoplasm**.

hypo- as a prefix in medical terms denotes below normal.

hypotension is a lower than normal blood pressure. However, since there is a considerable range of blood pressures for a population group, low blood pressure in itself may not denote any pathology. It is more normally seen as an acute medical condition due to excess loss of body fluids (eg in burns, vomiting and diarrhoea) or blood (eg haemorrhage). There are a number of other causes, including **myocardial infarction**, **pancreatitis**, Addison's disease, pulmonary embolism. Postural hypotension (othostatic hypotension) is a temporary fall in blow pressure when the subject rises from a supine position, and is due to impaired physiological compensatory reflexes. Many drugs can cause hypotension as either as part of a serious **adverse drug reaction** or as a minor side-effect. Many ANTIHYPERTENSIVES cause postural hypotension or periods of hypotension.

iatrogenic disease is produced as a result of medical or drug treatment, for instance, as a result of an **adverse reaction** to drug treatment.

idiosyncratic responses see **adverse drug reactions**

immunity is a state of protection against infection and disease through the activity of the immune system, comprising circulating **antibodies** and white blood cells. Therapeutically, IMMUNIZATION can be used to boost the immunity; active immunity can be stimulated by VACCINATION and passive immunity by administration of IMMUNOGLOBULINS.

immunocompromised is a term that refers to a person whose immune defences are very much lower than normal due to either a congenital (present at birth) or acquired condition. The commonest deficiencies are: of the white cells (neutrophils) which are the first line of defence in acute infections; of the white cells, macrophages, and T-lymphocytes, which are involved in cell-mediated killing of foreign or 'parasitized' host cells; and of the antibodies, which neutralize and bind to foreign antigens. Examples of immunocompromised hosts include: patients receiving immunosuppressant drugs to prevent rejection of transplanted organs; patients suffering from leukaemia, or being treated with high doses of cytotoxic drugs to treat cancer; and individuals with AIDS. In any of these circumstances 'opportunistic' infections are apt to occur where microbes which normally pose little threat to the healthy become highly invasive and pose a serious threat. Prophylaxis with ANTIBACTERIAL drugs may be required, and once infections are established they are much more difficult to eradicate, even with vigorous antibiotic treatment.

implant is a form of drug depot administration where a solid formulation of the drug is given at intramuscular or subcutaneous sites. The commonist used is for CONTRACEPTIVE hormone drugs.

in vitro is a term used to describe biological actions observed under artificial conditions in the on tissues or cells in laboratory glassware (eg organ-bath or culture-medium). See also **in vivo**.

in vivo is a term used to describe biological actions observed in the whole organism. See also **in vitro**.

inflammation is an acute or chronic bodily reaction to a chemical or physical injury, or to infection. It is characterized by the 'cardinal signs': calor (heat); rubor (redness); dolor (pain); and tumor (swelling). Although inflammation is initially protective, chronic inflammatory diseases can be incapacitating. See ANTI-INFLAMMATORY, ANTIRHEUMATICS and CORTICOSTEROIDS.

infusion is the continuous administration (by injection) of a drug or fluid over a period of minutes, hours or days. See also **routes of administration of drugs**.

injection of a drug or fluid is administration means of a needle and syringe. See also

routes of administration of drugs.

interaction see **drug interactions**

International Pharmacopoeia (Int. P) is the **pharmacopoeia** of the World Health Organization and is a **formulary** intended to meet international needs.

intolerance is when there is a greater than expected reaction to a drug. The term **hypersensitivity** is preferred.

intra- as a prefix, means within.

intradermal injections are made into the skin. See **routes of administration of drugs**.

intrathecal injections are made into the subarachnoid space of the spinal cord. This route is used to localize the actions of LOCAL ANAESTHETICS and ANALGESICS to certain segments of the body supplied by sensory nerves originating from the area of injection.

iontophoresis is a method of delivering drugs across the skin using an electrical current to drive electrically charged drug molecules.

isotonic solutions used in medicine normally have equal osmotic strength to human blood plasma or extracellular fluid. Solutions for injection are normally made up with an appropriate concentration of sodium chloride (0.9%) to achieve this, because they then cause less damage.

isotopes are atoms of the same element differing in the number of neutrons in the nucleus. They differ very little in chemical properties, but some unstable isotopes, radioisotopes, emit radiation, and can be used in medicine for a variety of purposes.

LD$_{50}$ denotes the lethal dose that kills 50% of a sample of experimental animals, and as such is a statistically acceptable measure of acute toxicity, though not necessarily a very meaningful medical measure.

leucopenia is a condition when there is a low level of leukocytes (white blood cells) in the bloodstream. It may be caused by an **adverse drug reaction**.

leukaemia is a **malignant** growth, a **cancer** where abnormal white blood cells proliferate in the bone marrow. There are four main types, and treatment for acute forms is available.

linctuses are medicated syrups that are thick and soothing enough to relieve sore throats or loosen a cough. However, a linctus is not the same thing as an EXPECTORANT, which is a drug that changes the viscosity of sputum, making it easier to cough up and so clear the lungs. Also, a linctus is not necessarily an **elixir**, which is a formulation that disguises a potentially unpleasant taste and is often a sweetening substance, such as glycerol, a sweetener or alcohol.

liniments are medicated lotions for rubbing into the skin. Many of them contain ALCOHOL and/or CAMPHOR, and are intended to relieve minor muscle aches and pains.

liposomes are a drug-delivery system, and are comprised of small vesicles of phopholipid-protein membrane with an aqueous drug-containing interior. They may allow absorption from the intestine of substances, such as the peptide insulin, that would otherwise be digested; also, liposomes may reduce the toxicity of substances given intravenously.

local action of drugs is where application or injection is such that drug action is limited to a certain area of the body; in contrast to **systemic** action where the drug passes into the blood circulation and thus has a general action.

lotions are medicated liquids used to bathe or wash skin, hair or eyes.

lozenges contain medicaments in a hard often sweetened and flavoured, base. They are intended to be slowly dissolved in the mouth to treat local irritation or infection.

lupoid syndrome (lupus erythematosus syndrome) is a chronic **autoimmune disease** that causes inflammation of connective tissue. Treatment is with ANTI-INFLAMMATORY drugs. The syndrome is also caused as an **adverse drug reaction** to a number of types of drugs, such as HYDRALAZINE, PROCAINAMIDE, ISONIAZID and SULPHASALAZINE.

lupus erythematosus is a chronic inflammatory condition of the connective tissue and is an **autoimmune disease**. Treatment is with NSAIDS and IMMUNOSUPPRESSANTS.

Lyme disease is caused by a bacterium (spirochaeta, Borrelia burgdorferi), which is transmitted by the bite of a tick that lives on deer and can also infest dogs. It causes acute inflammation at the site of the bite, and after a period, headache, lethargy, fever and muscle pain develop. There can be serious chronic symptoms. Treatment is with ANTIBIOTICS.

lymphoma is a **malignant** disease, a **cancer** arising in lymphoid tissue (mainly of the nodes and spleen), such as Hodgkin's disease.

malignant, in general, describes any condition in the body which if untreated may be a threat to health (eg malignant **hypertension**). Specifically, it describes a **tumour** that invades and destroys other cells or tissues, ie is cancerous (see **cancer**).

MCA see **Medicines Control Agency**

Medicines Control Agency (MCA) is part of the UK drugs regulatory system that administers the Medicines Act, acting on evidence received and advice from the **Committee on Safety of Medicines** (CSM).

meningitis is inflammation of the membranes covering the brain and spinal cord (meninges), commonly through infection by bacteria or viruses. Symptoms include severe headache, fever, stiff neck, nausea and vomiting, photophobia and other characteristic signs. In bacterial meningitis, there may also be a red blotchy skin rash. Infections by the viral form are usually mild, but those due to bacterial forms (meningococcal infection or Haemophilus influenza) can be serious. Vaccination against Haemophilus influenza is now in routine use in babies, and ANTIBIOTICS are used against the bacterial forms.

metabolism of drugs is the process whereby the body detoxifies chemicals and excretes them as metabolites. It can be divided into two phases of conversion.

methaemoglobin (methemoglobin in USA) is an oxidized form of haemoglobin that is not able to carry oxygen, so production of it can lead to toxic **anoxia**. Blood can be converted (normally reversibly) into this form by drugs and chemicals (eg nitrates, nitrofurantoin).

-mimetic as a suffix means to imitate or mimic. For example, SYMPATHOMIMETICS are agents that mimic the actions of the sympathetic nervous system.

MIMS (Monthly Index of Medical Specialities) is a comprehensive compendium of the drugs that are available to general practitioners, pharmacists and other health professionals.

misuse of drugs may be taken to refer to inappropriate use of drugs by doctors, for instance, overprescribing, inappropriate choice of drug and unethical uses of drugs. See also **abuse of drugs**.

modified-release preparations (sustained-release preparations), normally **tablets** or **capsules**, are designed to release their active constituents over a period of time, either for convenience or to minimize adverse effects.

molecular biology, literally, is the study of biology at the molecular level. Recently, it has taken on special meanings and is used particularly to denote the study of genes, gene products and sometimes pharmaceuticals produced by processes using genetic materials.

multidrug resistance is where pathogenic organisms have acquired resistance to ANTIBIOTIC or other ANTIBACTERIAL agents, each with a different mechanism of action, and thus are multidrug resistant.

multiple myeloma (myelomatosis) is a type of cancer of the bone marrow. It is characterized by proliferation and disorganized function of plasma cells (a type of B-lymphocyte, precursors of white blood cells) in the marrow. It is a condition first seen in middle age and in individuals possessing the 'Philadelphia chromosome'. It is treated with bone marrow transfusions and certain CYTOTOXIC drugs.

myasthenia gravis is a disorder characterized by skeletal muscle weakness, particularly drooping eyelids and weak speech. It is an **autoimmune disease** which causes impaired neurotransmission by acteylcholine at the neuromuscular junction, and can be treated with ANTICHOLINESTERASES.

myelomatosis see **multiple myeloma**

myelosuppression is a reduction in the production of blood cells by the bone marrow. It often occurs after cancer chemotherapy and may cause anaemia, abnormal bleeding or infection.

myocardial infarction (heart attack) is the sudden death of part of the heart muscle, characterized by severe unremitting pain. It is usually caused by **coronary thrombosis**, obstruction of the coronary arteries. Treatment, which should be immediate, is complex. **Arrhythmias** of the heart are treated with ANTIARRHYTHMIC drugs and electrical defibrillation. Associated formation of clots can be treated by FIBRINOLYTICS. Other drugs used include ANALGESICS, DIURETICS and BETA-BLOCKERS.

myocarditis is acute or chronic inflammation of the muscle of the heart (cardiac muscle). It may occur as an adverse side-effect of some drugs.

names of drugs are classified into three main types. The chemical name is the full name of the chemical that is the active component, but has the disadvantage in medical use that it is often very long and complex. The generic name is the official 'trivial' official name (eg paracetamol), and is used in normal medical prescribing and use. The proprietary name, the trade name, is always capitalized (eg Panadol), and is used for marketing purposes and commonly in packaging. See also **chemical name**; **generic drug name**.

narcolepsy is an extreme tendency to fall asleep in a quiet environment, although such individuals can be easily roused. STIMULANT drugs, such as DEXAMPHETAMINE, may be used in its treatment.

natriuretic means causing a sodium loss into the urine (which is a property of DIURETICS).

nebulizer see **aerosols**

neoplasm is any abnormal or new growth. Correctly, the term can be applied to relatively harmless swellings (**benign**) or cancerous (**malignant**) growths. Nevertheless, the term neoplastic disease is often loosely taken as synonymous with cancerous growth.

nephrosis (nephrotic syndrome) are the symptoms of damage to the glomeruli (the filtering units) of the kidney. There is often **proteinurea** and **oedema**. It may be caused by diabetes mellitus, hypertension, poisons (eg lead and carbon tetrachloride) or as an adverse reaction to some drugs .

neuropathy see **peripheral neuropathy**

neutropenia (granulocytopenia) is a decrease in the number of neutrophils (one of the types of white blood cells). It may be caused by a number of diseases or as an adverse reaction to certain drugs, and increases susceptibility to infection.

oedema is an abnormal accumulation of fluid in the body tissues, and may be localized (eg as a swelling) or generalized (eg after heart failure; 'dropsy'). It can be caused by injury as a component of inflammation, or as a symptom of various diseases (heart failure, cirrhosis of the liver or nephrotic syndrome). It may also be caused by a number of drugs (eg ORAL

CONTRACEPTIVES, CORTICOSTEROIDS and ANDROGENS). Treatment of oedema depends on the cause, but DIURETICS are commonly used.

oesophageal varices are widenings in the veins supplying the oesophagus (sometimes extending down to the stomach). They can develop as a result of portal hypertension (increased blood supply to the portal vein due to liver disease, including **cirrhosis**). The varices are thin-walled and may rupture causing life-threatening haemorrhage. Treatment is with VASOPRESSIN as a VASOCONSTRICTOR, together with a sclerosing agent to seal the veins, followed by surgery.

ointment is a general term that is used to describe a group of essentially greasy preparations which are insoluble in water and so do not wash off. They are used as bases for many therapeutic preparations for topical application (particularly in the treatment of dry lesions or ophthalmic complaints). Most ointments have a form of PARAFFIN as their base, but a few contain LANOLIN which may cause sensitivity reactions in a some people.

osteoarthritis is a type of arthritis (joint inflammation) in which there is degeneration of the cartilage that lines the joints. It is exacerbated by stress and characterized by creaking joints. Treatment of symptoms is by NSAIDS, CORTICOSTEROIDS or surgery. Osteoarthritis is different to **rheumatoid arthritis**.

osteoporosis is a loss of the bone tissue, leading to a tendency to become brittle and fracture. The cause can be infection, injury, as part of Cushing's syndrome, especially in long-term corticosteroid therapy, or in the elderly and women following the menopause. HRT may be used to minimize osteoporosis in postmenopausal women.

ototoxicity is toxic damage to the inner ear, including drug-induced damage to the nerve serving the inner ear (eighth cranial nerve) the cochlea and semicircular canals, so causing some degree of deafness or loss of the sense of balance. This is a common adverse effect seen with use of the antibiotic NEOMYCIN and related AMINOGLYCOSIDES.

pancreatitis is inflammation of the pancreas, and is commonly due to gallstones or alcohol abuse, though it can be caused by viral infection, **hyperlipidaemia** or a physical injury. A number of drugs may precipitate (normally acute) pancreatitis, including NSAIDS and ANTIBIOTICS, and also chronic use of PARACETAMOL.

parallel imports refers to the system whereby drugs are reimported for sale from a country where the drugs is sold at a cheaper price.

paralytic ileus is a condition of the gastrointestinal tract characterized by a failure of the normal peristaltic (see **peristalsis**) contractions, which leads to intestinal obstruction. It is usually seen after abdominal surgery and can be treated with drugs that stimulate the intestine, such as PARASYMPATHOMIMETICS or ANTICHOLINESTERASES.

parasuicide is attempted suicide in a setting that makes rescue possible, where they are believed to be calls for help from the subject.

parasympathetic nervous system see **autonomic nervous system**

parenteral means administration by any route other than the mouth. See also **routes of administration of drugs**.

pastille is a soft lozenge.

patents for drugs see **generic drug name**

pathogens are agents that cause disease, and are normally micro-organisms (including bacteria, viruses, protozoa and fungi).

pathological means relating to disease, or to pathology, the study of disease.

-pathy as a suffix denotes disease (eg neuropathy, encephalopathy, retinopathy).

Patient Information Leaflet (PIL) (or Product Information Leaflet) is the technical literature placed by the drug manufacturer in the packaging of medicines, and is intended to be read by the patient or carer. In the case of OTC (over-the-counter) drugs (medicines that can be bought without a prescription), these safety warnings are of particular importance.

peripheral neuropathy is disease of or damage to the peripheral nerves, and is characterized by numbness, tingling, pain or sometimes muscle weakness, particularly in the extremities. There are a number of possible causes (eg diabetic or alcoholic neuropathies). Poisoning with a number of chemicals (eg lead) may cause the syndrome and a number of drugs cause it as a side-effect (which is normally reversible on withdrawal of treatment).

603

peripheral vascular disease is a narrowing of the blood vessels in the legs and sometimes arms, causing pain and coldness in the extremities. There can be a number of causes, including **atheroma**, inadequately controlled diabetes mellitus, deep vein **thrombosis** and varicose veins. Sometimes it occurs without evident occlusion, eg Reynaud's disease and Brueger's disease.

peristalsis is the coordinated and rhythmic (involuntary) waves of muscular activity that move the contents of the intestines in the appropriate direction. It depends largely on intrinsic activity of the smooth muscle and the nerves within the wall of the gut, but is modulated from within the **central nervous system** via nerves of the **autonomic nervous system**. A wide variety of drugs affect peristalsis activity in the treatment of disease or as side-effects.

pessaries are formulations of drugs inserted into the vagina. See also **suppository.**

phaeochromocytoma is a type of growth of neuroendocrine glandular tissue of the type normally found in the adrenal medulla, leading to large and often dramatic release of adrenaline and noradrenaline. Treatment is with ALPHA-ADRENOCEPTOR ANTAGONISTS and BETA-BLOCKERS, prior to surgery. See also **carcinoid tumours**.

pharmacist is a practitioner of pharmacy, whether in the pharmaceutical industry, universities, hospital pharmacies or shops and high-street pharmacies.

pharmacodynamics is a term for the effects of drugs on the body, including mechanisms ('what the drug does to the body'). See also **pharmacokinetics**.

pharmacognosy is the study of botanical and other sources of drugs, and the properties of crude drugs.

pharmacokinetics is a term for the processes of absorption, distribution and metabolism of drugs ('what the body does to the drug'). See **pharmacodynamics**.

pharmacology is the science of drugs, the effect of chemical substances have on living processes. It can be divided into **pharmacodynamics** ('what the drug does to the body') and **pharmacokinetics** ('what the body does to the drug'). It is much concerned with the development of novel drugs.

pharmacopoeias lists official preparation of drugs. See also **British Pharmacopoeia**, **International Pharmacopoeia** and **European Pharmacopoeia**.

pharmacy is the preparation (formulation) and supply of medicines (and the place where it is done).

phenotype is the expression of characteristics (visual, biochemical or otherwise measurable) determined by the individual's genes (**genotype**) and their interaction with the environment. Two individuals with identical genotypes (eg identical twins) may express different phenotypes.

phenylketonuria is an inherited condition due to a deficiency of the enzyme that metabolizes the natural amino acid phenylalanine, which is a constituent of the protein in many foodstuffs. The condition is characterized by severe mental handicap unless the diet of affected infants is switched to special foods free of this amino acid.

photophobia is an intolerance to light to the extent that normal levels are uncomfortable. It occurs in some eye disorders (eg iriditis, corneal damage and chronic **glaucoma**), in some systemic infections (eg **meningitis**) or can be induced by drugs that dilate the pupil.

photosensitivity is abnormal reaction to sunlight (eg rash). Phototoxicity is where drug treatment lowers sensitivity of the skin to ultraviolet light, so that there is burning. One form is photoallergy where the drug combines with skin protein to form an **allergen**, to which the body reacts with an **allergic reaction**. Undesirable photosensitization is caused by a wide variety of drugs in standard usage (eg HYPOGLYCAEMICS, ORAL CONTRACEPTIVES, PHENOTHIAZINES, SULPHONAMIDES, SULPHONYLUREAS OR TETRACYCLINES). SUNSCREENS applied to the skin help in treatment.

pills are solid spherical or ovoid drug dose forms (originally made by a rolling process), which are now largely superseded by **tablets**. 'The Pill' is slang for oral contraceptives, which actually are in tablet form.

placebos are dummy treatments, having only psychological effects, used in **clinical trials**.

poisons "All things are poisonous and there is nothing that is harmless, the dose alone decides that something is no poison." Paracelsus (1493–1541). This statement still applies, indeed, many compounds previously regarded as poisons are today used as medicines (eg COLCHICINE from the autumn crocus (Colchicum autnale) and VINCA ALKALOIDS from the periwinkle (Vinca rosea)).

porphyria is one of a group of six uncommon disease states characterized by disturbed metabolism of the pigment haem (which occurs in the blood-pigment haemoglobin), leading to the accumulation in the body of porphyrins, causing red, brown or bluish urine. Aside from a number of porphyric disease states, some drug-induced porphyrias are known (eg that caused by TAMOXIFEN), and many drugs should not be used in individuals who suffer from porphyria.

postural hypotension see hypotension

potency of a drug is how strong it is, either in terms of the **dose** required to achieve a given effect, or the maximum effect that is achievable.

pre-eclampsia see eclampsia

Prescription-only Medicine (PoM) is one that must be prescribed by an appropriately qualified doctor on a proper prescription form, and can not be bought over-the-counter (OTC). Some drugs are subject to special restrictions, for instance, drugs on the Controlled Drugs List (eg OPIATES) or those used only in certain hospitals or clinics and on a 'named-patient-only' basis.

priapism is prolonged erection of the penis and is a painful condition requiring immediate treatment. It is caused by a failure of blood to drain from the spongy tissue of the penis. It can occur due to nerve damage, infection, as part of a variety of other disease stares and with blood clots. It can also occur as a side-effect incurred through the use of certain drugs, such as the PROSTAGLANDIN analogue ALPROSTADIL, when injected into the penis for the treatment of impotence.

pro-drug is a chemical form of a drug that is not in itself pharmacologically active, but is converted in the body to the active drug (eg ENALARIL to enalaprilat; phenacetin to PARACETAMOL). The pro-drugs may be chemically more stable or better absorbed than the active drugs.

proprietary name see names of drugs

proteinurea is the passage of increased amounts of protein in the urine. It can result

from a bacterial infection of the urinary tract, and a number of other disorders including pre-eclampsia (see **eclampsia**).

pruritus is itching, which, as well as occurring in several disease states, is a very common side-effect of certain drugs, especially those that release histamine in the body.

psoriasis is a chronic skin complaint characterized by thickened patches of itchy scaling skin. Treatment is problematical, but includes phototherapy, photodynamic therapy, and drugs including CORTICOSTEROIDS and METHOTREXATE.

pyelonephritis is an inflammation of the kidney, usually due to bacterial infection, and can occur in acute or chronic forms. Treatment of the acute form is usually with antibiotics.

pyloric stenosis is a narrowing of the pylorus (the small outlet of the stomach to the small intestine), which obstructs the passage of food. In adults it commonly results from scarring from chronic peptic ulcers, though it may also be caused by stomach cancer. Treatment is normally surgical.

pyrexia (fever) is a body temperature raised above normal, and is usually taken as indicating an infection. It is treated with ANTIPYRETIC drugs, such as PARACETAMOL and other NSAIDS.

pyrogens are substances that cause fever. They normally are produced as a result of microbial or other infection, with the result that the body's 'thermostat' in the brain is set too high. PROSTAGLANDINS are pyrogens, and NSAIDS, such as aspirin, that prevent their production are commonly used ANTIPYRETICS.

Raynaud's disease/syndrome see peripheral vascular disease

recombinant DNA technology introduces new genetic material (eg that of another species) or reorganized genetic material into host cells. When done by artificial techniques, it is a form of **genetic engineering**, and is used particularly in **biotechnology** to produce biopharmaceuticals, normally proteins (eg insulin, growth hormone).

reflux oesophagitis see gastro-oesophageal reflux

regimen is a systematic course of treatment.

Reye's syndrome which is seen in children, may be caused by ingestion of aspirin (though it may certainly have other causes). It is rare but serious, and is characterized by a fatty liver and brain damage. The link with aspirin is not entirely clear, but since 1986 aspirin bottles have been labelled as contraindicated in children under 12 years old, unless specifically indicated (as in juvenile arthritis).

rheumatoid arthritis is a type of arthritis (joint inflammation) in which the joints of the body, particularly of the fingers, wrists and toes, become, stiff, swollen, painful and eventually deformed. It is progressive, but periodic and quite different to **osteoarthritis**. Treatment is by NSAIDs, CORTICOSTEROIDS, IMMUNOSUPPRESSANTS and a number of other drugs.

rhinitis is an inflammation of the mucous membrane that lines the nose, resulting in nasal congestion and a running nose. Allergic rhinitis is associated with an **allergic reaction**, commonly to inhaled pollens (eg hay fever), and this can be treated with ANTIHISTAMINES, ANTI-ALLERGIC drugs and NASAL DECONGESTANTS, often in the form of nasal sprays or drops. There are a number of other forms of rhinitis characterized by a hypersensitivity (vasomotor rhinitis), and some of these may be precipitated by cold, foodstuffs, pregnancy and some drugs (eg NSAIDs and OESTROGENS, including ORAL CONTRACEPTIVES).

routes of administration of drugs are very varied. Some common routes include: intravascular injection or infusion (into the blood vessels) mainly intravenous (into veins) but sometimes intra-arterial (into arteries), intramuscular (injection into muscles), subcutaneous (injection beneath the dermis of the skin), intradermal (injection into the skin); transdermal (across the skin; eg from skin patches); topical (application to skin or mucous membranes), per rectum (by an ointment or suppository into the rectum), intravaginally (by an ointment or pessary into the vagina); intrathecal (by injection into the subarachnoid space of the spinal cord); intranasally (often as a spray or drops); orally (by mouth), by inhalation and many other routes.

sarcoma is a **malignant** type of **neoplasm**, a cancerous growth, which arises in the connective tissue in virtually any organ of the body. See also **carcinoma**.

electivity of drug action is where at a given concentration a given drug acts preferentially

on one receptor or tissue, and this helps minimize side-effects.

self-medication is the use of a medicine without the intervention of a doctor, though commonly with the advice of a pharmacist, normally with OTC (available 'over-the-counter') medicines.

sickle-cell disease (or sickle-cell anaemia) is a hereditary blood disease that occurs mostly in black people and some people of Mediterranean and Indian origin, and is caused in the child when both parents carry the defective gene. In this disease the red blood cells (erythrocytes) are abnormal, containing an abnormal form of haemoglobin (Hbs), and cause a serious form of ANAEMIA, where sickle-shaped erythrocytes are formed (sickling) when the blood is deprived of oxygen, and these cells are removed from the circulation causing jaundice and anaemia. Treatment is supportive, with supplements of FOLIC ACID, ANTIBIOTICS and oxygen therapy.

side-effect of a drug is an unwanted effect, but is dose-related and normally predictable (sometimes unavoidable). The term normally is used for relatively trivial unwanted actions of drugs (eg dry mouth) rather than potentially serious adverse-effects (see **adverse drug reactions**).

skeletal muscle is the type of striated muscle that makes up the majority of the musculature of the body. It is attached to the skeleton and is responsible for the movement of limbs, for breathing, etc. Nerve supply is by cholinergic fibres of the somatic (voluntary) nervous system, so the muscle is caused to contract by acetylcholine and blocked by ANTICHOLINERGIC drugs.

slow acetylators are individuals with an inherited condition where an enzyme that breaks down drugs within the body has low activity, so it is important that lower doses of such drugs (eg ISONIAZID) are taken by people with this disorder.

smooth muscle (involuntary muscle, plain muscle) unlike **striated muscle** has no cross-striations under the microscope, indicating an organization characteristic of muscle controlled by the **autonomic nervous system**, and reacting more slowly to neurotransmitters than the striated muscle of the voluntary nervous system.